ASSESSMENT OF AUTISM SPECTRUM DISORDER

Also Available

Handbook of Neurodevelopmental
and Genetic Disorders in Adults
Edited by Sam Goldstein and Cecil R. Reynolds

Handbook of Neurodevelopmental
and Genetic Disorders in Children, Second Edition
Edited by Sam Goldstein and Cecil R. Reynolds

A Parent's Guide to High-Functioning
Autism Spectrum Disorder, Second Edition:
How to Meet the Challenges and Help Your Child Thrive
*Sally Ozonoff, Geraldine Dawson,
and James C. McPartland*

Play Therapy Interventions to Enhance Resilience
*Edited by David A. Crenshaw, Robert Brooks,
and Sam Goldstein*

Assessment of AUTISM SPECTRUM DISORDER

SECOND EDITION

edited by

Sam Goldstein
Sally Ozonoff

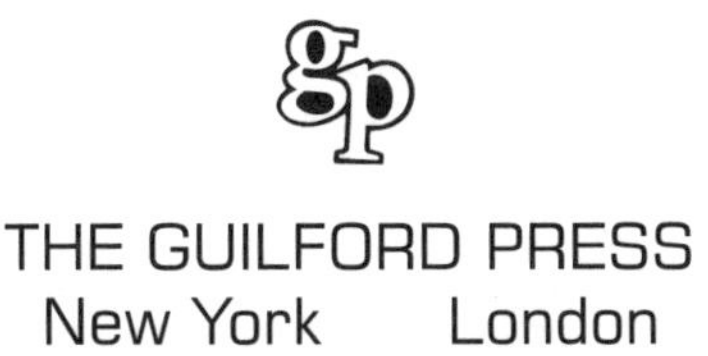

THE GUILFORD PRESS
New York London

A Division of Guilford Publications, Inc.
370 Seventh Avenue, Suite 1200, New York, NY 10001
www.guilford.com

Printed in the United States of America

This book is printed on acid-free paper.

Last digit is print number: 9 8 7 6 5 4 3 2

Library of Congress Cataloging-in-Publication Data

Names: Goldstein, Sam, 1952– editor. | Ozonoff, Sally, editor.
Title: Assessment of autism spectrum disorder / edited by Sam Goldstein, Sally Ozonoff.
Description: Second edition. | New York : The Guilford Press, [2018] | Revised edition of: Assessment of autism spectrum disorders / edited by Sam Goldstein, Jack A. Naglieri, Sally Ozonoff. 2009. | Includes bibliographical references and index.
Identifiers: LCCN 2017056101 | ISBN 9781462533107 (hardcover : alk. paper)
Subjects: LCSH: Autism in children—Diagnosis. | BISAC: PSYCHOLOGY / Psychopathology / Autism Spectrum Disorders. | MEDICAL / Psychiatry / Child & Adolescent. | SOCIAL SCIENCE / Social Work. | EDUCATION / Special Education / Social Disabilities.
Classification: LCC RJ506.A9 A867 2018 | DDC 618.92/85882—dc23
LC record available at *https://lccn.loc.gov/2017056101*

To the thousands of children with developmental challenges I have worked with, from whom I have learned much more, I believe, than they have learned from me

—Sam Goldstein

To autism professionals everywhere. We hope this volume will assist you in your quest to help children with autism thrive.

—Sally Ozonoff

To the memory of Lorna Wing (1928–2014). Professor Wing was an English psychiatrist, a pioneer in the field of childhood developmental disorders, and the author of 12 books on autism, including one of the first books written for parents, Autistic Children, *first published in 1964. Professor Wing did so very much to advance the cause of autism over the past half-century. It has been our great honor to know and work with her. She will be missed.*

—Sam Goldstein and Sally Ozonoff

About the Editors

Sam Goldstein, PhD, is Assistant Clinical Instructor in the Department of Psychiatry at the University of Utah School of Medicine and on staff at the University Neuropsychiatric Institute. He is also Clinical Director of the Neurology, Learning and Behavior Center in Salt Lake City. Dr. Goldstein is Editor-in-Chief of the *Journal of Attention Disorders* and serves on the editorial boards of six journals. He is author or editor of more than 50 books and 100 scholarly publications, as well as several psychological tests. He has lectured to thousands of professionals and the lay public in the United States, South America, Asia, Australia, and Europe.

Sally Ozonoff, PhD, is Endowed Professor and Vice Chair for Research in the Department of Psychiatry and the MIND Institute—a national center for the study and treatment of autism spectrum disorder (ASD)—at the University of California, Davis. Dr. Ozonoff is widely known for her research and teaching in the areas of early diagnosis and assessment of ASD. She is an actively practicing clinician and a strong advocate for parents and families. She is past Joint Editor of the *Journal of Child Psychology and Psychiatry*, serves on the editorial boards of six additional scientific journals, and has published over 150 empirical papers on related topics. Her work has been showcased on *60 Minutes*.

Contributors

Carolyn Thorwarth Bruey, PsyD, Lancaster–Lebanon Intermediate Unit, Lancaster, Pennsylvania

Kimberly M. Chambers, MA, Basis Charter School, Washington, DC

Katarzyna Chawarska, PhD, Child Study Center, Yale School of Medicine, New Haven, Connecticut

Blythe A. Corbett, PhD, Department of Psychiatry and Behavioral Sciences, Vanderbilt University Medical Center, Nashville, Tennessee

Lesley Deprey, PhD, MIND Institute, University of California Davis Medical Center, Sacramento, California

Florence D. DiGennaro Reed, PhD, Department of Applied Behavioral Science, University of Kansas, Lawrence, Kansas

Sam Goldstein, PhD, Department of Psychiatry, University of Utah School of Medicine, and Neurology, Learning and Behavior Center, Salt Lake City, Utah

Sandra L. Harris, PhD, Douglass Developmental Disabilities Center, Rutgers, The State University of New Jersey, New Brunswick, New Jersey

Susan H. Hedges, PhD, Frank Porter Graham Child Development Center, University of North Carolina at Chapel Hill, Chapel Hill, North Carolina

Perrine Heymann, BPhil, Child Study Center, Yale School of Medicine, New Haven, Connecticut

Kerry Hogan, PhD, Wilmington Psych, Wilmington, North Carolina

Yasmeen S. Iqbal, PhD, Department of Psychiatry and Behavioral Sciences, Vanderbilt University Medical Center, Nashville, Tennessee

Laura Grofer Klinger, PhD, TEACCH Autism Program, and Department of Psychiatry, University of North Carolina at Chapel Hill, Chapel Hill, North Carolina

Catherine Lord, PhD, Weill Cornell Medicine, Center for Autism and the Developing Brain, New York–Presbyterian Hospital, White Plains, New York

Lee M. Marcus, PhD, TEACCH Autism Program, Department of Psychiatry, University of North Carolina at Chapel Hill, Chapel Hill, North Carolina

Cynthia Martin, PsyD, Weill Cornell Medicine, Center for Autism and the Developing Brain, New York–Presbyterian Hospital, White Plains, New York

Mary E. McDonald, PhD, Department of Specialized Programs in Education, Hofstra University, Hempstead, New York

Keith D. McGoldrick, PhD, Neurology, Learning and Behavior Center, Salt Lake City, Utah

Gary B. Mesibov, PhD, Frank Porter Graham Child Development Center, University of North Carolina at Chapel Hill, Chapel Hill, North Carolina

Joanna L. Mussey, PhD, TEACCH Autism Program, and Department of Psychiatry, University of North Carolina at Chapel Hill, Chapel Hill, North Carolina

Jack A. Naglieri, PhD, Curry School of Education, University of Virginia, Charlottesville, Virginia

Sarah O'Kelley, PhD, Department of Psychology, University of Alabama at Birmingham, Birmingham, Alabama

Sally Ozonoff, PhD, Department of Psychiatry and Behavioral Sciences, MIND Institute, University of California Davis Medical Center, Sacramento, California

Mark Palmieri, PsyD, Center for Children with Special Needs, Glastonbury, Connecticut

Rhea Paul, PhD, Department of Speech–Language Pathology, Sacred Heart University, Fairfield, Connecticut

Lauren Pepa, PhD, Weill Cornell Medicine, Center for Autism and the Developing Brain, New York–Presbyterian Hospital, White Plains, New York

Kelly K. Powell, PhD, Child Study Center, Yale School of Medicine, New Haven, Connecticut

Cara E. Pugliese, PhD, Division of Neuropsychology, Center for Autism Spectrum Disorders, Children's National Medical Center, Washington, DC

Ifat Gamliel Seidman, PhD, Department of Psychology, The Hebrew University of Jerusalem, Jerusalem, Israel

Victoria Shea, PhD, TEACCH Autism Program, Department of Psychiatry, University of North Carolina at Chapel Hill, Chapel Hill, North Carolina

Isaac C. Smith, MS, Department of Psychology, Virginia Polytechnic Institute and State University, Blacksburg, Virginia

Katherine D. Tsatsanis, PhD, Child Study Center, Yale School of Medicine, New Haven, Connecticut

Susan W. White, PhD, Department of Psychology, Virginia Polytechnic Institute and State University, Blacksburg, Virginia

Tristyn Teel Wilkerson, PsyD, Neurology, Learning and Behavior Center, Salt Lake City, Utah

Kaitlyn P. Wilson, PhD, Department of Audiology, Speech–Language Pathology, and Deaf Studies, Towson University, Towson, Maryland

Nurit Yirmiya, PhD, Department of Psychology, The Hebrew University of Jerusalem, Jerusalem, Israel

Preface

One of evolution's greatest, and most important, gifts to our species is our capacity to socialize. Over thousands of generations, those of our ancestors demonstrating an affinity for socialization likely found an advantage for procreation. Evolution moved our species from isolated families into groups comprising many families, each supporting the others. Perhaps as a species we derive no greater benefits than those from socialization. The capacity to socialize provides us with the support of others, enhances our survival, serves as a source of pleasure—the sharing of knowledge, friendship, and love—and advances the procreation of the species. There is little doubt that our species evolved successfully through the support of and socialization with one another.

Thus, as a developmental disorder beginning during the prenatal period and continuing through the lifespan, autism represents one of the greatest challenges to any individual. Despite the significant increase in our understanding and knowledge of autism, it continues to be a complex, often difficult concept for professionals and the public alike to appreciate. Autism spectrum disorder (ASD), once thought to reflect the adverse outcome of cold and unaccepting parenting, is now recognized as a condition with strong genetic and biological roots. And as with all genetic phenomena, it is very clearly malleable through environmental experience. For individuals with ASD, genetics and biology, while affecting probability, do not speak to destiny. We now recognize the strong biological and genetic predisposition toward autism and the biopsychosocial forces that ultimately contribute to the individual course of the condition and life outcome.

From the time of its initial descriptions—Itard's reports of the wild boy of Aveyron's failure to use language or other forms of communication (Lane, 1977), Henry Maudsley's description in 1967, and Leo Kanner's first full scientific description in 1943—autism and the spectrum have fascinated researchers, mental health professionals, and the general public. Though it is a condition that occurs at a lower incidence than the common childhood conditions of attention-deficit/hyperactivity disorder, learning disability, depression, and anxiety, the atypical nature of the behavior, mannerisms, habits, cognitive development, and, most importantly, socialization of individuals with ASD continues to challenge many of the basic theories of child development and human behavior that guide our educational systems and methods of raising children. Many theories have come and gone, and autism is still enigmatic and perplexing with patterns of behavior, rates of development, and at times significant improvement or worsening of the condition that can be difficult to understand and explain.

As Kanner and Eisenberg (1956) pointed out over half a century ago, autism is a reflection of an inborn dysfunction underlying affective engagement that is now accepted as a lifelong condition. It is no longer a matter of helping the child with ASD through a particular developmental period but rather directing and engineering a child's transition through life to prepare him or her to function as an adult. It is thus more important now than ever that we possess valid, reliable, reasoned, and reasonable means of diagnosing, evaluating, and monitoring children with autism.

The first edition of this book arose from our interest in providing such an approach to the evaluation of autism. It focused on the assessment of autism and the spectrum of disorders that have been associated with it, reflecting dramatic growth in the field. That edition was the first text completely devoted to the evaluation of autism, providing a resource for understanding and assessment. With this much expanded and updated second edition, we believe we have set an important standard for researchers, clinicians, and caregivers, as well as a strong foundation for a consistent process of assessment and a thoughtful application of diagnostic criteria. Such a process ensures proper diagnosis and, most importantly, avoids the overstigmatization and pathologizing of normal variations in children's behavior.

The second edition includes five entirely new chapters, including one on the current diagnostic criteria of the fifth edition of the American Psychiatric Association's *Diagnostic and Statistical Manual of Mental Disorders* (DSM-5), as well as a chapter on the complex issue of assessment and diagnosis of early autism. We have also added a chapter on science and pseudoscience in autism, given the large volume of misinformation that still prevails concerning the disorder, as well as a chapter detailing comprehensive case studies and one on future directions in the assessment and treatment of ASD. As with the first edition, we have sought to bring together many of the best-known thinkers, scientists, and clinicians throughout the world in the field of autism. We are pleased that many of the authors of our first edition have added to and expanded their original chapters. Unfortunately, with the passing of the autism pioneer Dr. Lorna Wing, her epidemiology chapter addressing prevalence in our first edition could not be updated, and therefore is not included in this second edition. Incidence and prevalence issues are covered in other chapters.

One of the key goals in our initial volume was to bridge the available science to clinical practice. Since the publication of that edition, research on the assessment of ASD has continued in earnest. It is our intent in this second edition to emphasize valid and reliable methods of assessing this complex, often difficult-to-understand, condition. We have again broadly covered myriad comorbid conditions and problems that are present in many individuals on the spectrum. A broad assessment of comorbid conditions and development is critical given the high incidence of comorbidity between ASD and other behavioral, emotional, and developmental conditions. It is often these conditions that act catalytically in predicting the trajectory of a particular child's development.

The framework for *Assessment of Autism Spectrum Disorder* reflects Cohen and Volkmar's (1977) observation that there are "enormous differences among individuals with autism in their abilities and needs; among families, in their strengths and resources; and among communities and nations, in their own viewpoints and histories" (p. xvii). The second edition begins with a historical overview of autism. Our authors then address psychometric issues and current scales for assessing ASD. Since the publication of the first edition, a number of new scales have come to the marketplace; older scales have been revised and updated as well.

This volume continues by asking an important foundational question: Can a complex developmental disorder such as ASD be reliably and validly measured? We believe we answer this question affirmatively and then, along with our esteemed colleagues, proceed with chapters providing discussions of DSM-5, age-related issues and measurement of autism in very young children, assessment of social behavior, communication, and intellectual functioning. We then present chapters addressing the neuropsychological functioning of children with autism and, importantly, issues related to comorbid psychiatric conditions. The text continues with chapters addressing assessment of autism in the schools and a framework for applying assessment data to develop appropriate and individually targeted interventions.

This second edition concludes with three new chapters: the first addressing the diagnosis and assessment of ASD through case studies; a second chapter on distinguishing science and pseudoscience; and, finally, a third on future directions in the assessment and treatment of ASD.

This volume should serve the needs of a broad range of readers, from those new to the field (e.g., graduate students) to experienced clinicians and scientists across multiple disciplines. We believe this volume is also user-friendly for allied professionals and parents interested in learning about the valid and reliable assessment of autism. Along with our colleagues, it is our intent to provide a scholarly addition to the field. It is our hope that this volume will be widely used across multiple disciplines evaluating and treating ASD.

REFERENCES

Cohen, D. J., & Volkmar, F. R. (Eds.). (1997). *Handbook of autism and pervasive developmental disorders* (2nd ed.). New York: Wiley.

Kanner, L. (1943). Autistic disturbances of affective contact. *Nervous Child, 2*, 217–250.

Kanner, L., & Eisenberg, L. (1956). Early infantile autism, 1943–1955. *American Journal of Orthopsychiatry, 26*, 55–65.

Lane, H. (1977). *The wild boy of Aveyron*. London: Allen & Unwin.

Maudsley, H. (1967). Insanity of early life. In H. Maudsley (Ed.), *The physiology and pathology of the mind* (pp. 259–386). New York: Appleton.

Contents

If the brain were so simple we could understand it, we would be so simple we couldn't.

—LYALL WATSON

Disability doesn't make you exceptional, but questioning what you think you know about it does.

—STELLA YOUNG

Without deviation from the norm, progress is not possible.

—FRANK ZAPPA

CHAPTER ONE

Historical Perspective and Overview

Sam Goldstein

When the first edition of this volume was published in 2009, the singular consensus about the assessment of autism spectrum disorder (ASD), a condition characterized by patterns of atypical behavior and development, was acknowledged as complex. In the years between the publication of the first and second editions, great strides have been made in understanding, evaluating, and even treating ASD than likely in all the previous years. Yet, although there is a consensus that the definition and description of ASD is far less controversial than those of other childhood conditions (e.g., attention-deficit/hyperactivity disorder [ADHD]), they still involve their share of contradiction, uncertainty, and disagreement. As this book goes to press, it is still the case that the incidence of "autistic behaviors" in the general population is not fully understood—however, census-matched studies of autistic behaviors in the general population has yielded important new data (Goldstein & Naglieri, 2009). Nor has the positive and negative predictive power of specific behaviors related to ASD been thoroughly investigated (Matson & Goldin, 2013; Jeste & Geschwind, 2014). Although many parents of children with ASD are concerned about the social and communication development of their children at an early age, ASD still remains undiagnosed until the late preschool years or thereafter.

The fifth edition of *Diagnostic and Statistical Manual of Mental Disorders* (DSM-5; American Psychiatric Association, 2013) provides a revised and carefully crafted description of the symptom profile originally outlined in the DSM-IV-TR (American Psychiatric Association, 2000), related criteria, and impairment necessary to cross diagnostic thresholds. However, the application of these criteria through observation, checklists, and standardized tests continues to present numerous challenges (Volkmar, State, & Klin, 2009). It is still the case that ASD lacks a unifying genetic, biological, and behavioral theory. Although the data are progressively and "robustly" accumulating regarding the biological basis of ASD (Parellada et al., 2014; Volker & Lopata, 2008), it is still unclear whether ASD is a social, learning, behavioral, developmental, genetic, or cognitive problem, or some combination of these. Despite the significant increase in scientific research about ASD and the rapid and significant advances made, the efficient assessment of these conditions and their related problems continues to present challenges—as, most importantly, does effective intervention (Goldstein & Naglieri, 2013; Matson & Goldin, 2013). The combination of quantitative and qualitative research continues to seek a unifying theory combining genetics, biological variables, and behavior (Hoppenbrouwers, Vandermosten, & Boets, 2014).

It continues to be the case that researchers seek an evidence-based set of criteria to guide "practitioners in the selection, use and interpretation of assessment tools for ASD" (Ozonoff, Goodlin-Jones, & Solomon, 2005). Despite increasing data that the core features of ASD are highly genetic and reflect multifactorial risk likely interacting with changes in brain development, the diagnosis is reasonably stable, however, and certainly far from sufficiently precise. For example, Woolfenden, Sarkozy, Ridley, Coory, and Williams (2012) demonstrated through a systematic review of the diagnostic stability of ASD that in a combined sample of 23 studies and 1,466 participants, 53–100% of children still met the diagnostic criteria for ASD, yet many did not. These authors suggest that parents should be informed of the instability in the diagnosis, particularly in young children. In a review of methodological issues and differential diagnosis of ADHD, Matson, Nebel-Schwalm, and Matson (2007) describe the exponential growth in scales for differential diagnosis but note multiple limitations in currently used assessment tools.

The growth of a particular topic such as ASD is in part marked by the comprehensive, scientific, and clinical volumes published about it. Indeed, the field of ASD has grown to such an extent that texts related to specific issues (e.g., assessment, treatment) are now appearing. As the recognition and prevalence of ASD increases, the risks of over- and underdiagnosis increase in parallel. The need for carefully crafted guides for assessment have become paramount. We have created this second edition of our assessment volume primarily to serve as a desk reference and guide for clinicians. This first chapter begins with a historical discussion of autism and what has been referred to in the past as other ASD (e.g., Asperger syndrome). Then a short descriptive overview and the diagnostic criteria for ASD are presented, and the nature of comprehensive assessment related to early identification, differential diagnosis, comorbidity, related factors such as gender and ethnicity, and algorithmic models are discussed. The chapter concludes with three case studies exemplifying the complexities of assessment.

BRIEF HISTORY

Though the famous wild boy of Aveyron was thought to be a feral child living in the woods and purportedly raised by wolves in south central France at the end of the 18th century, it is more likely that he suffered from autism. The boy named Victor by the physician Jean Itard reportedly demonstrated classic signs of autism, particularly related to failure to use language or other forms of communication (Lane, 1977). In 1867, Henry Maudsley, in a text devoted to the physiology and pathology of the mind, described insanity in children. Some of his descriptions appeared consistent with today's symptoms of ASD. The qualities of stubborn, rigid, odd, and self-centered behavior have also been reported in historical figures throughout time. Interestingly, Frith (1989) hypothesized that a number of fictional characters, including Sherlock Holmes, may well have been given diagnoses and personalities consistent with autism.

The German word *autismus* was coined by the Swiss psychiatrist Eugen Bleuler (1911/1950). The word is derived from the Greek *autos* (self) and *ismos* (a suffix of action or of state). Bleuler, best remembered for his work in schizophrenia, first used this term to describe idiosyncratic, self-centered thinking that led to withdrawal into a private fantasy world. In 1943, Leo Kanner, in an article published in the journal *Nervous Child,* introduced the modern concept of "autism." Kanner borrowed the term from the field of schizophrenia as described by Bleuler. Kanner suggested that children with autism live in their own world, cut off from normal social intercourse, yet also hypothesized that autism is distinct from schizophrenia, representing a failure of development, not a regression. Kanner observed additional features reflecting problems with symbolization, abstraction, and understanding meaning in the clinical histories of these children. All had profound disturbances in communication.

In the 1943 article, Kanner described 11 children with "autistic disturbances of affective contact." He suggested that they had been born lacking the usual motivation for social interaction. Kanner described these disturbances in these children as reflecting the absence of the biological preconditions for psychologically metabolizing the social world and making it part of themselves. The condition was noted to lead to severe problems in social interaction and communication, as well as a need for sameness. Children with autism were described as rigid, inflexible, and reacting negatively to any change in their environment or routine. However, Kanner's first patient, Don Triplet, did not present to this level of extreme (Donovan & Zucker, 2010).

Kanner considered autism a genetically driven condition. He also observed that the parents of some of his patients were successful in the academic and vocational realms. Kanner suggested that autism, though a congenital condition, could be influenced by parenting. This led to the belief (which persisted for some time) that autism was caused by inappropriate parenting. In particular, those who espoused the psychoanalytic theory of the time came to believe that parents, particularly their child-rearing methods, were the causes of autism. That the interactional problems of autism arise from the child, and not the parents, has been well demonstrated in the research literature (Mundy, Sigman, Ungerer, & Sherman, 1986). The data today support the concept that biological and genetic factors convey the vulnerability to autism. Autism is also a condition that is typically observed across many generations and families. In 1956, Kanner and Eisenberg further elaborated on this theory, providing case observations collected between 1943 and 1955. During this period, it appears that Kanner's concept of the condition changed only minimally.

Kanner also suggested that many children with autism are not intellectually disabled, but are unmotivated to perform. A body of research now demonstrates that when developmentally appropriate tests are given, intelligence and developmental scores are in the range of intellectual disability for the nearly half majority of individuals with autism (Rutter, Bailey, Bolton, & Le Couteur, 1994; Centers for Disease Control, 2014). Yet as the concept of autism as reflecting primarily a social learning problem has become more widely accepted, the percentage of individuals on the autism spectrum who have normal intellectual abilities has increased. However, due to concerns that children with just social (pragmatic) language problems might be mistaken for youth with autism, DSM-5 now contains a social (pragmatic) communication disorder. This diagnosis was created in an effort to avoid providing diagnoses for children with pragmatic language problems absent marked patterns of atypical behavior. Though intellectual deficits were traditionally considered a key aspect of autism, current conceptualization has evolved to appreciate and recognize the differences between general intelligence on the one hand and the social learning problems characteristic of autism and other ASD on the other. These concepts are further discussed by Klinger, Mussey, and O'Kelley (see Chapter 8, this volume).

The year after publication of Kanner's (1943) original paper, Hans Asperger, a physician working in Vienna, proposed another autistic condition. Although Asperger was evidently unaware of Kanner's paper or its use of the word "autism," he used a similar term in his description of the social problems these children demonstrated. In 1944, Asperger described a syndrome he referred to as "autistic psychopathy." This condition was referred to as Asperger's disorder in DSM-IV-TR (it is also known as Asperger syndrome). His paper, published in German, was unavailable to English-speaking scientists until an account of his work was authored by Wing in 1981 and the paper was translated by Frith into English in 1991 (Asperger, 1944/1991; see also Frith, 1991).

Rutter et al. (1994) reported on Theodore Heller, a special educator in Vienna, who described an unusual condition in which children appeared normal for a number of years and then suffered a profound regression in functioning and development. This condition was originally known as "dementia infantilis" or "disintegrative psychosis." It was referred to as childhood disintegrative disorder in DSM-IV-TR. Another Austrian, Andreas Rett (1966), first observed females with an unusual developmental disorder characterized by a short period of normal development and a multifaceted form of intellectual and motor deterioration, with many symptoms similar to autism. In DSM-IV-TR, this condition was referred to as Rett's disorder (it is also known as Rett syndrome). Autism is also associated with many other genetic and medical conditions, occurring at a higher than expected rate in such disorders as fragile X syndrome, tuberous sclerosis, Williams syndrome, and neurofibromatosis (Gillberg, 1990). However, given the increasing literature demonstrating that autistic behaviors and ASD co-occur at a greater than chance rate in youth with a broad range of genetic disorders, the authors of DSM-5 attempted to improve positive and negative predictive power by eliminating the category of pervasive developmental disorder (PDD) and instead moving ASD into a category of neurodevelopmental disorders.

Until the 1970s, autism was considered a form of schizophrenia. In the first and second editions of DSM (American Psychiatric Association, 1952, 1968), only the term "childhood schizophrenia" was available to describe children with autism. It has become abundantly clear with further research that although young children with autism suffer in many other areas of their development, their behavior is very different from that seen in the psychotic disorders of later childhood or teenage years (Kolvin, 1971; see Cohen & Volkmar, 1997, for a review). The work of Cantwell, Baker, and Rutter (1980) and DeMyer, Hingtgen, and Jackson (1981) was influential in establishing the distinction between autism and schizophrenia. There is now a general consensus on the validity of autism as a separate diagnostic category, and on the majority of features central to its definition (Woolfenden et al., 2012). This consensus has been contributed to by the convergence of the two major diagnostic systems that include psychiatric and developmental disorders: DSM and the *International Classification of Diseases* (ICD; World Health Organization, 1993). Though there continue to be some differences between these two sets of diagnostic criteria, they have become more alike than different with each revision (Volkmar, 1998). In fact, autism probably has an excellent empirical basis for cross-cultural diagnostic criteria (Overton, Fielding, & de Alba, 2007).

In this book, we focus on ASD as defined by DSM-5. Autism was first included in DSM in its third edition (American Psychiatric Association, 1980), where it was called "infantile autism." The criteria were limited in their descriptions, specific symptoms were not outlined, and all criteria needed to be met for the diagnosis to be made were not defined (Volkmar, 1998). Major changes occurred in the revision of DSM-III, as Factor, Freeman, and Kardash (1989) noted. DSM-III-R (American Psychiatric Association, 1987) included detailed, concrete descriptions of specific behaviors and guidelines for number and patterns of symptoms that needed to be present, increasing the reliability of diagnosis. The lifelong nature of the disorder was also acknowledged, in the change in name from "infantile autism" to "autistic disorder." Deficits were defined in relation to a child's mental age, and subjective words and phrases (e.g., "bizarre," "gross deficits") that may have limited applicability to an older or higher-functioning individual were removed. Both verbal and nonverbal communication difficulties, including social use of language, were highlighted, rather than simply structural language deficits. The changes were much smaller from DSM-III-R to DSM-IV (American Psychiatric Association, 1994), but a major change was the inclusion for the first time of Asperger's disorder. The majority of these criteria remain the same but were reorganized for DSM-5 with the addition of sensory sensitivity as part of the diagnostic protocol.

DESCRIPTIVE OVERVIEW

Because of the unusual combination of behavioral weaknesses and a lack of well-proven biological models for this disorder, ASD is a most perplexing condition (Schopler & Mesibov, 1987). It is best conceptualized as a biologically determined set of behaviors that occurs with varying presentation and severity, probably as the result of varying causes. Autism occurs significantly more often in boys (Smalley, Asarnow, & Spence, 1988). It has been estimated that ASD affects at least 1% of the general population of school-age children with male to female ratios of about 3–4:1 in population cohorts and about 5–14:1 in clinical settings. In general, the highest gender ratios are reported for cognitively higher-functioning children with ASD (Baron-Cohen et al., 2009). Two population surveys (Lesinkienne & Puras, 2001; Mattila et al., 2007) report male to female ratios for Asperger's disorder at 1.6–2:1. Higher rates of clinically referred and assessed girls with ASD without learning disorder have also been reported (Sturm, Fernell, &

Gillberg, 2004). These findings have led to efforts to develop and validate instruments to better capture the female phenotype of ASD. Kopp and Gillberg (2011) report that behaviors such as avoiding demands, determination, careless about physical appearance and dress, and interacting with younger children may be more characteristic of females with ASD than males. ASD presents across all socioeconomic levels (Gillberg & Schaumann, 1982). It is estimated that one out of four children with autism experiences physical problems, including epilepsy (Rutter, 1970). Up to 75% were generally found to experience intellectual deficiencies, although this proportion has been dropping in recent years. Lotter (1974) first suggested that level of intellectual functioning and amount of useful language by 5 years of age were the best predictors of outcome, and these findings have been consistently supported by later research (Gillberg & Steffenburg, 1987; Howlin, Goode, Hutton, & Rutter, 2004; Venter, Lord, & Schopler, 1992).

Autism as commonly defined (Kanner's autism, DSM-IV-TR autistic disorder, DSM-5 ASD, etc.) is actually one point on a spectrum of disorders, along which individuals can present problems ranging from those that cause almost total impairment to others that allow some but not optimal function. Children on the autism spectrum experience a wide variety of developmental difficulties, involving communication, socialization, thinking, cognitive skills, interests, activities, and motor skills. Critics have suggested that DSM-IV-TR grouping of PDD, which includes ASD as discussed in this book, was poorly defined and inconsistent because it did not refer to all "pervasive developmental disorders" (e.g., intellectual disability). Because some children experience only specific or partial impairments (Gillberg, 1990), the category of PDD and the term "ASD" appear to equally define well the breadth and difficulties experienced by most of these children.

Rutter (1983) found that the pattern of cognitive disabilities in children with autism is distinctive, and different from that found in children with general intellectual disabilities. Language and language-related skills involving problems with semantics and pragmatics are present (Rutter, 1983). Other difficulties frequently include perceptual disorders (Ornitz & Ritvo, 1968), cognitive problems (Rutter, 1983), specific types of memory weaknesses (Boucher & Lewis, 1992), and impairment in social relations (Fein, Pennington, Markowitz, Braverman, & Waterhouse, 1986), many of which are described in detail in later chapters in this volume. Consistent with Kanner's (1943) description of autism, social impairments have been found to be the strongest predictors of receiving a diagnosis (Siegel, Vukicevic, Elliott, & Kraemer, 1989). Dimensionally measured variables such as those related to interpersonal relationships, play skills, coping, and communication are consistently impaired areas for youth with autism and other PDD. Hobson (1989) found that higher-functioning children with autism are unable to make social or emotional discriminations or read social or emotional cues well. These deficits appear to have an impact on social relations and are likely to stem from cognitive weaknesses. The inability to read social and emotional cues or to understand others' points of view leads to marked interpersonal difficulties (Baron-Cohen, 1989; MacDonald et al., 1989). Since Rutter's (1978) first description of social impairments without cognitive deficits in some higher-functioning youth with autism, diagnostic criteria for these conditions have expanded to include deficits in nonverbal behavior, peer relations, lack of shared enjoyment and pleasure, and problems with social and emotional reciprocity (American Psychiatric Association, 1994, 2000, 2013; World Health Organization, 1993). Relative to their cognitive abilities, children with these forms of ASD exhibit much lower than expected social skills, even compared with a group with intellectual disability (Volkmar et al., 1987). Delays in social skills are even stronger predictors of receiving a diagnosis of autism or another PDD than are delays in communication (Volkmar, Carter, Sparrow, & Cicchetti, 1993). Clearly, impairments in social skills among those receiving diagnoses of ASD are greater than expected relative to overall development (Loveland & Kelley, 1991).

CURRENT DIAGNOSTIC CRITERIA

DSM-5 reorganized DSM-IV-TR diagnostic criteria for autism into five categorical areas. Symptoms related to sensory sensitivity was the only new addition to these five areas.

The first area, Part A, describes persistent deficits in social communication and social interaction across multiple situations. A number of illustrative but not exhaustive descriptions are offered such as problems with social–emotional reciprocity and nonverbal communication, as well as deficits in developing, maintaining, and understanding relationships. Part B describes restrictive, repetitive patterns of behavior, interests, or activities, again manifested by two of a group of descriptions that are also offered as illustrative, not exhaustive. These include stereotypic or repetitive motor movements, use of objects or speech, lining up toys or flipping objects, and echolalia or idiosyncratic phrases, as well as insistence on sameness and an inflexible adherence to routine and rituals; fixated, abnormal interests; and hyper- or hyporeactivity to sensory input or unusual interest in sensory aspects of the environment. Part C suggests the symptoms must be present in the early developmental period but may not become fully manifest until environmental demands exceed limited capacity. Part D indicates that clinically significant impairment must be presented in social, occupational, or other important areas of current functioning. Finally, Part E suggests that these disturbances are not better explained by intellectual developmental disorder or global developmental delay. To make comorbid diagnoses of these two conditions, social communication should be below that expected for general developmental level.

The authors of DSM-5 provide explanation suggesting that "individuals with a well-established DSM-IV diagnosis of autistic disorder, Asperger's disorder or pervasive developmental disorder not otherwise specified should be given the diagnosis of autism spectrum disorder" (American Psychiatric Association, 2013, p. 51). However, for individuals with marked deficits in social communication but with symptoms that do not otherwise meet criteria for ASD, a new diagnosis—social (pragmatic) communication disorder—is recommended. Evaluators are asked to specify whether ASD presents with or without accompanying intellectual or language impairment, associated with a known medical condition or neurodevelopmental or behavioral disorder, and with or without catatonia. The severity of the condition is suggested on a level system with Level 1 reflecting the need for support; Level 2, the need for substantial support; and Level 3, the need for very substantial support. Evaluators are asked to provide levels for both social communication as well as restrictive, repetitive behaviors. DSM-5 suggests the prevalence of 1% in the population with environmental and genetic risk factors offered to explain possible risks for obtaining the diagnosis. In the section on differential diagnosis, evaluators are asked to consider the presence of Rett syndrome, selective mutism, social (pragmatic) communication disorder, intellectual development disorder, stereotypic movement disorder, ADHD, and schizophrenia.

THE NATURE OF A COMPREHENSIVE ASSESSMENT

As Cohen (1976) noted, the clinical provision of a diagnosis is but part of the overall diagnostic process—that is, comprehensive assessment is more than the simple application of a set of diagnostic criteria to a particular individual. It must provide an overview of the individual's history—relevant information about development (especially change over time), life course, and socialization—and, equally important, an overview of the environment in which the individual lives and functions. In short, as Cohen noted, the diagnostic process should provide a thorough overview of the individual's assets, liabilities, and needs. A thorough history is likely to be the best assessment tool. In most clinical assessments, history is often supported by checklists and standardized instruments. It is the rule rather than the exception that most evaluations for ASD also screen broadly for comorbid developmental, emotional, and behavioral problems. A comprehensive assessment for ASD thus typically evaluates a child's total functioning—intellectual, neuropsychological, communicative, behavioral, and emotional. Many of these issues are briefly reviewed below and covered in depth throughout this volume.

ASSESSMENT-RELATED ISSUES

Early Identification and Assessment of Young Children

Since the publication of the first edition of this volume, there have been a number of published studies demonstrating the relationship between early identification and a positive outcome over time (Dawson et al., 2010). As such, there is an increasing focus on identifying children at risk to receive a diagnosis of ASD or in fact those presenting with the full disorder at a very young age. This quest is primarily the result of encouraging results from intensive intervention programs for children under the age of 5 years (see Goldstein & Naglieri, 2013, for a review).

Matson, Wilkins, and Gonzalez (2008) review three methods of early detection and diagnosis, including well-developed assessment skills designed to identify behavioral differences at a young age between children experiencing ASD and genetic and biological studies that may provide markers for risk. Multiple research teams have focused on high-risk infants, including those presenting as preterm for risk of developing ASD (Zwaigenbaum et al., 2009). Single tools, such as the Modified Checklist for Autism in Toddlers (Yama, Freeman, Graves, Yuan, & Campbell, 2012), have demonstrated that tools such as these can be appropriately administered for children between 20 and 48 months of age. However, these authors note the importance of clinician expertise in verifying positive behavioral screens. The Autism Diagnostic Interview Schedule—Revised (Rutter, Le Couteur, & Lord, 2003) and the Autism Diagnostic Observation Schedule (Lord, Rutter, DiLavore, & Risi, 1999) have both been reported to assist in the identification of ASD at an early age. The second edition of the Autism Diagnostic Observation Schedule (Lord, Rutter, DiLavore, & Risi, 2012) has added a fifth module specifically for infants. Le Couteur, Haden, Hammal, and McConachie (2007) demonstrated that the combination of these two instruments provides good agreement and a complementary effect in aiding and confirming the diagnosis. Oosterling et al. (2009) examined three different screening instruments for ASD in toddlers (Early Screening of Autistic Traits Questionnaire, Social Communication Questionnaire, Communication and Symbolic Behavior Scales—Developmental Profile, and Infant Toddler Checklist) in an effort to identify key items presenting in youth with autism. In this study of children in two age groups (8–24 months and 25–44 months), none of these instruments nor individual items demonstrated satisfying power in discriminating ASD from non-ASD.

Among the critical issues is differentiating ASD from other developmental disabilities. Mitchell, Cardy, and Zwaigenbaum (2011) identified profiles of behavioral markers in the social realm by 12 months and in the communication realm by 18 months, which along with additional atypical motor behaviors, might distinguish ASD from a broader developmental delay. Ventola et al. (2006) combined multiple behavioral and observation tools in an effort to provide further differential diagnosis in a group of young children who failed a screening for ASD. These authors note that children with ASD had prominent and consistent impairments in socialization skills (especially joint attention) and were more impaired in some aspects of communication, play, and sensory processing than children with developmental delay. However, these authors also noted that the two groups shared multiple common features with a significant percentage demonstrating both conditions.

Finally, research groups have attempted to develop multistage screening approaches in an effort to avoid a high incidence of false-positive diagnoses (Oosterling et al., 2010). This research demonstrated that ASD was diagnosed 21 months earlier in an experimental population than in a control sample. Mean age of ASD diagnosis decreased by 19½ months from baseline in the experimental group. Interestingly, most of the early-diagnosed children had narrowly defined ASD with significant developmental delays. Stephens et al. (2012) utilized a three-stage screening process. They found that in a sample of over 500 infants, 20% had a single positive screen, 10% had a second positive screen, and 6% had two, but in only 1% were all three screens positive for a PDD.

Differential Diagnosis

As discussed in the previous section, particularly in young children, the differential diagnosis between ASD and developmental delay is a challenging issue. Differential diagnostic challenges overall reflect the broad presentation of comorbid disorders in children with ASD. Researchers have made efforts to differentiate ASD from pragmatic language impairment (Reisinger, Cornish, & Fombonne, 2011), ASD from broad language impairments (Matson et al., 2010), ASD from social phobia (Tyson & Cruess, 2012), ASD from social anxiety (Cholemkery, Mojica, Rohrmann, Gensthaler, & Freitag, 2013), ASD from schizophrenia (Solomon, Ozonoff, Carter, & Caplan, 2008), ASD from obsessive–compulsive disorder (Zandt, Prior, & Kyrios, 2009), and ASD from coordination disorders (Wisdom, Dyck, Piek, Hay, & Hallmayer, 2007).

By far, however, the most interesting differential diagnosis and diagnostic conundrum relates to differentiating or considering ADHD in the presence of ASD. In a census-matched sample of over 3,000 children,

Goldstein and Naglieri (2009) found symptoms of ADHD presented in an undifferentiated way between children with only ADHD and those with ASD. This finding has also been reported in smaller samples (Mayes, Calhoun, Mayes, & Molitoris, 2012). The overlap in impulsive, inattentive, and hyperactive symptoms in children absent ASD has generated a large volume of research and continued differing opinions about the diagnostic process. DSM-5 now recommends that ADHD can be diagnosed along with ASD. However, the distinction between these two conditions and the commonality of hyperactive, impulsive, and inattentive symptoms in children with ASD continues to beg the question as to whether this pattern of behavior should be part of the diagnostic criteria for ASD (Geurts, Verte, Oosterlaan, Roeyers, & Sergeant, 2004; Ghaziuddin, Welch, Mohiuddin, Lagrou, & Ghaziuddin, 2010; Hartley & Sikora, 2009).

It is also possible to question whether ASD extends to ADHD. There appears to be a subgroup of children with ADHD who demonstrate elevated ratings for core ASD symptoms not accounted for by ADHD or behavioral symptoms (Grzadzinski et al., 2011).

Geurts et al. (2004) demonstrated that pragmatic language problems in fact occurred in both youth with high-functioning autism and those with ADHD. It remains undetermined whether ADHD reflects a symptom profile independent of ASD or is also part of ASD. Very clearly there appears to be a high phenotypical overlap between ASD and ADHD with possible differing neurochemical pathways (dopaminergic vs. serotonergic; Sinzig, Walter, & Doepfner, 2009).

Comorbidity

Psychiatric and neurodevelopmental conditions co-occur commonly in children with ASD (Close, Lee, Kaufmann, & Zimmerman, 2012). These authors question whether changes in the diagnostic protocol for ASD are due to true etiological differences or shifts in diagnostic determination. It is still the case that there is no singular method for ensuring good sensitivity and specificity in identifying comorbid conditions in ASD (Matson, Beighley, & Turygin, 2012). Comorbidity in a variety of genetic disorders (tuberous sclerosis, fragile X, Down, neurofibromatosis, Angelman, Prader–Willi, Gilles de la Tourette, etc.) are well accepted. In these diagnostic situations, the clinician usually begins with the understanding and appreciation of the genetic condition and seeks to identify related comorbid problems, including ASD (Zafeiriou, Ververi, & Vargiami, 2007) and some researchers have suggested that certain genetic conditions such as fragile X are prognostic indicators in conditions like ASD (Brock & Hatton, 2010).

In a large, multisite study of over 2,500 children, children with a diagnosis of ASD and co-occurring psychiatric, neurological, or genetic conditions were more likely to be diagnosed or classified at a later age. Comorbidity is very clearly a risk for poor outcome over time. In a population-derived sample of children with ASD, 70% had at least one comorbid disorder and 41% had two or more. Most common diagnoses were social anxiety disorder (29.2%), ADHD (28.2%), oppositional defiant disorder (28.1%), and fetal alcohol syndrome (18%; Bishop, Gahagan, & Lord, 2007). Of those with ADHD, 84% received a second comorbid diagnosis. There were few associations between putative risk factors and psychiatric disorder (Simonff et al., 2008).

Some researchers have gone as far as to create a comorbidity interview developed to identify comorbid conditions within populations of youth with ASD (Mazefsky, Pelphrey, & Dahl, 2012). Finally, age-related differences in risk for and presentation of comorbidity continues to be an important area of research with emerging data very clearly demonstrating the prevalence and incidence of varying comorbitities as differing by age (Vasa et al., 2013).

Screening for Specific Risk Behaviors in ASD

There is an increasing interest in identifying from an algorithmic perspective certain behaviors that may be best at positive, and negative predictive power for the diagnosis as well as definitive risk over time and potential response to treatment (Gillis, Callahan, & Romanczyk, 2011; Karlsson, Rastam, & Wentz, 2013; Lam & Aman, 2007).

Factor Loadings

When behaviors associated with ASD as well as diagnostic criteria are examined, two- and three-factor domains emerge from exploratory factor analysis. Goldstein and Naglieri (2009) report, based on a census-matched sample, two factors in young children reflecting communication problems and atypical behavior with three factors reported in children between 5 and 18 years of age, reflecting the first two plus problems with self-regulation. Snow, Lecavalier, and Houts (2009) suggest that ASD can be statistically explained with a two-factor model using both exploratory and confirmatory factor analysis but acknowledge that two- and three-factor solutions are similar and slightly superior to a one-factor solution. These note that measures of functioning were not associated with domain scores in nonverbal children but negatively correlated with verbal children. Frazier, Youngstrom, Kubu, Sinclair, and Rezai (2008) also reported equal support for two- and three-factor models of ASD. A three-factor model separates peer relationships and play from other social and communicative behaviors. Absent in all but the Goldstein and Naglieri analyses are behaviors specifically addressing problems with attention, hyperactivity, impulsivity, and impaired self-regulation in children with ASD.

Sensitivity and Specificity of Assessment

Researchers have increasingly worked to develop valid and reliable instruments, many of which are built on algorithmic models (DeVincent & Gadow, 2009; Witwer & Lecavalier, 2007). Researchers have increasingly focused on measuring related phenomena that might be adversely impacted as the result of ASD such as adaptive behavior (Biederman et al., 2010; Gotham et al., 2008; Tomanik, Pearson, Loveland, Lane, & Shaw, 2006). Also, over the last 10 years multiple new assessment tools in addition to revisions of previous tools have come to the clinical marketplace (Chlebowski, Green, Barton, & Fein, 2010; Goldstein & Naglieri, 2009; Gotham, Risi, Pickles, & Lord, 2007; Schandling, Nowell, & Goin-Kochel, 2011; Ventola et al., 2006).

CASE STUDIES

The complexities and challenges of assessing ASD are reflected in the following three brief case studies. The issues raised in these studies, as well as many others, are further addressed and elaborated throughout this volume. The majority of assessments for autism are conducted with children; these three cases reflect issues at three different age levels (4, 9, and 13 years). These three cases are taken from our clinical practice—all three youth were referred because of questions about the presence of autism.

Joey

Four-year-old Joey came from a normally functioning family without any history of ASD or other developmental delays. At age 4, Joey demonstrated a number of idiosyncratic behaviors and stereotypic movements. He met many early developmental milestones within normal limits, but language was late in developing—he was also fearful of sitting on the toilet. Joey would point to make his needs known, but would not point on direction. He played in parallel with other children, but preferred to play alone—often in repetitive activities, lining up toys, and becoming distressed if even a single object was moved.

Parent responses to the Conners Early Childhood Rating Scales (Conners, 1997), a broad-spectrum questionnaire, noted mild attention challenges as well as difficulty with emotional lability absent significant disruptive behavior or developmental delay. Parent and preschool teacher responses to the Autism Spectrum Rating Scales (Goldstein & Naglieri, 2009) noted Joey's problems with conversational skills, avoidance of eye contact, inability to understand basic social behavior, and obsessive patterns. Nonetheless, Joey was able to smile appropriately and listen when spoken to, and he did not resist social interaction.

During a general developmental screening, Joey's overall development was deemed to be 1½ years below his chronological age. He could not complete even simple language measures, with estimated language skills at a 2- to 2½-year-old level. On Module 2 of the Autism Diagnostic Observation Schedule (Lord et al., 2012), Joey's speech was noted to have a rather atypical pattern of pitch, tone, and rhythm. Joey also struggled to maintain conversation and did not point consistently, but was capable of some shared enjoyment. His performance yielded a score of 8 for Language/Communication, a score of 9 for Reciprocal Social Interactions, and a total score of 17, well above the cutoff of 12 indicative of autism.

A DSM-5 diagnosis of ASD was provided, though it was noted that Joey possessed somewhat better-developed social engagement skills than other newly diagnosed 4-year-olds with autism. It appeared that Joey also demonstrated other developmental impairments (particularly significant language delays) that were further compounding his acquisition of developmental milestones and probably also contributing to his patterns of autistic behaviors.

John

Nine-year-old John was initially referred because of his problems with self-control and self-regulation. His parents wondered whether he might be autistic because he seemed uninterested in interacting with peers. There was no extended family history of ASD, but learning disabilities and emotional problems were present. John had been a difficult infant, irritable and hard to comfort. He spoke his first words by 9 months of age, but then stopped speaking. After pressure-equalization tubes were placed in his ears when he was 1½ years old, his language began to develop again. Toilet training was completed by 3½ years of age, although periodic daytime wetting was noted through 9 years of age. He was diagnosed at age 6 with ADHD, but responded adversely to stimulant medication. John was not doing well academically and did not appear particularly interested in the academic or social expectations of school. His parents noted that John "seems to not look at people as he is talking to them, and looks away talking quietly so you don't understand what he is saying."

Parent and teacher behavioral checklists (Autism Spectrum Rating Scale, Conners Comprehensive Behavior Rating Scale; Conners, 1997) noted John's problems with cognitive skills, inattention, restlessness, and social problems. He was not described as aggressive or disruptive. According to John's parents, he talked excessively about favorite topics that held limited interests for others, used certain words or phrases repetitively, interpreted conversation literally, asked irrelevant questions, struggled with conversational skills, avoided or limited eye contact with others, did not demonstrate much facial expression, did not appear to understand social behavior, and often missed social cues. John also demonstrated an extreme or obsessive interest in narrow subjects—his favorite topics of discussion were street signs and sprinkler heads. John's teacher at school noted that he was very passive but not a disruptive influence.

John's language skills were measured in the low average range, as was his overall intellectual ability. Measures of neuropsychological processes, however, noted John's very poor planning, attention, and simultaneous processing. He struggled to self-monitor, self-correct, use strategy efficiently, integrate information, and screen out detail. His motor and perceptual abilities appeared low average. His academic achievement appeared consistent with this overall neuropsychological profile. During a clinical interview, John's responses were tangential. He appeared to have difficulty sharing joint attention with the examiner and appreciating the ideas and thoughts of others. John's presentation on the Autism Diagnostic Observation Schedule—2 yielded a score crossing the autism criteria cutoff for his age range.

John's problems reflected a pervasive impairment in reciprocal social interaction, communication, interests, and activities. He also appeared impaired in the use of multiple nonverbal behaviors and, despite demonstrating adequate communicative speech, demonstrated impairment in pragmatic skills and in his ability to initiate and sustain conversation with others. Moreover, he demonstrated a pattern of interests that were mildly atypical in intensity and focus. The overall symptom profile was deemed to meet DSM-5 diagnostic criteria for ASD. Although a diagnosis of social (pragmatic) communication disorder was considered, John's patterns of obsessive and atypical behavior were deemed consistent with a full diagnosis of ASD. John was also provided with a diagnosis of ADHD—predominantly inattentive type. A significant percentage of children with ASD experience both conditions and suffer from elevated levels of impairments because of this (Goldstein & Schwebach, 2004). Issues related to comorbidity are explored by Deprey and Ozonoff in Chapter 10 of this volume.

Susan

Thirteen-year-old Susan had a history of slow overall development. As a preschooler, she had exhibited delayed language skills and had received speech–language services but still struggles with pragmatics. She had also been diagnosed in the past with the combined type of ADHD. During her educational career, a number of educators had raised questions as to whether Susan's problems reflected ASD. In particular, Susan demonstrated limited social interaction, was literal in interpreting conversation, frequently asked irrelevant questions, and struggled to maintain conversation. She also appeared not to understand basic social behavior, often missing social cues. Furthermore, at times she appeared to be obsessively interested in narrow subjects. Her current favorite subjects were the characters from the children's card game Yu-Gi-Oh!—she was an expert on each character's strengths and limitations.

At the time of assessment, Susan was in a self-contained classroom for youth with communication disorders. She was a number of grades behind her peers academically, but enjoyed reading for pleasure. She was not aggressive in the face of stress and could work for both short- and long-term rewards. There was also no extended family history of ASD or significant developmental delays. Though Susan's parents recognized and acknowledged her developmental impairments, they had never considered Susan to suffer from autism. They noted that she had enjoyed interacting with family members even as a young child. It was their impression that Susan did not demonstrate any of the symptoms they considered consistent with autism. Their responses on the Autism Diagnostic Interview—Revised (Rutter et al., 2003) did not strongly reflect the types of social context problems typically experienced by those with ASD. Instead, her parents attributed the majority of Susan's interpersonal difficulties to her cognitive and language impairments. Responses to the Autism Spectrum Rating Scale and Conners Comprehensive Behavior Rating Scale (Connners, 1997), completed by Susan's parents and teachers, noted symptoms of inattention, hyperactivity, impulsivity, and cognitive difficulty. Her language skills were measured in the borderline to low average range. Her intelligence was measured in the mild range of intellectual disability, as were her memory skills. A measure of nonverbal ability also yielded functioning in the mild range of intellectual disability. Neuropsychological processes such as planning, attention, and sequencing (Das, Naglieri, & Kirby, 1994) were also measured in this very low range. Her basic academic achievement appeared well below her age level, but consistent with expectations based upon this neuropsychological profile.

Susan's interaction with the examiner was immature. Module 3 of the Autism Diagnostic Observation Schedule—2 was administered. On this instrument, Susan showed neither echolalia nor marked speech abnormalities. She also demonstrated no excessive stereotypic behavior. However, she did not easily ask for or offer information. She did not easily report events, but could maintain a conversation in a simple way. Eye contact, though somewhat inconsistent, was not deemed to be inappropriate. Facial expression appeared generally normal, though immature. Susan could share enjoyment, but demonstrated some degree of limited insight and some difficulty sharing joint attention. Susan obtained a total score of 3 for Language/Communication (just at the autism cutoff) and 4 for Reciprocal Social Interactions (just at the cutoff for autism spectrum). Her total score of 7 was just at the cutoff reflecting autism spectrum.

Although Susan demonstrated a number of atypical symptoms consistent with ASD, her presentation did not meet the full diagnostic criteria. Moreover, differential diagnosis was clearly complicated by Susan's marked impairments in other areas of development, particularly language. Susan had also demonstrated improvement in some of her autistic symptoms, despite the fact that her development had continued to progress at a slow rate over the previous 4 years. Even with further discussion, Susan's parents found it difficult to accept that in part her problems may be related to ASD. Nonetheless, a provisional diagnosis of ASD was made. The combination of standardized historical and interactive assessment tools was helpful in understanding and appreciating Susan's symptoms and impairments (Risi et al., 2006). Clearly, Susan's comorbid problems caused by the combined type of ADHD and mild intellectual disability with language impairments presented as her greatest challenges. Later chapters in this volume address the assessment of many of these related issues, particularly intelligence, socialization, language, and neuropsychological functioning. Again, Chapter 10 thoroughly covers the issue of comorbid conditions and differential diagnosis.

SUMMARY

The assessment of ASD is complex, requiring a reasoned and reasonable appreciation of diagnostic criteria, assessment tools, and comorbid problems. A brief historical review reveals that autistic qualities are not simply manifestations of 20th- and 21st-century culture, but have probably presented challenges for individuals throughout human history. The current consensus on the majority of diagnostic criteria provides a good foundation for examining and evaluating individuals with possible ASD.

REFERENCES

American Psychiatric Association. (1952). *Diagnostic and statistical manual of mental disorders*. Washington, DC: Author.

American Psychiatric Association. (1968). *Diagnostic and statistical manual of mental disorders* (2nd ed.). Washington, DC: Author.

American Psychiatric Association. (1980). *Diagnostic and statistical manual of mental disorders* (3rd ed.). Washington, DC: Author.

American Psychiatric Association. (1987). *Diagnostic and statistical manual of mental disorders* (3rd ed., rev.). Washington, DC: Author.

American Psychiatric Association. (1994). *Diagnostic and statistical manual of mental disorders* (4th ed.). Washington, DC: Author.

American Psychiatric Association. (2000). *Diagnostic and statistical manual of mental disorders* (4th ed., text rev.). Washington, DC: Author.

American Psychiatric Association. (2013). *Diagnostic and statistical manual of mental disorders* (5th ed.). Arlington, VA: Author.

Asperger, H. (1991). "Autistic psychopathy" in childhood. In U. Frith (Ed. & Trans.), *Autism and Asperger syndrome* (pp. 37–92). Cambridge, UK: Cambridge University Press. (Original work published 1944)

Baron-Cohen, S. (1989). Do autistic children have obsessions and compulsions? *British Journal of Clinical Psychology, 28*(3), 193–200.

Baron-Cohen, S., Scott, F. J., Allison, C., Williams, J., Bolton, P., Matthews, F. E., et al. (2009). Prevalence of autismspectrum conditions: UK schoolbased population study. *British Journal of Psychiatry, 194*(6), 500–509.

Biederman, J., Petty, C. R., Fried, R., Wozniak, J., Micco, J. A., Henin, A., et al. (2010). Child Behavior Checklist Clinical Scales discriminate referred youth with autism spectrum disorder: A preliminary study. *Journal of Developmental and Behavioral Pediatrics, 31*, 485–490.

Bishop, S., Gahagan, S., & Lord, C. (2007). Re-examining the core features of autism: A comparison of autism spectrum disorder and fetal alcohol spectrum syndrome. *Journal of Child Psychology and Psychiatry, 48*(11), 1111–1121.

Bleuler, E. (1950). *Dementia praecox or the group of schizophrenias* (J. Zinkin, Trans.). New York: International Universities Press. (Original work published 1911)

Boucher, J., & Lewis, V. (1992). Unfamiliar face recognition in relatively able autistic children. *Journal of Child Psychology and Psychiatry, 33*, 843–860.

Brock, M., & Hatton, D. (2010). Distinguishing features of autism in boys with fragile x syndrome. *Journal of Intellectual Disability Research, 54*, 894–905.

Cantwell, D. P., Baker, L., & Rutter, M. (1980). Families of autistic children and dysphasic children: Family life and direction patterns. *Advances in Family Psychiatry, 2*, 295–312.

Centers for Disease Control. (2014). Prevalence of autism spectrum disorder among children aged 8 years—autism and developmental disabilities monitoring network, 11 sites, United States, 2010. *Morbidity and Mortality Weekly Report Surveillance Summaries, 63*, 1–21.

Chlebowski, C., Green, J. A., Barton, M. L., & Fein, D. (2010). Using the Childhood Autism Rating Scale to diagnose autism spectrum disorders. *Journal of Autism and Developmental Disorders, 40*(7), 787–799.

Cholemkery, H., Mojica, L., Rohrmann, S., Gensthaler, A., & Freitag, C. M. (2013). Can autism spectrum disorders and social anxiety disorders be differentiated by the social responsiveness scale in children and adolescents? *Journal of Autism and Developmental Disorders, 44*(5), 1168–1182.

Close, H. A., Lee, L. C., Kaufmann, C. N., & Zimmerman, A. W. (2012). Co-occurring conditions and change in diagnosis in autism spectrum disorders. *Pediatrics, 129*(2), 305–316.

Cohen, D. J. (1976). The diagnostic process in child psychiatry. *Psychiatric Annals, 6*, 29–56.

Cohen, D. J., & Volkmar, F. R. (Eds.). (1997). *Handbook of autism and pervasive developmental disorders*. New York: Wiley.

Conners, C. K. (1997). *Conners' Rating Scales—Revised*. North Tonawanda, NY: Multi-Health Systems.

Das, J. P., Naglieri, J. A., & Kirby, J. R. (1994). *Assessment of cognitive processes*. Needham Heights, MA: Allyn & Bacon.

Dawson, G., Rogers, S., Muson, J., Smith, M., Winter, J., Greenson, J., et al. (2010). Randomized control trial of an intervention for toddlers with autism: The Early Start Denver model. *Pediatrics, 125*(1), 17–23.

DeMyer, M. K., Hingtgen, J. N., & Jackson, R. K. (1981). Infantile autism reviewed: A decade of research. *Schizophrenia Bulletin, 7*, 388–451.

DeVincent, C. J., & Gadow, K. (2009). Relative clinical utility of three Child Symptom Inventory—4 scoring algorithms for differentiating children with autism spectrum disorder vs. attention-deficit/hyperactivity disorder. *Journal of Autism Research, 2*(6), 312–321.

Donovan, J., & Zucker, C. (2010). Autism's first child. *The Atlantic*. Retrieved from *www.theatlantic.com/magazine/archive/2010/10/autisms-first-child/308227/=*.

Factor, D. C., Freeman, N. L., & Kardash, A. (1989). A comparison of DSM-III and DSM-III-R criteria for autism. *Journal of Autism and Developmental Disorders, 19*, 637–640.

Fein, D., Pennington, B., Markowitz, P., Braverman, M., & Waterhouse, L. (1986). Towards a neuropsychological model of infantile autism: Are the social deficits primary? *Journal of the American Academy of Child Psychiatry, 25*, 198–212.

Frazier T. W., Youngstrom, E. A., Kubu, C. S., Sinclair, L., & Rezai, A. (2008). Exploratory and confirmatory factor analysis of the autism diagnostic interview-revised. *Journal of Autism and Developmental Disorders, 38*(3), 474–480.

Frith, U. (1989). *Autism: Explaining the enigma*. Oxford, UK: Blackwell.

Frith, U. (1991). Asperger and his syndrome. In U. Frith (Ed.), *Autism and Asperger syndrome* (pp. 1–36). Cambridge, UK: Cambridge University Press.

Geurts, H. M., Verte, S., Oosterlaan, J., Roeyers, H., & Sergeant, J. A. (2004). How specific are executive functioning deficits in attention deficit hyperactivity disorder and autism? *Journal of Child Psychology and Psychiatry, 45*(4), 836–854.

Ghaziuddin, M., Welch, K., Mohiuddin, S., Lagrou, R., & Ghaziuddin, N. (2010). Utility of the social and communication questionnaire in the differentiation of autism from ADHD. *Journal of Developmental and Physical Disabilities, 22*(4), 359–366.

Gillberg, C. (1990). Autism and pervasive developmental disorders. *Journal of Child Psychology and Psychiatry, 31*, 99–119.

Gillberg, C., & Schaumann, H. (1982). Social class and autism: Total population aspects. *Journal of Autism and Developmental Disorders, 12*, 223–228.

Gillberg, C., & Steffenberg, S. (1987). Outcome and prognostic factors in infantile autism and similar conditions: A population-based study of 46 cases followed through puberty. *Journal of Autism and Developmental Disorders, 17*, 273–287.

Gillis, J. M., Callahan, E. H., & Romanczyk, R. G. (2011). Assessment of social behavior in children with autism: The development of the Behavioral Assessment of Social Interactions in Young Children. *Research in Autism Spectrum Disorders, 5*, 351–360.

Goldstein, S., & Naglieri, J. A. (2008). *Autistic Rating Scales*. Toronto, ON, Canada: Multi-Health Systems.

Goldstein, S., & Naglieri, J. A. (2009a). *Autism Spectrum Rating Scale*. Toronto, ON, Canada: Multi-Health Systems.

Goldstein, S., & Naglieri, J. A. (2009b). Test review: Autism Spectrum Rating Scales. *Journal of Psychoeducational Assessment, 29*(2), 191–195.

Goldstein, S., & Naglieri, J. A. (2013). *Interventions for autism spectrum disorders.* New York: Springer.

Goldstein, S., & Schwebach, A. J. (2004). The comorbidity of pervasive developmental disorder and attention deficit hyperactivity disorder: Results of a retrospective chart review. *Journal of Autism and Developmental Disorders, 34*(3), 329–339.

Gotham, K., Risi, S., Dawson, G., Tager-Flusberg, H., Joseph, R., Carter, A., et al. (2008). A replication of the Autism Diagnostic Observation Schedule (ADOS) revised algorithms. *Journal of the American Academy of Child and Adolescent Psychiatry, 47*(6), 642–651.

Gotham, K., Risi, S., Pickles, A., & Lord, C. (2007). The Autism Diagnostic Observation Schedule: Revised algorithms for improved diagnostic validity. *Journal of Autism and Developmental Disorders, 37*(4), 613–627.

Grzadzinski, R., Di Martino, A., Brady, E., Mairena, M. A., O'Neale, M., Petkova, E., et al. (2010). Examining autistic traits in children with ADHD: Does the autism spectrum extend to ADHD? *Journal of Autism and Developmental Disorders, 41*(9), 1178–1191.

Hartley S. L., & Sikora, D. M. (2009). Sex differences in autism spectrum disorder: An examination of developmental functioning, autistic symptoms, and coexisting behavior problems in toddlers. *Journal of Autism and Developmental Disorders, 39,* 1715–1722.

Hobson, R. P. (1989). Beyond cognition: A theory of autism. In G. Dawson (Ed.), *Autism: Nature, diagnosis, and treatment* (pp. 22–48). New York: Guilford Press.

Hoppenbrouwers, M., Vandermosten, M., & Boets, B. (2014). Autism as a disconnection syndrome: A qualitative and quantitative review of diffusion tensor imaging studies. *Research in Autism Spectrum Disorders, 8,* 387–412.

Howlin, P., Goode, S., Hutton, J., & Rutter, M. (2004). Adult outcome for children with autism. *Journal of Child Psychology and Psychiatry, 45,* 212–229.

Jeste, S., & Geschwind, D. H. (2014). Disentangling the heterogeneity of autism spectrum disorder through genetic findings Nature reviews. *Neurology, 10*(2), 74–81.

Kanner, L. (1943). Autistic disturbances of affective contact. *Nervous Child, 2,* 217–250.

Kanner, L., & Eisenberg, L. (1956). Early infantile autism, 1943–1955. *American Journal of Orthopsychiatry, 26,* 55–65.

Karlsson, L., Rastam, M. R., & Wentz, E. (2013). The Swedish Eating Assessment for Autism Spectrum Disorders (SWEAA): Validation of a self-report questionnaire targeting eating disturbances within the autism spectrum. *Research in Developmental Disabilities, 34,* 2224–2233.

Kolvin, I. (1971). Studies in the childhood psychoses: I. Diagnostic criteria and classification. *British Journal of Psychiatry, 118,* 381–384.

Kopp S., & Gillberg, C. (2011) The Autism Spectrum Screening Questionnaire (ASSQ)-Revised Extended Version (ASSQ-REV): An instrument for better capturing the autism phenotype in girls?: A preliminary study involving 191 clinical cases and community controls. *Research in Developmental Disabilities, 32,* 2875–2888.

Lam, K. S. L., & Aman, M. G. (2007). The Repetitive Behavior Scale—Revised: Independent validation in individuals with autism spectrum disorders. *Journal of Autism and Developmental Disorders, 37,* 855–866.

Lane, H. (1977). *The wild boy of Aveyron.* London: Allen & Unwin.

Le Couteur, A., Haden, G., Hammal, D., & McConachie, H. (2007). Diagnosing autism spectrum disorders in preschoolers using two standardised assessment instruments: The ADI-R and the ADOS. *Journal of Autism and Developmental Disorders, 38*(2), 362–372.

Lord, C., Rutter, J., DiLavore, P. C., & Risi, S. (1999). *Autism Diagnostic Observation Schedule (ADOS)*. Los Angeles: Western Psychological Services.

Lord, C., Rutter, J., DiLavore, P. C., & Risi, S. (2012). *Autism Diagnostic Observation Schedule—Second Edition (ADOS-2)*. Los Angeles: Western Psychological Services.

Lotter, V. (1974). Factors related to outcome in autistic children. *Journal of Autism and Child Schizophrenia, 4,* 263–277.

Loveland, K. A., & Kelley, M. L. (1991). Development of adaptive behavior in preschoolers with autism and Down syndrome. *American Journal on Mental Retardation, 96*(11), 13–20.

Macdonald, H., Rutter, M., Howlin, P., Rios, P., LeConeur, A., Evered, C., et al. (1989). Recognition and expression of emotional cues by autistic and normal adults. *Journal of Child Psychology and Psychiatry, 30*(6), 865–877.

Matson, J. L., Beighley, J., & Turygin, N. (2012). Autism diagnosis and screening: Factors to consider in differential diagnosis. *Research in Autism Spectrum Disorders, 6,* 19–24.

Matson, J. L., & Goldin, R. L. (2013). Comorbidity and autism: Trends, topics and future directions. *Research in Autism Spectrum Disorders, 7,* 1228–1233.

Matson, J. L., Neal, D., Hess, J. A., Fodstad, J. C., Mahan, S., & Rivet, T. T. (2010). Reliability and validity of the Matson Evaluation of Social Skills with Youngsters (MESSY). *Behavior Modification, 34,* 539–558.

Matson, J. L., Nebel-Schwalm, M., & Matson, M. L. (2007). A review of methodological issues in the differential diagnosis of autism spectrum disorders in children. *Research in Autism Spectrum Disorders, 1*(1), 38–54.

Matson, J. L., Wilkins, J., & Gonzalez, M. (2008). Early identification and diagnosis in autism spectrum disorders in young children and infants: How early is too early? *Research in Autism Spectrum Disorders, 2,* 75-84.

Mattila, M. L., Kielinen, M., Jussila, K., Linna, S. L., Bloigu, R., Ebeling, H., et al. (2007). An epidemiological and diagnostic study of Asperger syndrome according to four sets of diagnostic criteria. *Journal of the American Academy of Child and Adolescent Psychiatry, 46*(5), 636–646.

Maudsley, H. (1867). Insanity of early life. In H. Maudsley (Ed.), *The physiology and pathology of the mind* (pp. 259–386). New York: Appleton.

Mayes, S. D., Calhoun, S. L., Mayes, R. D., & Molitoris, S. (2012). Autism and ADHD: Overlapping and discriminating symptoms. *Research in ASD, 6*(1), 277–285.

Mazefsky, C., Pelphrey, K. A., & Dahl, R. E. (2012). The need for a broader approach to emotion regulation research in autism. *Child Development Perspectives, 6*(1), 92–97.

Mitchell, S., Cardy, J. O., & Zwaigenbaum, L. (2011). Differentiating autism spectrum disorder from other developmental delays in the first two years of life. *Developmental Disabilities Research Reviews, 17*(2), 130–140.

Mundy, P., Sigman, M. D., Ungerer, J., & Sherman, T. (1986). Defining the social deficits of autism: The contribution of non-verbal communication measures. *Journal of Child Psychology and Psychiatry, 27,* 657–669.

Oosterling, I. J., Swinkels, S. H., van der Gaag, R. J., Visser, J. C., Dietz, C., &

Buitelaar, J. K. (2009). Comparative analysis of three screening instruments for autism spectrum disorder in toddlers at high risk. *Journal of Autism and Developmental Disorders, 39*(6), 897–909.

Oosterling, I. J., Wensing, M., Swinkels, S. H., van der Gaag, R. J., Visser, J. C., Woudenberg, T., et al. (2010). Advancing early detection of autism spectrum disorder by applying an integrated two-stage screening approach. *Journal of Child Psychology and Psychiatry, 51*(3), 250–258.

Ornitz, E. M., & Ritvo, E. R. (1968). Neurophysiological mechanisms underlying perceptual inconstancy in autistic and schizophrenic children. *Archives of General Psychiatry, 19*, 22–27.

Overton, T., Fielding, C., & de Alba, R. G. (2007). Differential diagnosis of Hispanic children referred for autism spectrum disorders: Complex issues. *Journal of Autism and Developmental Disorders, 37*(10), 1996–2007.

Ozonoff, S., GoodlinJones, B., & Solomon, M. (2005). Evidence based assessment of autism spectrum disorders in children and adolescents. *Journal of Clinical Child and Adolescent Psychiatry, 34*, 523–540.

Parellada, M., Penzol, M. J., Pina, L., Moreno, C., GonzálezVioquea, E., Zalsman, C., et al. (2014). The neurobiology of autism spectrum disorders. *European Psychiatry, 29*(1), 11–19.

Reisinger, L. M., Cornish, K. M., & Fombonne, E. (2011). Diagnostic differentiation of autism spectrum disorders and pragmatic language impairment. *Journal of Autism and Developmental Disorders, 41*(12), 1694–1704.

Rett, A. (1966). Uber ein eigenartiges hirnatrophisces Syndrome bei Hyperammonie im Kindersalter. *Wien Medizinische Wochenschrift, 118*, 723–738.

Risi, S., Lord, C., Gotham, K., Crosello, C., Chrysler, C., Szatmari, P., et al. (2006). Information from multiple sources in the diagnosis of autism spectrum disorders. *Journal of the American Academy of Child and Adolescent Psychiatry, 45*, 1094–1103.

Rutter, M. (1970). Autistic children: Infancy to adulthood. *Seminars in Psychiatry, 2*, 435–450.

Rutter, M. (1978). Diagnostic validity in child psychiatry. *Advances in Biological Psychiatry, 2*, 2–22.

Rutter, M., Bailey, A., Bolton, P., & Le Couteur, A. (1994). Autism in known medical conditions: Myth and substance. *Journal of Child Psychology and Psychiatry, 35*, 311–322.

Rutter, M., Le Couteur, A., & Lord, C. (2003). *Autism Diagnostic Interview—Revised.* Los Angeles: Western Psychological Services.

Rutter, R. (1983). Cognitive deficits in the pathogenesis of autism. *Journal of Child Psychology and Psychiatry, 24*(4), 513–531.

Schandling, G. T., Nowell, K. P., & Goin-Kochel, R. P. (2011). Utility of the Social Communication Questionnaire—Current and Social Responsiveness Scale as teacher-report screening tools for autism spectrum disorder. *Journal of Autism and Developmental Disorders, 42*(8), 1705–1716.

Schopler, E., & Mesibov, G. B. (Eds.). (1987). *Neurobiological issues in autism.* New York: Plenum Press.

Siegel, B., Vukicevic, J., Elliott, G. R., & Kraemer, H. C. (1989). The use of signal detection theory to assess DSM-III-R criteria for autistic disorder. *Journal of the American Academy of Child and Adolescent Psychiatry, 28*(4), 542–548.

Simonoff, E., Pickles, A., Charman, T., Chandler, S., Loucas, T., & Baird, G. (2008)

Psychiatric disorders in children with autism spectrum disorders: Prevalence, comorbidity, and associated factors in a population-derived sample. *Journal of the American Academy of Child and Adolescent Psychiatry, 47*, 921–929

Sinzig, J., Walter, D., & Doepfner, M. (2009). Attention deficit/hyperactivity disorder in children and adolescents with autism spectrum disorder: Symptom or syndrome? *Journal of Attention Disorders, 13*(2), 117–126.

Smalley, S., Asarnow, R., & Spence, M. (1988). Autism and genetics: A decade of research. *Archives of General Psychiatry, 45*, 953–961.

Snow, A. V., Lecavalier, L., & Houts, C. (2009). The structure of autism diagnostic interview-revised: Diagnostic and phenotypic implications. *Journal of Child Psychology and Psychiatry, 50*(6), 734–742.

Solomon, M., Ozonoff, S., Carter, C., & Caplan, R. (2008). Formal thought disorder and the autism spectrum: Relationship with symptoms, executive control and anxiety. *Journal of Autism and Developmental Disorders, 38*(8), 1474–1484.

Stephens, B. E., Bann, C. M., Watson, V. E., Sheinkopf, S. J., Peralta-Carcelen, M., Bodnar, A., et al. (2012). Screening for autism spectrum disorder in extremely preterm infants. *Journal of Developmental Pediatrics, 33*(7), 535–541.

Sturm, H., Fernell, E., & Gillberg, C. (2004). Autism spectrum disorders in children with normal intellectual levels: Associated impairments and subgroups. *Developmental Medicine and Child Neurology, 46*, 444–447.

Tomanik, S. S., Pearson, D. A., Loveland, K. A., Lane, D. M., & Shaw, J. B. (2006). Improving the reliability of autism diagnoses: Examining the utility of adaptive behavior. *Journal of Autism and Developmental Disorders, 37*(5), 921–928.

Tyson, K. E., & Cruess, D. G. (2012). Differentiating high-functioning autism and social phobia. *Journal of Autism and Developmental Disorders, 42(7)*, 1477–1490.

Vasa, A. J., Kalb, L., Mazurek, M. O., Kanne, S. M., Freedman, B., Keefer, A., et al. (2013). Age-related differences in the prevalence and correlates of anxiety in youth with autism spectrum disorders. *Research in Autism Spectrum Disorders, 7*(11), 1358–1369.

Venter, A., Lord, C., & Schopler, E. (1992). A follow-up study of high-functioning autistic children. *Journal of Child Psychology and Psychiatry, 33*, 489–507.

Ventola, P. E., Kleinman, J., Pandey, J., Barton, M., Allen, S., Green, J., et al. (2006). Agreement among four diagnostic instruments for autism spectrum disorders in toddlers. *Journal of Autism and Developmental Disorders, 36*(7), 839–847.

Volker, M. A., & Lopata, C. (2008). Autism: A review of biological bases, assessment, and intervention. *School Psychology Quarterly, 23*(2), 258–270.

Volkmar, F. (1998). Categorical approaches to the diagnosis of autism: An overview of DSM-IV and ICD-10. *Autism, 2*, 45–59.

Volkmar, F., Carter, A., Sparrow, S. S., & Cicchetti, D. V. (1993). Quantifying social development in autism. *Journal of the American Academy of Child and Adolescent Psychiatry, 32*(3), 627–632.

Volkmar, F. R., Sparrow, S. S., Goudreau, D., Cicchetti, D. V., Paul, R., & Cohen, D. J. (1987). Social deficits in autism: An operational approach using the Vineland Adaptive Behavior Scales. *Journal of the American Academy of Child and Adolescent Psychiatry, 26*(2), 156–161.

Volkmar, F. R., State, M., & Klin, A. (2009). Autism and autism spectrum disorders: Diagnostic issues for the coming decade. *Journal of Child Psychology and Psychiatry, 50*, 108–115.

Wing, L. (1981). Asperger's syndrome: A clinical account. *Psychological Medicine, 11,* 115–130.

Wisdom, S. N., Dyck, M. J., Piek, J. P., Hay, D., & Hallmayer, J. (2007). Can autism, language and coordination disorders be differentiated based on ability profiles? *European Child and Adolescent Psychiatry, 16*(3), 178–186.

Witwer, A. N., & Lecavalier, L. (2007). Autism screening tools: An evaluation of the Social Communication Questionnaire and the Developmental Behaviour Checklist—Autism Screening Algorithm. *Journal of Intellectual and Developmental Disabilities, 32*(3), 179–187.

Woolfenden, S., Sarkozy, V., Ridley, G., Coory, M., & Williams, K. (2012). A systematic review of two outcomes in autism spectrum disorder—epilepsy and mortality. *Developmental Medicine and Child Neurology, 54,* 306–312.

World Health Organization. (1993). *The ICD-10 classification of mental and behavioral disorders: Diagnostic criteria for research.* Geneva: Author.

Yama, B., Freeman, T., Graves, E., Yuan, S., & Campbell, M. K. (2012). Examination of the properties of the modified checklist for autism in toddlers (M-CHAT) in a population sample. *Journal of Autism and Developmental Disorders, 42*(1), 23–34.

Zafeiriou D. I., Ververi A., & Vargiami, E. (2007). Childhood autism and associated comorbidities. *Brain Development, 29*(5), 257–272.

Zandt, F., Prior, M., & Kyrios, M. (2009). Similarities and differences between children and adolescents with autism spectrum disorder and those with obsessive compulsive disorder. *National Autistic Society, 13*(1), 43–57.

Zwaigenbaum, L., Bryson, S., Lord, C., Rogers, S., Carter, A., Carver, L., et al. (2009). Clinical assessment and management of toddlers with suspected autism spectrum disorder: Insights from studies of high-risk infants [Review]. *Pediatrics, 123*(5), 1383–1391.

CHAPTER TWO

Psychometric Issues and Current Scales for Assessing Autism Spectrum Disorder

Jack A. Naglieri
Kimberly M. Chambers
Keith D. McGoldrick
Sam Goldstein

The study of any psychological disorder is dependent upon the tools that are used, as these tools directly influence what is learned about the subject in research as well as clinical practice. As in all areas of science, what we discover depends upon the quality of the instruments we use and the information they provide. Better-made instruments yield more accurate and reliable information. Instruments that uncover more information relevant to the subject being examined will have better validity, and ultimately will more completely inform both researchers and clinicians. The tools we use for diagnosis have a substantial impact on the reliability and validity of the information we obtain and the decisions we make. Simply put, the better the tool, the more valid and reliable the decisions, the more useful the information obtained, and the better the services that are eventually provided. In this chapter, the tools used for assessing the characteristics of children and adolescents who have autism spectrum disorder (ASD) are examined.

This chapter has two goals. First, we review the important psychometric qualities of test reliability and validity. The aim of this first section is to illustrate the relevance of reliability and validity for the decisions made by clinicians and researchers whose goal is to better understand ASD. We emphasize the practical implications these psychometric issues have for the assessment of ASD, and the implications they have for interpretation of results within and across instruments. Special attention is also paid to scale development procedures, particularly methods used to develop derived scores. The second section of this chapter focuses on the various measures used to assess ASD. The structure, reliability, and validity of each instrument are summarized. The overall aim of the chapter is to provide an examination of the relevant psychometric issues and the extent to which researchers and clinicians can have confidence in the tools they use to assess ASD.

PSYCHOMETRIC ISSUES

Reliability

The reliability of any variable, test, or scale is critical for clinical practice as well as research purposes. It is important to know the reliability of a test, so that the amount of accuracy in a score can be determined and used to calculate the amount of error in the measurement of the construct. The higher the reliability, the smaller the error, and the smaller the range of scores that are used to build the confidence interval around the estimated true score. The smaller the range, the more precision and confidence practitioners can have in their interpretation of the results.

Bracken (1987) provided levels for acceptable test reliability. He stated that individual scales from a test (e.g., a subtest or subscale) should have a reliability of .80 or greater, and that total tests should have an internal consistency of .90 or greater. The reason for testing and the importance of the decisions made could also influence the level of precision required—that is, if a score is used for screening purposes (where overidentification is preferred to underidentification), a .80 reliability standard for a total score may be acceptable. However, if decisions are made, for example, about special educational placement, then a higher reliability (e.g., .95) would be more appropriate (Nunnally & Bernstein, 1994).

Every score obtained from any test is composed of the true score plus error (Crocker & Algina, 1986). We can never obtain the true score, so we describe it on the basis of a range of values within which the person's score falls at a specific level of certainty (e.g., 90% probability). The range of scores (called the confidence interval) is computed by first obtaining the standard error of measurement (*SEM*) from the reliability coefficient and the standard deviation (*SD*) of the score in the following formula (Crocker & Algina, 1986):

$$SEM = SD \times \sqrt{1 - \text{reliability}}$$

The confidence interval should be used in practice, to better describe the range of scores that is likely to contain the true score. In practice, we say that a child earned an IQ score of 105 (±5), and state that there is a 90%

likelihood that the child's true IQ score falls within the range of 100–110 (105 ± 5).

The confidence interval is based on the *SEM*, which is the average *SD* of a person's scores around the true score. For this reason, we can say that there is a 68% chance (the percentage of scores contained within ±1 *SD*) that the person's true score is within that range. Recall that 68% of cases in a normal distribution fall within +1 and –1 *SD*. The *SEM* is multiplied by a *z* value of, for example, 1.64 or 1.96, to obtain a confidence interval at the 90 or 95% level, respectively. The resulting value is added to and subtracted from the obtained score to yield the confidence interval. So in the example provided above, the confidence interval for an obtained score of 100 is between 95 (100 – 5) and 105 (100 + 5). Figure 2.1 provides confidence intervals (95% level of confidence) for a standard score of 100 that would be obtained for measures with reliability of .50–.99. As would be expected, the range within which the true score is expected to fall varies considerably as a function of the reliability coefficient, and the lower the reliability, the wider the range of scores that can be expected to include the true score.

Technically, however, the confidence interval (and *SEM*) is centered on the estimated true score rather than the obtained score (Nunnally & Bernstein, 1994). In many published tests—for example, the Wechsler Intelligence Scale for Children, Fifth Edition (Wechsler, 2014) and the Cognitive Assessment System, Second Edition (Naglieri, Das, & Goldstein, 2014)—the confidence intervals are provided in the test manual's table for converting sums of subtest scores to standard scores, and the range is already centered on the estimated true score. The relationships among the various scores are illustrated in Table 2.1, which provides the obtained score, estimated true score, and lower and upper ranges of the confidence intervals

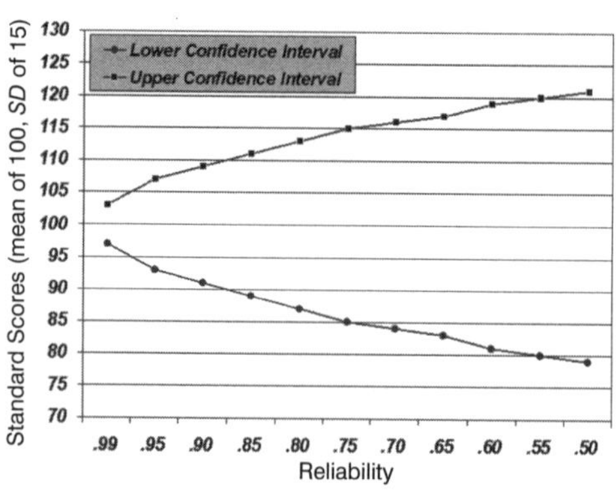

FIGURE 2.1. Relationships between reliability and confidence intervals.

for standard scores (mean of 100, *SD* of 15) for a hypothetical test with a reliability of .90 at the 90% level of confidence.

Examination of these scores shows that the confidence interval is equally distributed around a score of 100 (92 and 108 are both 8 points from the obtained score), but the interval becomes less symmetrical as the obtained score deviates from the mean. For example, ranges for standard scores that are below the mean are *higher* than the obtained score. As shown in Table 2.1, the range for a standard score of 80 is 74–90 (6 points below 80 and 10 points above 80). In contrast, ranges for standard scores that are above the mean are *lower* than the obtained score. The range for a standard score of 120 is 110–126 (10 points below 120 and 6 points above 120). This difference is the result of centering the range of scores on the estimated true score rather than the obtained score. Note that the size of the confidence interval is constant (±8 points) in all instances. Regardless of how the confidence intervals are constructed, the important point is that measurement error must be known and taken into consideration when scores from any measuring system are used. Confidence intervals, especially those that are based on the estimated true score, should be provided for all test scores including rating scales.

The importance of the *SEM* becomes most relevant when two scores are compared. The lower the reliability, the larger the *SEM*, and the more

TABLE 2.1. Relationships among Obtained Standard Scores, Estimated True Scores, and Confidence Intervals across the 40–160 Range

Obtained standard score	Estimated true score	True minus obtained score	Lower confidence interval	Upper confidence interval	Upper minus lower confidence interval
40	46	6	38	54	16
50	55	5	47	63	16
60	64	4	56	72	16
70	73	3	65	81	16
80	82	2	74	90	16
90	91	1	83	99	16
100	100	0	92	108	16
110	109	–1	101	117	16
120	118	–2	110	126	16
130	127	–3	119	135	16
140	136	–4	128	144	16
150	145	–5	137	153	16
160	154	–6	146	162	16

Note. This table assumes a reliability coefficient of .90 and a 90% confidence interval.

likely an individual's scores are to differ on the basis of chance. For example, when a child's score on a measure of self-regulation is compared with scores on a measure of social skills, the reliability of these measures will influence their consistency and therefore the size of the difference between them. The lower the reliability, the more likely they are to be different by chance alone. The formula for determining how different two scores need to be includes the *SEM* of each score and the *z* score associated with a specified level of significance. The difference can be computed by using the following formula:

$$Difference = Z \times \sqrt{SEM1_2 + SEM2_2}$$

The difference needed for significance when one is comparing two variables with reliability coefficients of .85 and .78, using an *SD* of 15, is easily calculated with the formula above. To illustrate, scores on measures of self-regulation (with a reliability of .85) and social skills (reliability of .78) would have to differ by 19 points (more than an entire *SD*) to be significant. Figure 2.2 provides the values that would be needed for comparing two scores with the same reliability, ranging from very good (.95) to very poor (.40) at the .05 level of significance, and a standard score that has an *SD* of 15. This figure shows that when one is comparing two scores with reliabilities of .70, differences of more than 20 points would be attributed to *measurement error alone*. Clearly, in both research and clinical settings, variables with high reliability are needed.

It is therefore important that researchers and clinicians who assess behaviors associated with ASD use measures that have a reliability coefficient of .80 or higher and composite score reliabilities of at least .90. If a test or rating scale does not meet these requirements, then its inclusion

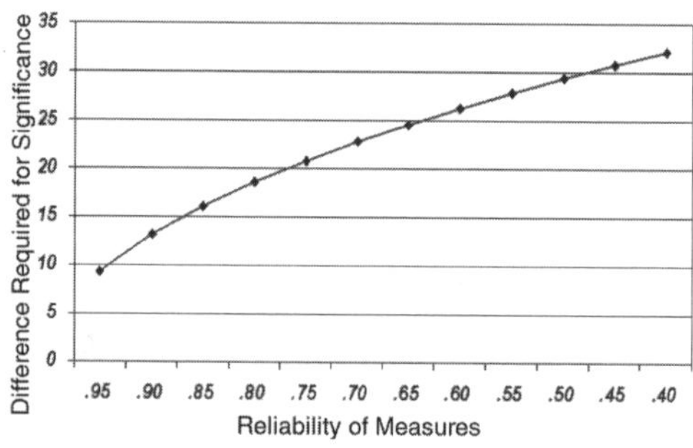

FIGURE 2.2. Relationships between reliability and the differences needed for significance when one is comparing two scores. Note that this figure assumes two variables with the same reliability and an *SD* of 15 at the 95% level of confidence.

in research should be questioned. This is particularly important in correlational research, because the extent to which two variables correlate is influenced by the reliability of each variable. Clinicians are advised not to use measures that do not meet reliability standards, because there will be too much error in the obtained scores to allow for reliable interpretation. This is especially important because the decisions clinicians make can have significant and long-lasting impact on the lives of examinees.

Validity

Although reliability is important, reliable measurement of a construct with little validity would be of limited utility to the clinician and researcher. Validity is described as the degree to which empirical evidence supports an interpretation of scores that represent a construct of interest. For example, a measure of ASD should contain carefully crafted questions that accurately reflect the disorder. Researchers who study ASD and authors who develop tools to be used during the diagnostic process are especially burdened with the responsibility to carefully and clearly define the behaviors associated with these disorders. When the behaviors and characteristics associated with a disorder are thoroughly operationalized, then further development of the dimensions or factors that can be used for diagnosis may be clarified. This depends, of course, on the extent to which the items have adequate reliability.

Given the fact that methods for evaluating ASD, as well as our understanding of the underlying aspects of these disorders, are evolving, we have a particular responsibility to provide validity evidence of the effectiveness of any method we choose (rating scales, tests, interviews, etc.). This is not as simple a task as demonstrating reliability, because validity is harder to demonstrate and the findings will be directly related to the content of the tools used to study ASD, as well as the methodology employed. For example, the items included in a rating scale define and limit the scope of the information that is obtained. This can provide a broad or truncated view of the behaviors associated with a disorder. Choosing the standard against which measures are validated is also not foolproof, because today's so-called diagnostic gold standard (i.e., the *Diagnostic and Statistical Manual of Mental Disorders, Fifth Edition* [DSM-5]; American Psychiatric Association, 2013) will undoubtedly evolve to reflect future research findings. Similarly, research methodology is also important, particularly when typical children are being compared with those who have ASD. Special attention should be made to ensure that research findings provide a sufficient number of control groups to determine how those with ASD differ from typical children, as well as from those with other types of disorders.

In summary, the very nature of our understanding of ASD is influenced by the psychometric quality of the tests and methods we use to study these disorders, as well as by the selection of variables we use in our research. Clinicians should be mindful, however, that until there is sufficient maturity in the scope and quality of the instruments used during the diagnostic process, a good understanding of the strengths and weaknesses of all the methods used is necessary. This includes a careful understanding of the manner in which any measure of ASD is constructed.

Development of Scales to Assess ASD

There is a need for a number of well-standardized measures of ASD that have demonstrated reliability and validity. At this writing, there are several behavior rating scales that have been used in both applied and research settings, as well as structured clinical interviews and direct assessments that have varying degrees of reliability and validity. This amplifies the need for practitioners and researchers to have a good understanding of the psychometric qualities and standardization samples associated with these methods. Researchers and practitioners should also be informed about the development of any scale used to aid in the diagnosis of ASD; the test's development should be carefully described by its authors. Development of any scale should follow a series of steps to ensure the highest quality and validity. The development of tools to help diagnose ASD is a task that demands well-known procedures amply described by Crocker and Algina (1986) and by Nunnally and Bernstein (1994). These are now summarized.

Initial test development should begin with a clear definition of the behaviors that represent autism and other ASD. These behaviors and other defining characteristics must be written with sufficient clarity that they can be assessed reliably over time and across raters. Behaviors should be included that represent the characteristics that define children with autism or other ASD as completely as possible, are specific to these disorders, and reflect current conceptualizations of the disorders (such as the behaviors included in DSM-5). Definitional clarity is *required* for good item writing.

The next step is to develop an initial pool of questions, followed by pilot testing of the items. Pilot tests are designed to evaluate the clarity of the instructions and items, as well as the structure of the form and other logistical issues. For instance, it is important to be cognizant of the ways items are presented on the page, size of the fonts, clarity of the directions, colors used on the form, position of the items on the paper, and so forth. Analyses of reliability and validity are typically not of interest at this point, because sample size usually precludes adequate examination of these issues. Instead, the goal of pilot testing is to answer essential questions such as these: Does the form seem to work? Do the users understand what they need to do? Are the items clear? Can the rater respond to each question?

In contrast, conducting experiments with larger samples that allow for an examination of the psychometric qualities of the items and their correspondence to the constructs of interest is the next important step. This effort is repeated until there is sufficient confidence that the items and the scales have been adequately operationalized. In each phase of the process, experimental evidence within the context of the practical demands facing clinical application should guide development, but some essential analyses such as the following should be conducted:

- Means and *SD*s, and *p* values (if dichotomous items are used), should be obtained for each item.
- Items designed to measure the same construct should correlate with a total score obtained from the sum of all those items designed to measure that same construct. If the correlations are low, their inclusion in the scale should be questioned.
- The contribution each item makes to the reliability of the scale(s) on which it is placed should be evaluated.
- An item designed to measure a particular construct should correlate more strongly with other items designed to measure that same construct than with items designed to measure different constructs. If this is not found, the item may be eliminated.
- The internal reliability of those items organized to measure each construct should be computed, as should the reliability of a composite score.
- The factor structure of the set of items may be examined to test the extent to which items or scales form groups, or factors, whose validity can be examined.

The procedures used at this phase are repeated until the scale is ready for standardization. The number of times these activities are repeated depends upon the (1) quality of the original concepts, (2) quality of the initial pool of items, (3) quality of the sampling used to study the instrument, and (4) consistency of the results that are obtained. The overall aim is to produce an experimental version of an instrument that is ready to be subjected to a larger-scale and more costly national standardization study. This would include sufficient data collection efforts to establish the reliability and validity of the final measure. Standardization requires that a sample of persons who represent the population of the country in which the scale will be used are administered the questions in a uniform manner, so that normative values can be computed. Standardization samples are ordinarily designed to be representative of the normal population, so that those that differ from normality can be identified and the extent to which they differ from the norm (50th percentile) can be calibrated as a standard score to reflect dispersion around the mean. Development of norms is an art as much as a science, and there are several ways in which this task can be accomplished (see Crocker & Algina, 1986; Nunnally & Bernstein, 1994; Thorndike, 1982). The next tasks at this stage are collection and analysis of data for establishing reliability (internal, test–retest, interrater, intrarater) and validity (e.g., construct, predictive, and content). Of these two, validity is more difficult to establish and should be examined by using a number of different methodologies, with emphasis on assessing the extent to which the scale is valid for its intended purposes.

There are many different types of validity, making it impossible for validity to be determined by a single study. According to the *Standards for Educational and Psychological Testing* volume (American Educational Research Association, American Psychological Association, & National Council on Measurement Education, 2014), evidence for validity is required to support interpretations of test scores for intended use. Additionally, validity is noted to be an open-ended process with evidence collected prior to initial use as well as further data analysis as the test is in operational use. The standards relating to validity issues are to be addressed by authors and test development companies. Some of the more salient issues include the need to provide evidence that supports the following:

- Interpretations based on the scores the instrument yields.
- The appropriate relationships between the instrument's scores and one or more relevant criterion variables.
- The utility of the measure across a wide variety of demographic groups, or its limitations based on race, ethnicity, language, culture, and so forth.
- The expectation that the scores provided differentiate between groups as intended.
- The alignment of the factorial structure of the items or subtests with the scale configuration provided by the authors.

There is wide variation in the extent to which test authors document the development, standardization, reliability, and validity of their measures in test manuals. Some manuals provide sufficient descriptions that bring out the strengths of the scale; others provide limited details. Readers interested in illustrative manuals might look at those developed for the Universal Nonverbal Intelligence Test (Bracken & McCallum, 1997); the

Kaufman Assessment Battery for Children, Second Edition (Kaufman & Kaufman, 2004); and the Cognitive Assessment System, Second Edition (Naglieri et al., 2014). These examples illustrate how to provide detailed discussion of the various phases of development, as well as instructions about how the scores should be interpreted for the various purposes for which the measures were intended.

Documentation of development may end with the writing of the sections in the manual that describe the construction, standardization, and reliability/validity of the instrument, but authors also have the responsibility to inform users about how the scores should be interpreted (American Educational Research Association, American Psychological Association, & National Council on Measurement Education, 2014). This includes how test scores should be compared with one another, and authors should especially provide the values needed for significance when the various scores a measure provides are compared. This information is critically important if clinicians are to interpret the scores from any instrument in a manner that is psychometrically defensible.

Researchers and clinicians have a responsibility to choose measures that have been developed according to the highest standards available, because important decisions will be made on the basis of the information these measures provide. We suggest that for a scale to be considered acceptable for clinical practice, in addition to being reliable, it must have a standardized administration and scoring format with norms based on a large sample that represents the country in which the scale is used. This includes ample documentation of methods used to develop the measure, as well as ample evidence of validity and explicit instructions for interpretation of the scores that are obtained.

Obtaining information about the psychometric characteristics of instruments that could be used as part of the diagnostic process is a time-consuming and sometimes confusing task. Manuals provide different types of information; sometimes the information is clear and concise, and at other times it is hard to ascertain enough details to fully evaluate the results being presented. Comparisons across instruments are complicated by this inconsistency and by the logistical task of collecting the information. In the next section, we provide a systematic examination of the scales used to assess the behaviors associated with ASD. Our goal is to be informative about the specific details associated with important issues, such as reliability, validity, and standardization samples. The discussion of each test includes a general description of the scale, as well as reliability and validity information provided by the authors of these instruments in their respective test manuals. We end this chapter with a commentary on the relative advantages of these scales.

DESCRIPTIONS OF SCALES USED TO ASSESS ASD

Autism Diagnostic Observation Schedule, Second Edition

Description

The Autism Diagnostic Observation Schedule, Second Edition (ADOS-2; Lord, Rutter, et al., 2012; Lord, Luyster, Gotham, & Guthrie, 2012) is a semistructured assessment of communication, social interaction, restricted and repetitive behaviors, and play/imaginative interaction in children or adults suspected of having ASD. A referred individual is assessed with one of the five modules contained in the ADOS-2. Each module can be administered in 40–60 minutes and is geared for a child or adult at a particular developmental and expressive language level. Each module consists of a variety of standard activities and materials that allow the examiner to observe an individual engaging in behaviors typical of persons with ASD within a standardized setting in order to aid diagnosis.

The Toddler Module and Module 1 are most appropriate for children who are preverbal or do not consistency use phrase speech (i.e., flexible use of non-echoed, three-word utterances, and spontaneous, meaningful word combinations). The Toddler Module is appropriate for children ages 12–30 months, whereas Module 1 is appropriate for those children ages 31 months and older. The Toddler Module consists of 11 activities, whereas Module 1 consists of 10 activities that focus on the playful use of toys. Module 2 also focuses on the playful use of toys and contains 14 separate activities geared toward individuals at the phrase speech language level. Module 3 is intended for children and young adolescents who are verbally fluent and focuses on social, communicative, and language behaviors through 14 different activities. Finally, Module 4 consists of 10 mandatory activities and five optional activities that also examine social, communication, and language behavior through unstructured conversation, structured situations, and interview questions. This module is used in the assessment of verbally fluent older adolescents and adults.

Examiners take notes during ADOS-2 administration, and ratings are made immediately following the administration. Guidelines for ratings are provided in each module, and algorithms are used to formulate diagnosis. Separate algorithms are used for the interpretation of each module. For the Toddler and Modules 1–3, the ADOS-2 uses an overall cutoff score, which is the sum of selected items from the algorithm domains (Social Affect and Restricted and Repetitive Behaviors). The Social Affect domain includes items related to communication and reciprocal social interaction. The Restricted and Repetitive Behaviors domain includes items pertaining to observed restricted and repetitive behaviors. Module 4 uses separate cutoff scores for the Communication and Social Interaction total scores and the Communication + Social Interaction total score. Although items related to stereotyped behaviors and restricted interests as well as imagination/creativity are presented on the form, they are not included in the algorithm for Module 4.

Although the ADOS-2 has many similarities to DSM-5 and the *International Classification of Diseases, Tenth Revision* (ICD-10; World Health Organization, 1992) models of diagnosing ASD, the ADOS-2 record form has a number of behaviors coded that are not included in the algorithms. In addition, the ADOS-2 does not include information about the age of onset or early history required for a DSM-5 or ICD-10 diagnosis. Last, the authors note, "In cases where ADOS-2 classification differs from the overall clinical diagnoses, clinical judgment should overrule the ADOS-2 classification in achieving a best-estimate clinical diagnosis" (Lord, Rutter, et al., 2012, p. 187). When overruling, clinicians need to specify how achieved scores do not adequately represent observed behaviors.

Description of the Comparison Group

The original validation sample of the ADOS consisted of 381 individuals, consecutively referred to the Developmental Disorders Clinic at the University of Chicago. The authors note the ADOS-2 items and codes are functionally identical to those of the original ADOS and that Module 4 was unchanged. Therefore, certain reliability and validity results from the ADOS continue to apply. As such, many of these individuals were also included in the ADOS-2 Extended Validation sample. The Extended Validation sample included 1,139 participants, with 325 participants having repeated ADOS assessments (between two and seven times), resulting in 1,620 assessments included in the sample. The Extended Validation sample was largely collected at the Developmental Disorders Clinic at the University of Chicago ($n = 926$). The remaining ($n = 213$) were obtained through a longitudinal study by the Treatment and Education of Autistic and Related Communication Handicapped Children (TEACCH) centers at the University of North Carolina, Chapel Hill, and University of Chicago, or in the University of Michigan Autism and Communication Disorders Clinic research studies. Last, the ADOS-2 replication sample ($N = 1,259$) was competed as a means to replicate the ADOS-2 algorithms. This sample was collected from 11 sites throughout the United States and Canada; data collected from the University of Michigan were excluded to develop an independent sample. In this sample, 23 participants had repeated assessments, all of which were included in the analysis.

For the three studies, samples were described in terms of (1) ASD, which encompasses all ASD diagnoses (e.g., autistic disorder, Asperger's disorder, pervasive developmental disorder not otherwise specified [PDD-NOS]); (2) autism (i.e., the more narrow diagnoses of autistic disorder; (3) non-autism

ASD (i.e., ASD diagnoses other than autism); and (4) non-spectrum (any other diagnosis that is not on the autism spectrum, such as language disorder or oppositional defiant disorder). It should be remembered the definitions used were based on *Diagnostic and Statistical Manual of Mental Disorders, Fourth Edition, Text Revision* (DSM-IV-TR; American Psychiatric Association, 2000).

The composition of the ADOS-2 Validation and Replication samples for each module are as follows:

- *Module 1—Few to No Words, Nonverbal Mental Age ≥ 15 Months*
  - Validation: autism (*n* = 69), non-autism ASD (*n* = 20), and non-spectrum (*n* = 16)
  - Replication: autism (*n* = 50) and non-spectrum (*n* = 5)
- *Module 1—Few to No Words, Nonverbal Mental Age ≥ 15 Months*
  - Validation: autism (*n* = 306), non-autism ASD (*n* = 51), and non-spectrum (*n* = 33)
  - Replication: autism (*n* = 245), non-autism ASD (*n* = 6), and non-spectrum (*n* = 46)
- *Module 1—Some Words*
  - Validation: autism (*n* = 201), non-autism ASD (*n* = 75), and non-spectrum (*n* = 76)
  - Replication: autism (*n* = 183), non-autism ASD (*n* = 21), and non-spectrum (*n* = 64)
- *Module 2—Younger Than 5 Years*
  - Validation: autism (*n* = 58), non-autism ASD (*n* = 49), and non-spectrum (*n* = 30)
  - Replication: autism (*n* = 53), non-autism ASD (*n* = 17), and non-spectrum (*n* = 18)
- *Module 2—Age 5 Years or Older*
  - Validation: autism (*n* = 126), non-autism ASD (*n* = 36), and non-spectrum (*n* = 30)
  - Replication: autism (*n* = 100), non-autism ASD (*n* = 9), and non-spectrum (*n* = 8)
- *Module 3*
  - Validation: autism (*n* = 129), non-autism ASD (*n* = 186), and non-spectrum (*n* = 83)
  - Replication: autism (*n* = 339), non-autism ASD (*n* = 45), and non-spectrum (*n* = 73)
- *Module 4*
  - Validation: autism (*n* = 16), non-autism ASD (*n* = 14), and non-spectrum (*n* = 15)
  - Replication: not completed, as no changes were made from original ADOS

For each sample and module, information within each diagnostic group of each module was further broken down by gender, chronological age, verbal mental age, and nonverbal mental age (this information is available in the test manual). The authors further report that the ethnicities of the participants for both studies were variable across modules and are provided in a range across groups. The ADOS-2 Validation sample ethnicity groups were as follows: white (71–91%), African American (4–27%), Asian American (1–5%), American Indian (0–0.8%), biracial (0–2.2%), and other or unknown race (0–0.6%); 3.4% of white participants were identified as Hispanic. The ADOS-2 Replication sample ethnicity groups were as follows: white (81–91%), multiracial (5–9%), African American (1.5–4%), Asian American (1–4%), American Indian (1%), and other or unknown race (1%); 2–7% of participants were identified as Hispanic.

The sample for the Toddler Module was collected on a total of 182 children ages 12–30 months who were seen for 360 assessments. The ASD group was seen between one and 14 times (mean [M] = 3.24, SD = 3.48) and the non-spectrum and typically developing groups were seen between one and 12 times (M = 2.43, SD = 2.68; M = 1.29, SD = 1.26, respectively). Children who were seen multiple times were participating in larger longitudinal studies. This sample consisted of children with ASD (n = 46), non-spectrum disorders (i.e., expressive language disorder, mixed receptive–expressive language disorder, nonspecific intellectual disability, and Down syndrome; n = 37), and typical development (n = 99). In this group, 76% were male and 24% female. Ethnicity groups for the Toddler sample were as follows: white (80%); Hispanic (4%); African American (2%); Asian American (2%); American Indian (1%); biracial, multiracial, or other (10%); and 1% did not report ethnicity. Information is further broken down by chronological age and socioeconomic status as measured by highest level of maternal educational attainment (this information is available in the test manual).

Reliability

In order to evaluate the reliability of individual items on the ADOS, the test authors obtained interrater reliability information for each module. As the authors purport the ADOS-2 items are functionally identical to the original ADOS items, reliability information from the original ADOS manual still apply. For Module 1, interrater reliability had a mean exact agreement of 91.5%, and all items had more than 80% exact agreement across raters. With the exception of items describing repetitive behaviors and sensory abnormalities, the mean weighted kappa coefficients exceeded .60 (M = .78). Items describing repetitive behaviors and sensory abnormalities were less frequently scored as abnormal within the autistic sample and proved more difficult to score. One item, "behavior when interrupted," was eliminated due to poor reliability.

The mean agreement for Module 2 items was 89%, and all items exceeded 80% agreement. Out of the 26 items, the kappa value for 15 items exceeded .60 (*M* = .70), and the kappa value for the remaining items equaled .50, with the exception of four items: "unusual sensory interest in play material/person," "unusually repetitive interests or stereotyped behaviors," "facial expressions directed to others," and "shared enjoyment in interaction" had kappa values ranging from .38 to .49, with agreements from 78 to 93%. These items were either edited or eliminated due to poor reliability.

For Module 3, the mean exact agreement was 88.2%. Many items (17) had kappa values of .60 or better (*M* = .65), and all but two items received 80% or more agreement. The item "stereotyped/idiosyncratic use of words or phrases" was rewritten, and "communication of own affect," "social distance," "pedantic speech," and "emotional gestures" were either eliminated or collapsed within another item due to poor reliability.

Module 4 had a minimum of 80% exact agreement, with kappa coefficients exceeding .60 for 22 of the items (*M* = .66), and the remaining items having kappa values of .50 or higher. "Excessive interest in or references to unusual or highly specific topics or objects or repetitive behavior" had a kappa value of .41, and "responsibility" had a kappa value of .48. The items were kept because the agreement for both equaled 85%. "Attention to irrelevant details" and "social disinhibition" were eliminated due to poor reliability.

Interclass correlations for Modules 1–3 were computed from a subsample of the ADOS-2 Validation sample that allowed for the algorithm subtotals and totals for each module and the combined modules. When data were collapsed across all modules, the interclass correlation coefficients for the Social Affect domain was .96, Restricted and Repetitive Behaviors was .84, and overall total had a coefficient of .96. The authors note that these calculations were not made for Module 4, as no changes were made. Interrater agreement for diagnostic classification for autism versus non-spectrum was examined. For Module 1, agreement was 95%; for Module 2, agreement was 98%; and for Module 3, agreement was 92%.

Test–retest reliability for the ADOS-2 was obtained from 87 participants who were administered the same ADOS module two times within an average of 10 months. The authors describe this sample as primarily young, high-functioning children. For Modules 1–3, reliability for Social Affect ranged from .81 to .92, for Restricted and Repetitive Behaviors from .68 to .82, and overall total from .83 to .87.

Finally, the Toddler Module reliability of individual items demonstrated out of 38 items, 30 items had weighted kappa values equal to or greater than

.60, whereas the remaining had weighted kappa values greater than .45. Interrater item reliability was accessed across five categories that included Language and Communication, Reciprocal Social Interaction, Play, Stereotyped Behaviors and Restricted Interests, and Other Behaviors. Of 41 items, 39 demonstrated exact agreement of 80% or greater, whereas the rest held at 71% or greater. The reliability of domain scores and algorithm classification correlations were generated for both the All Younger/Older with Few to No Words (n = 10) and Older with Some Words (n = 4) algorithms. For the combined algorithm groups, interclass correlations were .95 for overall total, .95 for Social Affect, and .90 for Restricted and Repetitive Behaviors. Correlations are provided for both algorithm types in the manual.

The test–retest reliability for the Toddler Module was assessed using 39 children who received two administrations within a 2-month span. The sample included 17 children with ASD, 11 children with non-spectrum disorders, and 11 children who were typically developing. The test–retest reliability for the All Younger/Older with Few to No Words (n = 31) algorithm demonstrated correlations of .83 for Social Affect, .75 for Restricted and Repetitive Behaviors, and .86 for overall total. The absolute mean difference across the two assessments was 1.29 points (SD = 3.55) for the total score and .90 points (SD = 3.14) and .39 points (SD = 1.54) for Social Affect and Restricted and Repetitive Behaviors, respectively. The Older with Some Words (n = 8) algorithm demonstrated interclass correlations for test–retest reliability of .94 for Social Affect, .60 for Restricted and Repetitive Behaviors, and .95 for overall total. The absolute means difference for this algorithm across the two assessments was .63 points (SD = 2.13) for the overall total score, and .38 points (SD = 2.77) and .25 points (SD = 1.04) for Social Affect and Restricted and Repetitive Behaviors, respectively.

Validity

The authors of the ADOS-2 have provided results from factor-analytic studies of their scale. They reported that items from the Social Interaction and Communication domains loaded highly on the first factor, and a second factor consisted of items dealing with speech and gesturing. Factor-analysis studies of ADOS-2 Expanded Validity were similar to those of the original ADOS. Social Affect and Restricted and Repetitive Behaviors factors were positively correlated. Comparisons of children with autism, those with PDD-NOS, and those not on the spectrum are provided in the manual for each ADOS module. Typically, children with autism earned significantly higher scores on those items included in the modules than those with PDD-NOS, and the lowest scores were obtained by those not on the spectrum. The sample sizes by module and by group were wide-ranging from a low of 14 to a high of 375.

A receiver operating characteristic (ROC) analysis with using the ADOS-2 Expanded Validity study for Modules 1–3 found sensitivity between autism and non-spectrum to range from 91 to 98% and specificity to range from 50 (Module 1—Few to No Words, Nonverbal Mental Age ≤ 15 Months) to 94%. When non-autism ASD was compared with non-spectrum, sensitivity ranged from 72 to 95%, while specificity ranged from 19 (Module 1—Few to No Words, Nonverbal Mental Age ≥ 15 Months) to 83%. When ROC analyses were also completed using the ADOS-2 Replication sample for Module 1—Few to No Words, Nonverbal Mental Age ≥ 15 Months; Module 1—Some Words; Module 2—Younger Than 5 Years; and Module 3, results differed. Sensitivity for autism and non-spectrum ranged from 82 to 94%, whereas specificity ranged from 80 to 100%. For the non-autism ASD group and non-spectrum group, sensitivity ranged from 60 to 95% and specificity ranged from 75 to 100%.

Comparisons of mean scores for the Toddler Module was highest for those with ASD, followed by non-spectrum and typically developing groups for both algorithm types. Sensitivity and specificity studies were conducted for each algorithm type and divided into "unique developmental groupings" and "all visits." Group sizes were wide-ranging from 11 to 153 participants. Overall sensitivity ranged from 83 to 91%, while specificity ranged from 86 to 94%.

Autism Diagnostic Interview, Revised

Description

The Autism Diagnostic Interview—Revised (ADI-R; Rutter, Le Couteur, & Lord, 2003) is an extended interview that produces information needed to diagnose autism and assist in assessing other ASD. The ADI-R consists of 93 questions focusing primarily on three domains: Language/Communication; Reciprocal Social Interactions; and Restricted, Repetitive, and Stereotyped Behaviors and Interests. This interview should be administered by an experienced clinician to an informant familiar with the assessed individual's behavior and development. The assessed individual must have a mental age of at least 2 years. The interview takes approximately 1½–2½ hours to complete.

The interviewer records and codes detailed responses to the 93 questions, using the interview protocol. The interviewer then scores the interview, using one or more of the five algorithm forms. Algorithms are used to code up to 42 of the interview items in order to produce formal and interpretable results. The algorithms consist of both Diagnostic and Current Behavior algorithms. Diagnostic algorithms are used for diagnosis and focus on the individual's developmental history at ages 4–5 years, whereas

Current Behavior algorithms reflect symptoms at the time of testing and can be used for treatment and/or educational planning.

Summary scores are calculated for each of four domains (Qualitative Abnormalities in Reciprocal Social Interactions; Qualitative Abnormalities in Communication; Restrictive, Repetitive, and Stereotyped Patterns of Behavior; and whether the manifestations of behavior were evident [i.e., before 36 months of age]) for the Diagnostic algorithms. Cutoff scores are then used to determine the presence of ASD. There is only one cutoff for ASD, rather than separate cutoffs for autism and ASD, as on the ADOS.

Description of the Comparison Group

The ADI-R comparison group was developed by administering the ADI-R to several hundred caregivers of individuals both with and without autism; the individuals' ages ranged from preschool to early adulthood. Interviews were conducted as initial clinical assessments and research evaluations. No further information is provided on this sample of several hundred.

Reliability

The ADI-R manual presents interrater and test–retest reliability coefficients. Weighted kappa values are provided for the behavioral items of the four Diagnostic algorithm domains. These coefficients are broken down by age and come from one of two studies. In a sample of 19 children 36–59 months of age, the weighted kappa coefficients ranged from .63 to .89. In a sample of 22 individuals ages 5–29 years, weighted kappa coefficients ranged from .37 to .95. Test–retest reliability coefficients are also presented from a study of 94 preschool children with a test–retest period of 2–5 months. Coefficients were provided for the behavioral items, including Reciprocal Social Interaction; Abnormalities in Communication; and Restricted, Repetitive, and Stereotyped Behaviors and Interests of the Diagnostic algorithm domains (excluding Age of First Manifestation). Intraclass correlation coefficients ranged from .93 to .97.

Validity

The associations between the ADI-R and the Social Communication Questionnaire (SCQ; Rutter, Bailey, & Lord, 2003; see the description of that instrument later in this chapter), which is essentially a short form of the ADI-R, were examined for a sample of children with developmental language disorders to assess concurrent validity (Bishop & Norbury, 2002). The ADI-R was scored to distinguish those students meeting full DSM-IV/ICD-10 criteria for autism (this applied to eight out of a total sample of 21 children and eight out of the 14 with ASD), as well as those qualifying for a broad designation of ASD (children meeting criteria for two out of the three domains). Of the eight children meeting the full criteria on the ADI-R, six children scored 15 or more on the SCQ. Intercorrelations between the ADI-R and SCQ for the three ADI-R domains were examined. The Reciprocal Social Interaction domain had a Pearson correlation of .92; the Language/Communication domain correlation was .73; and the Restricted, Repetitive, and Stereotyped Behaviors and Interests domain correlation was .89. Within the ADI-R and SCQ, the cross-correlations between the Reciprocal Social Interaction and Language/Communication domains were .77 for the SCQ and .70 for the ADI-R. The Restricted, Repetitive, and Stereotyped Behaviors and Interests correlations with the other two domains were .48 and .53 for the SCQ, and .41 and .54 for the ADI-R.

Item-by-item agreement between the ADI-R and SCQ was provided. The ADI-R items were classified as present if a score of 1, 2, or 3 was obtained, whereas a score of 1 indicated agreement on the SCQ. Agreement between the items on the two tests ranged from 45 to 85%, with an average of 70.8%.

Autism Spectrum Rating Scale

Description

The Autism Spectrum Rating Scale (ASRS; Goldstein & Naglieri, 2009) is an observer-completed rating scale designed to aid in the diagnosis of individuals who may have ASD. The ASRS is completed by parents (or similar caregivers) or teachers (or similar professionals) who rate behaviors characteristic of children ages 2–5 years (Early Childhood version) and older children ages 7–18 years (School-Age form). All forms ask the rater to consider behaviors during the past month. The items measure behaviors characteristic of ASD and are organized to yield both empirically and rationally defined scales. There are three empirically derived scales (Self-Regulation, Social/Communication, and Unusual Behaviors) and an ASRS total scale. In addition to the factorially derived scales, there are several scales developed on the basis of locally organized item groups: Adult Socialization, Attention, Behavioral Rigidity, Emotionality, Peer Socialization, Language, Sensory Sensitivity, and Unusual Interests. The score for each of these scales is a *T*-score with a normative mean of 50 and an *SD* of 10. In addition, a short Screening version of the ASRS is provided, consisting of 15 items.

The authors state that the ASRS was developed to measure ASD and autism-related problems, in order to allow clinicians to compare an individual to norm-based expectations in an objective and reliable manner. Because the ASRS items are linked to DSM-IV-TR symptoms of autistic disorder, Asperger's disorder, and PDD-NOS, the information provided can also facilitate the process of differential diagnosis. Used in combination with other assessment information, results from the ASRS provide valuable information to guide diagnostic decisions. The results can also be used to help form individualized intervention plans and suggest behaviors to target in treatment, as well as to evaluate an individual's response to treatment. Finally, the 15-item ASRS Screening scale is intended to be used in large-scale prevention programs.

Description of the Comparison Group

The ASRS was standardized on a large sample of children and adolescents who were selected to be representative of the United States, with a proportional sample from Canada. Two samples of data were collected—one for the Early Childhood version and one for the School-Age version—to create norms for parent and teacher raters. Equal numbers of males and females, who ranged in age from 2 years, 0 months, through 18 years, 11 months, were included.

The normative sample included a total of 1,280 parent and 1,280 teacher ratings; 2,560 total ratings. The two- to five-year-old sample consisted of 640 ratings, completed by parents (n = 320) and teachers (n = 320). The 6- to 18-year-old sample consisted of 1,920 ratings completed by parents (n = 960) and teachers (n = 960). Sample characteristics were based on the 2000 U.S. Census report. Race/ethnicity backgrounds for the ASRS Parent Normative samples included white (61%), Hispanic (15.6%), African American (14.8%), multinational/other (4.4%), and Asian (4.1%), whereas the ASRS Teacher Normative samples consisted of white (59.2%), Hispanic (16.1%), African American (14.9%), multinational/other (5.4%), and Asian (4.4%). The manual also provides further race/ethnicity backgrounds for each of the forms and by gender. Data for parent education level was collected only on parent forms and consisted of less then high school (10.8%), high school graduate (26.6%), some college (29.1%), and college or higher (33.3%), with .03% missing. Geographically, the ASRS Parent Normative data were collected from the South (31.3%), Northeast (24.5%), Midwest (21.4%), West (19.5%), and Canada (2.8%), with .4% missing. Similarly, the ASRS Teacher Normative data were collected from the Northeast (37.9%), South (23.5%), Midwest (22.2%), West (11.7%), and Canada (4.7%). The diagnostic disruption of children included in the 2- to 5-year-old sample consisted of those diagnosed with autism (0.6%), speech/language impairments (3.1%), and developmental delays (0.6%), totaling 4.4%. The 6- to 18-year-old diagnostic disruptions had those diagnosed with autism (0.5%), emotional disturbance (1.1%), attention-deficit/hyperactivity disorder (ADHD; 4%), and speech/language impairments (3%), providing a total of 8.7% of the sample having a clinical diagnosis.

Reliability

The internal reliability coefficients for the empirically based scales for the Early Childhood ASRS are as follows: Social/Communication (39 items; reliability of .94 and .95 for parents and teachers, respectively), and Unusual Behaviors (23 items; reliability of .91 for parents and .85 for teachers) with total scale reliability of .95 and .94 for parents and teachers, respectively. The internal reliability coefficients for the empirically based scales for the School-Age ASRS are as follows for parents and teachers, respectively: Social/Communication (19 items; reliability of .91 and .92), Unusual Behaviors (24 items; reliability of .93 for both parents and teachers), and Self-Regulation (17 items; reliability of .92 and .93) with total scale reliability of .97 for parents and teachers. The 15-item ASRS Screening scale's reliability coefficients are .87 and .90 for parents and teachers, respectively, on the Early Childhood version, and .89 and .90 for parents and teachers, respectively, on the School-Age form.

Validity

Scores from the general population were compared with those diagnosed with ASD and other clinical diagnoses that included anxiety disorders, depressive disorders, and language disorders. A separate group of those diagnosed with ADHD was also compared. The group for the Early Childhood version parent form consisted of those from the general population (n = 133), ASD (n = 133), and other clinical diagnosis (n = 67), whereas the Teacher/Childcare Provided consisted of those from the general population (n = 123), ASD (n = 122), and other clinical diagnosis (n = 72). The samples for the School-Age parent form consisted of those from the general population (n = 211), ASD (n = 211), ADHD (n = 122), and other clinical diagnosis (n = 52). The teacher form for the School-Age version consisted of those from the general population (n = 227), ASD (n = 228), ADHD (n = 147), and other clinical diagnosis (n = 69). The manual provides a breakdown of demographic characteristics for each of these groups. Mean score differences demonstrated those from the ASD group had values above the recommended cut score of 60, with the ASRS total score above 70 (more than 2 *SD* above the normative sample).

The authors assess the validity of the ASRS to evaluate the diagnostic efficiency. In comparing the ASD group with the general population, they found the overall correct classification rate to range from 89.4 to 91.4% for the total score on all forms with the ASRS scales ranging from 88 to 93.5% on the Social/Communication scale and 85.2 to 94.8% on the Unusual Behaviors scale. DSM-IV-TR scale ranged from 89.75 to 94.1%. Sensitivity for the total score ranged from 89.8 to 91.1%, whereas specificity ranged from 88.6 to 92.2%. The authors also provide efficiency statistics for the positive and negative predictive power, as well as the false-positive and false-negative rates and kappa score for the total score, ASRS scales, and DSM-IV-TR scale (see manual).

The manual provides several studies comparing the ASRS with other measures of ASD. These studies compared the *T*-score of the ASRS with the standard scores from the Gilliam Autism Rating Scale, Second Edition (GARS-2: Gilliam, 2006); and Gilliam Asperger's Disorder Scale (GADS; Gilliam, 2001); as well as the raw score from the Childhood Autism Rating Scale, Second Edition (CARS-2; Schopler, Van Bourgondien, Wellman, & Love, 2010). Correlations between the ASRS and GARS-2 ranged from .76 to 83, whereas the GADS ranged from .63 to .76. Correlations between the ASRS and CARS ranged from .06 to 50. The authors also compared the ASRS with the Cognitive Assessment System (CAS; Naglieri, Das, & Goldstein, 2013), which is based on A. R. Luria's conceptualization of major brain functions. The results found those with high ASRS total scores had mean standard scores ranging from 92.1 to 98.8 on the Planning, Simultaneous, and Successive scales, whereas the Attention scale had a mean score of 83.

Construct validity was assessed using several analyses to determine the extent to which the ASRS items form clusters that represent broad categories associated with the ASD diagnosis. Exploratory factory analysis suggested a two-factor solution was most suitable for the Early Childhood version, whereas a three-factor solution was most suitable for the School-Age version. For the Early Childhood version the exploratory factor analysis grouped behaviors related to socialization and communication into one factor and stereotypical and repetitive behaviors into a second factor. The School-Age version found socializing and communication problems loaded together on one factor, stereotypical and repetitive behaviors on a second factor, and self-regulatory behaviors on a third factor. Exploratory factor analysis also demonstrated consistency across genders, race/ethnicities, and clinical status.

Childhood Autism Rating Scale, Second Edition

Description

The Childhood Autism Rating Scale, Second Edition (CARS-2; Schopler et al., 2010) comprises three forms. The Childhood Autism Rating Scale, Second Edition, Standard Form (CARS2-ST) is for those ages 6 and younger, with an estimated IQ of 79 and lower. The CARS2-ST was formerly titled CARS in the original 1998 version. The Childhood Autism Rating Scale, Second Edition, High Functioning (CARS2-HF) version is designed for those ages 6 and older, with an estimated IQ of 80 or higher. These are 15-item behavior rating scales developed to help identify children with autism, to evaluate varying degrees of the disorder, and help determine whether a more comprehensive evaluation for ASD is warranted. The CARS-2 was also developed to differentiate children with autism from those with other developmental disorders, particularly those with moderate to severe intellectual disabilities. CARS-2 ratings are based on a clinician's observations or on parent report. Behaviors are rated on a scale of 1 (within normal limits), 2 (mildly abnormal), 3 (moderately abnormal), and 4 (severely abnormal for that age), based on a one- or two-sentence description of the behavior being evaluated. Item scores for the CARS2-ST and CARS2-HF are summed and categorized. Raw scores for the CARS2-ST that range between 15 and 29.5 are considered minimal-to-no symptoms of ASD, 30–36.5 is considered the range of mild to moderate ASD, and 37–60 is considered the severe ASD range. The CARS2-HF ranges are 15–27.5 for minimal symptoms of ASD, 28–33.5 for mild to moderate symptoms of ASD, and 34 and higher is considered the severe symptom range for ASD. There is also a CARS-2 Questionnaire for Parents or Caregivers (CARS2-QPC) version. The CARS2-OPC form is designed to assist in gathering information regarding behaviors related to ASD to help inform scoring of the CARS2-ST and CARS2-HF. The 15 items included in the CARS-2 are based on the diagnostic criteria from Kanner (1943), the nine dimensions by Creek (1961), Rutter's (1978) definition, criteria proposed by the National Society for Autistic Children (1978), and DSM-IV-TR.

Description of the Comparison Group

The CARS-2 comprises three samples: the original 1998 CARS sample (*N* = 1,606), the CARS2-ST Verification sample (*N* = 1,034), and the CARS2-HF Development sample (*N* = 994). The original CARS sample were children who were referred to the North Carolina TEACCH program. The 1998 manual noted this comparison group comprised a referred sample of children suspected of having autism who had CARS scores below 30 (46%). The remaining 54% were identified as having autism. About half of the sample with autism had CARS scores that fell in the mild to moderate range, and half met the criteria for severe autism. This sample consisted of 23% females and 72% males (5% were missing demographic information), whose racial background was white (62%), African American (28%), other (3%), and missing (7%). The authors describe the sample as predominantly from low socioeconomic levels, based on the Hollingshead–Redlich two-factor index. Almost one-fourth (23%) of the sample fell in the lowest socioeconomic category (V) identified by the index. The rest of the sample was distributed as follows: IV (29%), III (20%), II (8%), and I (8%); missing (12%). The sample was further described on the basis of IQ as follows: 52% ≤ 69, 12% = 70–84, and 10% = 85 and above, with 26% missing.

Finally, the children varied in age as follows: <6 years = 53%, 6–10 years = 30%, and 11 and above = 10%; missing = 6%. No data on the minimum or maximum ages of the children included in the sample, or other characteristics (e.g., parental education) were provided. The degree to which this sample represents a population of children with autism in the state of North Carolina or the country was not provided. Importantly, these data were collected from the late 1960s through the late 1980s, according to the CARS 1998 manual.

The CARS2-ST Verification sample (*N* = 1,034) consisted of those already diagnosed with autism in various clinical settings and collected from four demographic regions: South (43%), Northeast (29%), West (17%), and Midwest (11%). The authors' state that to maintain consistency with the demographics of individuals diagnosed with autism, the sample was 78% males and 22% females. Race/ethnicity backgrounds were white (60%), black/African American (16%), Hispanic/Latino (13%), Asian/Pacific Islander (7%), and other (4%). Socioeconomic status, provided as head of household years of education completed, were less than high school diploma (13%), high school graduate (34%), some college (13%), college graduate (20%), postgraduate (13%), and missing (7%). IQ descriptions for the sample were ≤70 (81%) and 80–85 (19%) and were intently skewed to represent those with lower cognitive functioning with the acknowledgment that ratings for higher-functioning individuals may also occur. Last, ages ranged from 2 to 36 years old, with age bands in years of 2–5 (30%), 6–10 (43%), 11–15 (20%), and 16–36 (7%). Information regarding methods previously used to diagnose autism was not provided, nor was the severity of autism symptoms. Although the U.S. Census figures for 2000 (U.S. Census Bureau, 2000) are provided, there are large discrepancies between the Verification sample and actual U.S. population.

For the CARS2-HF Development sample (*N* = 994), individuals had a verity of clinical diagnoses that included high-functioning autism (*n* = 248), Asperger's disorder (*n* = 231), PPD-NOS (*n* = 95), ADHD (*n* = 179), learning disorder (*n* = 111), and "other internalizing and externalizing clinical disorders" (*n* = 69). To verify an absence of symptoms on the CARS2-HF, a small group of general education (*n* = 21) and non-autistic special education (*n* = 40) students were included. This sample was collected from various clinical settings around the United States: South (48%), Midwest (21%), Northeast (20%), and West (10%). Similar to the CARS2-ST verification sample, the CARS2-HF consisted of 78% males and 22% females. Race/ethnicity backgrounds were white (73%), black/African American (14%), Hispanic/Latino (6%), Asian/Pacific Islander (3%), Native American (1%), and other (3%). Socioeconomic status, provided as head of household years of education completed, is broken into less than high school diploma (8%), high school graduate (30%), some college (15%), college graduate (17%), postgraduate (14%), and missing (16%). Ages ranged from 6 to 57 years old with age bands in years of 6–10 (35%), 11–15 (41%), and 16–57 (24%). The authors state that all individuals had an estimated IQ of 80 or higher—however, further information regarding IQ ranges is not provided.

Reliability

The CARS-2 manual presents internal, test–retest, and interrater reliability coefficients. In the CARS2-ST Verification sample (N = 1,034), internal reliability was estimated at an alpha coefficient of .93 with item-to-total correlations ranging from .43 to .81 (M = .69). The CARS2-HF Developmental sample (N = 994) obtained an estimated alpha coefficient of .96; item-to-total correlations ranged from .53 to .88 (M = .79).

Interrater reliability for the CARS (1998 version) was provided for the CARS2-ST. For the CARS, two trained independent raters evaluated 280 cases in the Development sample and obtained an estimated correlation of .71 with item correlations ranging from .55 to .93 (median = .71). Interrater reliability for the CARS2-HF was examined from two trained independent raters for 239 individuals in the Development sample. A correlation of .95 was obtained for total scores, whereas item correlations ranged from .53 to .93 (median = .73). Weighted kappa estimates were also calculated with a median level of agreement of .73, with items ranging from .51 to .90.

Information regarding test–retest reliability was provided only from the CARS (1998 version) Development sample, although the manual cites several external studies. The manual states 91 individuals assessed approximately 1 year apart resulted in an indication for the scale's stability over time—however, the correlation is not provided. Information is provided between the second and third evaluations, which the authors state is to avoid the effects of improvement in autistic behaviors frequently seen between the first and second assessment due to intensive treatment effort. Correlations between the second and third evaluation resulted in a correlation of .88 ($p < .01$) with means of 31.5 and 31.9 for the second and third evaluation, respectively; a kappa coefficient of .64 was also obtained. However, a time frame is not provided for the length between the first, second, and third evaluation. No test–rest reliability is provided for the CARS2-HF or updated for the CARS2-ST.

Validity

The authors assess internal structure of item ratings with the CARS2-ST using the Verification sample and the CARS2-HF using the Development sample. A similar pattern was observed between forms. The CARS2-ST correlations for item ratings ranged from .37 to .77; total raw score to item correlations ranged from .55 to .84. The CARS2-HF between-item rating correlations for individuals without ASD ranged from .57 to .85, total raw score to item correlations ranged from .76 to .92. The Autism sample ranged from .35 to .69, whereas total raw score to item correlations ranged from .66 to .85. Factor-analytic results for the CARS2-ST yielded two component factors accounting for 59% of the variance with the first factor related to communication and sensory issues and the second factor related to emotional issues. In a factor analysis of the CARS-HF for those with and without ASD, three factors accounted for 59% of the variances in the ratings. The first factor related to social and emotional issues, the second related to cognitive functioning and verbal ability, and the third related to sensory issues.

The authors provide a ROC analysis for the original CARS to identify those with and without ASD using the total raw scores and found a sensitivity value of .88 and specificity value of .86, resulting in a false-negative rate of 12% and false-positive rate of 14%. The authors report ratings obtained for the CARS2-ST Verification sample was consistent with the original findings. Several independent studies are provided in the manual that found similar results when a ROC analysis was conducted using the original CARS.

The Development sample of the CARS2-HF was examined for differences in total raw scores between diagnoses. They found those with high-functioning autism obtained a mean of 35.3 (SD = 6.9), followed by PPD-NOS (M = 33.6, SD = 7.2), Asperger's disorder (M = 32, SD = 6.1), mixed clinical (M = 24.8, SD = 7.7), ADHD (M = 19.6, SD = 5.1), nonverbal learning disorder (M = 19, SD = 6.4), learning disorder (M = 18.7, SD = 5.1), general education students (M = 17.3, SD = 2.1), and special education students (M = 17, SD = 2.6). The manual also provides mean scores for each item in these groups. A ROC analysis to distinguish the non-autistic and autistic groups found sensitivity to be .81 and specificity to be .87 with a corresponding false-positive rate of 11% and false-negative rate of 23%.

The authors assessed criterion-related validity for the original CARS by comparing total scores to clinical ratings obtained during the same diagnostic session ($r = .85$, $p < .001$). Total scores were also correlated with independent clinical assessments made by a child psychologist and a child psychiatrist. This was based on information obtained from referral records, parent interviews, and nonstructured clinical interviews ($r = .80$, $p < .001$).

The relationship between the CARS2-ST and CARS2-HF with other measures evaluating autism was compared. Comparing the CARS2-ST and the ADOS ($n = 37$) provided a correlation of .79, whereas comparing CARS2-HF and the ADOS ($n = 76$) provided a correlation of .77. Correlations between clinician-generated CARS-2 total scores and mothers' Social Responsiveness Scale (SRS) total scores ($n = 293$) resulted in a moderate relationship with a correlation of .38 for the CARS2-ST and .47 for the CARS2-HF. The authors purport the moderate relationship found is typically seen between clinician and parent ratings of children's behaviors. Several independent studies compared the original CARS with other measures of autism. Pilowsky, Yirmia, Shulman, and Dover (1998) reported 85.7% diagnostic agreement between the ADI-R and original CARS in a study of 83 children and adults with an overall kappa of .36. Another study found significant Pearson correlations on the original CARS scores and ADI-R that ranged from .60 on the ADI-R Communication subscale to .81 on the Social Impairment subscale and the CARS total score. Last, several studies compared the CARS with the Ritvo–Freeman Real Life Rating Scale (Ritvo et al., 2011) and Autism Behavior Checklist (Eaves, Campbell, & Chambers, 2000) with varying results.

Psychoeducational Profile, Third Edition

Description

The Psychoeducational Profile, Third Edition (PEP-3; Schopler, Lansing, Reichler, & Marcus, 2005) is an instrument designed to evaluate cognitive skills and behaviors typical of individuals characterized as having ASD and other developmental disabilities. This instrument is appropriate for children between the ages of 6 months and 7 years, for the purposes of planning educational programming and in the diagnosis of autism and other ASD. The test manual outlines four specific purposes of the PEP-3: to identify an individual's strengths and weaknesses, to aid in diagnosis, to establish developmental and adaptive level, and to serve as a research tool.

The PEP-3 has two major components: the Performance Part and the Caregiver Report. The Performance Part is administered through direct observation and testing, and consists of 10 subtests (six measuring developmental abilities and four measuring maladaptive behaviors) that form three composite scores: Communication, Motor, and Maladaptive Behavior. The Caregiver Report is completed by a parent or caregiver based on daily observations of the child. The Caregiver Report consists of two sections: (1) child's current developmental level and (2) degree of problems in different diagnostic categories. This information can be used to aid in clinical diagnosis. The Caregiver Report contains three subtests: Problem Behaviors, Personal Self-Care, and Adaptive Behavior.

Items on the PEP-3 are scored according to scoring criteria provided in the Examiner Scoring and Summary Booklet. Normative data are provided to facilitate a normative analysis, which allows the examiner to establish adaptive/developmental levels and make comparisons of the child to other children with autism. These scores can also be used in clinical analysis and provide information on a child's passing, emerging, or failing performance on individual items, as well as appropriate, mild, or severe performance on individual Maladaptive Behavior items.

Normative scores allow examiners to compare a child's developmental age to that of a typically developing sample. The test authors state that a child identified as having ASD characteristically has an uneven developmental profile in relation to the developmental subtests. This developmental profile can then be used for determining the child's strengths and weaknesses. Percentile ranks were determined based upon a comparison sample with ASD and are available for subtests (and composite scores for the developmental subtests). The manual provides interpretive guidelines for these scores. Percentile scores above 89 are considered to be at the adequate developmental/adaptive level, 75–89 at the mild level, 25–74 at the moderate level, and below 25 at the severe level. Percentile ranks for the Maladaptive Behavior composite can also be used in interpretation. The manual states that a score lower than the 90th percentile in this composite usually places a child on the autism spectrum. Scores on the Problem Behaviors and Adaptive Behavior subtests, as well as the Caregiver Report, can be used to reinforce this interpretation.

Description of the Comparison Group

A sample of 407 children with autism and other ASD, as well as 149 typically developing children, was used for the PEP-3 normative sample. In the group with ASD, 95% of the children were classified as having autism, 4% as having Asperger syndrome, and 1% as exhibiting a developmental delay. Children in the sample ranged from ages 2 to 21 years (2 years, n = 38; 3 years, n = 60; 4 years, n = 63; 5 years, n = 51; 6 years, n = 48; 7 years, n = 23; 8 years, n = 27; 9 years, n = 21; 10 years, n = 19; 11 years, n = 16; 12 years, n = 15; 13–21 years, n = 26). The sample closely matched the U.S. population with regard to geographic area, gender, race, Hispanic ethnicity, family income, and educational attainment of parents.

Individuals in the typically developing sample consisted of 149 children between the ages of 2 and 6 (2 years, n = 27; 3 years, n = 33; 4 years, n = 36; 5 years, n = 27; 6 years, n = 26). This sample was 53% female and 47% male. The normative population closely matched the U.S. population on the domains of geographic area, race, Hispanic heritage, family income, educational attainment, and disability status.

Reliability

Internal consistency was assessed in a sample of individuals with autism at 11 age intervals (ages 2–11). Average alpha coefficients for Performance Part subtests, Caregiver Report subtests, and composites ranged from .84

to .99. Coefficient alphas were also provided for six subgroups of individuals with autism and the normally developing sample. The six subgroups, and the range of their alpha values for the Performance Part subtests, Caregiver Report subtests, and composites, were as follows: white (.78–.99), black (.76–.99), other race (.80–.99), Hispanic (.79–.99), male (.77–.99), female (.81–.99), and the normally developing sample (.75–.97).

Test–retest reliability was also examined in a sample of 33 children with autism between the ages of 4 and 14 residing in California, Oklahoma, and Texas. The sample consisted of 28 males and five females, and was also broken down by race and Hispanic ethnicity (white = 24, black = 4, other race = 5, Hispanic ethnicity = 6). The correlation coefficients ranged from .94 to .99 for both Performance Part subtests and Caregiver Report subtests. Correlation coefficients could not be calculated for composite scores, as raw data were used. The time lapse between the first and second test was 2 weeks.

Interrater reliability was assessed by using polychoric correlations, because items on the Caregiver Report are ordered categorical data. The sample used in this reliability study consisted of 40 individuals ages 2–10 from seven different states. Of the 41 participants, 33 were male and seven were female, 32 were white, six were black, two were of other races, and one was Hispanic. Nine of the 40 children did not have a disability, 29 were diagnosed with autism, and two were diagnosed with Asperger syndrome. Two parents of each child independently completed the Caregiver Report, and polychoric correlations for the items on the Problem Behaviors, Personal Self-Care, and Adaptive Behavior subtests were computed. Polychoric correlations for the items on the Adaptive Behavior subtest ranged from .70 to .91 (M = .85), Personal Self-Care item correlations ranged from .65 to 1.00 (M = .90), and correlations for the Adaptive Behavior subtest items ranged from .52 to .90 (M = .78). It should be noted that one item on the Adaptive Behavior subtest was eliminated because it had a very low correlation.

Validity

Median item discrimination coefficients were calculated by the test authors for a sample of children with autism ages 2–12 to assess the degree to which an item would correctly differentiate among test takers. Such coefficients were calculated for 11 age intervals for each subtest of the Performance Part and the Caregiver Report. Item difficulty coefficients were also calculated at these 11 age intervals to determine the items that were too easy or too difficult and arrange them in order from least to most difficult.

In order to detect differential item function (DIF), a logistic regression procedure was applied to all PEP-3 subtest items. The sample of individuals with autism was used to make comparisons between these groups: male versus female, black versus non-black, and Hispanic versus non-Hispanic. Four of these comparisons were found to illustrate DIF at the .001 significance level. However, after reviewing these items, the test authors suggested that the four items exhibited benign DIF.

Criterion prediction validity was assessed in four studies by examining the relationship between the PEP-3 and four criterion measures. First, the authors examined the relationship between the PEP-3 and the original Vineland Adaptive Behavior Scales, Expanded Form (VABS; Sparrow, Balla, & Cicchetti, 1984) for a sample of 45 children with autism between the ages of 2 and 14. In general, the correlations were high, with only a few exceptions (e.g., Vineland Motor Skills with PEP-3 Problem Behaviors). The second study ($N = 68$) examined the correlations between the CARS and the PEP-3. Significant and large correlations were found. Similarly, the third study involved the correlations of the PEP-3 with the Autism Behavior Checklist, Second Edition (Krug, Arick, & Almond, 2008). The results for this sample of 316 children suggested that the two scales are highly correlated.

The test authors calculated correlations between all subtests and found that these correlations ranged from .39 to .90, with a mean of .68. The authors state that coefficients for the subtests range from moderate to very large, and that the mean coefficient falls within the large range. Because of this, they suggest that the PEP-3 subtests measure different skills or behaviors and that evidence thus exists for construct identification validity. These intercorrelations were further subjected to confirmatory factor analysis to test the degree to which the subtests' assignment to the three composites were supported by data from the standardization sample. The results indicated that the three composites (Communication, Motor, and Maladaptive Behavior) could be considered a viable structure for this instrument.

Social Communication Questionnaire

Description

The SCQ (Rutter, Bailey, et al., 2003) is a 40-item rating scale completed by parents to assess the symptoms associated with ASD. The content of the scale is the same as that of the ADI-R (Rutter, Le Couteur, at al., 2003), reviewed above, with items worded identically, but it is administered as a parent questionnaire rather than via an extended interview. The scale uses a yes/no format and, according to the test manual, takes approximately 10 minutes to complete and 5 minutes to score. Raw scores are summed to yield a total score, which is interpreted based on the form being used and recommended cutoff scores. The SCQ has two forms: Lifetime and Current

Behavior. The Lifetime form assesses the individual's entire developmental history, whereas the Current Behavior form assesses behavior in the most current 3 months. The Lifetime form is considered more useful for diagnosing or screening ASD, while the Current Behavior form can be beneficial for developing treatment plans.

According to the authors, the SCQ has three main uses. First, it can be used as a screening device for the presence of ASD. If a child is suspected of having ASD after being screened, further clinical assessment should be conducted. The SCQ is an alternative to the ADI-R for use when time does not permit a lengthy assessment, such as in screening; the questions are identical, so one or the other can be used, but not both. The subscores produced by the SCQ can also be used to match the domains of the ADI-R (Reciprocal Social Interaction; Language/Communication; and Restricted, Repetitive, and Stereotyped Behaviors and Interests). Although the production of subscores can be used for interpretation, the manual warns that these subscores have not been adequately researched. A second use of the SCQ is for research purposes; it can be used with groups of children diagnosed with ASD to compare symptoms across groups. A third identified use of the SCQ is its ability to identify severity of ASD symptoms or changes in severity of symptoms over time. This is accomplished through the use of the Current Behavior form.

Description of the Comparison Group

Raw scores from the SCQ are compared with those earned by a sample of 200 children who had participated in previous studies using the ADI-R. The children in this sample had a variety of developmental disabilities: 83 had autism, 49 had atypical autism, 16 had Asperger syndrome, seven had fragile X syndrome, five had Rett syndrome, 10 had conduct disorder, seven had language delay, 15 had intellectual disability, and eight had other clinical diagnoses.

Reliability

Information is provided on the internal consistency of the SCQ as a measure of reliability. Alpha coefficients were computed in two different ways. First, a sample of 214 children with both ASD and non-spectrum diagnoses was divided into five different groups. These groups consisted of a "no-language" group and four "language" groups divided by age. Alpha coefficients for these groups ranged from .84 to .93. Next, internal consistency was examined by dividing the 157 children in the language group into one of three diagnostic categories: autism, other ASD, and non-spectrum. Measures of internal consistency for these groups ranged from .81 to .92.

Validity

Of the 39 items scored on the SCQ, 33 showed statistical differentiation of children with ASD from those with other abnormalities. The items that did not show differentiation primarily concerned abnormal language features. These items had a relatively high frequency among children without ASD, but correlated with the total score (.64, .53, .45, and .57). Two items (self-injury and unusual attachment to objects) differentiated at the 7% significance level and showed more modest correlations with the total score (.37 and .27, respectively). Correlations were also calculated for the total score and domains (Reciprocal Social Interaction; Language/Communication; and Restricted, Repetitive, and Stereotyped Behaviors and Interests). All correlations were significant at the .0005 level within and across the domains and ranged from .31 to .71 (Berument, Rutter, Lord, Pickles, & Bailey, 1999).

Three- and four-factor solutions were explored for 39 items of the SCQ (items 2–40). Analysis suggested that a four-factor structure appeared to be an acceptable fit. Principal-component factoring with varimax rotation yielded four factors and explained 42.4% of the total variation of the SCQ data; 24.3% (eigenvalue = 9.7) was accounted for by a social interaction factor (1), 8.7% (eigenvalue = 3.38) by a communication factor (2), 5% (eigenvalue = 1.94) by an abnormal language factor (3), and 4.5% (eigenvalue = 1.74) by a stereotyped behavior factor (4). The alpha reliability was .90 for the total scale, .91 for factor 1, .71 for factor 2, .79 for factor 3, and .67 for factor 4. The individual item-to-total scores were positive and mainly substantial, with a range of .26–.73. The four factors mapped onto the three domains that were operationalized by the ADI-R algorithm criteria. Factor 1 coincided with the Reciprocal Social Interaction domain; factor 4 coincided with the Restricted, Repetitive, and Stereotyped Behaviors and Interests domain; and the Language/Communication domain items were mainly divided between factors 2 and 3 (Berument et al., 1999).

ROC analysis and a series of *t*-tests were used to assess the discriminative power of the SCQ (Berument et al., 1999). After examining the area under the curve (AUC), the authors reported that the SCQ was able to differentiate ASD (including autism) from non-ASD conditions, including intellectual disability (AUC = .86). The SCQ also effectively differentiated between autism and non-ASD conditions other than intellectual disability (AUC = .94), autism and intellectual disability (AUC = .92), and autism and other ASD (AUC = .74), although this last distinction was less clear-cut.

Analyses were then repeated, using an SCQ score that did not include the six items that failed to differentiate the groups at the 5% significance level. The authors reported that some improvement in discriminative validity was obtained. However, the discriminative validity between autism and other ASD was worse. The discriminative validity of the SCQ was then compared with that of the ADI-R. AUC results were contrasted for ASD versus non-ASD conditions (AUC = .88 and .87, respectively), autism versus intellectual disability (AUC = .93 and .96, respectively), and autism versus other ASD (AUC = .73 and .74, respectively).

The authors also reported that groups differed in IQ distribution, and considered that SCQ diagnostic differentiation could be due to this differentiation. In order to investigate this possibility, analyses were repeated within the identified IQ bands. Data came from various studies, and as a result, several different IQ tests were used to assess cognitive abilities. Results showed that in the comparison group, the SCQ score was the lowest (8.39) in the group with an IQ above 70 and highest in the group with severe intellectual disability (14.74), and that the SCQ score did not vary by IQ within the group with ASD. The diagnostic differentiation within the IQ bands was significant and clearest in the group with an IQ above 70.

Another set of analyses was conducted to examine whether individual behavioral domains of the SCQ provided better diagnostic information than that obtained with the total score. Items of the SCQ were placed in one of three domains determined by the equivalent items on the ADI-R. All three domains provided differentiation of ASD from other disorders (AUC ranged from .79 to .83), and differentiation on the total score was stronger (AUC = .90). The authors reported that the total score provided the best differentiation. This is supported by the finding that the Restricted, Repetitive, and Stereotyped Behaviors and Interests domain was not good at differentiating autism from intellectual disability (AUC = .70) or autism from other ASD (AUC = .59).

The authors reported that the ROC analysis for the total SCQ suggests a score of 15 or more as the cutoff for differentiating ASD from other diagnoses (sensitivity = .85, specificity = .75, positive predictive value = .55 for the sample). The authors also suggested that other cutoffs may be desirable for general population samples or other purposes. The cutoff of 15 or more had a sensitivity of .96 and a specificity of .80 for autism versus other diagnoses, excluding intellectual disability, and a sensitivity of .96 and a specificity of .67 for autism versus intellectual disability. Finally, a higher cutoff of 22 or more was required to differentiate autism from other ASD with a sensitivity of .75 and a specificity of .60.

As noted earlier, the relationships between the ADI-R and SCQ were examined in a sample of children with developmental language disorders to assess concurrent validity (Bishop & Norbury, 2002). See the "Validity" section in the ADI-R for the results of that study.

The relationships between the SCQ and ADI-R total scores were reported by the test authors for 81 children involved in an international genetics study. The correlation between the SCQ and ADI-R was .78 and the intercorrelations among domains ranged from .44 to .77 ($p < .01$). The authors reported that the intercorrelations did not vary by age, gender, or IQ. When scores of 1, 2, and 3 on the ADI-R were compared with SCQ scores of 1, agreement ranged from 36.6 to 91.9%, with an average of 69.8%. When the ADI-R scores of 0 and 1 were collapsed and contrasted with scores of 2 on the SCQ, agreements were very similar and had an average of 68.5%.

Social Responsiveness Scale, Second Edition

Description

The Social Responsiveness Scale, Second Edition (SRS-2; Constantino & Gruber, 2012) comprises four forms that allow for evaluation from ages 2 years, 5 months, through adulthood and includes the Preschool form (ages 2 years, 5 months, to 4 years, 5 months), School-Age form (ages 4–18 years), and Adult Self-Report and Adult Relative/Other-Report forms (ages 19 years and older). The forms consist of 65-item questionnaires that cover various dimensions of interpersonal behavior, communication, and repetitive/stereotypical behavior. Items on the scale focus on the behavior of the child or adult, and the rater's responses are given in a Likert-type format. Each form takes approximately 15 minutes to complete and 5–10 minutes to score.

The test authors recommend that the SRS-2 results be used in different ways, depending upon the goal of assessment. When the SRS is used as a broad screening tool for any ASD in general populations, a cutoff raw score of 70 is recommended. When the instrument is used for screening in clinical and educational settings for children suspected of having social development problems, a cutoff score of 85 is recommended. For all forms, when SRS-2 scores are converted to *T*-scores, a value of ≤ 59 is within normal limits and not associated with clinically significant ASD; 60–65 is considered to be in the mild range, indicating deficiencies in reciprocal social behaviors and generally attributed to other clinical reasons (e.g., ADHD, language delays); scores from 66 to 75 are in the moderate range and represent deficiencies in reciprocal social behaviors that are often seen in those with moderate ASD and social (pragmatic) communication disorder; scores ≤ 76 are in the severe range and are strongly associated with a clinical diagnosis of ASD. Two scales, with proposed alignment at the time the manual was written to DSM-5 criteria, are provided and include Social Communication and Interaction and Restrictive Interests and Repetitive Behaviors. Last, the SRS-2 also yields *T*-scores for five treatment subscales: Social Awareness, Social Cognition, Social Communication, Social Motivation, and Restrictive Interests and Repetitive Behaviors. The authors note that application of these treatment subscales should be limited to research of clinical investigation to target alleviation of symptoms as available evidence does not support individual interpretation of these subscales. Instructions for interpretation of DSM-5-compatible subscales and treatment subscales scores are provided in the test manual.

Description of the Comparison Group

The SRS-2 standardization included three independently collected samples. The School-Age standardization sample consisted of 1,014 children (ages 4–18) with 2,025 reports that included a parent/caretaker (n = 1,014) and teacher (n = 1,011) report for each child and was collected from four geographic regions: South (44.7%), West (23.2%), East (16.2%), and Midwest (15.9%). To maintain consistency with the 2009 U.S. Census (U.S. Census Bureau, 2009) figures, 51.2% were female and 48.7% were male. The racial composition of this normative group was as follows: white (59.5%), Hispanic/Latino (16.6%), black/African American (15.8%), Asian (5.7%), Native American (0.3%), and other (1.6%). Parental educational level included less then high school graduate (13.7%), high school graduate (26.1%), some college (24.8%), and 4 years of college or more (35.4%).

The Preschool standardization sample included 247 children with 474 reports that included a parent (n = 247) and teacher (n = 227) report for each child. Ratings were obtained when the children were between 30 and 54 months old with 58–70 children in each of the four age bands. The sample consisted of 51.4% male and 48.6% female from four geographic regions: South (29.6%), Midwest (27.5%), East (21.9%), and West (20.6%). Race/ethnic background consisted of white (64.4%), Hispanic/Latino (16.6%), black/African American (14.2%), Asian (1.6%), and other (2.2%). Educational level for parents included less then high school graduate (13.4%), high school graduate (32.4%), some college (23.5%), and 4 years of college or more (30%).

The Adult standardization sample involved 702 adults (ages 18–89) with 2,210 reports with at least three SRS-2 rating forms: Adult Self-Report and two Relative/Other-Report forms or three Relative/Other-Report forms if an Adult Self-Report form was not completed. Relative/Other-Report forms were completed by parents (n = 195), siblings or other relative (n = 519), spouse (n = 338), or close friend (n = 521). Of the sample, 54% were female and 46% were male. Geographic regions included South (37%), East (24.9%), Midwest (21.2%), and West (16.8%). The racial composition for the adult normative group was as follows: white (69.4%), black/African American (14.4%), Hispanic/Latino (13.8%), Asian (1.6%), Native American (0.1%), and other (0.7%). Educational attainment included less then high school graduate (14.5%), high school graduate (35.6%), some college (16%), and 4 years of college or more (32.5%). Data for the Adult standardization sample were collected from public and private schools, as well as church and other groups that the authors purport to be a broad cross-section of the local community.

A clinical sample (*N* = 7,921) was obtained from the Interactive Autism Network Research Database at Kennedy Krieger Institute and John Hopkins–Baltimore, dated February 14, 2011. This sample included clinical subjects (*n* = 4,891) who held a formal ASD diagnosis prior to completing the SRS-2 and unaffected siblings (*n* = 3,030). Subjects ranged from 4 to 18 years old, with the sample being predominantly younger in age. In the clinical sample, 82.7% were males and 17.3% were females, whereas the unaffected siblings were 53.2% males and 46.8% females. Additionally, the combined sample were predominantly white (82.7%), followed by multiple (4.7%), Hispanic/Latino (4.5%), black/African American (2.7%), other (1.6%), Asian (1%), and Native American (0.1%). Geographic regions for the total sample included South (33.8%), East (24.1%), Midwest (24%), and West (18%). The manual does not provide statistics on educational attainment.

Reliability

Internal consistency, construct temporal stability, and interrater agreement data are provided in the SRS-2 manual. For the School-Age form, parent and teacher ratings were broken down by age and gender. The alpha coefficient for internal consistency on parent data for males was .95 (*n* = 493) and for females was .95 (*n* = 518), with age-based alpha coefficients ranging from .92 to .97. In turn, the alpha coefficient for internal consistency with teacher data for the male population was .96 (*n* = 509) and for females was .95 (*n* = 505) with aged-based coefficients ranging from .92 to .97. Interrater agreement between parent and teacher forms was .61 for males (*n* = 467) and .60 for females (*n* = 476), and aged-based coefficients ranged from .42 to .77.

Internal consistency alpha coefficients for the Preschool parent form were .93 for males (*n* = 127) and .95 for females (*n* = 120), and age-based coefficients ranged from .93 to .95. The teacher form alpha coefficients for internal consistency were .94 for males (*n* = 116) and .96 for females (*n* = 111), and age-based coefficients ranged from .93 to .95. Interrater reliability coefficients between parent and teacher forms was .77 for both males (*n* = 116) and females (*n* = 111), and age-based coefficients ranged from .70 to .78.

The Adult Self-Report form yielded internal consistency alpha coefficients of .95 for males (*n* = 288) and .94 for females (*n* = 349), whereas the Relative/Other-Report form yielded .97 for males (*n* = 732) and .96 for females (n = 841). Age-based internal consistency alpha scores ranged from .93 to .96 for the Self-Report form and .94–.97 for the Relative/Other-Report form. Finally, interrater reliability coefficients were provided for self, mother, father, relative, spouse, and other. These ranged from .61 (self–other rater pairings) to .95 (other–mother pairings).

Internal consistency for the clinical sample yielded alpha coefficients of .95 for males and .94 for females for the clinical subjects, and .97 for both males and females of the unaffected siblings. Age-based internal consistency alpha scores for the clinical subjects ranged from .94 to .96 for males and from .96 to .97 for females of the unaffected siblings. For the clinical groups, internal consistency yielded alpha coefficients of .95 for all groups (i.e., autistic/autistic disorder, Asperger syndrome, PPD-NOS, PDD, and ASD).

Validity

The test authors used four independent samples to assess the factor structures of the SRS-2. These samples included the standardization subjects for the Preschool, School-Age, and Adult (Relative/Other-Report) forms, as well as a clinical sample. Results of the two-factor analysis of these samples indicated that a majority of items reflected autistic traits that fall under the Social Communication and Interaction scale, which comprises the treatment subscale items for Social Awareness, Social Cognition, Social Communication, and Social Motivation. The remaining items reflected a measure of the Restricted Interests and Repetitive Behaviors scale, which has a treatment subscale of the same name.

The authors report that a ROC analysis of the clinical sample revealed high degrees of sensitivity and specificity for the total raw scores. A total raw score of 60 was associated with a sensitivity of .93 and specificity of .91 for any ASD, whereas a total raw score of 75 was associated with a sensitivity of .84 and specificity of .94. The manual provides separate scores for males and females along with four total scores between 60 and 75.

In the manual, the authors cite more than 40 separate studies that represent over 30,000 independent administrations of the SRS-2 that evaluate assessment of autism and comorbid disorders, treatment effects, and validity with other instruments. The authors describe several independent studies from the United States and other countries that demonstrated similar findings in psychometric properties for mean differences, internal consistency, retest reliability and temporal stability, interrater reliability, and convergent validity, as well as sensitivity and specificity.

The authors describe a number of studies that investigated the comparison of the SRS-2 with other ASD-directed measures. The most widely investigated comparisons were between the SRS-2 with the SCQ. In studies of mixed samples, correlations ranged from .50 to .65 (Bölte, Poustka, & Constantino, 2008; Bölte, Westerwald, Holtmann, Freitag, & Poustka, 2011; Charman et al., 2007; Pine, Guyer, Goldwin, Towbin, & Leibenluft, 2008; Granader et al., 2010). Charman et al. (2007) also found in children identified as developmentally at risk that the SCQ produced a sensitivity of .86 and specificity of .78, whereas the SRS-2 produced a sensitivity of .78 and specificity of .67. Analyses of these differences found the SCQ demonstrated a stronger performance in those with lower intellectual functioning (IQ below 75) and performed similarly in a higher IQ subgroup.

In comparing the SRS-2 with the Children's Communication Checklist (CCC), Pine et al. (2008) found correlations of r = .49 and .72 with the two ASD-focused subscales of the CCC, whereas Charman et al. (2007) found a correlation of r = .75. In comparing the two measures between children with ASD and those without ASD, Charman et al. (2007) found the CCC to have a sensitivity of .93 and specificity of .46, whereas the SRS-2 sensitivity was .78 and specificity was .67. The authors note, as these findings suggest, that as a screening measure the CCC shows greater emphasis in identifying more children at risk, although with higher rates of false positives. However, they also state that the SRS-2 performs better when used in a clinical setting for diagnostic decision making.

The authors provide several studies comparing the SRS-2 with the ADOS and ADI-R, which uses a behavioral observation design to evaluate for ASD. In a small group of individuals diagnosed with ASD (n = 61), correlations between the SRS-2 and ADI-R ranged from .65 to .77 for mother reports, .60 to .74 for father reports, and .52 to .70 for teacher reports (Constantino & Todd, 2003). Lower findings were found in a subsequent larger sample with correlations ranging from .31 to .36 for parent reports and .26 to .40 for teacher reports (Constantino et al., 2007). The manual also provides several studies for European samples comparing the SRS-2 and ADI-R that demonstrated similar results. Comparing the SRS-2 and ADOS domain scores, correlations with parent scores ranged from .37 to .58, whereas teacher-report scores ranged from .15 to .35 (Constantino et al., 2007). Bölte et al. (2011) found a correlation of r = .48.

Studies were also presented that compared the SRS-2 with the Child Behavior Checklist (CBCL; Achenbach, 1991) and VABS (Sparrow et al., 1984). Constantino, Przybeck, Friesen, and Todd (2000; n = 84) and Bölte et al. (2008; n = 119) compared the CBCL with the SRS-2, reporting that the SRS-2 was more sensitive to behaviors associated with ASD, less sensitive to behaviors seldom seen in ASD, and greater sensitivity to behaviors not assessed by the CBCL. Both studies found moderate correlations on the SRS-2 and CBCL subscales ranging from .48 to .64. These correlations largely overlapped with the CBCL subscales Social Problems, Thought Problems, and Attention Problems. As expected, correlations were lower for those subscales not associated with behaviors seen in those diagnosed with ASD. Studies comparing the SRS-2 and VABS demonstrated a correlation of .44 for the VABS composite score (Charman et al., 2007). A study by Bölte et al. (2008) found a composite correlation of $r = .36$ and subscale correlations ranging from .34 to .43. The manual suggests these correlations with the VABS would be expected, given developmental impairments associated with ASD.

The manual authors conducted a study to evaluate the placement of the 65 SRS-2 items into five treatment subscales: Social Awareness, Social Cognition, Social Communication, Social Motivation, and Restricted Interests and Repetitive Behaviors. Expert judges ($N = 25$), including counselors, social workers, psychiatrists, pediatricians, and psychologists who had experience in working with ASD and PDD, were given the 65 items and asked to sort each item into one of the five groups. Each item was given an expert assignment based on the majority of placements. In order to compare the original placements with the expert placements, nominal scale cross-tabulation was used—there was a significant result ($\chi^2 = 94.24$, $p < .001$). Proportional-reduction-in-error statistics yielded Cohen's kappa of .585 and lambda = .506 (for both, $p < .001$).

The manual also reports that because subscales were not created as fully independent measures, there is a high degree of intercorrelation among them. Parent-report data from 168 cases were used to assess the consistency between the item-to-scale assignments. Alpha reliabilities were calculated for the set of items in each subscale. Values ranged from .60 in the Social Motivation subscale (11 items) to .72 for the Restricted Interests and Repetitive Behaviors subscale (12 items). In addition, the correlations of items with their subscale membership versus other subscales were examined. The authors concluded that there was support for the assignment of items to their respective scales.

Discriminant validity—the extent to which the SRS differentiates ASD from other psychiatric disorders—was assessed in several studies (Kalb, Law, Landa, & Law, 2010; Constantino et al., 2000; Charman et al., 2007; Coon et al., 2010; Bölte et al., 2008, 2011; Kamio et al., 2013; Pine et al., 2008; Towbin, Pradella, Gorrindo, Pine, & Leibenluft, 2005; Reiersen, Constantino, Volk, & Todd, 2007; Reiersen, Constantino, Grimmer, Martin, & Todd, 2008; Puleo & Kendall, 2011; Granader et al., 2010; Hilton et al., 2010; Hilton, Crouch, & Israel, 2008). The manual provides these mean scores and standard deviations, as well as descriptions for each study. The manual also provides a table demonstrating four largely nonoverlapping groups of the SRS-2 mean scores that demonstrate effectiveness in differentiating symptomatology. Groups of normal/typically developing males, females, and combined samples and control groups and normative data found mean total raw scores to range from 14.7 to 34. Those groups with behavioral and/or emotional diagnoses (e.g., ADHD, anxiety, major depression, mixed diagnoses, mood disorder) without ASD had mean scores that ranged from 40 to 69.2. Studies of those with other ASD, Asperger's, and PPD-NOS demonstrated mean scores from 77.6 to 101.47. Last, studies of those who were autistic provided mean scores from 89.9 to 116.1.

The SRS-2 Adult (Relative/Other-Report) and Adult (Self-Report) forms were evaluated for mean differences in four studies. Lyall (2011) reported controls with no ASD-related diagnoses had mean total scores of .19.4 (SD = 18), whereas those with ASD-related diagnoses had mean total scores of 98.8 (SD = 34). Those with ASD-related diagnoses were further evaluated for autistic (M = 110.5, SD = 31), Asperger's disorder (M = 93.4, SD = 33), and PPD-NOS (M = 99.6, SD = 35). On the SRS-2 Adult (Relative/Other-Report) form, Bolte (2011) provided information on 240 individuals in three groups: ASD (n = 20; M = 78.5, SD = 13.7), mixed psychiatric (n = 62; M = 63.4, SD = 15.4), and typically developing (n = 163; M = 55.5, SD = 9.9). In a large group (n = 250) of adults 18–36 years old diagnosed as autistic, Seltzer et al. (2011) reported a mean score of 94.6 (SD = 28.5). Another study (Mandell et al., 2012) comparing a group of individuals diagnosed with ASD (n = 14) and a mixed psychiatric sample (primarily schizophrenia; n = 127) found mean scores of 100.2 (SD = 32.7) and 76.5 (SD = 32.5), respectively. Mandell et al. (2012) also conducted a ROC analysis and found a sensitivity of .86 and specificity of .60.

In providing psychometric and validation evidence for the SRS-2 Preschool form, the authors note difficulties in collecting ASD-specific data due to the inherent problems of those who may not display symptoms of ASD until older. As no studies were conducted at the time of manual publication on those with clinical disorders (e.g., ASD, internalizing or externalizing disorders), the authors note that only results from the standardization study can serve as a reference point. One study found convergent validity with the CARS that provided interclass correlations to be .41 (n = 21, p < .002).

CONCLUSIONS

The information summarized in this chapter provides researchers and clinicians with important characteristics of methods used to assess behaviors associated with ASD, as well as a review of the psychometric qualities that such measures should possess. Table 2.2 provides a summary of the essential aspects of these instruments. As is apparent from examination of the table and the reviews provided earlier in this chapter, the authors of these rating scales differ considerably in their approach to instrument development. For instance, some of the scales are very short (e.g., the CARS-2 has

TABLE 2.2. Comparison of Essential ASD Rating Scale Characteristics

Behavior rating scale	No. of items	Age range	Comparison sample size	Comparison sample	Representative standardization sample	Scores for total scale	Scores for scales
Autism Diagnostic Interview—Revised (ADI-R)	93	2–*x* years	Exact *N* not given	Children with and without ASD, studies conducted by authors where interviews were administered as part of routine initial clinical assessment and systematic research evaluations	No	Raw score	Summary raw scores
Autism Spectrum Rating Scale (ASRS)	80	2–5 and 6–18 years	2,560	National standardization sample of children and youth in the United States and Canada	Yes	*T*-score	*T*-scores
Childhood Autism Rating Scale (CARS)	15	Exact ages not given	1,600	Children who were referred to the TEACCH program (see text)	No	Raw score	None
Social Communication Questionnaire (SCQ)	40	4–*x* years	200	A wide variety of individuals (persons with autism, atypical autism, Asperger syndrome, fragile X syndrome, Rett syndrome, conduct disorder, language delay, intellectual disability, and other clinical diagnoses)	No	Raw score	Raw scores
Social Responsiveness Scale (SRS)	65	4–18 years	1,636	Cases from five studies, combined into one sample (74% white, 11% black, 11% Hispanic, 2% Asian, 2% other)	No	*T*-score	*T*-scores

only 15 items), whereas others contain many items (e.g., 93 items in the ADI-R). Some authors provide only raw scores, which makes interpretation difficult, and only two scales (the ASRS and SRS-2) provide standard scores (*T*-scores). Although these two tests provide derived scores, only the sample upon which the ASRS was based was selected to represent the normal population. Basing standard scores on a national sample is greatly preferable to basing them on a sample of individuals who may have autism.

All the scales except the ASRS and SRS-2 use children with suspected or verified psychological disorders from either research studies or clinic settings as a comparison group. This method allows a clinician to determine whether an examinee is like other children with suspected or documented psychological problems, but comparing the score a child gets on a rating scale to the scores of other children who (1) were referred for evaluation, (2) had some diagnosis on the autism spectrum, or (3) participated in a study of children with autism has several problems. If an individual gets a *T*-score of 50, this would mean that he or she has evidenced behaviors like those of persons who may have ASD. This is not a diagnostic statement, however, for two reasons. First, there is no evidence that the samples used to create the comparison groups for each scale are representative of children with ASD or of the U.S. population. The samples may be limited in demographic characteristics, and therefore the comparison will be affected by the variability of that sample. The sample may be restricted or very heterogeneous, either of which will (1) be undetectable and (2) have a considerable effect on the quality of the comparison. Second, because it is unknown how well such a sample represents children and adolescents with ASD in the particular state in which the sample was collected, or any other state, generalization to clients in other states is limited.

Using a national sample to construct a norm conversion table provides a considerable advantage, for several reasons. First, a large sample allows for reliable calibration of derived scores. Second, comparison to that sample yields an understanding of how often behaviors associated with ASD are found within the typical population. Third, the comparison of a child's or adolescent's behavior to what is expected in the typically developing population provides for greater understanding of how far an individual may be from the norm. Fourth, having a well-normed score provides a means of calibrating how much response to intervention is needed to bring the individual's behavior into a range that can be considered typical.

The most glaring shortcoming of nearly all these scales is that they do not have standard scores that are based on a national standardization sample. This possesses a considerable liability for those who choose to use these measures, because it is imperative to know how different an examinee's behavior is from that of typical individuals, as well as how the behaviors compare with those of persons with ASD. The only way to know the rate at which typical children show behaviors associated with ASD is to have a national standardization group and to base norms on this sample. Clinicians can then make defensible statements about how far a child deviates from normality and to what extent the normative data support a diagnosis. Those measures that do not have a national standardization sample should be viewed with caution by clinicians, because interpretation of results across tests is made very difficult by the differences in the samples, and the stability of the norms cannot be determined. The use of well-developed, psychometrically sound assessments will greatly enhance the likelihood that accurate and valid information can be obtained.

REFERENCES

Achenbach, T. M. (1991). *Manual for the Child Behavior Checklist/4-18 and 1991 profile*. Burlington: University of Vermont, Department of Psychiatry.

American Educational Research Association, American Psychological Association, & National Council on Measurement in Education. (2014). *Standards for educational and psychological testing, 2014 edition*. Washington, DC: American Educational Research Association.

American Psychiatric Association. (2000). *Diagnostic and statistical manual of mental disorders* (4th ed., text rev.). Washington, DC: Author.

American Psychiatric Association. (2013). *Diagnostic and statistical manual of mental disorders* (5th ed.). Arlington, VA: Author.

Berument, S. K., Rutter, J., Lord, C., Pickles, A., & Bailey, A. (1999). Autism screening questionnaire: Diagnostic validity. *British Journal of Psychiatry, 175*, 444–451.

Bishop, D. V. M., & Norbury, C. F. (2002). Exploring the borderlands of autistic disorder and specific language impairment: A study using standardized diagnostic instruments. *Journal of Child Psychology and Psychiatry, 43*, 917–929.

Bölte, S., Poustka, F., & Constantino, J. N. (2008). Convergent and discriminant validation by the multitrait–multimethod matrix. *Psychological Bulletin, 56*, 81–105.

Bölte, S., Westerwald, E., Holtmann, M., Freitag, C., & Poustka, F. (2011). Autistic traits and autism spectrum disorders: The clinical validity of two measures presuming a continuum of social communication skills. *Journal of Autism and Developmental Disorders, 41*(1), 66–72.

Bracken, B. A. (1987). Limitations of preschool instruments and standards for minimal levels of technical adequacy. *Journal of Psychoeducational Assessment, 5*, 313–326.

Bracken, B. A., & McCallum, R. S. (1997). *Universal Nonverbal Intelligence Test*. Itasca, IL: Riverside.

Charman, T., Baird, G., Simonoff, E., Loucas, T., Chandler, S., Meldrum, D., et al. (2007). Efficacy of three screening instruments in the identification of autistic-spectrum disorders. *British Journal of Psychiatry, 191*(6), 554–559.

Constantino, J. N., Davis, S. A., Todd, R. D., Schindler, M. K., Gross, M. M., Brophy, S. L., et al. (2003). Validation of a brief quantitative genetic measure of autistic traits: Comparison of the Social Responsiveness Scale with the Autism Diagnostic Interview—Revised. *Journal of Autism and Developmental Disorders, 33*, 427–433.

Constantino, J. N., & Gruber, C. P. (2012). *Social Responsiveness Scale, Second Edition manual.* Torrance, CA: Western Psychological Services.

Constantino, J. N., LaVesser, P. D., Zhang, Y., Abbacchi, A. M., Gray, T., & Todd, R. D. (2007). Rapid quantitative assessment of autistic social impairment by classroom teachers. *Journal of the American Academy of Child and Adolescent Psychiatry, 46*(12), 1668–1676.

Constantino, J. N., Przybeck, R., Friesen, D., & Todd, R. D. (2000). Reciprocal social behavior in children with and without pervasive developmental disorders. *Journal of Developmental and Behavior Pediatrics, 21,* 2–11.

Constantino, J. N., & Todd, R. D. (2003). The genetic structure of reciprocal social behavior. *American Journal of Psychiatry, 157,* 2043–2045.

Coon, H., Villalobos, M. E., Robison, R. J., Camp, N. J., Cannon, D. S., Allen-Brady, K., et al. (2010). Genome-wide linkage using the Social Responsiveness Scale in Utah autism pedigrees. *Molecular Autism, 1*(1), 8.

Creek, M. (1961). Schizophrenia syndrome in childhood: Progress report of a working party. *Cerebral Palsy Bulletin, 3,* 501–504.

Crocker, L., & Algina, J. (1986). *Introduction to classical and modern test theory.* New York: Holt, Rinehart & Winston.

Eaves, R. C., Campbell, H. A., & Chambers, D. (2000). Criterion-related and construct validity of the Pervasive Developmental Disorders Rating Scale and the Autism Behavior Checklist. *Psychology in the Schools, 37*(4), 311–321.

Gilliam, J. (2001). *Gilliam Asperger's Disorder Scale manual.* Austin, TX: PRO-ED.

Gilliam, J. (2006). *GARS-2: Gilliam Autism Rating Scale* (2nd ed.). Austin, TX: PRO-ED.

Goldstein, S., & Naglieri, J. A. (2009). *Autism Spectrum Rating Scale.* Toronto, ON, Canada: Multi-Health Systems.

Granader, Y. E., Bender, H. A., Zemon, V., Rathi, S., Nass, R., & MacAllister, W. S. (2010). The clinical utility of the Social Responsiveness Scale and Social Communication Questionnaire in tuberous sclerosis complex. *Epilepsy and Behavior, 18*(3), 262–266.

Hilton, C. L., Crouch, M. C., & Israel, H. (2008). Out-of-school participation patterns in children with high-functioning autism spectrum disorders. *American Journal of Occupational Therapy, 62*(5), 554–563.

Hilton, C. L., Harper, J. D., Kueker, R. H., Lang, A. R., Abbacchi, A. M., Todorov, A., et al. (2010). Sensory responsiveness as a predictor of social severity in children with high functioning autism spectrum disorders. *Journal of Autism and Developmental Disorders, 40*(8), 937–945.

Kalb, L. G., Law, J. K., Landa, R., & Law, P. A. (2010). Onset patterns prior to 36 months in autism spectrum disorders. *Journal of Autism and Developmental Disorders, 40*(11), 1389–1402.

Kamio, Y., Inada, N., Moriwaki, A., Kuroda, M., Koyama, T., Tsujii, H., et al. (2013). Quantitative autistic traits ascertained in a national survey of 22,529 Japanese schoolchildren. *Acta Psychiatrica Scandinavica, 128*(1), 45–53.

Kanner, L. (1943). Autistic disturbances of affective contact. *Nervous Child, 2,* 217–250.

Kaufman, A. S., & Kaufman, N. L. (2004). *Kaufman Assessment Battery for Children, Second Edition manual.* Circle Pines, MN: American Guidance Service.

Krug, D. A., Arick, J. R., & Almond, P. J. (2008). *Autism Behavior Checklist, Second Edition.* Austin, TX: PRO-ED.

Lord, C., Luyster, R. J., Gotham, K., & Guthrie, W. (2012). *Autism Diagnostic Observation Schedule, Second Edition (ADOS-2) manual (Part II): Toddler Module.* Torrance, CA: Western Psychological Services.

Lord, C., Rutter, M., DiLavore, P. C., Risi, S., Gotham, K., & Bishop, S. L. (2012). *Autism Diagnostic Observation Schedule, Second Edition (ADOS-2) manual (Part I): Modules 1–4.* Torrance, CA: Western Psychological Services.

Mandell, D. S., Lawer, L. J., Branch, K., Brodkin, E. S., Healey, K., Witalec, R., et al. (2012). Prevalence and correlates of autism in a state psychiatric hospital. *Autism, 16*(6), 557–567.

Naglieri, J. A., Das, J. P., & Goldstein, S. (2014). *Cognitive Assessment System, Second Edition.* Itasca, IL: Riverside.

Naglieri, J. A., Das, J. P., & Goldstein, S. (2013). *Cognitive Assessment System* (2nd ed.). Austin, TX: PRO-ED.

National Society for Autistic Children. (1978). National Society for Autistic Children definition of the syndrome of autism. *Journal of Autism and Developmental Disorders, 8,* 132–137.

Nunnally, J. C., & Bernstein, I. H. (1994). *Psychometric theory.* New York: McGraw-Hill.

Pilowsky, T., Yirmia, N., Shulman, C., & Dover, R. (1998). The Autism Diagnostic Interview—Revised and the Childhood Autism Rating Scale: Differences between diagnostic systems and comparison between genders. *Journal of Autism and Developmental Disorders, 28*(2), 143–151.

Pine, D. S., Guyer, A. E., Goldwin, M., Towbin, K. A., & Leibenluft, E. (2008). Autism spectrum disorder scale scores in pediatric mood and anxiety disorders. *Journal of the American Academy of Child and Adolescent Psychiatry, 47*(6), 652–661.

Puleo, C. M., & Kendall, P. C. (2011). Anxiety disorders in typically developing youth: Autism spectrum symptoms as a predictor of cognitive-behavioral treatment. *Journal of Autism and Developmental Disorders, 41*(3), 275–286.

Reiersen, A. M., Constantino, J. N., Grimmer, M., Martin, N. G., & Todd, R. D. (2008). Evidence for shared genetic influences on self-reported ADHD and autistic symptoms in young adult Australian twins. *Twin Research and Human Genetics, 11*(6), 579.

Reiersen, A. M., Constantino, J. N., Volk, H. E., & Todd, R. D. (2007). Autistic traits in a population-based ADHD twin sample. *Journal of Child Psychology and Psychiatry, 48*(5), 464–472.

Ritvo, R. A., Ritvo, E. R., Guthrie, D., Rito, M. J., Hufnagel, D. Y., McMahon, W., et al. (2011). The Ritvo Autism Asperger Diagnostic Scale—Revised (RAADS-R): A scale to assist the diagnosis of autism spectrum disorder in adults: An international validation study. *Journal of Autism Developmental Disorders, 41*(8), 1076–1089.

Rutter, M. (1978). Diagnosis and definition of childhood autism. *Journal of Autism and Developmental Disorders, 8,* 139–161.

Rutter, M., Bailey, A., & Lord, C. (2003). *Social Communication Questionnaire.* Los Angeles: Western Psychological Services.

Rutter, M., Le Couteur, A., & Lord, C. (2003). *Autism Diagnostic Interview, Revised.* Los Angeles: Western Psychological Services.

Schopler, E., Lansing, M. D., Reichler, R. J., & Marcus, L. M. (2005). *Psychoeducational Profile, Third Edition.* Austin, TX: PRO-ED.

Schopler, E., Van Bourgondien, M. E., Wellman, G. J., & Love, S. R. (2010). *Childhood*

Autism Rating Scale, Second Edition. Torrance, CA: Western Psychological Services.

Seltzer, M. M., Greenberg, J. S., Taylor, J. L., Smith, L., Orsmond, G. I., Esbensen, A., et al. (2011). Adolescents and adults with autism spectrum disorder. In D. G. Amaral, G. Dawson, & G. Geschwind (Eds.), *Autism spectrum disorders* (pp. 242–252). New York: Oxford University Press.

Sparrow, S. S., Balla, D. A., & Cicchetti, D. V. (1984). *Vineland Adaptive Behavior Scales*. Circle Pines, MN: American Guidance Services.

Thorndike, R. L. (1982). *Applied psychometrics*. Boston: Houghton Mifflin.

Towbin, K. E., Pradella, A., Gorrindo, T., Pine, D. S., & Leibenluft, E. (2005). Autism spectrum traits in children with mood and anxiety disorders. *Journal of Child and Adolescent Psychopharmacology, 15*(3), 452–464.

U.S. Census Bureau. (2000). *Statically abstract of the United States: 2000*. Washington, DC: U.S. Government Printing Office.

U.S. Census Bureau. (2009). *Statically abstract of the United States: 2009*. Washington, DC: U.S. Government Printing Office.

Wechsler, D. (2014). *Wechsler Intelligence Scale for Children, Fifth Edition*. San Antonio, TX: Psychological Corporation.

World Health Organization. (1992). *The ICD-10 classification of mental and behavioral disorders: Clinical descriptions and guidelines*. Geneva, Switzerland: Author.

CHAPTER THREE

DSM-5 Diagnosis of Autism Spectrum Disorder

Cynthia Martin
Lauren Pepa
Catherine Lord

HISTORY OF THE DSM AS RELATED TO AUTISM: DSM-III TO DSM-IV-TR

The ways in which autism spectrum conditions are conceptualized, diagnosed, and researched have evolved substantially since pervasive developmental disorders (PDD) were first introduced in the third edition of the *Diagnostic and Statistical Manual of Mental Disorders* (DSM-III; American Psychiatric Association, 1980). Advances in research and clinical practice, combined with the availability of diagnostic measures, have allowed us to better understand symptoms of the autism spectrum across development. Over the last three decades, autism has expanded beyond earlier narrower definitions, to more current perspectives of autism as a spectrum of behaviors defined by a core set of social and behavioral symptoms that vary in form, severity, and level of impairment (Grzadzinski, Huerta, & Lord, 2013).

To briefly review the history of autism as a diagnosis, many of the behaviors consistent with autism were first described as early as the 1940s by Leo Kanner (1943) and Hans Asperger (1944). Autism was not introduced as a diagnosable condition until DSM-III in 1980, which used the term "infantile autism" to describe young children with profound social impairments and unusual behaviors. The inclusion of the term "infantile" was in recognition of the earlier onset of autism symptomology in comparison to schizophrenia and psychoses, the categories within which autistic symptoms had been included previously in diagnostic systems. It was also within the publication of DSM-III that the broader umbrella of PDD was introduced, to convey the lifelong and persistent nature of the new childhood disorders that were being described. At that time, the diagnostic criteria for infantile autism was specific to highly impacted children with intellectual disability (ID) with significant needs. Also under the umbrella of PDD were four other disorders characterized by behaviors similar to infantile autism, but which were meant to represent differences in the age of symptom onset as well as symptom severity. Given these distinctions, there were significant limitations in the clinical sensitivity and applicability of autism diagnostic criteria within the context of DSM-III (Volkmar, Cohen, & Paul, 1986).

Upon publication of DSM-III-R (American Psychiatric Association, 1987), the criteria for an autism diagnosis were expanded to include a wider range of symptoms, broadening the conceptualization of autism from the more limited "infantile autism" specification. Autism now comprises three core symptom domains: Qualitative Impairments in Social Interactions, Deficits in Verbal and Nonverbal Communication, and Restricted Interests and Repetitive Behaviors. In addition to this more expansive autism categorization, a clinical category for subthreshold manifestations of core symptoms, PDD not otherwise specified (PDD-NOS), was introduced within the same DSM-III-R revision. These changes within the DSM-III-R served to increase the sensitivity of autism criteria to better match how clinicians used the diagnosis in practice. However, specificity subsequently became a source of concern because so many children with developmental or psychological difficulties shared similar problems, thus resulting in substantial overlap among disorders, including children with severe cognitive and intellectual impairments, or significant psychiatric conditions with social challenges (Volkmar, Bregman, Cohen, & Cicchetti, 1988; Szatmari, 1992).

Within the field, the shift from overspecificity in DSM-III to oversensitivity in DSM-III-R criteria sparked a discussion about the most appropriate way to categorize and describe this group of core symptoms in childhood. As such, research began to focus directly on questions about the existence and nature of subtypes within PDD or what would be called "the autism spectrum" (Szatmari, 1992; Volkmar, Cicchetti, Bregman, & Cohen, 1992). Following the research literature, DSM-IV (American Psychiatric Association, 1994) and DSM-IV-TR (American Psychiatric Association, 2000a) then took on the goals of creating new criteria for this set of diagnoses. Specifically, the authors of the DSM-IV and the subsequent revision (DSM-IV-TR) sought to highlight the diversity within PDD and autism, while also increasing the specificity of each set of diagnostic criteria. This balance was achieved by introducing different subtypes of autism spectrum conditions under an overall diagnostic umbrella of PDD. Specifically, newly categorical diagnoses included autistic disorder, Asperger's disorder, Rett's disorder, and PDD-NOS.

RESEARCH SUPPORTING CLASSIFICATION/SUBTYPE CHANGES FOR DSM-5

Research over the next two decades has attempted to identify etiological and outcome differences among individuals diagnosed with the various autism-related PDD; specifically, autistic disorder, Asperger's disorder, and PDD-NOS. Originally, in DSM-IV, it had been anticipated that differential diagnoses between autistic disorder and Asperger's disorder could be made on the presence or absence of a history of language delay (American Psychiatric Association, 2000b). It was originally assumed that children who had delayed language early on would differ in outcome and presentation from children without language delays even at later ages. However, what constituted a language delay was not readily agreed upon (Mayes, Calhoun, & Crites, 2001; Tanguay, Robertson, & Derrick, 1998), thus making this differentiation more difficult. When language delay was defined as not meeting very early language milestones (i.e., first words by 24 months, sentences by 36 months), as determined by parent report, neither differences in outcome nor presentation were found when current levels of language skills were controlled (Eisenmajer et al., 1998). Evidence also emerged that parents' retrospective accounts of dates (i.e., for important language milestones), crucial for the classification of a language delay, are influenced by many factors that often result in reports of greater delays than are reflected in earlier records or testing (Hus, Taylor, & Lord, 2011). As such, the presence or absence of a reported early language delay did not serve as a useful differential criterion.

In addition to the difficulty with distinctions based on language delay, other diagnostic heuristics and patterns began to develop. For example, children with milder forms of autism symptoms or those who seemed to have "grown out" of some symptoms of autism as they reached adolescence or adulthood were given diagnoses of Asperger's disorder regardless of whether or not they had any degree of a language delay (Woodbury-Smith, Klin, & Volkmar, 2005). Further, many children who presented with significant symptoms of autism, but also had strengths in terms of language and cognitive abilities, were routinely given a diagnosis of PDD-NOS instead of autistic disorder (Lord et al., 2012). Research also suggested that, rather than differing in the criteria that defined the PDD subtypes in DSM-IV and DSM-IV-TR, diagnostic differences between autistic disorder, Asperger's disorder, and PDD-NOS were primarily accounted for by symptom severity, comorbid intellectual functioning, and current language abilities (Frith, 2004; Howlin, 2003; Macintosh & Dissanayake, 2004; Matson, Boisjoli, Gonzalez, Smith, & Wilkins, 2007; Ozonoff, South, & Miller, 2000; Snow & Lecavalier, 2011).

A large, multisite study across 12 university-based centers was conducted to determine the relationship between a child's presentation of symptoms and the clinical diagnosis of autistic disorder, Asperger's disorder, and PDD-NOS ultimately given (Lord et al., 2012). Results of this study suggested that diagnostic subtype classification was more often based on relatively idiosyncratic within-site hierarchies of criteria (IQ, language level, age, parent reports of severity) than on DSM-IV diagnostic standards. Within each clinical center, distinctions between autistic disorder, Asperger's disorder, and PDD-NOS were consistent and meaningful, but there was little consistency across the different clinics except that autistic disorder was more often diagnosed in children with greater overall symptom severity in social communication and/or lower IQs. As noted in other studies, the difference between "high-functioning autism"—a term used for individuals with autistic disorder but without ID or marked language delay—and Asperger's disorder was not meaningful except within the unique definitions of particular clinics or as a metric of severity (i.e., people given Asperger's disorder diagnoses often had less severe symptoms than those given autism diagnoses; Ozonoff et al., 2000: Lord et al., 2012).

Significant challenges to the specificity of PDD-NOS were also apparent (Lord & Bishop, 2015; Martinez-Pedraza & Carter, 2009; Towbin, 2005). Although PDD-NOS was supposed to be reserved for rare cases in which full emergence of autism symptoms was not present, the term became used to capture many children who had social challenges, both with and without autism symptomology (Chawarska, Klin, & Volkmar, 2010). Families frequently received first diagnoses of PDD-NOS, rather than autism, from professionals who were wary of bringing up the word "autism" or who were uncomfortable making a diagnosis in a young child. Parents often understood a diagnosis of PDD-NOS to mean that autism had been ruled out, rather than seeing it as a tentative marker of the need for further assessment and information (de Bruin, Ferdinand, Meester, de Nijs, & Verheij, 2007; Goin-Kochel, Mackintosh, & Myers, 2006). To complicate matters further, research using broad measures of social and communication deficits or repetitive behaviors in representative samples of typical children has shown that these features do exist in other populations (Constantino & Todd, 2003; Ronald, Edelson, Asherson, & Saudino, 2010). Sometimes PDD-NOS has been used to refer to children who have autistic traits (and who may have other disorders), but do not meet full criteria for autism. Thus, similar to the difficulties clarifying the differentiation between autistic disorder and Asperger's disorder, the same challenges applied to distinctions between PDD-NOS and the other disorders.

Other terms emerged as alternative ways to describe individuals with symptoms of autism, but without formally using an autism label, further complicating the diagnostic landscape. Specifically, terms such as "nonverbal learning disability," "auditory processing disorder," "sensory processing," and "semantic–pragmatic disorder" are examples of descriptions of difficulties that have not yet been shown to form reliably distinct, diagnosable disorders, but which are sometimes used to describe children with autism (Katz, Goldstein, & Beers, 2001; Chawarska et al., 2010; Tsur, Shalev, Manor, & Amir, 1995; Volden, 2013). Other than semantic–pragmatic disorder, which is now called social (pragmatic) communication disorder (SCD) in DSM-5 (American Psychiatric Association, 2013), the other terms have not yet been found to be discrete conditions. Rather, they may reflect cognitive, learning, and behavioral profiles that occur across a range of diagnostic categories and often co-occur with the social deficits that define autism (Klin, Volkmar, Sparrow, Cicchetti, & Rourke, 1996).

DSM-5 CHANGES TO DIAGNOSTIC CRITERIA

Given the abundance of research highlighting the difficulties in accurate and reliable differential diagnosis among the PDD categories, a different approach to diagnosis was introduced in DSM-5. In 2013, the fifth edition of the *Diagnostic and Statistical Manual of Mental Disorders* (American Psychiatric Association, 2013) initiated a significant change in the framework of autism, moving from the previous multicategorical model to a single diagnostic category of autism spectrum disorder (ASD; see Figure 3.1). ASD includes all individuals who received any of the former PDD diagnoses of autistic disorder, Asperger's disorder, and PDD-NOS, as well as childhood disintegrative disorder. Rett syndrome is diagnosed through genetic testing to identify abnormal sequencing and deletions/duplications of the *MECP2* gene or by meeting a specific set of clinical criteria, so is no longer included in DSM-5. ASD is not exclusive of Rett syndrome or other genetic or neurological disorders (such as fragile X or tuberous sclerosis), and may co-occur with any of them, if ASD criteria are also met. In such cases, the genetic or neurological disorder can be added as a *specifier* to the behaviorally defined diagnosis of ASD in DSM-5. Specifiers can also be added to indicate other sources of variability across individuals, such as whether language or intellectual impairments are evident. In this way, DSM-5 encompasses these variations within an individual's ASD diagnostic profile, rather than through the use of different categorical diagnoses such as autistic disorder or Asperger's disorder.

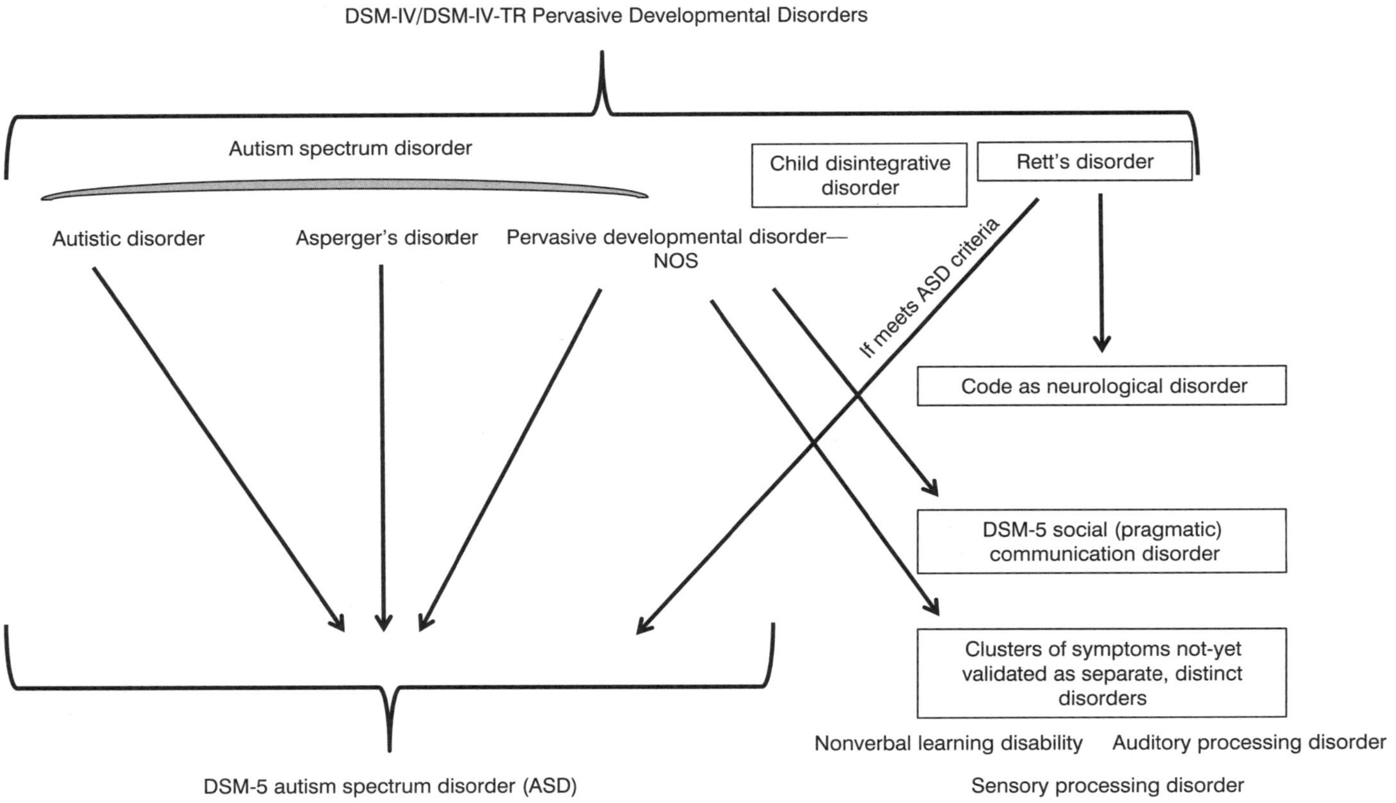

FIGURE 3.1. Changes in the diagnostic classification of pervasive developmental disorders in DSM-IV/DSM-IV-TR to autism spectrum disorder in DSM-5.

Changes were also made for comorbid diagnoses. Now, for example, the diagnosis of attention-deficit/hyperactivity disorder (ADHD) can be made along with ASD. (See Chapters 9 and 10 for more information about assessing and diagnosing ADHD within the context of ASD.)

A new diagnosis of SCD was also introduced within the category of communication disorders (not within ASD) to describe individuals who show impairments in social development and pragmatic language but do not have repetitive behaviors, thus excluding them from a diagnosis of ASD. The SCD diagnosis has some evidence supporting it (Gibson, Adams, Lockton, & Green, 2013) but has not yet been well validated (Swineford, Thurm, Baird, Wetherby, & Swedo, 2014). There may be developmental limitations as well. When assessing for pragmatic deficits, a child has generally acquired speech and language abilities. Therefore, a diagnosis of SCD in very young children is difficult to make and DSM-5 states that it is rarely found in children younger than 4 years of age.

Similar to the prior revisions of diagnostic criteria, changes in DSM-5 criteria reflect the current state of research on ASD (Lord & Bishop, 2015; Lord & Jones, 2012). Specifically, numerous studies showed that there were great overlaps among nonverbal communication deficits, impairments in reciprocal conversation, and the social impairments defined in DSM-IV-TR. Consequently, a two-domain diagnostic model has been proposed in DSM-5 (Guthrie, Swineford, Wetherby, & Lord, 2013; Harstad et al., 2015). While DSM-IV-TR contained three domains (Social Impairment, Communication Impairment, and Restricted and Repetitive Behaviors [RRB]), DSM-5 has collapsed the Social and Communication domains into one category. Moving forward, DSM-5 has a Social Communication domain, including three subdomains: Social Reciprocity, Nonverbal Communication, and Relationships, which includes understanding and maintaining relationships with others, as well as adjusting one's behavior to best suit the various social contexts of relationships. The other domain is Restricted, Repetitive Behaviors, which now includes four subdomains: Stereotyped or Repetitive Behaviors (including repetitive speech; moved out of DSM-IV category of Communication); Fixed and Restricted Interests, Rituals, and Resistance to Change; and a new subdomain of Unusual Reactions to Environmental (Sensory) Stimuli. A diagnosis of ASD requires meeting criteria currently and/or by history, in both Social Communication (presence of symptoms in all three subdomains) and RRB (symptoms in two of four subdomains), though how a child meets criteria within the different subdomains of each dimension can differ quite markedly (see Figure 3.2).

Another major change to DSM-5 was the reorganization of how language impairments are reflected in ASD criteria. Language and communication impairments are core features of ASD (Lord & Bishop, 2015), and

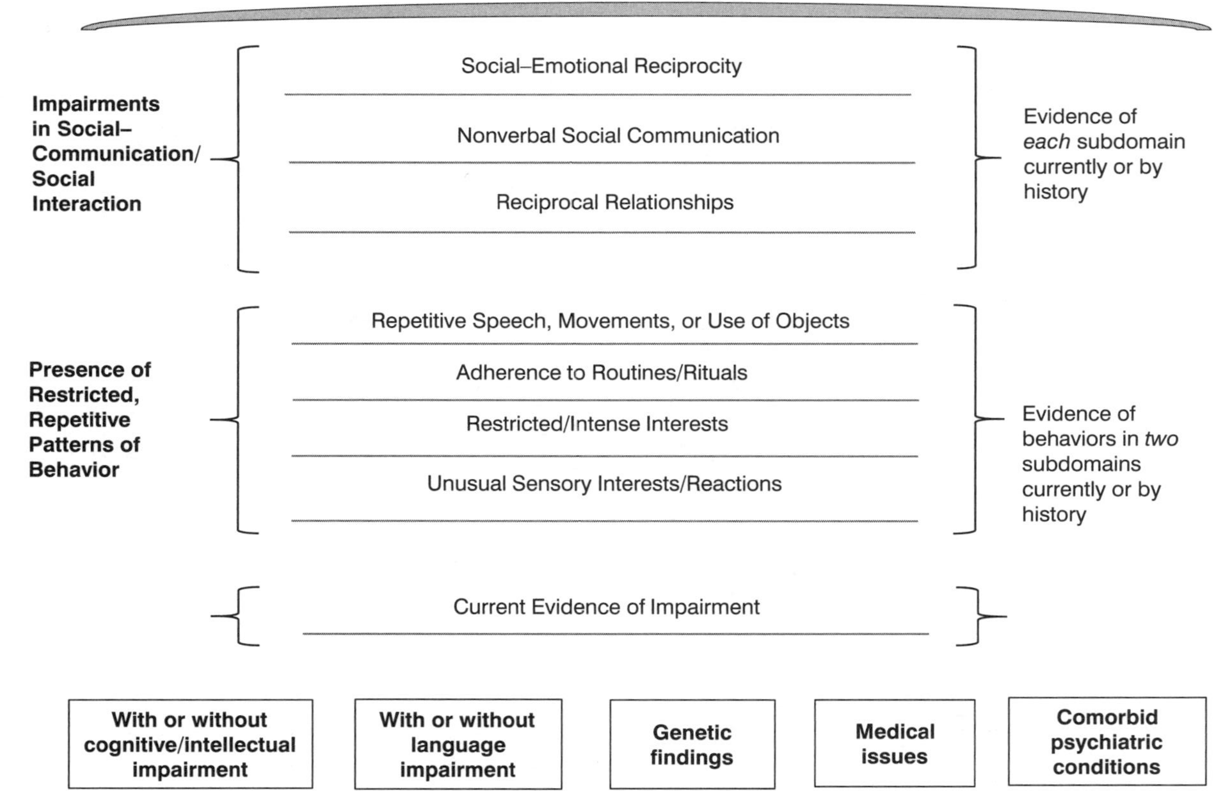

FIGURE 3.2. DSM-5 criteria for autism spectrum disorder.

often delays in expressive language are the reason why families first seek help. Expressive language level and verbal IQ during the preschool years are significant predictors of long-term prognosis, with the development of spoken language necessary but not sufficient for more favorable outcomes (Anderson, Liang, & Lord, 2014; Lord & Bishop, 2015). However, language delays occur in conjunction with many other disorders, and in the early years, may resolve themselves without treatment in typically developing children. In addition, some children with ASD meet standard language milestones (first words by 12–18 months, phrases by age 2). Overall, evidence does not support delayed language as a unique or universal feature of ASD, and thus is not part of the new ASD diagnostic criteria.

Nevertheless, the importance of language to the development and presentation of children and adults with ASD (and other disorders) cannot be underestimated. ASD features, such as poor turn taking in conversation, repetitive questioning, and unusual preoccupations, are all related to an individual's language level and must be considered within that context. For example, a child who has just begun to form simple sentences may use the same sentence structure (e.g., "More cookie" or "More jump") over and over; an adult whose expressive language level is like that of a 3-year-old is unlikely to have conversations with many turns on the same topic. On the other hand, an adult with ASD whose language is more like that of an 8-year-old should be able to talk about something not present and stay on topic in a conversation that is not only about his or her favorite interest for a few minutes. Consequently, when considering behaviors consistent with ASD, language level must be formally assessed and taken into account. (See Table 3.1 for a summary of DSM-5 changes.)

CLINICAL GUIDELINES FOR DIAGNOSING ASD

A goal of DSM-5 was to provide an updated framework that could be used by clinicians to organize and interpret diagnostic information relevant to ASD. DSM-IV and DSM-IV-TR had tried to use particular criteria, such as "lack of shared enjoyment" and "limited interactions with peers," to increase the specificity of the way in which autism was described. This was a reasonable approach at the time but had the consequence of being used in a dichotomous manner, where literal interpretations of the words "lack of" and "limited" were applied more exclusively to severe presentations, inadvertently excluding those with milder symptoms. Individuals who did not have a complete absence of the behaviors but nonetheless displayed inconsistencies in the quality or context (e.g., children who make direct eye contact in certain situations or have moments of shared enjoyment with their parents) could be dismissed as falling below the threshold of displaying

TABLE 3.1. Major Changes in DSM-5 Diagnosis of ASD

1. Consolidation of all PDD subtypes into a single diagnosis: ASD
2. Consolidation of three domains (Communication; Social Reciprocity; and Restricted, Repetitive Behaviors) from DSM-IV into two domains: Social Communication and Restricted, Repetitive Behaviors
3. Clarification that ASD is a behavioral diagnosis; anyone who meets criteria can have ASD, with or without an additional genetic or medical condition (which are now coded as specifiers)
4. Specification of use of history and/or current observation in diagnosis
5. Specification of need for some kind of impairment for a diagnosis
6. Shift from specific diagnostic criteria to statement of diagnostic principles, exemplified through clinician- and family-generated reports and observations
7. Requirement of examples of all three principles defining social communication deficits (social reciprocity, nonverbal communication, relationships/adjustments to social contexts) and two of the four subdomains in Restricted, Repetitive Behaviors
8. Addition of abnormal responses to sensory input in Restricted, Repetitive Behaviors
9. Movement of language delay from a criterion for ASD to a moderator
10. Movement of stereotyped speech from the Communication domain to the Restricted, Repetitive Behaviors domain
11. Elimination of a specific age for onset, but with the continued requirement that, to the degree possible to discern, onset of symptoms occurs during early childhood
12. Provision of dimensional severity scores based on the need for support or services
13. Creation of a newly proposed diagnosis within the Communication domain—social (pragmatic) communication disorder—to describe individuals who do not meet ASD criteria
14. Allowance of comorbid diagnoses of ASD and ADHD or other psychiatric disorders

ASD symptoms. Similarly, the criteria were often interpreted as appropriate only for specific age groups (e.g., toddlers do not yet necessarily have reciprocal friendships; older children with autism may share enjoyment in particular ways, especially with adults).

DSM-5 took a different approach, which was to state general principles of the nature of deficits and difficulties experienced by children and adults with autism across the age span. A clinician is then expected to use both observation and history to provide examples of the individual's ASD symptoms in each of the subdomains (American Psychiatric Association, 2013). Examples listed within DSM-5 criteria are now illustrative, not exhaustive. These changes allow for a better appreciation of the complexity of symptom manifestation in children and adults in clinical settings, in combination with allowing for more individualized phenotyping of children in research programs.

This is an important change for several reasons. Particularly because examples can come from history, it puts more of an onus on clinicians to find out about both past and present information about an individual child or adult seeking a diagnosis in order to conceptualize how his or her behavior fits into ASD. It also recognizes the tremendous individual differences both across people with ASD and also across time, even within the same person. It is hoped that this strategy, of broadly defined principles within the two domains, and the opportunity to operationalize these principles according to particular circumstances (strengths, challenges, culture, family context, experiences) of the individual with ASD, will result in better clinical care.

An additional change that has significant clinical implications, especially for providers who work with young children, is that there is no longer the "residual category" of PDD-NOS to use with children if the clinician is uncertain and/or has not gathered enough information to support an autism diagnosis. This is particularly relevant for very young children when a quick observation in a typical pediatric or neurology office visit may not give the clinician enough information to address the formal criteria for ASD. In addition, caregivers' informal descriptions of social and repetitive behaviors in very young children may be less helpful in arriving at an appropriate diagnosis, without some background or follow-up (Robins et al., 2014) than their responses to longer interviews or a more detailed observation of the child.

Very brief, nonspecific parent interviews that fail to ask parents in an understandable way about ASD symptoms, and the failure to use standardized diagnostic measures, lead to the risk of a clinician falsely concluding that a child does not have ASD (Lord & Bishop, 2015). Early field trials of DSM-5 criteria and other studies have encountered such problems, relying on parent report and brief child observations without the use of standard diagnostic measures (Matson, Kozlowski, Hattier, Horovitz, & Sipes, 2012; Mattila et al., 2011; McGuinness & Johnson, 2013; McPartland, Reichow, & Volkmar, 2012). In addition, if DSM-5 is interpreted to mean that symptoms must be fully present both by history and during observation/testing, some toddlers may not meet criteria, because RRB symptoms are less consistently reported by parents of young children and some of these behaviors overlap with ordinary somewhat repetitive play or language in toddlers (Barton, Robins, Jashar, Brennan, & Fein, 2013). The same issue is true of verbally skilled older children of average or even higher intelligence, where more subtle social and communicative deficits may be missed if the only information considered is the child's interactions with a parent, clinician, or other knowledgeable adult (such as a teacher). These are cases where systematic standardized observations, interviews, and questionnaires, and integrating information across sources, can help a clinician who is struggling to interpret what he or she saw or did not see (Corsello et al., 2007; Stronach & Wetherby, 2014).

The implication is that clinicians and researchers, if they have not gained enough information to evaluate each DSM-5 criterion, need to have the child return or refer the child for a more thorough or specialized evaluation, in order to reach a definitive diagnostic conclusion. Legally, children are entitled to early intervention without requiring a specific diagnosis, but practically, in many states, a child has to show clear deficits in several areas of development to receive services. Without the fallback of "PDD-NOS," clinicians will have to raise the possibility of ASD in making referrals, especially for children who do not have obvious language or other developmental delays but who do need ASD services.

A related concern is what will happen to people who demonstrated clear symptoms of autism in childhood but no longer show such behaviors later in development. In the past, such individuals often received diagnoses of Asperger's disorder or PDD-NOS later in life (even though this was not technically allowed by DSM-IV-TR), but in DSM-5 there are no "residual" categories of this type. In response to this concern, DSM-5 specifically indicates that criteria for any domain or subdomain can be met by history. The one immediate requirement is that the diagnosed individual must currently experience some level of impairment.

This means that someone who had clearly identifiable symptoms of ASD across the two dimensions as a child, meeting criteria for each subdomain in Social Communication and for two of four subdomains in RRB in the past, can still receive a diagnosis of ASD if he or she continues to need support or adaptations to an everyday environment. These supports might include a different work schedule, help in finding and keeping a job, medication to treat related comorbid difficulties (such as depression or social anxiety), or much more significant supports in residential living or employment. One approach to documenting impairment is to use adaptive scales because they typically measure what a person does every day as opposed to what he or she can do at his or her best (Bal, Kim, Cheong, & Lord, 2015). However, other indicators of impairment are appropriate too, including psychological distress in ordinary settings, the need for support in order to function at an expected level, or, in a young child, difficulties in everyday situations such as day care, preschool, going into the community (e.g., risk of wandering), or interactions with siblings.

Moreover, a DSM-5 diagnosis of ASD assumes that the clinician not only recognizes the presence or absence of ASD symptoms but also considers non-ASD factors such as IQ, language abilities, adaptive abilities, and comorbid disorders. While this is understandably a challenging endeavor for the clinician (Coury, 2013), it is well established that these other factors have significant impacts on responsiveness to treatment and long-term outcomes (Lord & Bishop, 2015). Cognitive impairments in the range of an ID are often associated with language delays (Matson & Shoemaker, 2009); greater severity of ASD symptoms, particularly RRB (Bishop, Richler, & Lord, 2006); and poorer prognostic outcomes (Anderson et al., 2014; Baghdadli et al., 2007; Bartak & Rutter, 1976; Thurm, Manwaring, Swineford, & Farmer, 2015; Elmose et al., 2014). Cognitive functioning is now considered a moderator of a DSM-5 diagnosis of ASD, as well as part of the criteria for ID.

As such, it is evident that including certain specifiers (IQ, language, etc.) within the ASD diagnosis will convey important information to families and professionals alike. Parents who understand their child's profile of strengths and challenges can better advocate for appropriate special education and treatment services (Kuhn & Carter, 2006). Difficulties in these areas, not specific to ASD, may change over time (e.g., the IQ of a 2-year-old is certainly not fixed, nor is the degree of language delay or activity level) and thus, it is important not only to include assessments of these factors in a diagnostic assessment but also to monitor how they change.

SEVERITY CODES

DSM-5, across all disorders, requires a description of dimensions of severity for each diagnosis. There was much concern in the autism clinical and research community about how these severity scores could be used because ASD is such a heterogeneous, multidimensional disorder that changes across development. A high level of severity in one aspect of ASD (e.g., very strong preoccupations or circumscribed interests) may be associated with a high degree of impairment in one person with ASD and associated with the development of strong, unique skills in another. Because language level and nonverbal IQ within the average range are necessary but not sufficient for independence without support, judging the "overall severity" of ASD has to be considered within the context of verbal and nonverbal abilities. In addition, much of what occurs in the life of an adult with ASD is dependent on the community and family in terms of opportunities afforded, including whether there is access to employment, residential systems (such as supported apartments), and social opportunities. This is also true for children, who do not all necessarily have access to individualized academic curricula, teaching of adaptive skills, or appropriate opportunities for peer interaction. Thus, there was skepticism from the committee reviewing neurodevelopmental disorders about the usefulness of a simple metric of ASD severity, separate from other factors and expectations.

In the end, the decision of the DSM-5 committee was to create very simple severity metrics that reflected the degree to which a child's or adult's behavior was dependent on support. The logic was that, in this way, severity scores are an indicator of how much support a person with ASD needs at any given time, rather than a severity rating of his or her ASD symptoms. Some research already suggests limitations in this approach (Weitlauf, Gotham, Vehorn, & Warren, 2014). DSM-5 severity codes for ASD must continue to be viewed and interpreted very cautiously.

THE ADDITION OF SCD

SCD is a new diagnosis in DSM-5 under the rubric of communication and language disorders; it is not considered an ASD (American Psychiatric Association, 2013). This new diagnosis was developed out of the concern that some individuals previously diagnosed with Asperger syndrome or PDD-NOS might no longer meet criteria for the revised ASD criteria due to an absence or only a single type of RRB. Furthermore, there were concerns that children with significant social communication deficits, who do not meet ASD criteria, will fall through the cracks without the availability of diagnoses of PDD-NOS or Asperger's disorder. Earlier analyses of children without formal ASD diagnoses, but who carried SCD diagnoses, suggested that many of them would meet ASD criteria (Norbury, 2014). Analyses of large research and clinical datasets that included many children with PDD-NOS diagnoses suggested that when there was a comprehensive assessment, including a comprehensive parent interview about history and present symptoms and a detailed observation, very few children (12 out of over 1,000) failed to meet ASD criteria (Huerta, Bishop, Duncan, Hus, & Lord, 2012). However, these datasets consisted mostly of children referred for possible ASD, not children seeking speech and language treatment, and so may have underestimated the proportion of children without ASD. Challenges in identifying separate ways of operationalizing the communication impairments inherent in core symptoms of ASD versus SCD have been documented in the research literature (Skuse, 2012), with some recent studies supporting the existence of a separate diagnosis (Gibson et al., 2013; Kim et al., 2014) and others not (Frith, 1996; Miller et al., 2015; Norbury, 2014; Reisinger, Cornish, & Fombonne, 2011; Tufan, 2014).

DSM-5 specifies that ASD must be thoroughly ruled out before SCD can be considered. The criteria for SCD indicates that a child must have impairments in four aspects of communication, including (1) the ability to use communication for social interactions; (2) adapting a communication system to the immediate context; (3) following the rules of conversation and staying on topic in conversation; and (4) understanding implicit, non-literal, and/or ambiguous language (see Chapter 7 for information on the assessment of language skills). The cumulative impairments in using verbal and nonverbal communication behaviors within a social context must be present without accompanying RRB in order to qualify for a diagnosis of SCD. As such, clinicians are encouraged to avoid using SCD as a residual or preliminary diagnosis for a child presenting with a diagnostic question of ASD. Given that subtle RRB may be more difficult to observe and for parents to report, as discussed earlier, there is a concern that SCD could be used as a replacement for PDD-NOS when there is not sufficient information or a clinician is reluctant to bring up ASD (Lord & Jones, 2012). However, again, DSM-5 specifies that SCD can be diagnosed only after ASD is ruled out.

COMORBID DIAGNOSIS OF ADHD

Individuals with ASD are at increased risk for comorbid disorders, at an estimated rate of two to four times greater than their typically developing peers (Matson, Gonzales, Wilkins, & Rivet, 2008). ADHD has been recognized as one of the most frequent comorbidities with ASD (Aman, Farmer, Hollway, & Arnold, 2008; Hanson et al., 2013; Simonoff et al., 2008; Sinzig, Walter, & Doepfiner, 2009).

In DSM-IV, concurrent diagnoses of ADHD and ASD were expressly forbidden because of concern about overdiagnosis of ADHD due to inattention or high activity levels associated with social deficits or repetitive behaviors in ASD. With DSM-5, this is no longer true.

Exactly how to define when a comorbid diagnosis of ASD and ADHD should be made is not clear (Hanson et al., 2013). Measuring symptoms of inattention, impulsivity, and hyperactivity in individuals with ASD can be difficult, particularly if a child or adult with ASD is in an environment that is not sufficiently structured or developmentally appropriate. Scores on broadband scales, such as the Child Behavior Checklist (Havdahl, von Tetzchner, Huerta, Lord, & Bishop, 2016), and narrower measures, such as the Conners Attention Scales (Craig et al., 2015), are often elevated in ASD even when children do not seem to evidence ADHD symptoms by other metrics. Clinical observation, parent, and teacher report may provide different sets of information, with parents being more likely to report higher frequencies of ADHD symptoms and teachers, less so, likely due to the structured and routine nature of classroom settings (Hanson et al., 2013).

As such, there is large variation in estimated comorbidity associated with different methods and interpretation of data.

Nonetheless, it is commonly recognized that a subset of children with ASD do have significant challenges with attention, impulsivity, and activity level. When children with ASD have comorbid ADHD symptoms, their overall functioning level is reduced and complicated by higher levels of social deficits and adaptive impairments (Hazell, 2007; Holtmann, Boltm, & Poustka, 2007; Sinzig, Bruning, Morsch, & Lehmkuhl, 2008). Taken together, while further research is needed in the overlap between ASD and ADHD, individuals with ASD and high activity levels and/or inattention or impulsive behaviors are at risk of co-occurring behavior problems, greater deficits in social functioning and behavior, poorer adaptive scores, and in the long run, less positive outcomes, even in those with average or greater intelligence (Anderson et al., 2014; Konst, Matson, Goldin, & Rieske, 2014; Reiersen & Todd, 2008; Sprenger et al., 2013).

SUMMARY OF THE IMPLICATIONS OF DSM-5 FOR ASD CLINICAL DIAGNOSES AND ASSESSMENT

It is hoped that DSM-5 criteria will make the diagnosis of ASD more straightforward and reliable for children and adults across clinicians and across time. By leaving room for multiple sources of information—family- and clinician-generated examples of subdomains; use of historical information as well as current reports and observations; and incorporation of specifiers and moderators such as language level, IQ, and comorbidities—the job of the clinician has not become easier. As well, a higher proportion of children with ASD do not have intellectual disabilities in research prevalence estimates. This is encouraging, but also makes diagnosis more difficult because of the ways in which more able children can compensate for their deficits (Skuse et al., 2009). To make matters more difficult, the increased public awareness of ASD, which is good, is also sometimes accompanied by perceptions by families that children and adults will receive more help with an ASD diagnosis than with other developmental or psychiatric disorders. This may affect the validity of caregiver reports of symptoms (Lord & Jones, 2012). Finally, assessing RRB through parent interviews can be challenging for even the skilled clinician (Lord & Bishop, 2015; Harstad et al., 2015; Schaaf & Lane, 2015), especially when the parents are not expressing their own concerns about their child potentially having ASD.

There remains great hope that, with the increase in neurobiological data and more sophisticated methods of collection and interpretation of behavioral data, we will be able to be more efficient and more accurate in making diagnoses of ASD in the future. The move toward dimensionalization of the features of ASD, particularly if it can take into account other factors such as age and developmental levels, may also yield important information about social communication deficits and RRB in ASD and in other populations (Lord & Bishop, 2015).

Research and clinical experience have shown that it is not enough to read a list to caregivers asking whether a child meets diagnostic criteria, or to hand them a checklist without consideration of the context in which they are viewing it (e.g., families seeking services, screening populations where no concern has been expressed, families with existing diagnoses participating in research; Stenberg et al., 2014; Weitlauf et al., 2014). Standardized parent-report measures, such as the Social Communication Questionnaire (SCQ) (Berument, Rutter, Lord, Pickles, & Bailey, 1999); Social Responsiveness Scale, Second Edition (SRS-2) (Constantino & Gruber, 2012); and Autism Diagnostic Interview—Revised (ADI-R) (Rutter, Le Couteur, & Lord, 2003) provide relatively broad accounts of autism-related symptomatology. However, relying only on parent report can significantly decrease the accuracy of an ASD diagnosis (Taylor, Vehorn, Noble, Weitlauf, & Warren, 2014), resulting in both false positives (Charman et al., 2007; DiGuiseppi et al., 2010; Hus, Bishop, Gotham, Huerta, & Lord, 2013) and false negatives (Taylor et al., 2014; Mazefsky, Kao, & Oswald, 2011; Eaves, Wingert, & Ho, 2006).

Observing the child across a variety of contexts is an important part of an evaluation (Lord & Bishop, 2015). Using standardized diagnostic measures that directly assess the child's social, communication, play, and behavioral functioning within the context of common social situations is recommended (Lord & Jones, 2012). To date, the Autism Diagnostic Observation Schedule, Second Edition (ADOS-2) has the highest sensitivity and specificity to an ASD clinical diagnosis when administered by a clinician who is trained and reliable in the measure (Gotham, Risi, Pickles, & Lord, 2007; Hus & Lord, 2014; Kim & Lord, 2012), but it requires skill and practice. The Screening Tool for Autism in Two-Year-Olds (Stone & Ousley, 1997; Stone, Coonrod, & Ousley, 2000), appropriate for young preschool children, is shorter and easier to administer (Stone, Coonrod, Turner, & Pozdol, 2004; Stone, McMahon, & Henderson, 2008). The Childhood Autism Rating Scales, Second Edition (CARS-2) (Schopler, Van Bourgondien, Wellman, & Love, 2010) is another commonly used observational measure that can provide a useful summary of information, but is confounded with language level and IQ and not particularly concordant with DSM-5 (Magyar & Pandolfi, 2007).

In the end, no one source of information is perfect, and diagnoses appear to be more reliable across clinicians and time when a combination of direct observation and caregiver report are used, as is proposed in DSM-5.

Perhaps with larger datasets available using the standard instruments and with more sophisticated analyses in which age and developmental level can be taken into account, one day we will have more automated algorithms combining different sources of information to quantify the dimensions that define ASD and the factors that influence how these dimensions are manifested. For now, this is the role of the assessing clinician. We remain dependent on clinical astuteness to make sense of the behaviors portrayed in DSM-5 criteria and, we hope, use this information to make judicious recommendations.

REFERENCES

Aman, M. G., Farmer, C. A., Hollway, J., & Arnold. L. E. (2008). Treatment of inattention, overactivity, and impulsiveness in autism spectrum disorders. *Child and Adolescent Psychiatric Clinics of North America, 17*(4), 713–738.

American Psychiatric Association. (1980). *Diagnostic and statistical manual of mental disorders* (3rd ed.). Washington, DC: Author.

American Psychiatric Association. (1987). *Diagnostic and statistical manual of mental disorders* (3rd ed., rev.). Washington, DC: Author.

American Psychiatric Association. (1994). *Diagnostic and statistical manual of mental disorders* (4th ed.). Washington, DC: Author.

American Psychiatric Association. (2000a). *Diagnostic and statistical manual of mental disorders* (4th ed., text rev.). Washington, DC: Author.

American Psychiatric Association. (2000b). Task force on DSM-IV. *Diagnostic and statistical manual of mental disorders: DSM-IV-TR*. Washington, DC: Author.

American Psychiatric Association. (2013). *Diagnostic and statistical manual of mental disorders* (5th ed.). Arlington, VA: Author.

Anderson, D. K., Liang, J. W., & Lord, C. (2014). Predicting young adult outcome among more and less cognitively able individuals with autism spectrum disorders. *Journal of Child Psychology and Psychiatry, 55*(5), 485–494.

Asperger, H. (1944). Die sutistischen psychopathen im kindesalter. *Archives für Psychiatrie, 117,* 76–137.

Baghdadli, A., Picot, M.-C., Michelon, C., Bodet, J., Pernon, E., Burstezjn, C., et al. (2007). What happens to children with PDD when they grow up?: Prospective follow-up of 219 children from preschool age to mid-childhood. *Acta Psychiatrica Scandinavica, 115,* 403–412.

Bal, V. H., Kim, S. H., Cheong, D., & Lord, C. (2015). Daily living skills in individuals with autism spectrum disorder from 2 to 21 years of age. *Autism, 19*(7), 1–11.

Bartak, L., & Rutter, M. (1976). Differences between mentally retarded and normally intelligent autistic children. *Journal of Autism and Childhood Schizophrenia, 6*(2), 109–120.

Barton, M. L., Robins, D. L., Jashar, D., Brennan, L., & Fein, D. (2013). Sensitivity and specificity of proposed DSM-5 criteria for autism spectrum disorder in toddlers. *Journal of Autism and Developmental Disorders, 43*(5), 1184–1195.

Berument, S. K., Rutter, M., Lord, C., Pickles, A., & Bailey, A. (1999) Autism screening questionnaire: Diagnostic validity. *British Journal of Psychiatry, 175,* 444–451.

Bishop, S. L., Richler, J., & Lord, C. (2006). Association between restricted and repetitive behaviors and nonverbal IQ in children with autism spectrum disorders. *Child Neuropsychology, 12*(4–5), 247–267.

Charman, T., Baird, G., Simonoff, E., Loucas, T., Chandler, S., Meldrum, D., et al. (2007). Efficacy of three screening instruments in the identification of autistic-spectrum disorders. *British Journal of Psychiatry, 191*(6), 554–559.

Chawarska, K., Klin, A., & Volkmar, F. R. (2010). *Autism spectrum disorder in infants and toddlers: Diagnosis, assessment, and treatment.* New York: Guilford Press.

Constantino, J. N., & Gruber, C. P. (2012). *Social responsiveness scale (SRS).* Torrance, CA: Western Psychological Services.

Constantino, J. N., & Todd, R. D. (2003). Autistic traits in the general population: A twin study. *Archives of General Psychiatry, 60*(5), 524–530.

Corsello, C., Hus, V., Pickles, A., Risi, S., Cook, E. H., Jr., Leventhal, B. L., et al. (2007). Between a ROC and a hard place: Decision making and making decisions about using the SCQ. *Journal of Child Psychology and Psychiatry, 48*(9), 932–940.

Coury, D. L. (2013). DSM-5 and autism spectrum disorders: Implications for families and clinicians. *Journal of Developmental and Behavioral Pediatrics, 34*(7), 494–496.

Craig, F., Lamanna, A. L., Margari, F., Matera, E., Simone, M., & Margari, L. (2015). Overlap between autism spectrum disorders and attention deficit hyperactivity disorder: Searching for distinctive/common clinical features. *Autism Research, 8*(3), 328–337.

de Bruin, E. I., Ferdinand, R. F., Meester, S., de Nijs, P. F., & Verheij, F. (2007). High rates of psychiatric co-morbidity in PDD-NOS. *Journal of Autism and Developmental Disorders, 37*(5), 877–886.

DiGuiseppi, C., Hepburn, S., Davis, J. M., Fidler, D. J., Hartway, S., Lee, N. R., et al. (2010). Screening for autism spectrum disorders in children with Down syndrome. *Journal of Developmental and Behavioral Pediatrics, 31*(3), 181–191.

Eaves, L. C., Wingert, H., & Ho, H. H. (2006). Screening for autism: Agreement with diagnosis. *Autism, 10*(3), 229–242.

Eisenmajer, R., Prior, M., Leekam, S., Wing, L., Ong, B., Gould, J., et al. (1998). Delayed language onset as a predictor of clinical symptoms in pervasive developmental disorders. *Journal of Autism and Developmental Disorders, 28*(6), 527–533.

Elmose, M., Trillingsgaard, A., Jørgensen, M., Nielsen, A., Bruhn, S. S., & Sørensen, E. U. (2014). Follow-up at mid-school age (9–13 years) of children assessed for autism spectrum disorder before the age of four. *Nordic Journal of Psychiatry, 68*(5), 362–368.

Frith, U. (1996). Social communication and its disorder in autism and Asperger syndrome. *Journal of Psychopharmacology, 10*(1), 48–53.

Frith, U. (2004). Emanuel Miller lecture: Confusions and controversies about Asperger syndrome. *Journal of Child Psychology and Psychiatry, 45*(4), 672–686.

Gibson, J., Adams, C., Lockton, E., & Green, J. (2013). Social communication disorder outside autism?: A diagnostic classification approach to delineating pragmatic language impairment, high functioning autism, and specific language impairment. *Journal of Child Psychology and Psychiatry, 54*(11), 1186–1197.

Goin-Kochel, R. P., Mackintosh, V. H., & Myers, B. J. (2006). How many doctors does it take to make an autism spectrum diagnosis? *Autism, 10*(5), 439–451.

Gotham, K., Risi, S., Pickles, A., & Lord, C. (2007). The Autism Diagnostic Observation

Schedule: Revised algorithms for improved diagnostic validity. *Journal of Autism and Developmental Disorders, 37*(4), 613–627.

Grzadzinski, R., Huerta, M., & Lord, C. (2013). DSM-5 and autism spectrum disorders (ASDs): An opportunity for identifying ASD subtypes. *Molecular Autism, 4*(1), 12.

Guthrie, W., Swineford, L. B., Wetherby, A. M., & Lord, C. (2013). Comparison of DSM-IV and DSM-5 factor structure models for toddlers with autism spectrum disorder. *Journal of the American Academy of Child and Adolescent Psychiatry, 52*(8), 797–805.e2.

Hanson, E., Cerban, B. M., Slater, C. M., Caccamo, L. M., Bacic, J., & Chan, E. (2013). Brief report: Prevalence of attention deficit/hyperactivity disorder among individuals with an autism spectrum disorder. *Journal of Autism and Developmental Disorders, 43*(6), 1459–1464.

Harstad, E. B., Fogler, J., Sideridis, G., Weas, S., Mauras, C., & Barbaresi, W. J. (2015). Comparing diagnostic outcomes of autism spectrum disorder using DSM-IV-TR and DSM-5 criteria. *Journal of Autism and Developmental Disorders, 45*(5), 1437–1450.

Havdahl, K. A., von Tetzchner, S., Huerta, M., Lord, C., & Bishop, S. L. (2016). Utility of the child behavior checklist as a screener for autism spectrum disorder. *Autism Research, 9*(1), 33–42.

Hazell, P. (2007). Drug therapy for attention-deficit/hyperactivity disorder-like symptoms in autistic disorder. *Journal of Paediatrics and Child Health, 43*(1–2), 19–24.

Holtman, M., Bölte, S., & Poustka, F. (2007). Autism spectrum disorders: Sex differences in autistic behaviour domains and coexisting psychopathology. *Developmental Medicine and Child Neurology, 49*(5), 361–366.

Howlin, P. (2003). Outcome in high-functioning adults with autism with and without early language delays: Implications for the differentiation between autism and Asperger syndrome. *Journal of Autism and Developmental Disorders, 33*(1), 3–13.

Huerta, M., Bishop, S. L., Duncan, A., Hus, V., & Lord, C. (2012). Application of DSM-5 criteria for autism spectrum disorder to three samples of children with DSM-IV diagnoses of pervasive developmental disorders. *American Journal of Psychiatry, 169,* 1056–1064.

Hus, V., Bishop, S., Gotham, K., Huerta, M., & Lord, C. (2013). Factors influencing scores on the Social Responsiveness Scale. *Journal of Child Psychology and Psychiatry, 54*(2), 216–224.

Hus, V., & Lord, C. (2014). The Autism Diagnostic Observation Schedule, module 4: Revised algorithm and standardized severity scores. *Journal of Autism and Developmental Disorders, 44*(8), 1996–2012.

Hus, V., Taylor, A., & Lord, C. (2011). Telescoping of caregiver report on the Autism Diagnostic Interview—Revised. *Journal of Child Psychology and Psychiatry, 52*(7), 753–760.

Kanner, L. (1943). Autistic disturbances of affective contact. *Nervous Child, 2,* 217–250.

Katz, L. J., Goldstein, G., & Beers, S. R. (2001). Concluding thoughts. In *Learning disabilities in older adolescents and adults: Clinical utility of the neuropsychological perspective* (pp. 179–183). New York: Springer.

Kim, S. H., & Lord. C. (2012). Combining information from multiple sources for the diagnosis of autism spectrum disorders for toddlers and young preschoolers from

12 to 47 months of age. *Journal of Child Psychology and Psychiatry, 53*(2), 143–151.

Kim, Y. S., Fombonne, E., Koh, Y. J., Kim, S. J., Cheon, K. A., & Leventhal, B. L. (2014). A comparison of DSM-IV pervasive developmental disorder and DSM-5 autism spectrum disorder prevalence in an epidemiologic sample. *Journal of the American Academy of Child and Adolescent Psychiatry, 53*(5), 500–508.

Klin, A., Volkmar, F. R., Sparrow, S. S., Cicchetti, D. V., & Rourke, B. P. (1996). Validity and neuropsychological characterization of Asperger syndrome: Convergence with nonverbal learning disabilities syndrome. *Annual Progress in Child Psychiatry and Child Development, 36*, 241–259.

Konst, M. J., Matson, J. L., Goldin, R., & Rieske, R. (2014). How does ASD symptomology correlate with ADHD presentations? *Research in Developmental Disabilities, 35*(9), 2252–2259.

Kuhn, J. C., & Carter, A. S. (2006). Maternal self-efficacy and associated parenting cognitions among mothers of children with autism. *American Journal of Orthopsychiatry, 76*(4), 564–575.

Lord, C., & Bishop, S. L. (2015). Recent advances in autism research as reflected in DSM-5 criteria for autism spectrum disorder. *Annual Review of Clinical Psychology, 11*, 53–70.

Lord, C., & Jones, R. M. (2012). Annual research review: Re-thinking the classification of autism spectrum disorders. *Journal of Child Psychology and Psychiatry, 53*(5), 490–509.

Lord, C., Petkova, E., Hus, V., Gan, W., Lu, F., Martin, D. M., et al. (2012). A multisite study of the clinical diagnosis of different autism spectrum disorders. *Archives of General Psychiatry, 69*(3), 306–313.

Macintosh, K. E., & Dissanayake, C. (2004). Annotation: The similarities and differences between autistic disorder and Asperger's disorder: A review of the empirical evidence. *Journal of Child Psychology and Psychiatry, 45*(3), 421–434.

Magyar, C. I., & Pandolfi, V. (2007). Factor structure evaluation of the Childhood Autism Rating Scale. *Journal of Autism and Developmental Disorders, 37*(9), 1787–1794.

Martínez-Pedraza, F. D. L., & Carter, A. S. (2009). Autism spectrum disorders in young children. *Child and Adolescent Psychiatric Clinics of North America, 18*(3), 645–663.

Matson, J. L., Boisjoli, J. A., Gonzalez, M. L., Smith, K. R., & Wilkins, J. (2007). Norms and cut off scores for the autism spectrum disorders diagnosis for adults (ASD-DA) with intellectual disability. *Research in Autism Spectrum Disorders, 1*(4), 330–338.

Matson, J. L., Gonzalez, M. L., Wilkins, J., & Rivet, T. T. (2008). Reliability of the Autism Spectrum Disorder—Diagnostic for Children (ASD-DC). *Research in Autism Spectrum Disorders, 2*(3), 533–545.

Matson, J. L., Kozlowski, A. M., Hattier, M. A., Horovitz, M., & Sipes, M. (2012). DSM-IV vs DSM-5 diagnostic criteria for toddlers with autism. *Developmental Neurorehabilitation, 15*(3), 185–190.

Matson, J. L., & Shoemaker, M. (2009). Intellectual disability and its relationship to autism spectrum disorders. *Research in Developmental Disabilities, 30*(6), 1107–1114.

Mattila, M. L., Kielinen, M., Linna, S. L., Jussila, K., Ebeling, H., Bloigu, R., et al. (2011). Autism spectrum disorders according to DSM-IV-TR and comparison with DSM-5 draft criteria: An epidemiological study. *Journal of the American Academy of Child and Adolescent Psychiatry, 50*(6), 583–592.e11.

Mayes, S. D., Calhoun, S. L., & Crites, D. L. (2001). Does DSM-IV Asperger's disorder exist? *Journal of Abnormal Child Psychology, 29*(3), 263–271.

Mazefsky, C. A., Kao, J., & Oswald, D. P. (2011). Preliminary evidence suggesting caution in the use of psychiatric self-report measures with adolescents with high-functioning autism spectrum disorders. *Research in Autism Spectrum Disorders, 5*(1), 164–174.

McGuinness, T. M., & Johnson, K. (2013). DSM-5 changes in the diagnosis of autism spectrum disorder. *Journal of Psychosocial Nursing and Mental Health Services, 51*(4), 17–19.

McPartland, J. C., Reichow, B., & Volkmar, F. R. (2012). Sensitivity and specificity of proposed DSM-5 diagnostic criteria for autism spectrum disorder. *Journal of the American Academy of Child and Adolescent Psychiatry, 51*(4), 368–383.

Miller, M., Young, G. S., Hutman, T., Johnson, S., Schwichtenberg, A. J., & Ozonoff, S. (2015). Early pragmatic language difficulties in siblings of children with autism: Implications for DSM-5 social communication disorder? *Journal of Child Psychology and Psychiatry, 56*(7), 774–781.

Norbury, C. F. (2014). Practitioner review: Social (pragmatic) communication disorder conceptualization, evidence and clinical implications. *Journal of Child Psychology and Psychiatry, 55*(3), 204–216.

Ozonoff, S., South, M., & Miller, J. N. (2000). DSM-IV-defined Asperger syndrome: Cognitive, behavioral and early history differentiation from high-functioning autism. *Autism, 4*(1), 29–46.

Reiersen, A. M., & Todd, R. D. (2008). Co-occurrence of ADHD and autism spectrum disorders: Phenomenology and treatment. *Expert Review of Neurotherapeutics, 8*(4), 657–669.

Reisinger, L. M., Cornish, K. M., & Fombonne, E. (2011). Diagnostic differentiation of autism spectrum disorders and pragmatic language impairment. *Journal of Autism and Developmental Disorders, 41*(12), 1694–1704.

Robins, D. L., Casagrande, K., Barton, M., Chen, C. M. A., Dumont-Mathieu, T., & Fein, D. (2014). Validation of the Modified Checklist for Autism in Toddlers, Revised with Follow-Up (M-CHAT-R/F). *Pediatrics, 133*(10), 37–45.

Ronald, A., Edelson, L. R., Asherson, P., & Saudino, K. J. (2010). Exploring the relationship between autistic-like traits and ADHD behaviors in early childhood: Findings from a community twin study of 2-year-olds. *Journal of Abnormal Child Psychology, 38(2),* 185–196.

Rutter, M., Le Couteur, A., & Lord, C. (2003). *Autism diagnostic interview—revised.* Los Angeles: Western Psychological Services.

Schaaf, R. C., & Lane, A. E. (2015). Toward a best-practice protocol for assessment of sensory features in ASD. *Journal of Autism and Developmental Disorders, 45,* 1380–1395.

Schopler, E., Van Bourgondien, M. E., Wellman, G. J., & Love, S. R. (2010). *CARS 2—Childhood autism rating scale.* Los Angeles: Western Psychological Services.

Simonoff, E., Pickles, A., Charman, T., Chandler, S., Loucas, T., & Baird, G. (2008). Psychiatric disorders in children with autism spectrum disorders: Prevalence, comorbidity, and associated factors in a population-derived sample. *Journal of the American Academy of Child & Adolescent Psychiatry, 47*(8), 921–929.

Sinzig, J., Bruning, N., Morsch, D., & Lehmkuhl, G. (2008). Attention profiles in autistic children with and without comorbid hyperactivity and attention problems. *Acta Neuropsychiatria, 20*(4), 207–215.

Sinzig, J., Walter, D., & Doepfner, M. (2009). Attention deficit/hyperactivity disorder in children and adolescents with autism spectrum disorder: Symptom or syndrome? *Journal of Attention Disorders, 13*(2), 117–126.

Skuse, D. H. (2012). DSM-5's conceptualization of autistic disorders. *Journal of the American Academy of Child and Adolescent Psychiatry, 51*(4), 344–346.

Skuse, D. H., Mandy, W., Steer, C., Miller, L. M., Goodman, R., Lawrence, K., et al. (2009). Social communication competence and functional adaptation in a general population of children: Preliminary evidence for a sex-by-verbal IQ differential risk. *Journal of the American Academy of Child and Adolescent Psychiatry, 48*(2), 128–137.

Snow, A. V., & Lecavalier, L. (2011). Comparing autism, PDD-NOS, and other developmental disabilities on parent-reported behavior problems: Little evidence for ASD subtype validity. *Journal of Autism and Developmental Disorders, 41*(3), 302–310.

Sprenger, L., Bühler, E., Poustka, L., Bach, C., Heinzel-Gutenbrunner, M., Kamp-Becker, I., et al. (2013). Impact of ADHD symptoms on autism spectrum disorder symptom severity. *Research in Developmental Disabilities, 34*(10), 3545–3552.

Stenberg, N., Bresnahan, M., Gunnes, N., Hirtz, D., Hornig, M., Lie, K. K., et al. (2014). Identifying children with autism spectrum disorder at 18 months in a general population sample. *Paediatric and Perinatal Epidemiology, 28*, 255–262.

Stone, W. L., Coonrod, E. E., & Ousley, O. Y. (2000). Brief report: Screening tool for autism in two-year-olds (STAT): Development and preliminary data. *Journal of Autism and Developmental Disorders, 30*(6), 607–612.

Stone, W. L., Coonrod, E. E., Turner, L. M., & Pozdol, S. L. (2004). Psychometric properties of the STAT for early autism screening. *Journal of Autism and Developmental Disorders, 34*(6), 691–701.

Stone, W. L., McMahon, C. R., & Henderson, L. M. (2008). Use of the Screening Tool for Autism in Two-Year-Olds (STAT) for children under 24 months: An exploratory study. *Autism, 12*(5), 557–573.

Stone, W. L., & Ousley, O. Y. (1997). *STAT manual: Screening tool for autism in two-year-olds.* Unpublished manuscript, Vanderbilt University, Nashville, TN.

Stronach, S., & Wetherby, A. M. (2014). Examining restricted and repetitive behaviors in young children with autism spectrum disorder during two observational contexts. *Autism, 18*(2), 127–136.

Swineford, L. B., Thurm, A., Baird, G., Wetherby, A. M., & Swedo, S. (2014). Social (pragmatic) communication disorder: A research review of this new DSM-5 diagnostic category. *Journal of Neurodevelopmental Disorders, 6*(1), 41.

Szatmari, P. (1992). The validity of autistic spectrum disorders: A literature review. *Journal of Autism and Developmental Disorders, 22*(4), 583–600.

Tanguay, P. E., Robertson, J., & Derrick, A. (1998). A dimensional classification of autism spectrum disorder by social communication domains. *Journal of the American Academy of Child and Adolescent Psychiatry, 37*(3), 271–277.

Taylor, C. M., Vehorn, A., Noble, H., Weitlauf, A. S., & Warren, Z. E. (2014). Brief report: Can metrics of reporting bias enhance early autism screening measures? *Journal of Autism and Developmental Disorders, 44*(9), 2375–2380.

Thurm, A., Manwaring, S. S., Swineford, L., & Farmer, C. (2015). Longitudinal study of symptom severity and language in minimally verbal children with autism. *Journal of Child Psychology and Psychiatry, 56*(1), 97–104.

Towbin, K. (2005). Pervasive developmental disorder not otherwise specified. In F. R. Volkmar, R. Paul, A. Klin, & D. J. Cohen (Eds.), *Handbook of autism and pervasive developmental disorders* (3rd ed., pp. 165–200). New York: Wiley.

Tsur, V. G., Shalev, R. S., Manor, O., & Amir, N. (1995). Developmental right-hemisphere syndrome clinical spectrum of the nonverbal learning disability. *Journal of Learning Disabilities, 28*(2), 80–86.

Tufan, E. (2014). The relationship between social communication disorder (SCD) and broad autism phenotype (BAP). *Journal of the American Academy of Child and Adolescent Psychiatry, 53*(10), 1130.

Volden, J. (2013). Nonverbal learning disability. *Handbook of Clinical Neurology, 111*, 245–249.

Volkmar, F. R., Bregman, K., Cohen, D. J., & Cicchetti, D. V. (1988). DSM-III and DSM-III-R diagnoses of autism. *American Journal of Psychiatry, 145*, 1404–1408.

Volkmar, F. R., Cicchetti, D. V., Bregman, J., & Cohen, D. J. (1992). Three diagnostic systems for autism: DSM-III, DSM-III-R, and ICD-10. *Journal of Autism and Developmental Disorders, 22*(4), 483–492.

Volkmar, F. R., Cohen, D. J., & Paul, R. (1986). An evaluation of DSM-III criteria for infantile autism. *Journal of the American Academy of Child Psychiatry, 25*(2), 190–197.

Weitlauf, A. S., Gotham, K. O., Vehorn, A. C., & Warren, Z. E. (2014). Brief report: DSM-5 "levels of support": A comment on discrepant conceptualizations of severity in ASD. *Journal of Autism and Developmental Disorders, 44*(2), 471–476.

Woodbury-Smith, M., Klin, A., & Volkmar, F. (2005). Asperger's syndrome: A comparison of clinical diagnoses and those made according to the ICD-10 and DSM-IV. *Journal of Autism and Developmental Disorders, 35*(2), 235–240.

CHAPTER FOUR

Assessment and Diagnosis of Infants and Toddlers with Autism Spectrum Disorder

Kelly K. Powell
Perrine Heymann
Katherine D. Tsatsanis
Katarzyna Chawarska

Science examining etiological factors contributing to autism spectrum disorder (hereafter referred to as ASD or "autism") implicates a biological basis for the neurodevelopmental disorder as documented by burgeoning research, including prospective studies of younger siblings of those with confirmed diagnoses of ASD as well as twin studies (Jeste & Geschwind, 2014). Prospective studies of infants at risk for developing autism estimate that 18.7% of siblings develop ASD themselves by the age of 36 months (Ozonoff et al., 2011) and approximately 76–88% of identical twins both meet criteria for ASD (Ronald & Hoekstra, 2011). Although genetic influences are highly implicated in the expression of ASD, a specific biological marker present across all cases has yet to be identified; there is no medical test to signify the presence or absence of the disorder. Therefore, the diagnosis of ASD continues to be based solely on clinical observations involving the confluence of delays and/or aberrations from typical developmental trajectories in the domains of Social Communication and Interaction, as well as the presence of restricted, repetitive patterns of behavior, interests, or activities (RRBIAs; DSM-5; American Psychiatric Association, 2013).

Among the behavioral abnormalities that define ASD, the constellation of symptoms across individuals is often highly heterogeneous—this notion of heterogeneity holds true even when comparing children with similar cognitive and language profiles (Matson & Shoemaker, 2009). The unique and often broad constellation of symptoms of ASD can vary in the overall number of symptoms falling within each diagnostic criterion as well as the severity of each symptom and the degree of functional impairment caused by the observed delays and atypical behaviors. As such, the presence of an accompanying intellectual disability, language impairment, and attentional impairments (Miller et al., 2015; Johnson, Gilga, Jones, & Charman, 2015), as well as symptoms of anxiety (van Steensel, Bögels, & Perrin, 2011), adds another layer of diagnostic complexity. Recent estimates suggest that approximately 30% of children with autism are classified in the range of intellectual disability (IQ score ≤70; Centers for Disease Control and Prevention, 2016), approximately 40% meet criteria for an anxiety disorder (van Steensel et al., 2011), and 20% meet criteria for attention-deficit/hyperactivity disorder (ADHD; Russell, Rodgers, & Ukoumunne, 2014). When considering these co-occurring disorders (see also Chapter 10), there is an added challenge to assess how a child's social disability exceeds delays in other impaired domains (e.g., verbal or nonverbal domains) and to what extent they are altered by emerging attentional or affective problems.

While high rates of co-occurring developmental delays are documented within cohorts of toddlers who receive diagnoses of ASD, common diagnostic rule-outs in young children suspected of having ASD are global developmental delays and language delays. Therefore, it is important for professionals to differentiate delays and atypicalities in social engagement and reciprocity, as well as the presence of repetitive behaviors due to emerging cognitive profiles of intellectual disability or specific language impairment from those resultant from ASD. It is important to highlight that the presence of global developmental delays during early childhood does not dictate persisting cognitive impairments later in life nor does an early language delay predict a long-term language impairment (Charman et al., 2005; Chawarska, Klin, Macari, & Volkmar, 2009; Lord et al., 2006; Magiati, Charman, & Howlin, 2007; Magiati, Moss, Charman, & Howlin, 2011; Kim, Macari, Koller, & Chawarska, 2016). Longitudinal investigations of young children with ASD between 2 and 3 years of age indicate that the rate of progress is often variable, particularly in regard to language and cognitive abilities, with some toddlers making remarkable gains and others making slower progress (Bryson et al., 2007; Chawarska et al., 2009; Kim et al., 2016). While the absence of co-occurring cognitive and/or language delays at the time of first diagnosis is generally understood as a positive prognostic marker, the presence of marked delays does not necessarily predict that the toddler will have persisting cognitive and/or language impairments during later developmental periods (Chawarska et al., 2009; Kim et al., 2016). Conversely, autism may also be overlooked in children with average and above-average cognitive or language abilities. Unusual behaviors or abnormalities in development in these children, especially in very young children, may be dismissed as mild or transient.

Additionally, accumulating evidence from over a decade of prospective studies examining the emergence of readily *observable* behavioral symptoms related to ASD highlights that the defining features of the disorder are not yet reliably discernable in infants 6 months and younger (Young, Merin, Rogers, & Ozonoff, 2009; Rozga et al., 2011; Zwaigenbaum et al., 2005; Ozonoff et al., 2010; Bryson et al., 2007) but emerge sometime thereafter (Ozonoff et al., 2010; Rogers, 2009). Moreover, infants later diagnosed with ASD appear to have no major developmental delays in the areas of nonverbal functioning, language, or motor skills as captured by the Mullen Scales of Early Learning (Chawarska, Macari, & Shic, 2013; Landa & Garrett-Mayer, 2006; Ozonoff et al., 2010; Zwaigenbaum et al., 2005). Though recently, subtle motor deficits, including poor postural control, have been observed at 6 months (Flanagan, Landa, Bhat, & Bauman, 2012), possibly foreshadowing the motor difficulties described in older children with ASD (Fournier, Hass, Naik, Lodha, & Cauraugh, 2010). While a subset of children may in fact evidence symptoms within the first year of life, a more common pattern of symptom expression involves an early course of rather typical development or mild delays followed by a loss of skills (usually language and/or social) paired with the emergence of ASD-related atypical behaviors including repetitive behaviors and atypical object exploration (Nadig et al., 2007; Kim & Lord, 2010; Ozonoff, Heung, Byrd, Hansen, & Hertz-Picciotto, 2008; Paul, Fuerst, Ramsay, Chawarska, & Klin, 2011). A new perspective on patterns of symptom onset in autism suggests that some behaviors (e.g., eye contact and social smiling) may show a gradual decrease in frequency from 6 to 18 months, whereas others (e.g., social vocalizations) may fail to increase at the rate observed in normative samples (Ozonoff et al., 2010). These findings suggest that the models of symptom onset might be best captured by a multidimensional approach, as it is plausible that the departure from typical trajectories in specific domains may follow different patterns (i.e., plateau or regression) and take place during different developmental periods.

Given the notion that the protracted developmental progression of ASD may not necessarily be evident for months or potentially several years, compounded by the inherent phenotypic heterogeneity, it is difficult to diagnose autism in the first year of life; rather than observing the full constellation of symptoms, we are likely detecting the subtle unfolding symptoms of social and communicative dysfunction. However, if significant developmental concerns are identified in infancy, clinicians are advised to recommended intervention for the documented delays (e.g., social, language, cognitive) and provide close monitoring of the child's development, including a reevaluation within 3–6 months.

Despite the variability of syndrome expression and the developmental nature of the disorder, particularly during the first year of life, research suggests that early *comprehensive* and *interdisciplinary* assessment leads to reliable diagnosis made during the second year of life. The majority of children who receive a diagnosis in this second year continue to do so at 3–4 years of age, with rates ranging from 80 to 100% (Lord et al., 2006; Chawarska, Klin, Paul, & Volkmar, 2007; Chawarska et al., 2009; Guthrie, Swineford, Nottke, & Wetherby, 2013; Kim et al., 2016; Ozonoff et al., 2015) with similar longer-term stability estimates at school age (Charman et al., 2005; Lord et al., 2006; Turner, Stone, Pozdol, & Coonrod, 2006). Comparable rates of stability are also found in high-risk children with ASD outcomes (Zwaigenbaum et al., 2016; Ozonoff et al., 2015). However, studies also show that there is a subset of children who receive an ASD diagnosis at their 3-year visit who were not initially identified at 2 years of age (Ozonoff et al., 2015). Therefore, for toddlers at risk for ASD due to familial factors (e.g., having an older sibling with ASD), follow-up is essential, even if diagnostic criteria are not met at early initial assessments. While the number of children diagnosed with ASD by the age of 3 years is growing, many are not formally identified as having ASD until they enter preschool or thereafter (Filipek et al., 1999; Werner, Dawson, Osterling, & Dinno, 2000; Woods & Wetherby, 2003; Mandell, Novak, & Zubritsky, 2005). The Centers for Disease Control and Prevention (2016) estimates the median age of identification is over 4 years. Factors associated with earlier diagnosis include male sex, IQ within the range of intellectual disability, and an onset pattern of developmental regression (Shattuck et al., 2009). Unfortunately, delayed diagnoses are even more common for children from underrepresented minority groups and lower socioeconomic status (Begeer, Bouk, Boussaid, Terwogt, & Koot, 2008; Thomas, Ellis, McLaurin, Daniels, & Morrissey, 2007). These delays, which inherently lengthen the interval between symptom onset and initiation of intervention, further narrow the window for early and intensive intervention during periods when the human brain is the most plastic and amenable to modifying the atypical developmental course (Fenske, Zalenski, Krantz, & McClannahan, 1985; Lovaas & Smith, 1988; Rogers, 1996; Wolff et al., 2012).

COMPLEXITIES OF EARLY IDENTIFICATION AND DIAGNOSIS

In addition to the protracted course of symptom emergence and phenotypic heterogeneity, early identification and diagnosis of ASD is accompanied by a number of other complexities. First, the expression of ASD-related behaviors changes over time and symptom presentation typically differs across different developmental periods. For example, a toddler with ASD may present with severely delayed language, lack of social interest, poor functional play, and atypical communication patterns such as hand-over-hand gestures. In contrast, the same child in preschool may evidence verbosity, inappropriate social overtures toward peers, or all-encompassing interests in a specific topic or activity, accompanied by emerging executive dysfunction and anxiety symptoms. Relatedly, language, social, and behavioral expectations progress rapidly over the first few years of life and behaviors that were once considered developmentally appropriate for an infant or young toddler (e.g., production of undirected vocalizations [in the form of vocal play or babbling to oneself], exploration of sensory features of objects, or the demonstration of whole-body movements when excited) become atypical if they persist past the normative period of development.

Second, early identification of ASD is further complicated because many of the early markers or "red flags" depend on the *absence* of appropriate developmental behaviors, such as *not* pointing to objects to show interest, *reduced* eye contact, *not* responding to one's name when called, *decreased* frequency or *lack* of showing and/or giving items for purely social purposes such as to share, and so forth. Research indicates that the absence or delay in development of more typical social behaviors are in fact better predictors of ASD in young children (Barton, Dumont-Mathieu, & Fein, 2012). Even though toddlers with ASD may demonstrate more severe and/or frequent repetitive actions with objects, motor mannerisms, sensory interests, and nonspeech vocalizations compared with children with developmental delays and typically developing children (Kim & Lord, 2010; Schoen, Paul, & Chawarska, 2011; Watt, Wetherby, Barber, & Morgan, 2008), these behaviors are also sometimes observed in other disorders (Baranek, 1999; Lord, 1995). Unfortunately, diagnoses based on the reduced frequency and quality or complete absence of behaviors are commonly more challenging for parents and practitioners to identify in comparison to the presence of aberrant behaviors that may be seen as more atypical, disruptive, or interfering.

Last, other factors that need to be considered in early identification and diagnosis of ASD that are more difficult to elucidate include the potential emergence of prodromal features of disorders that typically manifest later in development (e.g., anxiety, ADHD). While less is known about the profile of symptom emergence in these specific disorders, particularly among children with autism, research indicates that the majority of children with ASD will also meet criteria for one or more comorbid disorders by school age (Simonoff et al., 2008; Doshi-Velez, Ge, & Kohane, 2014). This may be particularly relevant when assessing siblings of children with autism; these children are at greater risk for autism as well as for a range of other delays and/or aberrant behaviors (Ozonoff et al., 2014; Bora, Aydın, Saraç, Kadak, & Köse, 2016; Messinger et al., 2013; Zwaigenbaum et al.,

2007; Yirmiya & Ozonoff, 2007). Therefore, careful consideration of the potential impact of the prodromal phases of later-developing comorbid diagnostic outcomes needs to be considered, although, as noted, research examining these factors is more limited. Taken together, the presentation of social abnormalities early in life should be interpreted in the context of the child's mental and chronological age, an understanding of typical development, as well as knowledge of the child's medical and family history.

GUIDING PRINCIPLES OF COMPREHENSIVE DIAGNOSTIC ASSESSMENT

Comprehensive Assessment Model

Diagnostic practices vary in regard to the scope and depth of assessment procedures as well as the team of professionals involved. Common practice involves primary reliance on parent report coupled with behavioral observations during traditional office visits to formulate a diagnosis. However, best-practice guidelines for young children recommend a comprehensive evaluation that often involves a team of professionals assessing various developmental domains (Zwaigenbaum et al., 2009; Johnson & Meyers, 2007; Risi et al., 2006; Steiner, Goldsmith, Snow, & Chawarska, 2012). The aim of a comprehensive diagnostic evaluation is fourfold: (1) elucidating the child's unique profiles of strengths and weaknesses; (2) providing diagnostic clarification; (3) providing recommendations for treatment planning; and (4) identifying additional evaluations that are needed such as genetics, neurology, and/or vision and hearing exams, as well as referrals for additional specialists (e.g., feeding, sleeping).

A comprehensive evaluation preferably takes on a multi- or interdisciplinary approach. Various professionals, including psychologists, social workers, speech and language pathologists—and where possible or as needed—occupational therapists, psychiatrists, developmental pediatricians, and/or neurologists, are involved. Whereas an interdisciplinary approach typically entails a team of professionals working together to provide a single coherent view of the child's strengths, weaknesses, and diagnostic presentation, a multidisciplinary evaluation follows similar procedures but is not integrative because each discipline conducts its own separate evaluation. Although the multi- or interdisciplinary approach is recommended because a response to the diagnostic questions involves consideration of multiple domains, if unattainable, it is recommended that the expert clinician responding to the diagnostic question gathers information across multiple domains (e.g., history; developmental abilities; speech, language, and communication skills; autism symptomatology; adaptive behavior; and a screening for comorbidities).

Assessment Process

Given the breadth and scope of the comprehensive diagnostic evaluation, a number of methods are used to collect the necessary and pertinent information. In order to develop a complete picture, it is important that information pertaining to the child's development and functioning is garnered from a variety of settings and sources such as the clinic, home, day care or school, and community. Data are collected via a combination of parent/caregiver interviews, record review, standardized assessments, behavioral questionnaires, and informed observation. In addition, information gathered from early interventionists as well as teachers/day care providers through the completion of behavioral questionnaires and interviews is recommended when feasible. Once all pertinent information is collected, the clinician(s) meet to discuss and integrate findings in an effort to provide a coherent conceptualization of the child, noting the areas of strengths and vulnerability that contribute to his or her behavioral and diagnostic presentation. This conceptualization is then used to provide recommendations for intervention. Results of the evaluation are shared with families via in-person feedback meetings and the approach to delivering the information is tailored to the needs of the family. In addition, the details of the evaluation are provided in a written report. Given parental consent, communication with the child's day care, interventionists, and outside providers is suggested to facilitate the implementation of the recommendations, as coordination of care is imperative in the successful treatment of children with ASD.

Characteristics of Young Child Assessments

Children, particularly young children suspected of having developmental delays, may demonstrate different behavioral presentations across different people, contexts, and even points in time. Therefore, the comprehensive assessment should include an opportunity to observe and interact with the toddler in a variety of settings and during activities wherein the evaluators can vary the degree of scaffolding and support they provide in order to more closely understand the child's profile of strengths and weaknesses and better inform recommendations for treatment. Behaviors observed across settings are highly informative given the different behavioral expectations demanded under various conditions. For example, developmental assessments are generally highly structured; they occur at a table or a designated spot on the floor, involve adult-directed activities, and generally require some degree of emerging ability to learn skills including sitting, attending, and monitoring an adult's actions. Although most typically developing toddlers are able to sit and attend for intervals of time, breaks between tasks and provision of reinforcements are often needed to maintain attention and engagement; some degree of off-task behavior and noncompliance falls within normative expectations. Conversely, while many young children with autism may demonstrate interest in the assessment materials presented and show goal-directed behavior, their capacity to sit at or stand near the assessment table, comply with adult directives, and benefit from modeling and instruction of tasks is often limited, particularly if they have not yet received intervention. In such circumstances, a flexible approach to assessment administration is necessitated while at the same time maintaining testing fidelity (e.g., not altering standardized administration of the test items); this may involve the use of behavioral momentum strategies, first–then contingencies, planned breaks, and so forth. For those children who do not yet possess foundational skills such as shared joint attention, imitation, a pointing response, and so on, they may require even more flexible testing parameters wherein the clinician may set out materials and observe how the child manipulates them independently. Other assessments, such as those intended to measure communication and social engagement, often utilize less structured testing parameters, because the frequency and quality of spontaneous behaviors elicited under more naturalistic conditions are under primary examination. While many of these assessment tools are also standardized (e.g., Autism Diagnostic Observation Schedule, Second Edition; Lord et al., 2012), the semistructured format lends itself to observing a different subset of behaviors with a greater reliance on spontaneous communication and social engagement. Furthermore, observations occurring outside of the formal assessment context are made in waiting rooms during transitions between activities and separation from a caregiver during parent interviews and/or feedback meetings; these situations also provide valuable information that may contribute to the diagnostic formulation process.

The assessment context is also informative to further elucidate the nature of the child's observed skills. In this regard, a distinction is made between *capacity* (e.g., demonstration of skill set given optimal conditions) and *consistency* (e.g., use of skill set consistently across settings and people and in functional and/or predictable ways). For example, it is common for a toddler to demonstrate a skill such as the ability to use blocks purposefully to replicate simple constructions (e.g., a tower) during one assessment but then not complete this same activity using another set of blocks with a different clinician during another session. When such inconsistencies in performance are observed, it is an opportunity to examine why the discrepancy occurred. For example, the variability may be driven by poor generalization of skills (e.g., the toddler learned to stack blocks with one set of blocks but cannot do so with a novel set), variability in the degree of self-directed behavior exhibited by the child, fatigue from the assessment process, inattention, and/or differing degrees of scaffolding (e.g., differences in the number of preteaching methods used, variability in utilization of first–then contingencies). In turn, clinicians may decide to "test the limits" and provide additional opportunities for modeling and/or prompting (including full physical hand-over-hand methodologies) to preteach a skill. While the toddler will not be awarded credit for successfully completing testing items that required this level of support, the child's responsivity toward these intervention techniques can be informative in regard to the types of treatment strategies he or she may benefit from.

Caregiver Involvement

Parent/caregiver involvement in the evaluation is crucial as caregivers know their child most intimately and can provide a more complete picture of the toddler's behaviors in the home and the community. While parental perspective may be biased, their reflections and input are very useful and sufficiently reliable (Lord, Rutter, & Couteur, 1994). Concerns identified by parents, particularly in high-risk cohorts, can also help improve earlier recognition of ASD (Sacrey et al., 2015). Caregivers also offer information pertaining to history including medical and developmental histories, which are necessary components of the evaluative process.

Given the young age of the toddler, a parent or caregiver is often present during the assessment procedures. It is common and natural for parents to be anxious and eager to see their child perform well and they may have difficulty taking a "backseat" during the assessment, wanting to provide the customary level of scaffolding and support they do while at home and in the community. However, this level of involvement can mask weaknesses and/or invalidate assessment findings, particularly if the standardized assessments call for specific administrative procedures. By providing parents with explicit information regarding the instruments utilized, standardized assessment practices, and the degree of parental involvement invited during administration of testing items, the clinician can attempt to maintain environmental control over the evaluation. Parents should be encouraged to offer commentary regarding behaviors they expected to see but did not and vice versa; caregivers can also remark on skills the child displayed during the evaluation that he or she has not demonstrated previously and/or are considered emerging yet inconsistently exhibited skills. Explanations and observations about levels of effort and compliance are valuable as parents can compare their toddler's performance during the current evaluation to more typical presentations. Furthermore, the assessment process can be viewed as the first step in the treatment process. Parents' observations mediated by clinician input during the evaluation may aid in their personal understanding and acceptance of the validity of the assessment findings and subsequent recommendations, which typically involve a highly intensive program.

Parental consent for the clinician(s) to communicate with current interventionists and/or day care personnel is recommended. This form of communication is relevant to symptom presentation but also when recommendations for intervention are considered, as the diagnostic clinicians will want a broad understanding of the interventions that have previously proved to be effective and those that have been less efficacious. A collaborative approach should be a hallmark feature embedded within diagnostic processes and procedures (Zwaigenbaum et al., 2009).

DOMAINS OF ASSESSMENT FOR INFANTS AND TODDLERS

The comprehensive diagnostic evaluative model described involves an intimately integrated, and in some capacity, overlapping, set of procedures intended to collect data necessary for diagnostic clarification and for delineating a comprehensive profile of the toddler's strengths and vulnerabilities in efforts to inform the design and implementation of an individualized and intensive intervention program. As noted, the following domains should be considered: (1) history; (2) developmental functioning; (3) speech, language, and communication skills; (4) ASD-related behaviors; (5) adaptive functioning; and (6) screening for comorbidities.

History

The first component involves a detailed history including prenatal and birth, postnatal medical, developmental, behavioral, educational, treatment/interventions, and family histories. Histories can be gathered from a clinical interview with a parent/caregiver and via comprehensive record review. Social workers, psychologists, psychiatrists, or developmental pediatricians commonly conduct the detailed history. Obtaining a thorough history is important for both formulation of an ASD diagnosis and for differential diagnostic purposes. Through this process the clinical team establishes the onset and course of symptom emergence and identifies any pertinent complicating variables (e.g., medical, family history).

Developmental Functioning

Direct assessment of the toddler's developmental abilities provides a foundational understanding of his or her current level of functioning. The term "cognitive development" refers to the ability to think and understand. Infants learn about the world first through touching, mouthing, looking, manipulating, and listening—then the learning process becomes more thoughtful and complex. Toddlers begin to form mental images for things, actions, and concepts. They begin to understand the relationship between objects and show emerging nonverbal and verbal problem solving. Therefore, typically included in the developmental evaluation is a broad measure of the toddler's nonverbal problem solving and motor abilities (fine and/or gross motor), as well as a basic assessment of receptive and expressive language.

An important reminder, as noted above, is that the results of a developmental assessment do not necessarily predict future levels of cognitive functioning. Results offer a benchmark against which behavioral observations as well as performance across assessment instruments are compared. Preliminary results from the developmental assessment may indicate the need for a more in-depth evaluation of particular domains of function—for example, occupational and/or physical therapy evaluations to more thoroughly examine motor skills. Information gleaned from the developmental assessment can also reveal developmental strengths and identify gaps in skill sets across domains, as well as inform decisions as to appropriate treatment goals and types of interventions the child may benefit from.

The developmental profiles of very young children with autism can be quite variable across developmental domains. For example, approximately 75% of toddlers with ASD present with significant delays in at least one developmental domain (Akshoomoff, 2006). Even for those children with delays across multiple areas of development, uneven strengths and weaknesses may exist (Chawarska et al., 2009; Weismer, Lord, & Esler, 2010). One common toddler profile is characterized by weaker verbal skills compared with nonverbal skills (Akshoomoff, 2006; Chawarska et al., 2009; Joseph, Tager-Flusberg, & Lord, 2002; Paul, Chawarska, Cicchetti, & Volkmar, 2008). In addition, many young toddlers with autism display more significant deficits in their understanding of and responsivity to language as compared with their spoken language as reflected in significantly lower receptive versus expressive language scores (Weismer et al., 2010).

Motor skills are typically evaluated as part of a developmental assessment. Broadly speaking, gross motor abilities involve the use and coordination of large muscles (e.g., arms, legs, feet, or entire body such as walking, jumping). In contrast, fine motor skills involve the movement of smaller muscles (e.g., hands, wrists, and fingers) and visual–motor development, including fine motor coordination, planning, and control, as well as graphomotor abilities.

Motor impairments in cohorts of children with ASD include deficits in gross and fine motor control as well as motor learning deficits (Esposito & Paşca, 2013) and are present early in life (Leary & Hill, 1996; Landa, Gross, Stuart, & Faherty, 2013). Even when motor abilities are within average limits based on standardized assessments, many children may appear clumsy and have poor motor coordination. As described by Kanner (1943) in his initial case series, these abnormalities were referred to as "clumsiness in gait and motor performances." Others may have the motor control to successfully complete a test item but have difficulty imitating the actions of the clinician and therefore do not receive credit for skills they may actually possess. All such factors should be considered during diagnostic formulation and treatment planning.

There are a number of standardized assessment tools available to measure developmental skills. The Mullen Scales of Early Learning (MSEL; Mullen, 1995); the Bayley Scales of Infant and Toddler Development, Third Edition (Bayley–III; Bayley, 2005); the Battelle Developmental Inventory, Second Edition (BDI-2; Newborg, 2005); the Developmental Assessment of Young Children, Second Edition (DAY-C; Voress & Maddox, 1998); and the Hawaii Early Learning Profile 0–3 years (HELP: 0–3 years; Parks, 2007) are commonly used instruments. (See Table 4.1 for a detailed description of each.) While these tools differ across a variety of dimensions, including the use of parent report to score specific items, they all measure key facets of development including nonverbal problem solving, fine and gross motor skills, and verbal abilities. In addition, the Bayley–III, BDI-2, DAY-C, and HELP: 0–3 Years provide an assessment of social–emotional and/or self-help behavior. The MSEL is the most commonly cited developmental assessment within the autism research literature, although other measures are often utilized by early intervention agencies, academic institutions, and hospitals, as well as practitioners in community and private settings. While pros and cons are debated, the Bayley–III, HELP: 0–3 Years, and DAY-C currently provide the most updated norms and materials (published between 2005 and 2007) in comparison to the MSEL, which was published in 1995. The BDI-2 normative update (Newborg, 2016) was released in 2016.

Speech, Language, and Communication Skills

An essential component of a comprehensive diagnostic evaluation is a speech, language, and communication assessment. Particularly during early developmental periods, communication is inextricably linked to social development. In fact, many early emerging "social skills"—including joint attention, reciprocity, and imitation—are also considered foundational skills for later-developing communicative abilities. Given this overlapping relationship, speech, language, and/or communication skills are commonly impaired in children with ASD, and therefore represent an essential piece of the comprehensive diagnostic assessment and possibly the most central and crucial area of intervention (Wetherby, Prizant, & Schuler, 2000; Prizant, Wetherby, & Rydell, 2000). Additionally, first concerns reported by parents generally involve delayed speech and language abilities (De Giacomo & Fombonne, 1998).

TABLE 4.1. Assessment Instruments for Comprehensive Evaluation of Infants and Toddlers Suspected of ASD

Name	Abbreviation	Age range	Type of assessment	Description
		Developmental/cognitive		
Mullen Scales of Early Learning	MSEL	Birth–68 months	Direct assessment; 35–60 minutes	Assessment that evaluates gross and fine motor abilities, expressive and receptive language, and visual reception.
Bayley Scales of Infant and Toddler Development—3rd Edition	Bayley–III	1–42 months	Direct assessment and parent questionnaire; 30–90 minutes	Measures cognitive skills, adaptive behavior, fine and gross motor abilities, expressive and receptive language, and social–emotional functioning.
Battelle Developmental Inventory—2nd Edition	BDI-2	Birth–7 years, 11 months	Structured observation, play-based activities, and caregiver interview; full: 60–90 minutes	Evaluates cognitive level, communication, and motor abilities through direct assessment, as well as adaptive and social–emotional functioning through a parent interview.
Developmental Assessment of Young Children—2nd Edition	DAY-C	Birth–5 years, 11 months	Direct assessment, observation, and parent interview; 10–20 minutes per subset	Measures cognitive skills, language, adaptive behaviors, physical development, and social–emotional development to help identify delays.
Hawaii Early Learning Profile 0–3 years	HELP: 0–3 years	Birth–3 years	Direct assessment, observation, and parent interview; 45–90 minutes	Assesses cognitive abilities, language, gross and fine motor, social–emotional, and self-help development.

		Speech, language, and communication		
Preschool Language Scales—5th Edition	PLS-5	Birth–7 years, 11 months	Direct assessment and parent questionnaire; 45–60 minutes	Assessment of auditory comprehension and expressive language with supplemental screeners for articulation, language sample, and a home communication questionnaire.
Communication and Symbolic Behavior Scales	CSBS-DP	6 months–6 years	Direct assessment and parent questionnaire; 60 minutes	Screener for early social communication, expressive language, and symbolic functioning delays through seven clusters: communicative functions, gestural communication, vocal communication means, verbal communication, reciprocity, social–affective signaling, and symbolic behavior. Allows for early identification of delays in social communication, expressive language, and symbolic functioning delays.
MacArthur–Bates Communicative Development Inventories—2nd Edition	CDI	8–37 months	Parent questionnaire; 5–10 minutes	Parent report of child's understanding of early words and gesture production.
Language Use Inventory	LUI	18–47 months	Parent questionnaire; 5–10 minutes	Parent questionnaire that measures the child's communication in a variety of settings and functions through 14 subscales.
Rossetti Infant– Toddler Language Scale	Rossetti	Birth–3 years, 11 months	Direct assessment, parent questionnaire, and free-play session; <45 minutes	Evaluates mastery of items in interaction attachment, pragmatics, gestures, play, and language comprehension. This assessment does not have standard norms for comparison.

(continued)

TABLE 4.1. *(continued)*

Name	Abbreviation	Age range	Type of assessment	Description
			ASP-related behaviors	
Autism Diagnostic Observation Schedule—2nd Edition	ADOS-2	12 months–adulthood	Structured play-based assessment; 40–60 minutes	Play-based assessment that is divided into four modules based on age and language abilities. This assessment measures social communication and play behaviors. An algorithm and severity score is given.
Autism Diagnostic Interview—Revised	ADI-R	Children and adults with mental age above 2 years	Parent interview; 1½–2½ hours	Semistructured parent interview that measures the child's functioning; communication; and restricted, repetitive behaviors. Can be used to diagnose and distinguish ASD from other developmental disorders.
Childhood Autism Rating Scale—2nd Edition	CARS-2	2 years and up	Direct observation and parent questionnaire; 5–10 minutes	Brief observation to determine symptom severity through quantifiable ratings.
Autism Observation Scale for Infants	AOSI	6–18 months	Direct assessment; 20 minutes	Currently serves as a research tool to help detect and monitor early signs of ASD. Mostly used with high-risk (HR) siblings.
			Adaptive behavior	
Vineland Adaptive Behavior Scales—3rd Edition	VABS-III	Birth–90 years	Interview or parent questionnaire; 20–90 minutes	Structured interview about the child's current functioning in four domains: communication, daily living, socialization, and motor skills.

				Considered to be the "gold standard" for adaptive functioning measures.
Adaptive Behavior Assessment System—2nd Edition	ABAS-II	Birth–89 years	Parent, teacher, or caregiver questionnaire; 12–20 minutes	Assesses adaptive functioning in three areas: conceptual, social, and practical, and 10 adaptive skills. Two of the five rating forms are appropriate for early assessment: the Parent/Primary Caregiver Form (0–5 years) and the Teacher/Daycare Provider Form (2–5 years).
		Behavioral/psychiatric comorbidities		
Child Behavior Checklist—1½–5 years	CBCL	18 months–5 years	Parent questionnaire; 10–20 minutes	Parents rate 99 questions and describe problems, disabilities, and what concerns them the most. Questions cover the following: emotional reactiveness, withdrawal, anxiety/depression, attention problems, somatic complaints, and aggressive behaviors.
Behavior Assessment System for Children—Third Edition	BASC-3	2–21 years, 11 months	Parent and teacher questionnaires; 10–30 minutes	Designed to help implement treatment plans by facilitating a differential diagnosis and educational clarification through examining emotional and behavioral difficulties.
Early Childhood Behavior Questionnaire	ECBQ	18–36 months	Parent questionnaire; 10–20 minutes	Questionnaire designed to assess temperament in toddlers through 16 categories.

Communication is a broad construct that involves a range of behaviors (verbal and nonverbal) used for delivering a message between a sender and receiver. Nonverbal communication encompasses behaviors such as gaze, facial expression, body posture, gestures, physical approach, and so forth. Verbal communication involves directed spoken language (expressive language), including non-word vocalizations such as single-syllable sounds, babbling, and jargon, as well as meaningful single or combined words. Another component of language is receptive language, which involves the ability to understand or comprehend language. Precursors to language comprehension include attention to language and object use. Receptive language also involves skills such as understanding the use of gestures, vocabulary words, and simple directions. Thus, there is an important distinction to be made between *language* and *communication,* particularly when making the differential diagnosis between a language disorder and ASD. Expressive language delays can take the form of limited vocalizations, babbling, first words, naming objects, and being able to put thoughts to words and sentences in a way that is grammatically accurate. Expressive communication further involves vulnerabilities in the use of gestures and the integration of verbal and nonverbal communicative functions (e.g., eye gaze, facial expressions, body language).

Children with ASD show atypical communication patterns, particularly during the toddler years. Although some children show delays in development of vocalizations in infancy (Paul et al., 2011), by their second birthday, their communication deficits are usually more pronounced (Chawarska et al., 2009; Chawarska & Volkmar, 2005; Paul et al., 2008). These deficits include difficulty understanding gestures and verbal communication of others, diminished initiation of communicative acts, and as mentioned, weaker verbal in comparison with nonverbal abilities. Expressively, there may be less directed vocalization, atypical intonation, and fewer consonants, word combinations, and inventory of overall words produced. Toddlers with ASD tend not to compensate for their lack of spoken language with nonverbal forms of communication such as gaze and/or gesture use. There may be reduced use of nonverbal behaviors in general, including lack of pointing, showing, and giving. In addition, aberrant language and communication behaviors may be present that are often not observed in typical development including echolalia, odd intonation patterns, scripting, and the use of hand over hand (e.g., taking someone's hand and leading the person to objects of interest, taking someone's finger and using it to point, putting someone's hand on an object; generally, all described hand-over-hand behaviors are unaccompanied by coordinated eye gaze). Given the variable yet core impairments in speech, language, and communication, a comprehensive assessment of these skills is needed.

There are a number of assessment tools that were developed and standardized for use with young children, including toddlers. Commonly used measures in autism research include the Preschool Language Scales, now in its fifth edition (PLS-5; Zimmerman, Steiner, & Pond, 2011), and the Communication and Symbolic Behavior Scales (CSBS; Wetherby & Prizant, 2002). The PLS-5 is a standardized evaluation used to assess auditory comprehension and expressive communication skills in young children from birth to 6 years of age. The CSBS is another standardized evaluation but it measures seven language predictors including emotion and eye gaze, communication, gestures, sounds, words, understanding, and object use. While less commonly used in autism research and more typically utilized in early intervention assessment batteries, the Rossetti Infant–Toddler Language Scale (Rossetti, 1990) offers another measurement of language and communication. Additionally, there are a variety of questionnaires parents/caregivers can complete including the MacArthur–Bates Communicative Development Inventories, Second Edition (CDI; Fenson et al., 2007) and the Language Use Inventory (LUI; O'Neill, 2002), a measure of pragmatic communication, among others. See Table 4.1 for a description of measures.

ASD-Related Behaviors

The fourth facet of the comprehensive diagnostic evaluative process involves the assessment of core behaviors related to ASD, including delays and aberrations in the domains of Social Communication and Interaction (including play) as well as the presence of RRBIAs. The provision of a detailed description of the core features of ASD is clearly necessary to provide a diagnostic label, but also important in informing recommendations for treatment related to increasing the frequency and quality of delayed skills and/or reducing the presence of deviant or atypical behaviors associated with autism.

There are often questions regarding how to systematically apply the diagnostic features outlined in DSM-5 to very young children. This diagnostic symptom challenge is not unique to the most recent rendition of DSM—this was also a weakness within the DSM-IV classification system. This is particularly salient given that some of the required criteria for a diagnosis of ASD describe behaviors that are not yet developed or demonstrated in even typically developing young children. For example, the third symptom within domain A is "deficits in developing, maintaining, and understanding relationships." Examples provided include difficulties sharing imaginative play and the desire for friendships. Advice is offered within the text of DSM-5 (American Psychiatric Association, 2013, p. 54), with a description of how these deficits may manifest in young children, stating, "These difficulties are particularly evident in young children, in whom there is often a lack of shared social play and imagination (e.g., age-appropriate flexible pretend play) . . . rules." However, the term "young children" is likely not meant to include toddlers (particularly those with delays in verbal and/or nonverbal skills), as shared imaginative play typically does not emerge until 36 months of age (Göncü, 1993).

Furthermore, there are questions about how RRBIAs may manifest in very young children. Previous research suggested that RRBIAs generally do not differentiate children with ASD from those with delayed or typical development early in life (Baranek, 1999; Lord, 1995), and are relatively common in cohorts of very young children without autism (Evans et al., 1997; Sallustro & Atwell, 1978; Thelen, 1979). Some research suggests that RRBIAs may emerge over a prolonged developmental period and show full expression only later in childhood (Richler, Bishop, Kleinke, & Lord, 2007). However, more recent findings indicate that high-risk 12-month-olds who are later diagnosed with ASD show more stereotyped motor mannerisms and repetitive manipulation of objects relative to their low- and high-risk counterparts who do not go on to develop ASD (Elison et al., 2014). As such, more research is needed to better understand the developmental expression of RRBIAs in children with and without ASD and how this relates to DSM-5 criteria.

Clinicians may need to think carefully about the kinds of behaviors at different ages that provide evidence of a certain DSM symptom being met. The following framework conceptualizes ASD-related behaviors into separate but intrinsically related social communicative functions such as behaviors used for *attending and/or responding* to others and *initiating* interactions, as well as the ability to *sustain the interactions*. There is growing clinical and research interest to conceptualize ASD-related behaviors in regard to the presence of delays in skills that are observed in typical development (negative symptoms), as well as the presence of atypical behaviors (positive symptoms; Foss-Feig, McPartland, Anticevic, & Wolf, 2016)—this conceptual model is highly applicable for young children. Therefore, additional consideration is made for behaviors that involve the reduced frequency, quality, or absence of expected behaviors, as well as those that are viewed as more atypical or aberrant as they are generally not observed in typically developing toddlers (see Table 4.2).

Domain A: Social Communication and Social Interaction Impairments

ATTENDING AND/OR RESPONDING

Reference is made to attending and/or responding skills within domain A—criterion A1: deficits in social–emotional reciprocity. Toddlers with ASD often demonstrate negative symptoms—that is, a lack of or significant reduction in behaviors that would be expected in typical development. Examples include reduced abilities to share joint attention for an object or activity, poor observational/imitative learning, failure to respond to name when called, and limited or inconsistent responses to others' social overtures. For some toddlers with ASD it is particularly difficult to secure their attention and shift it to a shared activity. An overfocus on nonsocial stimuli in the environment (e.g., toys, objects such as a doorstop, small details within visual scenes) can be the catalyst for inconsistent responsivity. In other instances, the child's overall attention, attunement, and responsiveness to language is so impoverished that it is difficult to gain his or her attention. When a child's attention is captured and child-directed speech is used, he or she may demonstrate a limited social response and fail to vocalize or smile in turn. For slightly older toddlers and/or those with intact core language abilities, while the aforementioned behaviors may still apply, other common impairments include providing an off-topic verbal response to a posed question and ignoring social bids made by others. Within nonverbal communication (criterion A2: deficits in nonverbal communicative behaviors used for social interaction), reduced or inconsistent response to joint attention bids made by others, including shifts in gaze or following a point, are common, as are limited responses to social smiling at them. When given a toy to share in play the child may be unresponsive to the bid, or if he or she does welcome the offering, the child may play in isolation or orient his or her body away from the adult.

INITIATING INTERACTIONS

Many toddlers with ASD demonstrate impairments in social communicative initiations, including reduced directed vocalizations (e.g., single-syllable sounds, babble, jargon, words). If directed spontaneous vocalizations are present, they may occur in a limited number of contexts (e.g., restricted to requesting behaviors or seeking comfort, rather than to share interest or enjoyment). These behaviors can be considered to fall under criterion A1: deficits in social–emotional reciprocity. This is also true for nonverbal communicative behaviors (criterion A2: deficits in nonverbal communicative behaviors used for social interaction). While children with ASD may use eye gaze or demonstrate an emerging repertoire of gestures (e.g., reach, use of functional signs), the contexts in which they utilize these nonverbal strategies is similarly restricted. Additionally, the frequency, quality, and type of gesture use may be limited (e.g., only reaching and not shaking head yes or no; reaching only for the purpose of requesting vs. for more social purposes). Eye contact is inconsistent, avoidant, and/or poorly integrated with other forms of communication. Other behaviors within this domain include restricted range of facial expressions, and/or limited sharing of affect (e.g., directing facial expressions toward others). Reduced sharing of interests via holding items up to show, giving for the purpose of sharing, and utilizing three-point gaze shifts to draw attention to objects in the environment or

TABLE 4.2. Common ASD Symptoms in Toddlers: Framework for Using DSM-5 Criteria

Attending/responding to others	Initiating interactions	Sustaining interactions
Reduction or lack of behavior • Poor observational/imitative learning (A1 | A2) • Reduced ability to share joint attention on shared activity or object (A1) • Failure or significant inconsistency in responding to name when called (A1) • Limited or inconsistent responses to others' social overtures (e.g., walking away when fun toy is introduced) (A1 | A3) • Reduced or inconsistent response to joint attention bids made by others (A2) • Difficulties obtaining the toddler's attention (A1) • At times less attentive to someone talking than nonspeech sounds (toy) (A1) Presence of atypical behaviors • Stereotyped responses or phrases (A1) • Attention and focus may be more on objects in environment than people (A1) • Verbal toddlers may start talking about something off topic in response to a question (A1)	Reduction or lack of behavior • Little or no initiation of social interaction (A1) • Reduced directed vocalizations (A1) • Limited number of contexts for initiating interactions (e.g., restricted to acquiring help and/or comfort and less so to initiate a shared game or activity) (A1) • Limited drive to share experiences with others as seen via reduced directed facial expression (e.g., when feeling happy, sad, afraid, frustrated), reduced showing, giving to share, and pointing (A1 | A2) • Reduced initiations of joint attention (A1 | A2) • Reduced use of appropriate eye contact (A2) • Poor use of gestures (e.g., frequency), type (e.g., descriptive, conventional, and idiosyncratic), purpose (e.g., request rather than direct attention), and/or integration with other communicative functions (A2) • Inconsistent use of integrated behaviors (e.g., pairing eye contacts with gestures) (A2)	Reduction or lack of behavior • Limited or absent repertoire of communicative skills to maintain playful interactions (e.g., passive waiting for the adult to take action, bring and drop toy) (A1) • Preference for solitary activities (A3) • Decreased level of engagement (A1) • Inconsistently spontaneously engaged or adult has to work hard to keep the interaction going (A1) Presence of atypical behaviors • Use atypical strategies to maintain interaction (e.g., hand over hand) (A2) • Verbal toddlers may start talking about something off topic in response to a question (A1)

	Presence of atypical behaviors
	• Increased frequency of undirected vocalization (A1) • Atypical requesting strategies (e.g., hand over hand) (A2) • Atypical approaches (e.g., frequent "docking" into parent's lap, hand-over-hand guiding parents) • Odd speech intonation (A2) • Echolalia and scripting (B1)

Play	RRBIAs
• Exploratory (e.g., visual inspection, banging, mouthing) • Functional (e.g., using toys for their intended purpose such as pushing a train on a track, rolling a ball, stacking blocks) • Imaginative (e.g., feeding a baby doll, pretending to eat food) • Simple social (e.g., parallel play, turn taking) • Complementary/reciprocal social (e.g., reversal/imitation of play action of others) • Shared imaginative play (e.g., following the lead of another, building on each other's creative play themes)	• Stereotyped or repetitive motor movements, use of objects or speech • Hand, finger, or complex motor mannerisms • Lining up toys • Echolalia and/or idiosyncratic phrases • Insistence on sameness or ritualized verbal or nonverbal behaviors • Difficulties with transitions • Extreme distress at small changes • Ritualized greetings • Highly restricted or fixated interests • Preoccupations • Unusual attachment to object • Atypical sensory behaviors • Visual peering • Adverse/unusual responses to sounds, smells, or touch

Note. Some children may demonstrate overall delays in reaching play milestones. If play appears developmentally appropriate given age and developmental functioning, presence of nonfunctional use of objects (RRBIA), repetitive play schemes (RRBIA), and inflexibility in play (RRBIA) may be observed.

toward toys that the child is engaging with, are also common features of ASD that are expressed in toddlers. As mentioned, the latter nonverbal communicative behaviors may also be considered deficits in social–emotional reciprocity. The use of another's body as a tool (e.g., leading someone to a desired object without coordinated eye contact, positioning another's hand into a point to be used to show or select) is also considered an atypical nonverbal communicative behavior, which often occurs in the absence of paired eye contact. For toddlers who are older and/or demonstrate intact language skills, the abovementioned behaviors are also applicable. Atypical behavior not often demonstrated in typical development includes undirected vocalizations that do not serve a communicative or pragmatic purpose. Often the vocalizations produced (including production of repetitive nonmeaningful sounds—although considered a repetitive behavior) have atypical prosodic features (e.g., singsong, flat, mechanical, high pitched).

SUSTAINING INTERACTIONS

Sustaining interactions refers to utilizing a variety of behaviors to maintain or continue an interaction. These can be considered interactions that the child has spontaneously initiated or those that were started by others. As such, common impairments in regard to sustaining or maintaining interactions include limited strategies to continue enjoyable routines (e.g., peek-a-boo, familiar songs, bubble activities). For example, a toddler may passively wait for the adult to take action to continue the activity or he or she may utilize less sophisticated strategies including bringing the toy over and dropping it near the adult without coordinated eye contact. Additionally, difficulty taking simple turns in play is common; relinquishing a toy even for a short while is often problematic. It is important to consider that attending/responding and/or initiating behaviors are inherently related to one's ability to sustain interactions; it is nearly expected that impairments in these domains would impact abilities to maintain interactions. Yet, for some children with ASD, familiar routines provide a context wherein they are better able to utilize social communicative behaviors. As such, a toddler may demonstrate improved attending/responding and/or initiating behaviors within familiar routinized interactions (e.g., motor-based songs, routines with objects). The challenge for toddlers who demonstrate relatively robust attending/responding and/or initiating behaviors lies in sustaining or maintaining the dyadic interaction. For example, a toddler may approach an adult to bring over a toy for help and pair a vocalization, gesture, and eye contact, but once his or her immediate need is met, the child retreats from the interaction and plays alone. Verbal toddlers or young children may demonstrate difficulty providing a contingent comment or produce frequent off-topic responses to posed questions.

PLAY SKILLS

While play skills are also related to the aforementioned social communication and interaction deficits outlined, it is often clinically useful to evaluate and describe play behaviors separately. Within this domain we can consider the toddler's exploratory, functional, imitative, imaginative, and shared play. Children with ASD may demonstrate significant delays in play and use toys only in exploratory and/or sensory-seeking fashions (e.g., visual inspection, banging, mouthing). Others may demonstrate emerging functional play (e.g., using toys for their intended purpose such as pushing a train on a track, rolling a ball, stacking blocks) but have difficulty engaging in simple pretend play actions (e.g., feeding a baby doll, pretending to eat food). While emerging social play (e.g., parallel play), simple social play (e.g., turn taking), and complementary/reciprocal social play (reversal/imitation of the play action of others) generally emerge by age 24 months, some toddlers demonstrate the aforementioned foundational play skills but have trouble playing interactively. Additionally, if play skills appear scant, repetitive actions/schemes may be salient features of the toddler's play. While some standardized assessment procedures may offer different guidelines (e.g., ADOS-2 Module 1 and Toddler Module evaluate play skills in comparison to chronological age expectations, not developmental level or estimated expressive language skills), it is also important to evaluate play skills relative to the child's level of language and overall developmental functioning.

RELATIONSHIPS AND PEER INTERACTIONS

An interest in peers and engagement in parallel play is not fully expected until a toddler is approximately 2 years old, and even so, we would not anticipate robust peer interactions at this age. However, a lack of interest in other children and a passivity in peer interactions, as well as atypical approaches such as consistent aggressive behavior in a social context, should be considered during the diagnostic conceptualization process, which is captured under criterion A3: deficits in developing, maintaining, and understanding relationships.

In all, the spontaneity, quality, context, and frequency of social communication, including the ability to integrate various social communicative behaviors, needs to be considered. While many toddlers may not utilize these skills spontaneously, there are strategies that may facilitate the use of these skills such as the provision of choice and/or the use of expectant waiting. Information gleaned from dyadic interactions supported in this way can again provide important information regarding treatment approaches.

Domain B: Restricted, Repetitive Patterns of Behavior, Interests, or Activities

Along with impairments in social interaction and communication, the diagnosis of ASD also involves the presence of RRBIAs. Within DSM-5, this domain is further divided into four separate criteria, wherein at least two of the four criteria must be met. Some repetitive behaviors are typical of early childhood (e.g., echolalia used for early language learning strategies, repetitive play with objects, carrying around attachment objects)—thus, typically, if a RRBIA is identified, it is due to the presence of an atypical behavior that is not generally seen during toddlerhood (e.g., it is a positive symptom). These include criteria B1: stereotyped or repetitive motor movements, use of objects, or speech; B2: insistence on sameness or ritualized verbal or nonverbal behaviors; B3: highly restricted or fixated interests; and B4: atypical sensory behaviors (seeking and/or aversions). While some young children demonstrate a constellation of RRBIAs, they may be very subtle and/or not present in every context. These behaviors may be emerging but not fully expressed in infants and toddlers (Richler et al., 2007). RRBIAs that may present very early include B1: hand, finger, or complex motor mannerisms, lining up toys, presence of echolalia, and/or idiosyncratic phrases; B2: difficulties with transitions, extreme distress at small changes, and ritualized greetings; B3: preoccupations, and unusual attachment to objects; and B4: visual fixations (e.g., close inspection of or peering at objects) and adverse/unusual responses to sounds, smells, or touch.

There are a number of diagnostic instruments available that provide standardized opportunities to observe specific behaviors pertaining to a diagnosis of autism and/or provide frameworks to conceptualize symptoms. These measures should be utilized to collect information about ASD-related behaviors, but again, should not be used in isolation. Moreover, in the final analysis, incorporating clinical judgment is required to interpret observed behaviors.

Measures such as the Autism Diagnostic Observation Schedule, now in its second edition (ADOS-2) and the Autism Diagnostic Interview—Revised (ADI-R; Rutter, Le Couteur, & Lord, 2003 are generally referred to as the "gold standard" instruments. While these assessment tools are informative, clinicians utilizing them need to be aware of the limitations, particularly when used in populations of toddlers with a nonverbal age ≤15 months because sensitivity of the instrument is strong but its specificity is lower in younger children (Lord et al., 2000; Risi et al., 2006; Chawarska et al., 2007). However, the newly published ADOS-2 Toddler Module demonstrates improved sensitivity and specificity as compared with Module 1, in which children 30 months of age and younger do not yet speak in phrases (Luyster et al., 2009). Other assessment tools used to measure

ASD-related behaviors in clinical or research settings include the Childhood Autism Rating Scale, Second Edition (although the minimum age is 2 years; CARS-2; Schopler, Van Bourgondien, Wellman, & Love, 2010), and the Autism Observation Scale for Infants (AOSI; Bryson, McDermott, Rombough, Brian, & Zwaigenbaum, 2000). See Table 4.1 for a description of measures.

Adaptive Functioning

Adaptive behavior includes those skills necessary for personal and self-sufficiency in real-life situations/independent living. While this may sound like an inappropriate construct to consider for toddlers, adaptive behaviors in this age group are demonstrated by their functional adjustment in day-to-day situations. Decades of research have shown that older children with ASD have adaptive skill deficits as compared to their level of cognitive functioning (Fenton et al., 2003; Paul et al., 2004; Tomanik, Pearson, Loveland, Lane, & Shaw, 2007; Carter et al., 1998; Volkmar et al., 1987). The discrepancy between intellectual ability and consistency in utilizing skills in naturalistic settings can be pronounced even for toddlers (Klin, Volkmar, & Sparrow, 1992). While some children fail to achieve skills that are typically attained in the first few months of life (Klin et al., 1992), this discrepancy persists into the second year of life (Stone, Ousley, Hepburn, Hogan, & Brown, 1999; Paul, Loomis, & Chawarska, 2014).

Research examining adaptive behavioral profiles in toddlers with ASD is emerging—as a group young children with autism tend to have lower adaptive functioning abilities compared with chronological and mental-age-matched controls. While some findings suggest delays across communication, socialization, daily living, and motor functioning (Ventola et al., 2007), others report weaker scores in the socialization and communication domains, as well as significant discrepancies between adaptive behavior and mental age (Stone et al., 1999) in cohorts of toddlers with ASD. Moreover, a common adaptive profile in toddlers with autism involves motor skills → daily living skills → socialization → communication abilities. Of note, overall scores in the Social Communication domain can be misleading as a result of inflated scores on the "written" subdomain, given that in this age bracket such skills refer primarily to interest in and knowledge of letters and numbers, which is often observed in young children with autism. Thus, it is important to carefully analyze subdomain profiles, and, in many cases, to conduct a more thorough item analysis.

The most common adaptive functioning measure used in autism research is the Vineland Adaptive Behavior Scales; the third edition was published in 2016 (Sparrow, Cicchetti, & Balla, 2016). Other instruments include the Scales of Independent Behavior—Revised (Bruininks,

Woodcock, Weatherman, & Hill, 1996) and the Adaptive Behavior Assessment System, Second Edition (Harrison & Oakland, 2003). Additionally, as mentioned above, components of some developmental assessments—including the Battelle and the Bayley–III—provide screening for adaptive/self-help behavior. See Table 4.1 for a description of measures.

Screening for Comorbidities

Screening for comorbidities is recommended as part of the comprehensive assessment, particularly those that are most often affected in children with ASD and are related to self-regulation, such as the presence of disruptive/noncompliant behaviors, anxiety symptoms, difficulties regulating attention, overactivity, sleep difficulties, feeding problems, and so on. While there is currently no single measure that assesses for common comorbidities associated with ASD in toddlers, a number of social–emotional screening tools are available for young children. Examples of screening instruments include the Child Behavior Checklist—1½–5 Years (CBCL; Achenbach, 2000) and the Behavior Assessment System for Children, Third Edition (BASC-3; Reynolds & Kamphaus, 2015). Additionally, questionnaires assessing temperament, such as the Early Childhood Behavior Questionnaire (ECBQ; Putnam, Garstein, & Rothbart, 2006), provide valuable information that may elucidate the presence of comorbid symptoms and interfering behaviors. As noted, while it is unlikely that a full constellation of symptoms will be present to warrant an official comorbid diagnosis, these symptoms should be considered in the diagnostic conceptualization and creation of treatment recommendations. See Table 4.1 for a description of measures.

CONCLUSIONS

Clinical presentation of young children with ASD is marked by high variability in the severity of autism symptoms, language and cognitive profiles, and presence of the prodromal features of later-developing comorbid disorders involving emotional, attentional, and behavioral regulatory control problems. A growing number of behavioral assessment instruments are now available that have been calibrated for children in their second and third year of life, and comprehensive diagnostic strategies such as those described in this chapter have been developed and tested in university-based clinical settings. Despite the heterogeneity of syndrome expression and a dynamic developmental picture, early comprehensive evaluation leads to stable and reliable diagnosis, shortening the interval between symptom onset and implementation of early intervention and improving the prospect for enhanced quality of life of the affected children and their families.

REFERENCES

Achenbach, T. M. (2000). *Manual for the Child Behavior Checklist 1½–5*. Burlington: University of Vermont, Department of Psychiatry.

Akshoomoff, N. (2006). Use of the Mullen Scales of Early Learning for the assessment of young children with autism spectrum disorders. *Child Neuropsychology, 12*, 169–277.

American Psychiatric Association. (2013). *Diagnostic and statistical manual of mental disorders* (5th ed.). Washington, DC: Author.

Baranek, G. T. (1999). Autism during infancy: A retrospective video analysis of sensory–motor and social behaviors at 9–12 months of age. *Journal of Autism and Developmental Disorders, 29*(3), 213–224.

Barton, M. L., Dumont-Mathieu, T., & Fein, D. (2012). Screening young children for autism spectrum disorders in primary practice. *Journal of Autism and Developmental Disorders, 42*(6), 1165–1174.

Bayley, N. (2005). *Bayley Scales of Infant and Toddler Development, Third Edition.* San Antonio, TX: Pearson.

Begeer, S., Bouk, S. E., Boussaid, W., Terwogt, M. M., & Koot, H. M. (2008). Underdiagnoses and referral bias of autism in ethnic minorities. *Journal of Autism and Developmental Disorders, 39*(1), 142–148.

Bora, E., Aydın, A., Saraç, T., Kadak, M. T., & Köse, S. (2016). Heterogeneity of subclinical autistic traits among parents of children with autism spectrum disorder: Identifying the broader autism phenotype with a data-driven method. *Autism Research, 10*(2), 321–326.

Bruininks, R. H., Woodcock, R. W., Weatherman, R. F., & Hill, B. K. (1996). *Scales of Independent Behavior Revised: Manual.* Boston: Riverside.

Bryson, S. E., McDermott, C., Rombough, V., Brian, J., & Zwaigenbaum, L. (2000). *The Autism Observation Scale for Infants*. Unpublished scale, Toronto, Ontario, Canada.

Bryson, S. E., Zwaigenbaum, L., Brian, J., Roberts, W., Szatmari, P., Rombough, V., et al. (2007). A prospective case series of high-risk infants who developed autism. *Journal of Autism and Developmental Disorders, 37*(1), 12–24.

Carter, A. S., Volkmar, F. R., Sparrow, S. S., Wang, J.-J., Lord, C., Dawson, G., et al. (1998). The Vineland Adaptive Behavior Scales: Supplementary norms for individuals with autism. *Journal of Autism and Developmental Disorders, 28*(4), 287–302.

Centers for Disease Control and Prevention. (2016). Prevalence and characteristics of autism spectrum disorder among children aged 8 years—autism and developmental disabilities monitoring network, 11 sites, United States, 2012. *Morbidity and Mortality Weekly Report Surveillance Summaries, 65*(3), 1–23.

Charman, T., Taylor, E., Drew, A., Cockerill, H., Brown, J., & Baird, G. (2005). Outcome at 7 years of children diagnosed with autism at age 2: Predictive validity of assessments conducted at 2 and 3 years of age and pattern of symptom change over time. *Journal of Child Psychology and Psychiatry, 46*(5), 500–513.

Chawarska, K., Klin, A., Paul, R., Macari, S., & Volkmar, F. (2009). A prospective study of toddlers with ASD: Short-term diagnostic and cognitive outcomes. *Journal of Child Psychology and Psychiatry, 50*(10), 1235–1245.

Chawarska, K., Klin, A., Paul, R., & Volkmar, F. (2007). Autism spectrum disorder in the second year: Stability and change in syndrome expression. *Journal of Child Psychology and Psychiatry, 48*(2), 128–138.

Chawarska, K., Macari, S., & Shic, F. (2013). Decreased spontaneous attention to social scenes in 6-month-old infants later diagnosed with autism spectrum disorders. *Biological Psychiatry, 74*(3), 195–203.

Chawarska, K., & Volkmar, F. (2005). Autism in infancy and early childhood. In F. R. Volkmar, R. Paul, A. Klin, & D. J. Cohen (Eds.), *Handbook of autism and pervasive developmental disorders* (3rd ed., pp. 223–246). Hoboken, NJ: Wiley.

De Giacomo, A. D., & Fombonne, E. (1998). Parental recognition of developmental abnormalities in autism. *European Child and Adolescent Psychiatry, 7*(3), 131–136.

Doshi-Velez, F., Ge, Y., & Kohane, I. (2014). Comorbidity clusters in autism spectrum disorders: An electronic health record time-series analysis. *Pediatrics, 133*(1) e54–e63.

Elison, J. T., Wolff, J. J., Reznick, J. S., Botteron, K. N., Estes, A. M., Gu, H., et al. (2014). Repetitive behavior in 12-month-olds later classified with autism spectrum disorder. *Journal of the American Academy of Child and Adolescent Psychiatry, 53*(11), 1216–1224.

Esposito, G., & Paşca, S. P. (2013). Motor abnormalities as a putative endophenotype for autism spectrum disorders. *Frontiers in Integrative Neuroscience, 7,* 43.

Evans, D. W., Leckman, J. F., Carter, A., Reznick, J. S., Henshaw, D., King, R. A., et al. (1997). Ritual, habit, and perfectionism: The prevalence and development of compulsive-like behavior in normal young children. *Child Development, 68*(1), 58.

Fenske, E. C., Zalenski, S., Krantz, P. J., & McClannahan, L. E. (1985). Age at intervention and treatment outcome for autistic children in a comprehensive intervention program. *Analysis and Intervention in Developmental Disabilities, 5*(1–2), 49–58.

Fenson, L., Marchman, V. A., Thal, D. J., Dale, P. S., Rexnick, J. S., & Bates, E. (2007). *MacArthur Bates Communicative Development Inventories* (2nd ed.). Baltimore: Brookes.

Fenton, G., D'Ardia, C., Valente, D., Vecchio, I. D. V., Fabrizi, A., & Bernabei, P. (2003). Vineland adaptive behavior profiles in children with autism and moderate to severe developmental delay. *Autism, 7*(3), 269–287.

Filipek, P. A., Accardo, P. J., Baranek, G. T., Cook, E. H., Dawson, G., Gordon, B., et al. (1999). The screening and diagnosis of autistic spectrum disorders. *Journal of Autism and Developmental Disorders, 29*(6), 439–484.

Flanagan, J. E., Landa, R., Bhat, A., & Bauman, M. (2012). Head lag in infants at risk for autism: A preliminary study. *American Journal of Occupational Therapy, 66*(5), 577–585.

Foss-Feig, J., McPartland, J., Anticevic, A., & Wolf, J. (2016). Re-conceptualizing ASD within a dimensional framework: Positive, negative, and cognitive feature clusters. *Journal of Autism and Developmental Disorders, 46*(1), 342–351.

Fournier, K. A., Hass, C. J., Naik, S. K., Lodha, N., & Cauraugh, J. H. (2010). Motor coordination in autism spectrum disorders: A synthesis and meta-analysis. *Journal of Autism and Developmental Disorders, 40*(10), 1227–1240.

Göncü, A. (1993). Development of intersubjectivity in social pretend play. *Human Development, 36*(4), 185–198.

Guthrie, W., Swineford, L. B., Nottke, C., & Wetherby, A. M. (2013). Early diagnosis of autism spectrum disorder: Stability and change in clinical diagnosis and symptom presentation. *Journal of Child Psychology and Psychiatry, 54*(5), 582–590.

Harrison, P. L., & Oakland, T. (2003). *Adaptive Behavior Assessment System* (2nd ed.). San Antonio, TX: Harcourt Assessment.

Jeste, S. S., & Geschwind, D. H. (2014). Disentangling the heterogeneity of autism spectrum disorder through genetic findings. *Nature Reviews Neurology, 10*(2), 74–81.

Johnson, C. P., & Myers, S. M. (2007). Identification and evaluation of children with autism spectrum disorders, *Pediatrics, 120*(5), 1183–1215.

Johnson, M. H., Gilga, T., Jones, E., & Charman, T. (2015). Annual research review: Infant development, autism, and ADHD—early pathways to emerging disorders. *Journal of Child Psychology and Psychiatry, 56*(3), 228–247.

Joseph, R. M., Tager-Flusberg, H., & Lord, C. (2002). Cognitive profiles and social–communicative functioning in children with autism spectrum disorder. *Journal of Child Psychology and Psychiatry, 43*(6), 807–821.

Kanner, L. (1943). Autistic disturbances of affective contact. *Nervous Child, 2,* 217–250.

Kim, S. H., & Lord, C. (2010). Restricted and repetitive behaviors in toddlers and preschoolers with autism spectrum disorders based on the Autism Diagnostic Observation Schedule (ADOS). *Autism Research, 3*(4), 162–173.

Kim, S. H., Macari, S., Koller, J., & Chawarska, K. (2016). Examining the phenotypic heterogeneity of early autism spectrum disorder: Subtypes and short-term outcomes. *Journal of Child Psychology and Psychiatry, 57,* 93–102.

Klin, A., Volkmar, F. R., & Sparrow, S. S. (1992). Autistic social dysfunction: Some limitations of the theory of mind hypothesis. *Journal of Child Psychology and Psychiatry, 33*(5), 861–876.

Landa, R., & Garrett-Mayer, E. (2006). Development in infants with autism spectrum disorders: A prospective study. *Journal of Child Psychology and Psychiatry, 47*(6), 629–638.

Landa, R. J., Gross, A. L., Stuart, E. A., & Faherty, A. (2013). Developmental trajectories in children with and without autism spectrum disorders: The first 3 years. *Child Development, 84,* 429–442.

Leary, M. R., & Hill, D. A. (1996). Moving on: Autism and movement disturbance. *Mental Retardation, 34,* 39–53.

Lord, C. (1995). Follow-up of two-year-olds referred for possible autism. *Journal of Child Psychology and Psychiatry, 36*(8), 1365–1382.

Lord, C., Risi, S., DiLavore, P. S., Shulman, C., Thurm, A., & Pickles, A. (2006). Autism from 2 to 9 years of age. *Archives of General Psychiatry, 63*(6), 694–701.

Lord, C., Risi, S., Lambrecht, L., Cook, E. H., Leventhal, B. L., DiLavore, P. C., et al. (2000). The Autism Diagnostic Observation Schedule—Generic: A standard measure of social and communication deficits associated with the spectrum of autism. *Journal of Autism and Developmental Disorders, 30*(3),205–223.

Lord, C., Rutter, M., & Couteur, A. L. (1994). Autism Diagnostic Interview—Revised: A revised version of a diagnostic interview for caregivers of individuals with possible pervasive developmental disorders. *Journal of Autism and Developmental Disorders, 24*(5), 659–685.

Lord, C., Rutter, M., DiLavore, P. C., Risi, S., Gotham, K., & Bishop, S. (2012). *Autism Diagnostic Observation Schedule: ADOS-2.* Los Angeles: Western Psychological Services.

Lovaas, O. I., & Smith, T. (1988). Intensive behavioral treatment for young autistic children. *Advances in Clinical Child Psychology, 11,* 285–324.

Luyster, R., Gotham, K., Guthrie, W., Coffing, M., Petrak, R., Pierce, K., et al. (2009). The Autism Diagnostic Observation Schedule—Toddler Module: A new module of a standardized diagnostic measure for autism spectrum disorders. *Journal of Autism and Developmental Disorders, 39*(9), 1305–1320.

Magiati, I., Charman, T., & Howlin, P. (2007). A two-year prospective follow-up study of community-based early intensive behavioral intervention and specialist nursery provision for children with autism spectrum disorders. *Journal of Child Psychology and Psychiatry, 48*(8), 803–812.

Magiati, I., Moss, J., Charman, T., & Howlin, P. (2011). Patterns of change in children with autism spectrum disorders who received community based comprehensive interventions in their pre-school years: A seven year follow-up study. *Research in Autism Spectrum Disorders, 5*(3), 1016–1027.

Mandell, D. S., Novak, M. M., & Zubritsky, C. D. (2005). Factors associated with age of diagnosis among children with autism spectrum disorders. *Pediatrics, 116*(6), 1480–1486.

Matson, J. L., & Shoemaker, M. (2009). Intellectual disability and its relationship to autism spectrum disorders. *Research in Developmental Disabilities, 30*(6), 1107–1114.

Messinger, D., Young, G. S., Ozonoff, S., Dobkins, K., Carter, A., Zwaigenbaum, L., et al. (2013). Beyond autism: A baby siblings research consortium study of high-risk children at three years of age. *Journal of the American Academy of Child and Adolescent Psychiatry, 52*(3), 300–308.

Miller, M., Iosif, A. M., Young, G. S., Hill, M., Phelps Hanzel, E., Hutman, T., et al. (2015). School-age outcomes of infants at risk for autism spectrum disorder. *Autism Research, 9*(6), 632–642.

Mullen, E. M. (1995). *Mullen Scales of Early Learning* (AGS ed.). San Antonio, TX: Pearson.

Nadig, A. S., Ozonoff, S., Young, G. S., Rozga, A., Sigman, M., & Rogers, S. J. (2007). A prospective study of response to name in infants at risk for autism. *Archives of Pediatrics and Adolescent Medicine, 161*(4), 378.

Newborg, J. (2005). *Battelle Developmental Inventory* (2nd ed.). Rolling Meadows, IL: Riverside.

Newborg, J. (2016). *Battelle Developmental Inventory* (2nd ed., normative update). Boston: Houghton Mifflin Harcourt.

O'Neill, D. K. (2002). *Language Use Inventory for Young Children: An assessment of pragmatic language development.* Unpublished document, University of Waterloo, Ontario, Canada.

Ozonoff, S., Heung, K., Byrd, R., Hansen, R., & Hertz-Picciotto, I. (2008). The onset of autism: Patterns of symptom emergence in the first years of life. *Autism Research, 1*(6), 320–328.

Ozonoff, S., Iosif, A., Baguio, F., Cook, I. C., Hill, M. M., Hutman, T., et al. (2010). A prospective study of the emergence of early behavioral signs of autism. *Journal of the American Academy of Child and Adolescent Psychiatry, 49*(3), 256–266.

Ozonoff, S., Young, G. S., Belding, A., Hill, M., Hill, A., Hutman, T., et al. (2014). The broader autism phenotype in infancy: When does it emerge? *Journal of the American Academy of Child and Adolescent Psychiatry, 53*(4), 398–407.

Ozonoff, S., Young, G. S., Carter, A., Messinger, D., Yirmiya, N., Zwaigenbaum, L., et al. (2011). Recurrence risk for autism spectrum disorders: A baby siblings research consortium study. *Pediatrics, 128*(3), 488–495.

Ozonoff, S., Young, G. S., Landa, R. J., Brian, J., Bryson, S., Charman, T., et al. (2015). Diagnostic stability in young children at risk for autism spectrum disorder: A baby siblings research consortium study. *Journal of Child Psychology and Psychiatry, and Allied Disciplines, 56*(9), 988–998.

Parks, S. (2007). *Hawaii Early Profile (HELP) strands (0–3).* Palo Alto, CA: Vort.

Paul, R., Chawarska, K., Cicchetti, D., & Volkmar, F. (2008). Language outcomes of toddlers with autism spectrum disorders: A two-year follow-up. *Autism Research, 1*, 97–107.

Paul, R., Fuerst, Y., Ramsay, G., Chawarska, K., & Klin, A. (2011). Out of the mouths of babes: Vocal production in infant siblings of children with ASD. *Journal of Child Psychology and Psychiatry, 52*(5), 588–598.

Paul, R., Loomis, R., & Chawarska, K. (2014). Adaptive behavior in toddlers under two with autism spectrum disorders. *Journal of Autism and Developmental Disorders, 44*(2), 264–270.

Paul, R., Miles, S., Cicchetti, D., Sparrow, S., Klin, A., Volkmar, F., et al. (2004). Adaptive behavior in autism and pervasive developmental disorder—not otherwise specified: Microanalysis of scores on the Vineland Adaptive Behavior Scales. *Journal of Autism and Developmental Disorders, 34*(2), 223–228.

Prizant, B. M., Wetherby, A. M., & Rydell, P. J. (2000). Communication intervention issues for young children with autism spectrum disorders. In A. M. Wetherby & B. M. Prizant (Eds.), *Autism spectrum disorders: A transactional developmental perspective* (pp. 193–224). Baltimore: Brookes.

Putnam S. P., Garstein, M. A., & Rothbart, M. K. (2006). Measurement of fine-grained aspects of toddler temperament: The Early Childhood Behavior Questionnaire. *Behavior and Development, 29*(3), 386–401.

Reynolds, C. R., & Kamphaus, R. W. (2015). *Behavior Assessment System for Children* (3rd ed.). Circle Pines, MN: American Guidance Service.

Richler, J., Bishop, S. L., Kleinke, J. R., & Lord, C. (2007). Restricted and repetitive behaviors in young children with autism spectrum disorders. *Journal of Autism and Developmental Disorders, 37*(1), 73–85.

Risi, S., Lord, C., Gotham, K., Corsello, C., Chrysler, C., Szatmari, P., et al. (2006). Combining information from multiple sources in the diagnosis of autism spectrum disorders. *Journal of the American Academy of Child and Adolescent Psychiatry, 45*(9), 1094–1103.

Rogers, S. J. (1996). Brief report: Early intervention in autism. *Journal of Autism and Developmental Disorders, 26*(2), 243–246.

Rogers, S. J. (2009). What are infant siblings teaching us about autism in infancy? *Autism Research, 2*(3), 125–137.

Ronald, A., & Hoekstra, R. A. (2011). Autism spectrum disorders and autistic traits: A decade of new twin studies. *American Journal of Medical Genetics Part B: Neuropsychiatric Genetics, 156*(3), 255–274.

Rossetti, L. (1990). *The Rossetti Infant–Toddler Language Scale: A measure of communication and language.* East Moline, IL: LinguiSystems.

Rozga, A., Hutman, T., Young, G. S., Rogers, S. J., Ozonoff, S., Dapretto, M., et al. (2011). Behavioral profiles of affected and unaffected siblings of children with autism: Contribution of measures of mother–infant interaction and nonverbal communication. *Journal of Autism and Developmental Disorders, 41*(3), 287–301.

Russell, G., Rodgers, L. R., Ukoumunne, O. C., & Ford, T. (2014). Prevalence of parent-reported ASD and ADHD in the UK: Findings from the Millennium Cohort Study. *Journal of Autism and Developmental Disorders, 44,* 31–40.

Rutter, M., Le Couteur, A., & Lord, C. (2003). *Autism Diagnostic Interview—Revised.* Los Angeles: Western Psychological Service.

Sacrey, L. A., Zwaigenbaum, L., Bryson, S., Brian, J., Smith, I. M., Roberts, W., et al. (2015). Can parents' concerns predict autism spectrum disorder? A prospective study of high-risk siblings from 6 to 36 months of age. *Journal of the American Academy of Child and Adolescent Psychiatry, 54*(6), 470–478.

Sallustro, F., & Atwell, C. W. (1978). Body rocking, head banging, and head rolling in normal children. *Journal of Pediatrics, 93*(4), 704–708.

Schoen, E., Paul, R., & Chawarska, K. (2011). Phonology and vocal behavior in toddlers with autism spectrum disorders. *Autism Research, 4*(3), 177–188.

Schopler, E., & Van Bourgondien, M. E., Wellman, G. J., & Love, S. R. (2010). *Childhood Autism Rating Scale—Second Edition (CARS-2).* New York: Irvington.

Shattuck, P. T., Durkin, M., Maenner, M., Newschaffer, C., Mandell, D. S., Wiggins, L., et al. (2009). Timing of identification among children with an autism spectrum disorder: Findings from a population-based surveillance study. *Journal of the American Academy of Child and Adolescent Psychiatry, 48*(5), 474–483.

Simonoff, E., Pickles, A., Charman, T., Chandler, S., Loucas, T., & Baird, G. (2008). Psychiatric disorders in children with autism spectrum disorders: Prevalence, comorbidity, and associated factors in a population-derived sample. *Journal of the American Academy of Child and Adolescent Psychiatry, 47*(8), 921–929.

Sparrow, S. S., Cicchetti, D. V., & Balla, D. A. (2016). *Vineland Adaptive Behavior Scale* (3rd ed.). Circle Pines, MN: American Guidance Service.

Steiner, A. M., Goldsmith, T. R., Snow, A. V., & Chawarska, K. (2012). Practioner's guide to assessment of autism spectrum disorders in infants and toddlers. *Journal of Autism and Developmental Disorders, 42,* 1183–1196.

Stone, W. L., Ousley, O. Y., Hepburn, S. L., Hogan, K. L., & Brown, C. S. (1999). Patterns of adaptive behavior in very young children with autism. *American Journal of Mental Retardation, 104*(2), 187–199.

Thelen, E. (1979). Rhythmical stereotypies in normal human infants. *Animal Behavior, 27,* 699–715.

Thomas, K. C., Ellis, A. R., McLaurin, C., Daniels, J., & Morrissey, J. P. (2007). Access to care for autism-related services. *Journal of Autism and Developmental Disorders, 37*(10), 1902–1912.

Tomanik, S. S., Pearson, D. A., Loveland, K. A., Lane, D. M., & Shaw, J. B. (2007). Improving the reliability of autism diagnoses: Examining the utility of adaptive behavior. *Journal of Autism and Developmental Disorders, 37*(5), 921–928.

Turner, L. M., Stone, W. L., Pozdol, S. L., & Coonrod, E. E. (2006). Follow-up of children with autism spectrum disorders from age 2 to age 9. *Autism, 10*(3), 243–265.

van Steensel, F. J., Bögels, S. M., & Perrin, S. (2011). Anxiety disorders in children and adolescents with autistic spectrum disorders: A meta-analysis. *Clinical Child and Family Psychology Review, 14*(3), 302–317.

Ventola, P., Kleinman, J., Pandey, J., Wilson, L., Esser, E., Boorstein, H., et al. (2007). Differentiating between autism spectrum disorders and other developmental disabiliteis in children who failed a screening instrument for ASD. *Journal of Autism and Devleopmental Disorders, 37*(3), 425–436.

Volkmar, F. R., Sparrow, S. S., Goudreau, D., Cicchetti, D. V., Paul, R., & Cohen, D. J. (1987). Social deficits in autism: An operational approach using the Vineland

Adaptive Behavior Scales. *Journal of the American Academy of Child and Adolescent Psychiatry, 26*(2), 156–161.

Voress, J. K., & Maddox, T. (1998). *Developmental assessment of young children.* Los Angeles: Western Psychological Services.

Watt, N., Wetherby, A. M., Barber, A., & Morgan, L. (2008). Repetitive and stereotyped behaviors in children with autism spectrum disorders in the second year of life. *Journal of Autism and Developmental Disorders, 38*(8), 1518–1533.

Weismer, S. E., Lord, C., & Esler, A. (2010). Early language patterns of toddlers on the autism spectrum compared to toddlers with developmental delay. *Journal of Autism and Developmental Disorders, 40*(10), 1259–1273.

Werner, E., Dawson, G., Osterling, J., & Dinno, N. (2000). Brief report: Recognition of autism spectrum disorder before one year of age—a retrospective study based on home videotapes. *Journal of Autism and Developmental Disorders, 30*(2), 157–162.

Wetherby, A. M., & Prizant, B. M. (2002). *Communication and Symbolic Behavior Scales developmental profile.* Baltimore: Brookes.

Wetherby, A. M., Prizant, B. M., & Schuler, A. L. (2000). Understanding the nature of communication and language impairments. In A. M. Wetherby & B. M. Prizant (Eds.), *Autism spectrum disorders: A transactional developmental perspective* (pp. 109–142). Baltimore: Brookes.

Wolff, J. J., Gu, H., Gerig, G., Elison, J. T., Styner, M., Gouttard, S., et al. (2012). Differences in white matter fiber tract development present from 6 to 24 months in infants with autism. *American Journal of Psychiatry, 169,* 589–600.

Woods, J. J., & Wetherby, A. M. (2003). Early identification of and intervention for infants and toddlers who are at risk for autism spectrum disorder. *Language, Speech, and Hearing Services in Schools, 34,* 180–193.

Yirmiya, N., & Ozonoff, S. (2007). The very early phenotype of autism. *Journal of Autism and Developmental Disorders, 37*(1), 1–11.

Young, G. S., Merin, N., Rogers, S. J., & Ozonoff, S. (2009). Gaze behavior and affect at 6 months: Predicting clinical outcomes and language development in typically developing infants and infants at risk for autism. *Developmental Science, 12*(5), 798–814.

Zimmerman, I. L., Steiner, V. G., & Pond, R. E. (2011). *Preschool Language Scales* (5th ed.). San Antonio, TX: Pearson.

Zwaigenbaum, L., Bryson, S. E., Brian, J., Smith, I. M., Roberts, W., Szatmari, P., et al. (2016). Stability of diagnostic assessment for autism spectrum disorder between 18 and 36 months in a high-risk cohort. *Autism Research, 9*(7), 790–800.

Zwaigenbaum, L., Bryson, S., Lord, C., Rogers, S., Carter, A., Carver, L., et al. (2009). Clinical assessment and management of toddlers with suspected autism spectrum disorder: Insights from studies of high-risk infants. *Pediatrics, 123*(5), 1383–1391.

Zwaigenbaum, L., Bryson, S., Rogers, T., Roberts, W., Brian, J., & Szatmari, P. (2005). Behavioral manifestations of autism in the first year of life. *International Journal of Developmental Neuroscience, 23*(2–3), 143–152.

Zwaigenbaum, L., Thurm, A., Stone, W., Baranek, G., Bryson, S., Iverson, J., et al. (2007). Studying the emergence of autism spectrum disorders in high-risk infants: Methodological and practical issues. *Journal of Autism and Developmental Disorders, 37*(3), 466–480.

CHAPTER FIVE

Age-Related Issues in the Assessment of Autism Spectrum Disorder

Susan H. Hedges
Victoria Shea
Gary B. Mesibov

Although the universal goal of assessing autism spectrum disorder (ASD) is obtaining information that will in some way benefit each individual and his or her family, the specific focus and tools for assessment of ASD vary markedly, depending on the age of the person being assessed. In this chapter, we discuss age-related issues in ASD assessment in five developmental stages: early childhood (up to age 3 years), preschool (ages 3–5 years), elementary school (ages 6–11 years), middle school and high school (ages 12–17 years), and adulthood (ages 18 years and beyond).

Many assessments for ASD take place through local developmental clinics or agencies, public schools, small teams, or individual clinicians. The assessment models described by most researchers—involving large university-based interdisciplinary teams, analysis of video footage, multiple assessment sessions, home visits, or observation of the target child with other children—may not be available or affordable for many families. Nevertheless, given the availability of good assessment tools for diagnosis and skill measurement, along with training in ASD, it is possible for clinicians in a variety of settings to perform meaningful, appropriate evaluations for individuals across the age range (Ozonoff, Goodlin-Jones, & Solomon, 2005).

FOCUS OF ASSESSMENT AT DIFFERENT DEVELOPMENTAL STAGES

We begin with a discussion of the ways the focus and nature of assessment change depending on the individual's age. As a general rule, assessments of young children tend to focus on establishing a diagnosis, whereas assessments at later ages tend to focus on measuring skills.

Early Childhood and Preschool Age

Although assessment tools exist to reliably diagnose ASD by the age of 2 (Jeans, Santos, Laxman, McBride, & Dyer, 2013; Ozonoff et al., 2015), the average age of diagnosis is still around 4 years of age (Centers for Disease Control and Prevention, 2016). Despite the recommendation of the U.S. Preventive Services Task Force against universal screening for autism (*www.uspreventiveservicestaskforce.org/Page/Document/RecommendationStatementFinal/autism-spectrum-disorder-in-young-children-screening*), the American Academy of Pediatrics (AAP) has reiterated their recommendation that all children be screened for ASD at 18 and 24 or 30 months using standardized measures. The AAP provides a toolkit to professionals to help guide them through that process (*www.aap.org/en-us/advocacy-and-policy/aap-health-initiatives/pages/Caring-for-Children-with-Autism-Spectrum-Disorders-A-Resource-Toolkit-for-Clinicians.aspx*). The typical focus of assessment at these stages is on answering the underlying question "Is it autism?" and then "What can be done to help the child?"

Many parents come to the assessment having observed, suspected, or been told by someone that their child's development is delayed or disordered. Others may be stunned by a diagnosis having thought that their child, although somewhat socially immature, was developmentally precocious or gifted. Some parents have had to wait and worry for months before the assessment appointment, while others come by the suspected diagnosis unexpectedly at a medical appointment or a well-baby checkup. Whenever it occurs, most parents are devastated by hearing an ASD diagnosis for the first time. Professionals who tell parents that their child has ASD, and perhaps intellectual disability as well, must be both honest and compassionate as they present information and answer questions (Mesibov, Shea, & Schopler, 2005). Accurate diagnostic terms should be used and explained, and questions about the child's future developmental course should be answered as fully as possible. Emotional support, kindness, and empathy are essential during such sessions with the parents.

As discussed by Hogan and Marcus in Chapter 12 of this volume, information about educational and treatment options should usually be part of the initial diagnostic assessment. Parents may or may not be ready to hear details about local programs, theories of intervention, or the like—however, making basic recommendations (such as good books and websites about ASD), providing contact information for the early intervention system, and offering suggestions for handling pressing behavioral concerns are often the most meaningful outcomes of assessment at this stage of development.

Elementary School Age

Assessments (which are often reassessments) for children of elementary school age occasionally focus on making or confirming the diagnosis of ASD, but are more likely to focus on the underlying question "Will he or she be able to . . . ?" Assessments during this stage thus move away from diagnostic issues to periodic evaluation of a child's skills. During the elementary school years, the child's intellectual, language, academic, and adaptive skills and potential typically become clear, based on increased cooperation with standardized testing procedures, trends in test scores over the years, and reports of the child's response to stimulation and instruction.

Because an important function of assessment at this stage is to support a wide range of interventions, scores on standardized tests in isolation are not very useful, although they may indicate specific instructional needs. In addition to needs in the areas of cognitive, language, and academic instruction, however, many children with ASD have significant problems with activities of daily living and social skills, both at school and at home—these often require qualitative assessment.

School-based skills and behaviors that may need instruction and intervention include behavior on the school bus, making transitions throughout the school day, and remaining calm and engaged during activities in high-stress locations such as the cafeteria and gym. Various home-based daily living skills may also need assessment and intervention: aspects of getting ready for school in the morning (e.g., dressing, eating breakfast, brushing teeth, and leaving home on time) and after-school routines (e.g., doing homework or playing constructively, eating dinner, bathing, brushing teeth, and going to bed on time).

For children at this age with significant cognitive impairment, aspects of toilet training may still require assessment and intervention, both at home and at school. For more cognitively capable students, support is often needed with more organizationally based tasks such as writing down assignments, taking materials home, completing the work, taking the work back to school, and turning it in to the teacher. Also, assessment of social skills is important for ascertaining children's intervention needs in terms of playing near or with other children (including siblings), sharing materials, taking turns, initiating and accepting social bids to and from peers, and beginning to learn social behaviors through observation and imitation (see Seidman & Yirmiya, Chapter 6, this volume).

Some elementary school-age children with ASD may not yet have been identified as having ASD or at least as having special needs. These students often have strong academic skills, particularly in math, science, and aspects of reading, so that they may not be considered by school systems to need special services (although in the later years of elementary and secondary school, difficulties with school-related skills such as organization of materials, time management, handwriting, and inferential reading usually become evident). Recent research suggests that some females with autism without intellectual disability may go undiagnosed as they may be better able to "camouflage" their autistic symptoms (Lehnhardt et al., 2016).

When parents seek assessments that yield a diagnosis of ASD at this age, they sometimes ask, "Should we tell the school?" As a general principle, we believe that providing accurate and complete information to school systems is the most effective way to obtain appropriate supports and services. Rather than not disclosing the diagnosis because of stereotypes (such as "All students with ASD are lacking in intelligence and nonverbal") or inappropriate tracking (such as "All students with ASD are placed in self-contained special education classrooms"), it is almost always preferable to share information with the school system and the individualized education program (IEP) team (with additional professional and advocacy support as needed), and then to work collaboratively to design an individualized program of supports and services based on the student's assessed needs.

Middle School and High School Age

Reassessments for children of middle and high school age may focus on several related questions: "What does he or she need now in the way of instruction or supports?"; "What services and supports may be needed in the future?"; and "For what services is he or she eligible?" Assessment thus typically includes both developing school-based programs and helping develop plans for adulthood. For children with ASD and significant cognitive impairments, assessment may be needed as part of the application process for publicly funded programs, such as Medicaid and Medicaid waiver programs (*www.medicaid.gov*), Supplemental Security Income (*www.ssa.gov/ssi*), and vocational rehabilitation services administered by each state. For some students, assessment of ASD-related special needs may be used as part of the process of selecting and applying to colleges (Palmer, 2006), including obtaining modified administration of college admissions tests (*www.collegeboard.org/students-with-disabilities/typical-accommodations, www.act.org/content/act/en/products-and-services/the-act/taking-the-test/services-for-examinees-with-disabilities.html*).

Parents of an undiagnosed child who arrives at middle or high school have typically experienced years of academic and social difficulties, emotional distress, and diagnostic confusion by the time of the ASD assessment and diagnosis. Their underlying question is often a frustrated "What's wrong with him or her?" and their reaction to the diagnosis may be, in effect, a relieved "Aha, so that's it!" Even though the diagnosis of ASD may be hard to hear, at this stage parents are often grateful to have an explanation for the difficulties they have lived with, and to receive recommendations for addressing behavioral and social problems and obtaining appropriate accommodations in their child's school program.

Adulthood

Reassessment for the purpose of answering the multifaceted question "What public services and funds are available for him or her?" continues to be typical for adults with ASD, who may need such supports as supplemental income, room and board, supervision and instruction in self-care and community living skills, job training and supported employment, medical care, and transportation. These and other publicly funded services have specific guidelines in terms of assessment tools and documentation of functional deficits (*www.benefits.gov/benefits/browse-by-category/category/DIA*).

Individuals whose first assessment for ASD occurs in adulthood usually fall into two categories: those with severe developmental delays who are screened for autism in institutional settings, and those with high cognitive and adaptive functioning. These latter individuals may refer themselves for assessment because of employment-related difficulties and/or social/interpersonal problems, they may have come to suspect their diagnosis in conjunction with the ASD assessment of one of their children, or they may be assessed in forensic or outpatient psychiatric settings (Nylander & Gillberg, 2001; Murrie, Warren, Kristiansson, & Dietz, 2002).

AGE-BASED TOOLS FOR DIAGNOSTIC ASSESSMENT

Because the behavioral characteristics of ASD differ over the course of development, different approaches to assessment for the purpose of diagnosis are needed at various ages.

Early Childhood: First Year

As discussed in more detail in Chapter 4 of this volume (Powell, Heymann, Tsantsanis, & Chawarska), there is currently a great deal of research interest in identifying characteristics of ASD in children below the age of 12 months (Gammer et al., 2015; Jones, Gliga, Bedford, Charman, & Johnson, 2014). In addition, several assessment tools are currently under development and showing promising results, including the Autism Observation Scale for Infants (Bryson, Zwaigenbaum, McDermott, Rombough, & Brian, 2008; Gammer et al., 2015), which is a semistructured play-based measure, and the First Year Inventory (Turner-Brown, Baranek, Reznick, Watson, & Crais, 2013), which is a parent-report instrument.

Using these and other measures, several research groups have identified a large number of behaviors or characteristics that differentiate *groups* of very young children who are eventually diagnosed with ASD from control groups of children with either typical development or various other types of developmental disabilities—however, no standardized assessment tools are available yet for *individual* diagnosis of children younger than 12 months of age. Behaviors in the first year of life that have been reported to be strongly associated with later diagnoses of autism include decreased social responsiveness (e.g., responding to name, looking at people, joint attention behaviors) and atypical sensory–regulatory behaviors (e.g., increased mouthing of objects, unusual visual attention patterns, increased irritability; Bryson et al., 2008; Jones et al., 2014). Other standardized assessment tools that have been used to differentiate a group of children 1 year of age or less are the MacArthur–Bates Communicative Development Inventories—Infant Form (Fenson et al., 2007) and the Mullen Early Learning Scales (Mullen, 1995). Zwaigenbaum et al. (2005) reported that on the MacArthur–Bates Infant Form at 12 months of age, a group of youngsters later diagnosed with autism used significantly fewer gestures and understood fewer phrases than controls—Landa and Garrett-Mayer (2006) reported that such children had significantly lower scores than control group children on all subscales of the Mullen except Visual Reception.

Early Childhood: Second Year

The "gold standard" direct observation measure for diagnosis of *some* children beginning in the second year of life is the Autism Diagnostic Observation Schedule, Second Edition (ADOS-2; Lord et al., 2012). According to its authors, the ADOS can be used with children who have a nonverbal developmental age of at least 12 months through adulthood (*www.wpspublish.com/store/p/2648/autism-diagnostic-observation-schedule-second-edition-ados-2*). The ADOS is widely acknowledged to be the most sophisticated and psychometrically sound direct observation tool for ASD (McCrimmon & Rostad, 2014)—however, it is expensive to purchase and time-consuming to learn, administer, and score.

Screening tools for ASD beginning in the second year of life include both Level 1 screens (screening for ASD or other developmental problems in the general population of young children) and Level 2 screens (screening for ASD in groups of children for whom developmental concerns have already been raised). Setting a cutoff score on a screening test involves weighing the importance of sensitivity (low rate of false negatives) versus specificity (low rate of false positives); the lower the cutoff score, the higher the sensitivity but the lower the specificity, and vice versa (Coonrod & Stone, 2005). Sensitivity rates of ASD screening tests for young children are lowered both by the phenomenon of regression that occurs in some children after the age of screening, and also by the difficulty of identifying children with less severe ASD symptomology. Specificity rates are affected by the overlap of ASD with other developmental disabilities, particularly intellectual disability and developmental language disorders (Coonrod & Stone, 2005; Eaves, Wingert, & Ho, 2006; Scambler, Hepburn, & Rogers, 2006).

For young children 12 months and older, several screening assessments for ASD are either published in the professional literature or commercially available. The Modified Checklist for Autism in Toddlers (M-CHAT; Pandey et al., 2008; Robins & Dumont-Mathieu, 2006) is widely used. Another well-known screening instrument for children at this age is the Screening Tool for Autism in Two-Year-Olds (STAT; Stone, Coonrod, & Ousley, 2000) and requires that a clinician briefly observe the child in a play-based environment. The Bayley Scales of Infant and Toddler Development, Third Edition (Bayley–III; Bayley, 2005), administered by a trained examiner, is considered a gold standard for assessing developmental delays in children from 12 to 42 months (Scattone, Raggio, & May, 2011).

Behaviors on these instruments that are most often associated with a later diagnosis of ASD include absence or limited frequency of responding to name, following a point or a gaze, pointing for reasons other than making a request, and engaging in pretend play (Chawarska & Volkmar, 2005; Scambler et al., 2006; Ventola et al., 2007). A newly developed parent-completed screening tool for ASD that is showing promise for children beginning at age 12 months through adulthood is the Mobile Autism Risk Assessment (MARA; Duda, Daniels, & Wall, 2016). It is delivered by electronic platform and consists of only seven items related to communication, social skills, and behaviors.

Early Childhood: Ages 2–3 Years

The ADOS continues to be the gold standard observational instrument for both clinical and research purposes in the toddler years. An alternative observational measure beginning at age 2 years that is less expensive and less complicated than the ADOS is the Childhood Autism Rating Scale, Second Edition (CARS-2; Schopler, Van Bourgondien, Wellman, & Love, 2010), which has strong psychometric properties (Lord & Corsello, 2005; Perry, Condillac, Freeman, Dunn-Geier, & Belair, 2005).

The gold standard parent-report measure for diagnosis beginning at developmental age 2 years is the Autism Diagnostic Interview—Revised (ADI-R; Rutter, Le Couteur, & Lord, 2003). Its administration time is approximately 2 hours (Lord & Corsello, 2005), which makes it cumbersome to use in many clinical settings. Similar to the ADI-R, the Diagnostic Interview for Social Communication Disorders (DISCO; Wing, Leekham, Libby, Gould, & Larcombe, 2002), popular in the United Kingdom, takes 2–3 hours to complete and requires highly trained clinical interviewers. Unfortunately, alternative parent interview measures for diagnosis are limited.

At age 2, most studies indicate that a diagnosis of ASD based on the clinical judgment of an experienced professional is the best single predictor of later diagnostic status, although Lord et al. (2006) demonstrated that the ADOS and the ADI-R make additional important contributions to diagnosis, particularly in the direction of increasing sensitivity (i.e., reducing false negatives). In general, diagnoses of autism at age 2 are highly likely to be confirmed later in life (Ozonoff et al., 2015) or associated with some other form of developmental disorder (Charman & Baird, 2002; Eaves & Ho, 2004; Moore & Goodson, 2006; Sutera et al., 2007).

In addition to making a diagnosis of autism, assessing intellectual ability beginning around age 2 can be helpful, as many individuals with ASD have impaired cognitive functioning. However, this assessment can be complicated by communication deficits and behavioral issues (Grondhuis & Mulick, 2013). It may be necessary to use several cognitive measures to gain a clearer picture of intellectual ability, including a nonverbal measure such as the Leiter International Performance Scale—Third Edition (Leiter–3; Roid, Miller, Pomplun, & Koch, 2013; Grondhuis & Mulick, 2013).

Preschool Age

For preschool-age children, the ADOS, ADI-R, and the CARS-2 continue to be the standard measures for diagnosis. Most studies indicate that a diagnosis of ASD made at age 3 years is very stable (Charman & Baird, 2002; Ozonoff et al., 2015; Turner, Stone, Pozdol, & Coonrod, 2006).

For screening and research purposes beginning at age 4 years (except for children with severe or profound intellectual disability), the Social Communication Questionnaire (SCQ; Rutter et al., 2003) can be used (Eaves, Wingert, & Ho, 2006; Eaves, Wingert, Ho, & Mickelson, 2006; Howlin & Karpf, 2004; Wetherby, Watt, Morgan, & Shumway, 2007). The SCQ is a 40-item parent-report measure using the items from the ADI-R that were found to be most discriminative of ASD. Because of its questionnaire format and brevity compared with the full ADI-R, it is more practical than the ADI-R for use in typical clinical settings.

The Vineland Adaptive Behavior Scales, Second Edition (Vineland–II; Sparrow, Cicchetti, & Balla, 2005) is a parent/caregiver rating form that is used to assess adaptive behavior beginning at age 2 through adulthood. Behavior assessment is essential in planning interventions, therapies, and support programs for individuals with ASD (Yang, Paynter, & Gilmore, 2016) and can be repeated to measure progress.

Elementary School Age

As previously noted, most children with severe symptoms of ASD are now diagnosed before elementary school age—however, many children with milder symptoms are not identified until much later (McConachie, LeCouteur, & Honey, 2005). In addition to the standard ASD assessment tools previously mentioned (i.e., the ADOS, ADI-R, and CARS-2), several assessment tools for those children who present with milder characteristics of ASD beginning at elementary age are being used. These include the Child Behavior Checklist (CBCL; Achenbach & Rescorla, 2001) and the Social Responsiveness Scale, Second Edition (SRS-2; Constantino, 2012). The CBCL is a questionnaire designed to assess behavior and emotional problems in children in general but has been found to do a good job at picking up possible ASD and thus prompting a more formalized ASD assessment (Mazefsky, Anderson, Conner, & Minshew, 2011). The SRS-2 (Constantino, 2012) has strengths as a measure of the social deficits associated with ASD in children ages 4–18 years.

Middle School and High School Age

The assessment tools just discussed for elementary school-age children can also be used for middle and high school students.

Two helpful skill assessments for adolescents and adults with ASD are the Supports Intensity Scale (SIS; Thompson et al., 2016) and the Instrument for Classification and Assessment of Support Needs (I-CAN; Arnold, Riches, & Stancliffe, 2014). The SIS was designed to help guide caregivers of individuals with developmental disabilities in promoting independence to improve quality of life (Mehling & Tasse, 2016). The I-CAN was designed to identify support needs for current and future planning for the individual (Mehling & Tasse, 2016). Both assessments are completed by teachers, parents, or other caregivers. These assessments can be especially helpful in planning and preparing for the transition to adulthood.

As self-awareness increases during adolescence for all teens, so too can social–emotional problems. For teens with ASD, the rates of anxiety and depression are much higher than they are for typical peers (White, Oswald, Ollendick, & Scahill, 2009), thus screening for comorbid mental health issues is suggested.

Adulthood

For individuals who can report on their own experiences, the adult version of the Autism-Spectrum Quotient (AQ; Baron-Cohen, Wheelwright, Skinner, Martin, & Clubley, 2001a, 2001b) can be used as a place to start on the path to a diagnosis. The AQ and other self-report ASD diagnostic tools are freely available on the Internet. Although many adolescents and adults are using these to diagnose themselves, it is important to have the diagnosis confirmed by a professional (either psychologist or psychiatrist) who can also provide recommendations for resources and supports to help manage any symptoms that may be interfering with quality of life.

AGE-RELATED ISSUES IN SKILL ASSESSMENT

As discussed in the preceding section, diagnoses of ASD made at or after 2 years of age by experienced professionals using clinical judgment and standardized diagnostic tools are generally stable. Skills on developmental tests, on the other hand, are more variable over time. The most obvious factor accounting for this is that all children develop and learn new skills as they age. In addition to this universal upward trajectory, the developmental trajectory of children with autism is particularly variable. Low scores on developmental tests at age 2 are *not* stable or predictive in many cases (Charman et al., 2005; Turner et al., 2006), with significant numbers of children either making marked developmental progress or cooperating better with testing (or both) during the preschool years (Rapin, 2003). In general, after the preschool years mean verbal IQ scores of groups tend to either remain stable or increase, and behavioral symptoms often decrease through childhood, adolescence, and even adulthood, particularly for individuals without intellectual disability (Howlin, 2005; McGovern & Sigman, 2005; Sigman & Ruskin, 1999; Shattuck et al., 2007). However, group means may mask *individual* differences: Some people make marked progress, while others' cognitive scores and general functioning decline in adolescence or adulthood (Shea & Mesibov, 2005). Furthermore, academic and vocational skills and independence in daily life often do not develop to the same extent as IQ and language skills, so that in adulthood the majority of individuals diagnosed with ASD as children require some combination of family support and social services (Howlin, 2005; Klin et al., 2007; Shattuck et al., 2012).

Specific age-related aspects of assessing the skills of individuals with ASD are discussed below.

Early Childhood

Before the age of 3 years, skill assessment generally does not require intentional cooperation on the part of a child with ASD—it relies instead on observation of the child's exploration of standardized materials and reactions to events in the assessment setting or on parent report.

Preschool Age

Evaluations of preschool-age children with both ASD and significant developmental delays must continue to rely on the observational and parent-report techniques used with younger children, but some children at this age can cooperate with requests to perform tasks with standardized test materials (such as those described in this volume: Paul & Wilson in Chapter 7 on language and communication; Klingeret, Mussey, & O'Kelley in Chapter 8 on intelligence; and Corbett & Iqbal in Chapter 9 on neuropsychological functioning). When test items become too difficult, however, behaviors such as leaving the table, having tantrums, or giving perseverative answers are often seen. Returning to developmentally earlier items is a useful method for assessing whether the behavioral difficulties are related to the developmental level of the tasks.

Accurate assessment requires engaging a child's attention and motivation to demonstrate his or her skills (Koegel, Koegel, & Smith, 1997; Ozonoff, Rogers, & Hendren, 2003). One way to do this is to use visual structure that shows the child how many tasks he or she will be asked to complete before receiving a small reward. For example, a word-processing program can be used to create rows of blank boxes, with a shaded box at the end of each row to represent a treat (see Figure 5.1). Each blank box represents one test item—when the child attempts or completes it, the examiner says something like "Good job. Check," and puts a check in the box. This procedure is used for *each* question or test item, regardless of the child's success, so that the reward reflects cooperation, not correct performance. The child can see that he or she is making progress along each row toward the shaded box, as well as progress down the page. When the examiner senses that the child needs a break, a special line or the word "Break" can be written at the end of a row. Multiple pages may be needed for testing with many items—it is advisable to have more than enough pages prepared and visible to the child since it is better to end early than to present additional test items that the child is not expecting.

(Item 1)	*(Item 2)*	*(Item 3)*	*(Item 4)*	
(Item 5)	*(Item 6)*	*(Item 7)*	*(Item 8)*	
(Etc.)				

FIGURE 5.1. Sample of visual support sheet for standardized testing. The shaded box at the end of each row represents a treat as a reward for cooperation.

Elementary School Age

Most elementary school-age children with ASD can cooperate with testing requests (as long as test items are not too developmentally challenging)—but sometimes children are older than norms of tests at their functioning level, so test results must be reported carefully (see Klinger et al., Chapter 8, this volume). For students who are delayed, the grid in Figure 5.1 can still be used. More developmentally advanced students can typically work for longer periods (i.e., with more columns before the column of shaded reward boxes), and some may like to choose a reward from options that are written in each shaded box. These more advanced students may also benefit from seeing a list of subtests checked off.

Middle School Age, High School Age, and Adulthood

For individuals with ASD in adolescence and into adulthood, checking off a list of subtests, though not absolutely necessary, may reduce anxiety about how long testing will last and what it will consist of.

Accurately diagnosing ASD and assessing skills and behaviors are central to providing good services. Assessment should be an ongoing, carefully designed process, although it is sometimes taken for granted or not implemented with the rigor that it requires.

Individuals with ASD differ greatly from one another in terms of their cognitive skills, communication ability, interests, behaviors, and social understanding, among other factors. Assessment enables professionals to understand each person as an individual and to develop appropriate intervention strategies and programs. Furthermore, in addition to individual differences, developmental changes occur as each person with ASD grows and matures. At different ages, there are different skills to be taught and different challenges to be addressed. For this reason, assessment strategies and instruments change as people with ASD move through the lifespan.

Although the field of ASD includes a wide variety of theories and treatment strategies, it is universally agreed that the population is enormously varied in terms of skills, interests, and behaviors. The implementation of age-appropriate diagnostic and skills assessment strategies is essential for any theoretical approach to working with these students to be effective. Our goal in writing this chapter has been to contribute to the understanding, strategies, and instruments that will advance this process for individuals with ASD at different ages.

REFERENCES

Achenbach, T. M., & Rescorla, L. A. (2001). *Manual for the ASEBA school-age forms AND profiles: An integrated system of mult-informant assessment.* Burlington: University of Vermont, Research Center for Children, Youth and Families.

Arnold, S., Riches, V., & Stancliffe, R., (2014). I-CAN: The classification and prediction of support needs. *Journal of Applied Research in Intellectual Disabilities, 27*(2), 97–111.

Baron-Cohen, S., Wheelwright, S., Skinner, R., Martin, J., & Clubley, E. (2001a). The Autism-Spectrum Quotient: Evidence from Asperger syndrome/high functioning autism, males and females, scientists and mathematicians. *Journal of Autism and Developmental Disorders, 31,* 5–17.

Baron-Cohen, S., Wheelwright, S., Skinner, R., Martin, J., & Clubley, E. (2001b). Errata. *Journal of Autism and Developmental Disorders, 31,* 603.

Bayley, N. (2005). *Bayley Scales of Infant and Toddler Development, Third Edition (Bayley–III).* San Antonio, TX: Harcourt Assessment.

Bryson, S. E., Zwaigenbaum, L., McDermott, C., Rombough, V., & Brian, J. (2008). The Autism Observation Scale for Infants: Scale development and reliability data. *Journal of Autism and Developmental Disorders, 38*(4), 731–738.

Centers for Disease Control and Prevention. (2016). Prevalence and characteristics of autism spectrum disorder among children aged 8 years—Autism and Developmental Disabilities Monitoring Network, 11 sites, United States, 2012. *Morbidity and Mortality Weekly Report Surveillance Summaries, 65,* 1–23.

Charman, T., & Baird, G. (2002). Practitioner review: Diagnosis of autism spectrum disorder in 2- and 3-year-old children. *Journal of Child Psychology and Psychiatry, 43,* 289–305.

Charman, T., Taylor, E., Drew, A., Cockerill, H., Brown, J., & Baird, G. (2005). Outcome at 7 years of children diagnosed with autism at age 2: Predictive validity of assessments conducted at 2 and 3 years of age and pattern of symptom change over time. *Journal of Child Psychology and Psychiatry, 46,* 500–513.

Chawarska, K., & Volkmar, F. R. (2005). Autism in infancy and early childhood. In F. R. Volkmar, R. Paul, A. Klin, & D. Cohen (Eds.), *Handbook of autism and pervasive developmental disorders: Vol. I* (3rd ed., pp. 223–246). Hoboken, NJ: Wiley.

Constantino, J. (2012). *Social Responsiveness Scale* (2nd ed.). Torrance, CA: Western Psychological Services.

Coonrod, E. E., & Stone, W. L. (2005). Screening for autism in young children. In F. R. Volkmar, R. Paul, A. Klin, & D. Cohen (Eds.), *Handbook of autism and pervasive developmental disorders: Vol. 2* (3rd ed., pp. 707–729). Hoboken, NJ: Wiley.

Duda, M., Daniels, J., & Wall, D. (2016). Clinical evaluation of a novel and mobile autism risk assessment. *Journal of Autism and Developmental Disorders, 46*(6), 1953–1961.

Eaves, L. C., & Ho, H. H. (2004). The very early identification of autism: Outcome to age 4½–5. *Journal of Autism and Developmental Disorders, 34,* 367–378.

Eaves, L. C., Wingert, H., & Ho, H. H. (2006). Screening for autism: Agreement with diagnosis. *Autism, 10,* 229–242.

Eaves, L. C., Wingert, H., Ho, H. H., & Mickelson, E. C. R. (2006). Screening for autism spectrum disorders with the Social Communication Questionnaire. *Journal of Developmental and Behavioral Pediatrics, 27*(Suppl. 2), S95–S103.

Fenson, L., Marchman, V. A., Thal, D. J., Dale, P. S., Reznick, J. S., & Bates, E. (2007). *MacArthur–Bates Communicative Development Inventories (CDIs) Second Edition.* Baltimore: Brookes.

Gammer, I., Bedford, R., Elsabbagh, M., Garwood, H., Pasco, G., Tucker, L., et al. (2015). Behavioural markers for autism in infancy: Scores on the Autism Observational Scale for Infants in a prospective study of at-risk siblings. *Infant Behavior and Development, 38,* 107–115.

Grondhuis, S. N., & Mulick, J. A. (2013). Comparison of the Leiter International Performance Scale—Revised and the Stanford–Binet Intelligence Scales, 5th Edition, in children with autism spectrum disorders. *American Journal on Intellectual and Developmental Disabilities, 118*(1), 44–54.

Howlin, P. (2005). Outcomes in autism spectrum disorders. In F. R. Volkmar, R. Paul, A. Klin, & D. Cohen (Eds.), *Handbook of autism and pervasive developmental disorders: Vol. 1* (3rd ed., pp. 201–230). Hoboken, NJ: Wiley.

Howlin, P., & Karpf, J. (2004). Using the Social Communication Questionnaire to identify "autism spectrum" disorders associated with other genetic conditions: Findings from a study of individuals with Cohen syndrome. *Autism, 8,* 175–182.

Jeans, L. M., Santos, R. M., Laxman, D. J., McBride, B., & Dyer, W. J. (2013). Early predictors of ASD in young children using a nationally representative data set. *Journal of Early Intervention, 35,* 303–331.

Jones, E., Gliga, T., Bedford, R., Charman, T., & Johnson, M. H. (2014). Developmental pathways to autism: A review of prospective studies of infants at risk. *Neuroscience and Biobehavioral Reviews, 39,* 1–33.

Klin, A., Saulnier, C. A., Sparrow, S. S., Cicchetti, D. V., Volkmar, F. R., & Lord, C. (2007). Social and communication abilities and disabilities in higher functioning individuals with autism spectrum disorders: The Vineland and the ADOS. *Journal of Autism and Developmental Disorders, 37,* 748–759.

Koegel, L. K., Koegel, R., & Smith, A. (1997). Variables related to differences in standardized test outcomes for children with autism. *Journal of Autism and Developmental Disorders, 27,* 233–243.

Landa, R., & Garrett-Mayer, E. (2006). Development in infants with autism spectrum disorders: A prospective study. *Journal of Child Psychology and Psychiatry, 47,* 629–638.

Lehnhardt, F., Falter, C. M., Gawronski, A., Pfeiffer, K., Tepest, R., Franklin, J., et al. (2016). Sex-related cognitive profile in autism spectrum disorders diagnosed late in life: Implications for the female autistic phenotype. *Journal of Autism and Developmental Disorders, 46*(1), 139–154.

Lord, C., & Corsello, C. (2005). Diagnostic instruments in autistic spectrum disorders. In F. R. Volkmar, R. Paul, A. Klin, & D. Cohen (Eds.), *Handbook of autism and pervasive developmental disorders: Vol. 2* (3rd ed., pp. 730–771). Hoboken, NJ: Wiley.

Lord, C., Risi, S., DiLavore, P., Shulman, C., Thurm, A., & Pickles, A. (2006). Autism from 2 to 9 years of age. *Archives of General Psychiatry, 63,* 694–701.

Lord, C., Rutter, M., DiLavore, P., Risi, S., Gotham, K., & Bishop, S. (2012). *Autism Diagnostic Observation Schedule* (2nd ed.). Torrance, CA: Western Psychological Services.

Mazefsky, C. A., Anderson, R., Conner, C. M., & Minshew, N. (2011). Child Behavior Checklist scores for school-aged children with autism: Preliminary evidence of patterns suggesting the need for referral. *Journal of Psychopathology and Behavioral Assessment, 33*(1), 31–37.

McConachie, H., Le Couteur, A., & Honey, E. (2005). Can a diagnosis of Asperger syndrome be made in very young children with suspected autism spectrum disorder? *Journal of Autism and Developmental Disorders, 35,* 167–176.

McCrimmon, A., & Rostad, K. (2014). Review of Autism Diagnostic Observation Schedule, Second Edition (ADOS-2) manual (Part II): Toddler module and Autism Diagnostic Observation Schedule, Second Edition. *Journal of Psychoeducational Assessment, 32*(1), 88–92.

McGovern, C. W., & Sigman, M. (2005). Continuity and change from early childhood to adolescence in autism. *Journal of Child Psychology and Psychiatry, 46,* 401–408.

Mehling, M. H., & Tassé, M. J. (2016). Severity of autism spectrum disorders: Current conceptualization, and transition to DSM-5. *Journal of Autism and Developmental Disabilities, 46*(6), 2000–2016.

Mesibov, G. B., Shea, V., & Schopler, E. (with Adams, L., et al.). (2005). *The TEACCH approach to autism spectrum disorders.* New York: Kluwer Academic/Plenum.

Moore, V., & Goodson, S. (2006). How well does early diagnosis of autism stand the test of time?: Follow-up study of children assessed for autism at age 2 and development of an early diagnostic service. *Autism, 7,* 47–63.

Mullen, E. M. (1995). *Mullen Scales of Early Learning: AGS Edition.* Circle Pines, MN: American Guidance Service.

Murrie, D. M., Warren, J. I., Kristiansson, M., & Dietz, P. E. (2002). Asperger syndrome in forensic settings. *International Journal of Forensic Mental Health, 1,* 59–70.

Nylander, L., & Gillberg, C. (2001). Screening for autism spectrum disorders in adult psychiatric outpatients: A preliminary report. *Acta Psychiatrica Scandinavica, 103,* 428–434.

Ozonoff, S., Goodlin-Jones, B. L., & Solomon, M. (2005). Evidence-based assessment of autism spectrum disorders in children and adolescents. *Journal of Clinical Child and Adolescent Psychology, 34,* 523–540.

Ozonoff, S., Rogers, S. J., & Hendren, R. L. (2003). *Autism spectrum disorders: A research review for practitioners.* Washington, DC: American Psychiatric Publishing.

Ozonoff, S., Young, G. S., Landa, R. J., Brian, J., Bryson, S., Charman, T., et al. (2015). Diagnostic stability in young children at risk for autism spectrum disorder: A baby siblings research consortium study. *Journal of Child Psychology and Psychiatry, 56,* 988–998.

Palmer, A. (2006). *Realizing the college dream with autism or Asperger syndrome.* London: Kingsley.

Pandey, J., Verbalis, A., Robins, D. L., Boorstein, H., Klin, A. M., Babitz, T., et al. (2008). Screening for autism in older and younger toddlers with the Modified Checklist for Autism in Toddlers. *Autism, 12*(5), 513–535.

Perry, A., Condillac, R. A., Freeman, N. L., Dunn-Geier, J., & Belair, J. (2005). Multisite study of the Childhood Autism Rating Scale (CARS) in five clinical groups of young children. *Journal of Autism and Developmental Disorders, 35,* 625–634.

Rapin, I. (2003). Value and limitations of preschool cognitive tests, with an emphasis on longitudinal study of children on the autistic spectrum. *Brain and Development, 25,* 546–548.

Robins, D. L., & Dumont-Mathieu, T. M. (2006). Early screening for autism spectrum disorders: Update on the Modified Checklist for Autism in Toddlers. *Journal of Developmental and Behavioral Pediatrics, 27*(Suppl. 2), S111–S119.

Roid, G. H., Miller, L. J., Pomplun, M., & Koch, C. (2013). *Leiter International Performance Scale—Third Edition.* Wood Dale, IL: Stoelting.

Rutter, M., Le Couteur, A., & Lord, C. (2003). *The Autism Diagnostic Interview—Revised: WPS Edition.* Los Angeles: Western Psychological Services.

Scambler, D. J., Hepburn, S. L., & Rogers, S. J. (2006). A two-year follow-up on risk status identified by the Checklist for Autism in Toddlers. *Journal of Developmental and Behavioral Pediatrics, 27*(Suppl. 2), S104–S110.

Scattone, D., Raggio, D. J., & May, W. (2011). Comparison of the Vineland Adaptive Behavior Scales, Second Edition, and the Bayley Scales of Infant and Toddler Development, Third Edition. *Psychological Reports, 109*(2), 626–634.

Schopler, E., Van Bourgondien, M., Wellman, J., & Love, S. (2010). *Childhood Autism Rating Scale—Second Edition (CARS-2): Manual.* Los Angeles: Western Psychological Services.

Shattuck, P. T., Narendorf, S. C., Cooper, B., Sterzing, P. R., Wagner, M., & Taylor, J. L. (2012). Postsecondary education and employment among youth with an autism spectrum disorder. *Pediatrics, 129*(6), 1042–1049.

Shattuck, P. T., Seltzer, M. M., Greenberg, J. S., Orsmond, G., Bolt, D., Kring, S., et al. (2007). Change in autism symptoms and maladaptive behaviors in adolescents and adults with an autism spectrum disorder. *Journal of Autism and Developmental Disorders, 37,* 1735–1747.

Shea, V., & Mesibov, G. B. (2005). Adolescents and adults with autism. In F. R. Volkmar, R. Paul, A. Klin, & D. Cohen (Eds.), *Handbook of autism and pervasive developmental disorders: Vol. 1* (3rd ed., pp. 288–311). Hoboken, NJ: Wiley.

Sigman, M., & Ruskin, E. (1999). Continuity and change in the social competence of children with autism, Down syndrome, and developmental delays. *Monographs of the Society for Research in Child Development, 64*(1, Serial No. 256).

Sparrow, S. S., Cicchetti, D., & Balla, D. (2005). *Vineland Adaptive Behavior Scales, Second Edition (Vineland–II).* Circle Pines, MN: American Guidance Service.

Stone, W. L., Coonrod, E. E., & Ousley, O. Y. (2000). Screening Tool for Autism in Two-Year-Olds (STAT): Development and preliminary data. *Journal of Autism and Developmental Disorders, 30,* 607–612.

Sutera, S., Pandey, J., Esser, E. L., Rosenthal, M. A., Wilson, L. B., Barton, M., et al. (2007). Predictors of optimal outcome in toddlers diagnosed with autism spectrum disorders. *Journal of Autism and Developmental Disorders, 37,* 98–107.

Thompson, J. R., Wehmeyer, M. L., Hughes, C., Shogren, K. A., Seo, H., Little, T. D., et al., (2016). *Supports Intensity Scale—Children's Version: User's manual.* Washington, DC: American Association on Intellectual and Developmental Disabilities.

Turner, L. M., Stone, W. L., Pozdol, S. L., & Coonrod, E. E. (2006). Follow-up of children with autism spectrum disorders from age 2 to age 9. *Autism, 10,* 243–265.

Turner-Brown, L. M., Baranek, G. T., Reznick, J. S., Watson, L. R., & Crais, E. R. (2013). The First Year Inventory: A longitudinal follow-up of 12-month-old to 3-year-old children. *Autism, 17*(5), 527–540.

Ventola, P., Kleinman, J., Pandey, J., Wilson, L., Esser, E., Boorstein, H., et al. (2007). Differentiating between autism spectrum disorders and other developmental disabilities in children who failed a screening instrument for ASD. *Journal of Autism and Developmental Disorders, 37,* 425–436.

Wetherby, A. M., Watt, N., Morgan, L., & Shumway, S. (2007). Social communication profiles of children with autism spectrum disorders late in the second year of life. *Journal of Autism and Developmental Disorders, 37,* 960–975.

White, S. W., Oswald, D., Ollendick, T., & Scahill, L. (2009). Anxiety in children and adolescents with autism spectrum disorders. *Clinical Psychology Review, 29*(3), 216–229.

Wing, L., Leekham, S. R., Libby, S. J., Gould, J., & Larcombe, M. (2002). The Diagnostic Interview for Social and Communication Disorders: Background, inter-rater reliability and clinical use. *Journal of Child Psychology and Psychiatry, 43,* 307–325.

Yang, S., Paynter, J. M., & Gilmore, L. (2016). Vineland Adaptive Behavior Scales II profile of young children with autism spectrum disorder. *Journal of Autism and Developmental Disorders, 46*(1), 64–73.

Zwaigenbaum, L., Bryson, S., Rogers, T., Roberts, W., Brian, J., & Szatmari, P. (2005). Behavioral manifestations of autism in the first year of life. *International Journal of Developmental Neuroscience, 23,* 143–152.

CHAPTER SIX

Assessment of Social Behavior in Autism Spectrum Disorder

Ifat Gamliel Seidman
Nurit Yirmiya

The diathesis–stress or transactional model of development suggests that genetic and environmental regulators of behavior transact continuously over time and thus constantly mutually influence each other (Sameroff, 2000). Typically developing infants are born with the genetic predisposition or preparedness that endows them to learn and acquire certain behaviors quite easily (Seligman, 1970). In typical development, for example, infants become social very early. They identify their mothers by 1 week of age, and by 3 months they recognize photographs of their mothers and prefer them over photographs of strangers (Barrera & Maurer, 1981; Pascalis, de Schonen, Morton, Deruelle, & Fabre-Grenet, 1995). They also begin very early to imitate, which is a powerful mechanism for learning. Some researchers have suggested that even newborns at 2 days of age are able to imitate adults' facial movements, such as tongue protrusion and mouth opening (Meltzoff & Moore, 1977, 1999); most researchers agree that by 1 year of age, infants are able to use imitation to learn new behaviors quite easily and flawlessly. Thus, typically developing infants engage in nonverbal social-communicative behaviors and are able to synchronize or attune their affective and arousal states to those of their partners from a very early period (Feldman, 2007). The intact newborn develops normatively and progresses through major developmental cornerstones in all realms of development, including the social realm. These achievements are attributed to biological maturational processes and to a good enough environmental experience, as suggested by the transactional diathesis–stress model.

In contrast to typically developing children, children diagnosed with autism spectrum disorder (ASD), and some children even prior to receiving such diagnoses, experience difficulties in achieving milestones and displaying behaviors easily achieved by their typically developing peers. A major area of these difficulties is social—the social behavior of children, adolescents, and adults with ASD differs qualitatively from that of their typically developing agemates. Indeed, impairments in social behavior constitute one of the three general areas of impairments required for an ASD diagnosis.

For example, the diagnostic criteria for ASD in the fifth edition of the *Diagnostic and Statistical Manual of Mental Disorders* (DSM-5; American Psychiatric Association, 2013) describe behaviors and impairments in two domains, one of which pertains to the focus of the current chapter: deficits in social communication and social interaction. According to DSM-5 (American Psychiatric Association, 2013, p. 50), the diagnostic criteria for impairment in the Social and Communicative Behaviors domain are as follows:

> Qualitative impairment in social interaction, as manifested by all three of the following:
> 1. Deficits in social–emotional reciprocity.
> 2. Deficits in nonverbal behaviors used to regulate social interaction.
> 3. Deficits in developing, maintaining, and understanding social relationships.

The other diagnostic domain focuses on restricted, repetitive, and stereotyped patterns of behavior, interests, and activities.

In this chapter, we adopt a developmental framework and review the cardinal findings and assessment measures pertaining to social behavior in children and adolescents with ASD.

IDENTIFYING SOCIAL DIFFICULTIES IN THE EARLY YEARS

The earliest evidence for social difficulties of children later diagnosed with ASD comes from two lines of research. The first consists of retrospective investigations, such as retrospective parental interviews or the investigation of home movies videotaped during the first year of life (or soon after) of children who later receive an ASD diagnosis. The second comprises prospective studies of infants who are at risk for ASD.

The early ontogeny of autism has often been examined via retrospective analyses of home videos of infants who were later diagnosed with the disorder (e.g., Adrien et al., 1991, 1993; Baranek, 1999; Clifford & Dissanayake, 2008; Clifford, Young, & Williamson, 2007; Losche, 1990; Maestro et al.,

2002, 2005; Osterling & Dawson, 1994; Osterling, Dawson, & Munson, 2002; Ozonoff et al., 2011; Werner, Dawson, Osterling, & Dinno, 2000). This body of literature has revealed evidence of early impairments in social engagement among such infants. For example, in comparison to a group of typically developing children, infants who were later diagnosed with autism revealed impairments in sensory–motor development, joint social activities, and symbolic play (Losche, 1990); impairments in social interaction, social smiling, and facial expressions, combined with hypoactivity and poor attention (Adrien et al., 1993); and significantly less eye contact and less responsiveness to their names being called (Osterling & Dawson, 1994). Comparing children later diagnosed with autism to children later diagnosed with developmental delays, Baranek (1999) validated that only the children who were later diagnosed with autism demonstrated impairments in response to their names and in orientation to visual stimuli, as well as aversion to touch. Clifford and Dissanayake (2008) also investigated early development of infants later diagnosed with autism during the first 2 years of life, by using retrospective parental interviews and analyses of home videos. They suggested that abnormalities in dyadic behaviors—such as poor quality of eye contact, impairment in the use of smiling, and inappropriate affect—may be detected in home videos even before the first birthday.

In contrast to retrospective studies with children who were later diagnosed with ASD, the strategy of prospective studies has been to employ groups of children known to be at risk for ASD, and to follow their development from close to birth until they reach the age of 2–3 years or older, at which time their outcome diagnosis of ASD or non-ASD becomes known (Jones, Gliga, Bedford, Charman, & Johnson, 2014; Yirmiya & Ozonoff, 2007). Researchers working with at-risk samples employ various observations and screening measures, as well as experimental methods. Great effort has been invested in producing predictive measures for ASD and for related difficulties among young infants (Barbaro & Dissanayake, 2013). Some of these screening measures are designed as "Level 1" screeners—that is, brief instruments used to identify children at risk for ASD in the general population, and administered mostly by primary care physicians and general practitioners. In contrast, "Level 2" screeners (Hampton & Strand, 2015) are used to identify risk for ASD versus other types of developmental delays among selected groups of children who are already considered as being at risk (e.g., younger siblings of children with ASD, or children referred with various developmental concerns and delays). These latter screeners are usually more time-consuming instruments, and are administered more often by trained professionals other than general practitioners (Robins & Dumont-Mathieu, 2006).

In the next section, we describe instruments that involve parental reports, observations and testing by health care professionals, or both, as these pertain to the assessment of social behavior in young infants and toddlers and early identification of ASD, as well as to the assessment of social behavior in older children, adolescents, and adults. We present these measures chronologically, from those that are suitable for the youngest of infants to those relevant for toddlers, older children, adolescents, and adults. It is important to note that different measures are used for different purposes. Some measures are most appropriate for developmental surveillance or Level 1 screening, some for Level 2 screening, and some for diagnosis and/or research. Although a clinician should never base a formal diagnosis of ASD on any of this set of measures alone, especially without actually seeing a child, some of the assessments described in this next section do provide cost-effective means of achieving a current perspective on a child's difficulties at any particular time. (See Naglieri, Chambers, McGoldrick, & Goldstein, Chapter 2, this volume, for further information about diagnosis vs. screening.)

ASSESSMENT AND DIAGNOSTIC MEASURES FOR SOCIAL BEHAVIOR

The Autism Observation Scale for Infants (AOSI; Bryson, McDermott, Rombough, Brian, & Zwaigenbaum, 2000), as its name indicates, is a short observational assessment designed to detect and monitor putative signs of ASD in infants ages 6–18 months. After a short interaction and observation, the attending professional uses a checklist for 18 specific behavioral risk markers for autism, including visual attention and attention disengagement, coordination of eye gaze with action, imitation, affect, behavioral reactivity, social-communicative behaviors, and sensory–motor development. Using the AOSI, Zwaigenbaum et al. (2005) compared a group of high-risk infants (siblings of children with autism) with a group of low-risk infants, and found that several behaviors observed at 12 (but not at 6) months predicted a future Autism Diagnostic Observation Schedule (ADOS) classification of autism at 24 months for the high-risk group. At 12 months, these behaviors included impairments in eye contact, visual tracking, disengagement of visual attention, orienting to name, imitation, social smiling, reactivity, social interest, and sensory-oriented behaviors. Similar results were reported in an independent sample by Gammer and colleagues (2015), who found that the AOSI distinguished children with ASD outcomes at 14 months, but not at 7 months. Bryson, Zwaigenbaum, McDermott, Rombough, and Brian (2008) reported good to excellent reliability and called for further investigation of the AOSI's ability to discriminate high-risk infants who will eventually develop ASD. Recently, Yaari et al. (2016) examined early ASD risk in preterm infants using the AOSI at 8 and 12 months. These researchers found that the percentage of preterm infants who identified at risk for ASD decreased over time, suggesting that children "grew out" of risk over time, thus emphasizing the importance of prospective, longitudinal designs in at-risk cohorts.

In contrast to the AOSI, which is administered and coded by a trained professional, the First Year Inventory (FYI; Reznick, Baranek, Reavis, Watson, & Crais, 2007) is a questionnaire administered to infants' caregivers to identify 12-month-olds in the general population who are at risk for atypical development in general, but with a special focus on infants whose risk patterns are most predictive of a future ASD diagnosis. The target behaviors depicted by the various items are based on retrospective and prospective studies that suggested risk markers in infancy for an eventual diagnosis of autism. In this 63-item checklist, parents are asked to describe their children on two major domains: Social and Communicative Behaviors (i.e., social orienting, receptive communication, social affective engagement, imitation, and expressive communication) and Sensory and Regulatory Behaviors (i.e., sensory processing, regulatory patterns, reactivity, and repetitive behavior). A retrospective version of the FYI was administered to parents of preschool children with ASD, children with other developmental disabilities, and children with typical development, to strengthen the validity of the FYI and to improve its utility for prospective screening of both infants from the general population and infants at risk (Turner-Brown, Baranek, Reznick, Watson, & Crais, 2012; Watson et al., 2007).

The Early Screening of Autistic Traits Questionnaire (ESAT; Swinkels et al., 2006), designed as a general population screener for 14- to 15-month-old infants, is a two-stage, 14-item questionnaire administered to health practitioners and caregivers. Four items were identified as having good discriminability for ASD: readability of emotions, reaction to sensory stimuli, and two play behaviors—interest in different toys and varied play. The authors suggest that these four items could be used as a quick prescreening instrument, to limit the number of children who need to be further screened with the full version of the ESAT (Swinkels et al., 2006). In a large population study (Dietz, Swinkels, van Daalen, van Engeland, & Buitelaar, 2006), 14- to 15-month-old infants were prescreened by physicians using these four items. Infants with positive results on the prescreening were then evaluated at home by a trained professional using the full ESAT, and were also invited for a complete psychiatric examination, as well as for follow-up examinations at 24 and 42 months. Dietz et al. (2006) underscored the large number of false-positive results in both the prescreening (first stage) and the administration (second stage) of the ESAT for a later diagnosis of ASD—therefore, this screener should be used with caution. However, it can assist clinicians who are considering referrals for a more comprehensive diagnostic evaluation of ASD.

The Communication and Symbolic Behavior Scales (CSBS; Wetherby & Prizant, 1993) and its shortened version, the Communication and

Symbolic Behavior Scales Developmental Profile (CSBS-DP; Wetherby & Prizant, 2002), are standardized tools designed as evaluation procedures for early identification of communication disorders in children between 12 and 24 months of age. The CSBS-DP actually consists of three measures: the Infant–Toddler Checklist, which is a 14-item screening questionnaire that can be completed quickly by a parent at the physician's office; a Caregiver Questionnaire; and a Behavior Sample, which is a semistructured observation of the child interacting with a parent and clinician, when the child is being presented with a series of "communication temptations" such as interesting toys and other play opportunities. Three composites may be derived from the Infant–Toddler Checklist and Behavior Sample: Social (emotion, eye gaze, and communication), Speech (sounds and words), and Symbolic (understanding and object use). The CSBS-DP has been standardized to have a mean of 10 and standard deviation of 3 for each composite, and a mean of 100 and standard deviation of 15 for the total score. Good evidence for reliability and validity supports the use of the Infant–Toddler Checklist and Behavior Sample as appropriate screening and evaluation tools for identifying young children with developmental delays at 12–24 months of age (Wetherby, Allen, Cleary, Kublin, & Goldstein, 2002; Wetherby, Goldstein, Cleary, Allen, & Kublin, 2003), with promising results regarding the identification of later ASD as well (Wetherby et al., 2004).

The CSBS-DP has also been used as a standardized measure for assessing social, communication, and play behavior of 14- to 24-month-old infants with high and low risk for autism, in a prospective longitudinal study investigating developmental trajectories of children with early and later diagnosis of ASD (Landa, Holman, & Garrett-Mayer, 2007). In Wetherby et al.'s (2004) prospective longitudinal study of a large population-based sample of children between 12 and 24 months of age, the CSBS-DP was utilized to detect early indicators of ASD ("red flags") in the second year of life, which could differentiate children later diagnosed with ASD from children diagnosed with developmental delays and children with typical development. Some of these red flags included indicators of atypical early social development, such as lack of sharing enjoyment or interest and lack of response to name. Furthermore, Wetherby, Watt, Morgan, and Shumway (2007) investigated the "social communication phenotype" late in the second year of life among children later diagnosed with ASD. Their research highlighted five pivotal social communication skills detected by the CSBS-DP: communicative intentions, conventional behaviors, representation, social referencing, and rate of communication.

The Checklist for Autism in Toddlers (CHAT; Baron-Cohen, Allen, & Gillberg, 1992) is one of the first screening measures designed to identify toddlers from the general population who are at risk for ASD, by detecting abnormalities in early social orienting behaviors such as joint attention and pretend play. The CHAT is a 14-item yes/no checklist completed by both parents and a home health visitor. Five key items describing protodeclarative pointing, gaze monitoring, and pretend play were found to have the best discriminability as early as 18 months for a later diagnosis of autism (Baird et al., 2000; Baron-Cohen et al., 1996). The Modified CHAT (M-CHAT; Robins, Fein, Barton, & Green, 2001; Robins et al., 2014) omits the CHAT's observational section but includes additional parent-report items, for a total of 23 items. It may be administered to parents as well as to pediatricians and family practitioners to detect early features of autism in children ages 16–30 months. A follow-up interview is administered to parents of children who obtain positive results on the M-CHAT to review their answers on all failed items, before the children are referred for full ASD evaluation. Items regarding early social development include "Does your child enjoy playing peek-a-boo/hide-and-seek?" and "Does your child look at your face to check your reaction when faced with something unfamiliar?" Six critical items of the M-CHAT were identified as offering the best discriminability for ASD: taking interest in other children, using index finger to point and to indicate interest in something, bringing objects over to show the parent, imitating, responding to name when called, and following pointing across the room.

Robins et al. (2001) suggested that M-CHAT screening with 24-month-olds rather than 18-month-olds improves the instrument's sensitivity and acceptability to health care providers. In a replication study, Kleinman et al. (2008) confirmed the validity of the M-CHAT in detecting possible ASD in low-risk and high-risk samples of children ages 16–30 months. Furthermore, along with other screening measures, the M-CHAT was used successfully as a screener for possible ASD in a group of children with the genetic syndrome of molecularly confirmed 22q11.2 deletions (Fine et al., 2005).

The Screening Tool for Autism in Two-Year-Olds (STAT; Stone & Ousley, 1997) is a Level 2 screener designed to differentiate young children with ASD from other children already identified as being at risk (i.e., children with language and/or developmental delays), ranging in age from 24 through 35 months. The STAT is an observational measure consisting of a 20-minute play-based interactive session that provides a standard context for eliciting and observing early social-communicative behaviors. Twelve items assess behaviors in four social-communicative domains: Play, Requesting, Directing Attention, and Motor Imitation. Reports on the STAT's psychometric properties indicate high sensitivity, specificity, and predictive values, as well as acceptable levels of reliability and concurrent validity with the ADOS (Stone, Coonrod, Turner, & Pozdol, 2004). Using the STAT, McDuffie, Yoder, and Stone (2005) investigated the associations between early prelinguistic social-communicative behaviors in 2- and 3-year-old children with ASD (i.e., attention following, motor imitation, commenting, and requesting) and later language development. Surprisingly, commenting behavior predicted language comprehension, and both commenting and motor imitation of actions without objects predicted language production, thus suggesting their important potential as intervention targets (McDuffie et al., 2005).

In contrast to the aforementioned observations and screeners, the Early Social Communication Scales (ESCS; Mundy, Hogan, & Doehring, 1996; Seibert, Hogan, & Mundy, 1982) is a research-based procedure that enables assessment of children's initiating and responding to nonverbal communication acts, including joint attention behaviors, social play behaviors, and requesting behaviors. This 20-minute structured observation is appropriate for typically developing children between the ages of 6 and 30 months; it is commonly used for children with ASD who do not speak yet, to assess their nonverbal social-communicative abilities. A set of eliciting play and interactive situations using turn-taking tasks, social games, and interesting toys is presented to encourage social interaction between child and adult. The ESCS yields frequency-of-behavior scores in five categories: Initiating Social Interaction, Responding to Social Interaction, Initiating Joint Attention, Responding to Joint Attention, and Initiating Behavior Requests. Children with ASD show significant delays in their joint attention and requesting behaviors on the ESCS, compared with participants without ASD (Mundy, Sigman, Ungerer, & Sherman, 1986). Furthermore, performance on the ESCS in the preschool years has been found to predict language acquisition in middle childhood for children with ASD (Mundy & Gomes, 1998; Mundy, Sigman, & Kasari, 1990; Sigman & Ruskin, 1999).

We next describe the common diagnostic battery for children suspected of having ASD. This diagnostic battery typically involves standardized assessments specific to ASD, plus a developmental or intelligence test and a language test (language assessments are more fully discussed by Paul & Wilson, Chapter 7, this volume) based on a child's age and abilities, as well as an assessment of daily living skills. The two gold standard diagnostic systems for research purposes are the Autism Diagnostic Interview—Revised (ADI-R; Rutter, LeCouteur, & Lord, 2003) and the Autism Diagnostic Observation Schedule, Second Edition (ADOS-2; Lord et al., 2012), which are based on DSM-5 (American Psychiatric Association, 2013) criteria for ASD, including specific items relating to social abilities.

The ADI-R is a semistructured interview that is completed with a child's caregivers. The Reciprocal Social Interactions items of the ADI-R include questions regarding peer relationships (e.g., imaginative play/group play with peers, interest in/response to other children), sharing enjoyment (e.g., showing and directing attention, offering/seeking to share), and social–emotional reciprocity (e.g., quality of social overtures, offering comfort). Due to its considerable length and training requirements, the ADI-R is not an ideal measure for use in clinical settings—but as stated above, it is primarily for research.

The ADOS-2 is a semistructured, standardized observational assessment that provides a number of opportunities for interaction (e.g., play, turn-taking games, looking at books). The Social Affect items of the ADOS-2 include such behaviors as unusual eye contact, deficit in directing facial expression to others, accompanying spoken language with nonverbal communication (e.g., gaze, facial expression, gesture), showing shared enjoinment in the interaction, communicating affect, and understanding of others' emotions.

A cognitive and developmental evaluation is an essential component of the diagnostic process for ASD. Most IQ tests include at least some subscales that assess social understanding. For example, the Wechsler Intelligence Scale for Children—Fifth Edition (WISC-V; Wechsler, 2014) contains the Comprehension subtest, in which children are asked to explain their understanding of various social situations. Individuals with autism are notorious for their low scores on the Wechsler subtests (and subtests of other IQ tests) that pertain to social understanding and behavior (e.g., Ehlers et al., 1997; Happé, 1994; Li, Du, Luan, Li, & Ousley, 2017); Mayes & Calhoun, 2003, 2004; Siegel, Minshew, & Goldstein, 1996). In all of these studies, the mean WISC Comprehension subtest score was lower than the mean scores on the other subtests that compose the Verbal Comprehension Index.

The Vineland Adaptive Behavior Scales, Second Edition (Vineland–II; Sparrow, Cicchetti, & Balla, 2005), a well-known instrument assessing daily living skills, is used in clinical, educational, and research settings. It assesses four broad adaptive behavior domains: Communication, Daily Living Skills, Socialization, and Motor Skills. The Vineland–II is administered as an interview or a rating scale for parents/caregivers and teachers; it was designed to assess daily functioning of individuals with a variety of disorders and disabilities, such as intellectual disability, ASD, and other developmental delays. The four domain composite scores are all standard scores with a mean of 100 and a standard deviation of 15. Together, they make up the Adaptive Behavior Composite score. Furthermore, the Vineland–II may yield scaled scores for subdomains (a mean of 15 and a standard deviation of 3), percentile ranks, and age equivalents. The Socialization domain comprises three subdomains: Interpersonal Relationships (e.g., "meets with friends regularly"), Play and Leisure Time (e.g., "takes turns without being asked"), and Coping Skills (e.g., "chooses not to taunt, tease, or bully").

A typical profile found on the Vineland–II in young children with ASD includes (1) a low score on the Socialization domain, including low scores on its three subdomains; (2) a low score on the Expressive subdomain of the Communication domain; and (3) significant discrepancies between domain scores (Yang, Paynter, & Gilmore, 2016).

Research on social abilities as measured by the original Vineland revealed that individuals with autism obtained lower scores on interpersonal skills than either individuals with Down syndrome (Rodrigue, Morgan,

& Geffken, 1991) or individuals with developmental delays matched on chronological age, gender, and IQ (Volkmar et al., 1987). Researchers have also investigated Vineland scores associated with diagnostic procedures, age, and IQ. Tomanik, Pearson, Loveland, Lane, and Shaw (2007) have suggested that assessment of an individual's adaptive functioning using the original Vineland (including the Socialization domain score) may improve ASD diagnostic accuracy, especially when the ADI-R and ADOS classifications are not congruent. Klin et al. (2007) demonstrated that levels of social ability in high-functioning individuals with ASD (as measured by the Vineland Socialization domain) decreased markedly with age, suggesting that these high-functioning individuals become increasingly socially impaired relative to their agemates through later childhood and into adolescence. Interestingly, verbal IQ scores as well as social difficulties as measured by the ADOS were unrelated to the Vineland Socialization domain score, thus suggesting that cognitive competency and/or fewer social disabilities may not contribute to functioning in the real world (Klin et al., 2007).

Another instrument specifically designed to assess the social domain is the Social Responsiveness Scale, Second Edition (SRS-2; Constantino, 2012). This instrument was developed as a general measure of social responsiveness and is applicable to a wide continuum of people, including those who are not diagnosed with ASD. The SRS-2 is a 65-item rating scale administered to caregivers that focuses on a child's ability to engage in emotionally appropriate reciprocal social interaction and communication. It measures the severity of ASD symptoms as they occur in natural social settings (i.e., social awareness, social information processing, capacity for reciprocal social communication, social anxiety/avoidance, and autistic preoccupations and traits). In addition to a total score, the SRS-2 generates scores for five subscales: Receptive, Cognitive, Expressive, and Motivational aspects of social behavior, as well as Autistic Preoccupations. The SRS has also been used to investigate the social endophenotype in siblings of children with autism (Constantino et al., 2006) and in families with two or more probands with autism (Duvall et al., 2007), as well as in other populations at risk, and in the general population (Constantino et al., 2004; Reiersen, Constantino, Volk, & Todd, 2007). Furthermore, the SRS has been used in evaluating responses to intervention programs in children with ASD (Freitag et al., 2016).

The Social Communication Questionnaire (SCQ; Rutter, Bailey, & Lord, 2003), formerly the Autism Screening Questionnaire (ASQ; Berument, Rutter, Lord, Pickles, & Bailey, 1999), designed as a screening instrument for children age 4 years and above to evaluate autism spectrum symptoms, has a cutoff score that can be used to indicate the likelihood that a child has ASD. The SCQ is made up of 40 items from the ADI-R (Rutter, LeCouteur, & Lord, 2003). It offers two algorithms: a lifetime diagnosis, which refers to behavior throughout the child's lifetime, and a current algorithm, which focuses on the most recent 3-month period. Social items include questions such as "Does he or she have any particular friends or a best friend?" or "Does he or she ever try to comfort you when you are sad or hurt?" The SCQ was reported to have good discriminative validity with respect to the separation of ASD from non-ASD diagnoses at all IQ levels (Berument et al., 1999), although more recent studies (Barnard-Brak, Brewer, Chesnut, Richman, & Schaeffer, 2016) suggest that sensitivity and specificity are lower than initially reported. Other researchers have suggested different cutoff points for different populations (i.e., younger vs. older children, verbal vs. nonverbal children, clinical vs. nonclinical populations) and pointed to the importance of adjusting cutoff scores depending on research or screening goals (Baird et al., 2006; Corsello et al., 2007; Eaves, Wingert, & Ho, 2006a; Eaves, Wingert, Ho, & Mickelson, 2006b; Lee, David, Rusyniak, Landa, & Newschaffer, 2007).

Additional instruments have been specifically developed to measure symptom severity in individuals with high-functioning autism and individuals with Asperger syndrome. For example, the Childhood Asperger Syndrome Test (CAST; Scott, Baron-Cohen, Bolton, & Brayne, 2002) was designed as a screening questionnaire to identify children at risk for Asperger syndrome and related conditions from a general population. Caregivers rate their children on 37 items describing behaviors on the autism continuum, and a cutoff of 15 reflects possible risk for Asperger syndrome and ASD. Social items include questions regarding peer relationships (e.g., "Does he or she join in playing games with other children easily?") and play activities (e.g., "Does he or she prefer imaginative activities such as play-acting or storytelling, rather than numbers or lists of facts?"). The CAST has shown good to moderate test–retest reliability in various samples (e.g., nonclinical, high scoring; Allison et al., 2007; Williams et al., 2006), and good sensitivity and specificity (Scott et al., 2002; Williams et al., 2005). It was also used to measure autism-like traits in a nonclinical twin study (Dworzynski et al., 2007; Ronald, Happé, Bolton, et al., 2006; Ronald, Happé, Price, Baron-Cohen, & Plomin, 2006).

Another screening measure for individuals with high-functioning autism and individuals with Asperger syndrome is the Asperger Syndrome Screening Questionnaire (ASSQ; Ehlers, Gillberg, & Wing, 1999), designed to identify symptom characteristics of Asperger syndrome and other high-functioning ASD in school-age children. The ASSQ has been used in population samples and in clinical settings (Guo et al., 2011; Mattila et al., 2012; Posserud, Lundervold, & Gillberg, 2006); however, a later version, the Autism Spectrum Screening Questionnaire—Revised Extended Version (ASSQ-REV; Kopp & Gillberg, 2011), has been proposed, with special attention to females with ASD.

Some rating scales have also been designed to detect autism-like traits, which are useful in assessing the broad phenotype of autism in at-risk samples or in other populations of interest, and which address the social domain as well. For example, the Autism-Spectrum Quotient (AQ; Baron-Cohen, Wheelwright, Skinner, Martin, & Clubley, 2001) is a self-administered questionnaire designed to measure the degree to which an adult with normal intelligence has traits associated with autism in five domains: Social Skills, Attention Switching, Attention to Detail, Communication, and Imagination. The AQ was found to have good discriminative validity in differentiating a group with high-functioning ASD from randomly selected controls (Baron-Cohen et al., 2001; Woodbury-Smith, Robinson, Wheelwright, & Baron-Cohen, 2005), but results regarding cross-cultural reliability have been mixed (Ketelaars et al., 2008; Kurita, Koyama, & Osada, 2005; Wakabayashi, Baron-Cohen, Wheelwright, & Tojo, 2006). Furthermore, gender differences were detected on the AQ (i.e., where men scored higher than women in a nonclinical sample; Austin, 2005), and the examination of parents of children with autism revealed no significant differences from parents of children with typical development (Scheeren & Stauder, 2008).

Similarly, the Broader Phenotype Autism Symptoms Scale (BPASS; Dawson et al., 2007; Bernier, Gerdts, Munson, Dawson, & Estes, 2012) is an instrument for assessing autism-related traits in children and adults with ASD, as well as in parents and nonaffected siblings. This measure assesses such traits not only through informant interview but also through the observation made during the interaction with a clinical examiner, thus enabling the direct assessment of social behaviors characteristic to autism. The BPASS measures four separate domains of autism-related traits: Social Motivation, Social Expressiveness, Conversational Skills, and Repetitive/Restricted Behaviors.

The Friendship Questionnaire (FQ; Baron-Cohen & Wheelwright, 2003) is a self-report questionnaire designed to assess an individual's ability to enjoy close, empathic, and supportive friendships and interest in interacting with others. Baron-Cohen and Wheelwright (2003) reported that women scored significantly higher on the FQ than men, and that adults with Asperger syndrome or high-functioning autism scored significantly lower than both men and women with typical development. Thus, the FQ may reflect sex differences in the style of friendship in the general population and "may help us understand conditions like autism or [Asperger syndrome] not as qualitatively different from anything else we are familiar with but, instead, simply as an extreme of the normal quantitative variation we see in any sample" (Baron-Cohen & Wheelwright, 2003, p. 514).

As the present review has made clear, social impairment—one of the three hallmarks of ASD—is indeed assessed in every screening and diagnostic instrument for possible ASD. The social difficulties inherent in ASD are also evident in the relationships that individuals with ASD have with other people in their daily lives. In the next two sections, we discuss the social relationships that children with ASD have with significant others in their lives—their attachment to parents and their friendships with agemates. We end this chapter with a short presentation of the deficits in "theory of mind" (ToM) and the recently discovered dysfunction in mirror neurons that are associated with the social deficits in ASD.

ATTACHMENT

Both the ill-conceived notion that children with autism do not differentiate between their caregivers and other adults, and Kanner's (1949) claim that autism has a psychogenic origin, led to scanty research regarding the attachment patterns of children with autism (Yirmiya & Sigman, 2001). More recently, however, researchers within the fields of both autism and attachment have begun to revive interest in parent–child interactions in general, and in attachment in particular, among families of children with autism. "Attachment" is defined as the affectional bond that an infant forms between him- and herself and his or her caregiver (Ainsworth, Blehar, Waters, & Wall, 1978), and it is thought to be fundamental for later development of social relationships and cognitive skills (Weinfield, Sroufe, Egeland, & Carlson, 1999). Behaviors that maintain proximity and contact between the child and caregiver are defined as "attachment behaviors" (Bowlby, 1969). Ainsworth and her colleagues (Ainsworth, 1979; Ainsworth et al., 1978) designed the Strange Situation paradigm as a working model to assess the attachment patterns of children between the ages of 12 and 18 months. This paradigm involves an unfamiliar setting in which the child can play in the presence of his or her mother, and includes 3-minute-long separations from the mother in the presence of an unfamiliar woman. The child's reactions to the separation from the mother, and especially to the reunion with her, are coded for the child's pattern of attachment. This pattern may be classified as indicative of secure attachment or of one of three insecure attachment categories: ambivalent, avoidant, or disorganized.

A child with a secure attachment pattern of behavior is one for whom the mother presents a secure base for investigating the unfamiliar surroundings and new toys, while maintaining eye contact with her. When the mother leaves the room, the secure child typically shows signs of distress; when she returns, the child clearly shows joy and relief, and then quickly returns to exploration and play. A child with an insecure–ambivalent pattern of attachment tends to remain close to the mother and is less willing to explore the unfamiliar room. When the mother leaves, the child tends to cry bitterly, showing extensive signs of distress. When the mother returns, the child typically rejects her attempts at reassurance—for instance, by rejecting the mother's attempts to pick him or her up. A child with an insecure–avoidant pattern of attachment shows apparent signs of ignoring the mother, both during the play session in her presence and when she leaves the room. The child also shows no apparent awareness of her return, but physiological measurement has clearly revealed that these children experience the greatest amount of stress in the Strange Situation (Ainsworth, 1979). Finally, the disorganized pattern of insecure attachment is characteristic of a child who does not show a consistent pattern of behavior in the Strange Situation, but exhibits a confused and even contradictory array of responses (Main & Solomon, 1990).

Bowlby's (1969) description of attachment behaviors suggests that the development of attachment can be disrupted by various conditions that limit or impair the child's behavior. Most important, the different patterns of attachment are considered to be responses to the behaviors of the caregivers. Mothers of children classified as securely attached were shown to display more sensitive caregiving behaviors toward their children than mothers of children classified as insecurely attached (e.g., Weinfield et al., 1999).

Several groups of researchers have investigated attachment patterns in children with autism (Dissanayake & Crossley, 1996, 1997; Oppenheim, Koren-Karie, Dolev, & Yirmiya, 2009; Rogers, Ozonoff, & Maslin-Cole, 1991, 1993; Shapiro, Sherman, Calamari, & Koch, 1987; Sigman & Mundy, 1989; Sigman & Ungerer, 1984; van IJzendoorn et al., 2007; Yirmiya & Sigman, 2001). Most of these studies suggest that the majority of children with ASD form secure attachments with their mothers. In contrast, Rutgers, Bakermans-Kranenburg, van IJzendoorn, and van Berckelaer-Onnes (2004), using both a narrative approach and a meta-analytic approach, examined two questions: whether children with autism have the same chance as children without autism to form a secure attachment relationship with their parents, and whether security of attachment is correlated with mental development and chronological age. Furthermore, these researchers were interested in exploring possible differences in attachment security between children diagnosed with pervasive developmental disorder not otherwise specified (PDD-NOS) and those diagnosed with autistic disorder. In contrast to previous findings and a previous narrative summary (Yirmiya & Sigman, 2001), which suggested that children with autism do form secure attachments to their parents, Rutgers et al.'s meta-analysis revealed that when all studies were pooled together by meta-analytic procedures, (1) children with autism scored about one-half of a standard deviation lower on attachment security than did children without autism (with other diagnoses or with typical development); and (2) low-functioning children with autism showed less security in their attachment than higher-functioning children with autism. These authors suggested that children with autism experience difficulties in their relationship with their parents from very early on.

The same research group (van IJzendoorn et al., 2007) examined parental sensitivity and attachment in a group of children with ASD and concluded that these children showed more attachment disorganization and were less involved with their parents than the other groups of children studied. Several methodological and analytic issues may limit the generalizability of these results, however. First, due to power-related issues, the authors compared the attachment security of the children with ASD with that of *all* other study participants (typically developing children and those with developmental delays were combined in one group). In addition, analyses were uncorrected for multiple comparisons—group differences were marginally significant (e.g., *p*'s = .04–.08) and effect sizes were low. These researchers concluded, in sharp contrast to the authors of previous studies, that children with ASD are less securely attached than are other children. Further investigation and replication are needed to confirm this conclusion. Later studies found that cognitive abilities play a significant role when measuring attachment among young children with ASD (Grzadzinski, Luyster, Gunn Spencer, & Lord, 2012), and that children's attachment security was associated with maternal resolution and insightfulness (Oppenheim, Koren-Karie, Dolev, & Yirmiya, 2012). At the present time, based on the great majority of empirical studies, we suggest that most children with ASD, just like most children with other diagnoses or most typically developing children, are securely attached to their parents—however, we urge the field to continue to explore this important area.

SOCIAL INTERACTIONS WITH PEERS

Following Kanner's (1943) description that the principal deficit of autistic disorder was social, or in his words "extreme autistic aloneness" (p. 242) and/or "the inability to relate themselves in the ordinary way to people and situations," (p. 242) persons with autism have been characterized as exhibiting withdrawal, aloofness, indifference, passivity, lack of cooperation, and lack of engagement in the activities of others. Such social deficits are clearly displayed—from a young age, individuals with autism reveal an inability and/or lack of desire to interact with peers, poor appreciation of social cues, and socially and emotionally inappropriate responses. These characteristics may vary in such individuals, on a continuum from total withdrawal to the ability to communicate and socialize actively (but awkwardly).

In research regarding social interactions with peers, assessments have mainly targeted school-age children with autism, with some tests measuring perceived social relationships and others measuring interactions more directly (Sigman & Ruskin, 1999; Travis & Sigman, 1998). Studies using self-reports, interviews, and projective tests of children's general perceptions of friendship and loneliness, as well as the children's specific perception of their own personal social relationships, demonstrated that higher rates of loneliness were reported by high-functioning children with autism than by children with typical development (Bauminger & Kasari, 2000; Bauminger, Shulman, & Agam, 2003, 2004). Furthermore, high-functioning children with autism who perceived their social relationship with a friend as close, safe, and supportive also perceived themselves as less lonely, similarly to typically developing children (Bauminger et al., 2004).

Other studies using more naturalistic observations of children with autism in their everyday peer relations, during school activities such as free play or lunchtime, detected very few interactions with peers in group settings. The few interactions that did occur were characterized as awkward and unsuccessful, and the children exhibited difficulties in both initiating and responding to the initiations of other children (Hauck, Fein, Waterhouse, & Feinstein, 1995; Stone & Caro-Martinez, 1990; Travis & Sigman, 1998). Sigman and Ruskin (1999) investigated the social interactions with peers of several groups of children with developmental disabilities, including children with autism; they used observations in natural settings (more and less structured), and such measures as the Peer Play Scale (Howes, 1980), as well as teacher reports. Sigman and Ruskin reported that the children with autism were less socially engaged, and more infrequently initiated and accepted play bids with classmates, than either children with Down syndrome or children with developmental delays. Furthermore, using a longitudinal design to detect predictors and correlates of peer competence among individuals with autism, Sigman and Ruskin found that early language and cognitive development, especially joint attention, play, and emotional responsiveness, were associated with later social development and peer interactions.

Cooperative social behavior, fairness, and other interpersonal strategies displayed by individuals with autism have been investigated in various settings and with various procedures. In one study, children with autism did not differ significantly from other groups of children without autism (youngsters with attention-deficit/hyperactivity disorder, oppositional defiant disorder, and typical development) in their cooperative behavior, level of emotional understanding, and aloof behavior (Downs & Smith, 2004). However, the group with autism did show deficits in identifying emotions and displaying socially appropriate behavior (Downs & Smith, 2004; Sally & Hill, 2006). A possible explanation for the null findings was that the participants with autism may have received social skills training, thus making it more difficult to distinguish them from the other groups.

Several studies have investigated social problem-solving ability, considered to be associated with the social difficulties in everyday lives of individuals with ASD. Cognitive processes such as executive functions and ToM abilities (see below), as well as real-life experiences, contribute to everyday problem solving. Such problem-solving capacities include the ability to identify appropriate goals, generate potential courses of action, and make reasoned comparative judgments by looking ahead and evaluating the potential future consequences. Social problem-solving ability can be assessed by using short stories that describe a problem and then ask for possible resolutions of the problem situation. The solutions produced by individuals with Asperger syndrome in this task were shorter and less detailed, as well as less effective, than those of controls without ASD (Goddard, Howlin, Dritschel, & Patel, 2007). Furthermore, adolescents with Asperger syndrome who attempted a novel problem-solving task (videotaped scenarios of awkward everyday situations) had more difficulties in retrieving and recounting pertinent facts and in selecting preferred and efficient solutions than typically developing adolescents did—these findings thus suggested impairment in social appropriateness (Channon, Charman, Heap, Crawford, & Rios, 2001).

Empathy is essential for the ability to socialize and interact adequately, and several reports have highlighted difficulties in empathy as part of the impairment in the social–emotional domain in autism. In one study, children with high-functioning autism performed less well than typically developing children on empathy measures—however, their performance was surprisingly better than expected (Yirmiya, Sigman, Kasari, & Mundy, 1992). Empathy was measured by using videotaped stories about children experiencing different events and emotions; children were asked about their own feelings after watching each story. In more recent research, the empathic ability of high-functioning adults with autism did not significantly differ from that of typically developing participants, as measured during a conversation with a typically developing stranger (Ponnet, Buysse, Roeyers, & De Corte, 2005). In this naturalistic task of dyadic interaction, assessments of empathy tapped both the partner's overt behavioral characteristics (i.e., verbalizations, gazes, positive affect, gestures, and interpersonal distance) and the partner's covert thoughts and feelings (i.e., self-reported unexpressed thoughts and affects). Both groups revealed similar levels of empathic accuracy in inferring the thoughts and feelings of the interaction partner.

Baron-Cohen and Wheelwright (2004) designed the Empathy Quotient (EQ), a 60-item self-report scale including such items as "It is hard for me to see why some things upset people so much" or "I find it easy to put myself in somebody else's shoes." These authors found that adults with Asperger syndrome or high-functioning autism scored significantly lower on the EQ than individuals with typical development matched for age and gender; in the typical development group, women scored significantly higher than men. Lawrence, Shaw, Baker, Baron-Cohen, and David (2004) reported on the EQ's psychometric properties. The EQ was inversely correlated with two domains of the AQ (Baron-Cohen et al., 2001): Social Sensitivity and Sensitive Communication, both of which require empathy. Furthermore, the EQ was positively correlated with the FQ (Baron-Cohen & Wheelwright, 2003), which assesses empathy in the context of close relationships, thus suggesting concurrent validity support for the instrument. Lawrence et al. (2004) indicated the need for future exploration of the EQ's sensitivity and specificity.

The suggestion that the social impairments in individuals with ASD result from an inability to know about the inner world of other people is one of the leading hypotheses regarding the core deficits of autism, termed difficulties in ToM. In the next section, we briefly touch upon this topic.

THEORY OF MIND

One of the current hypotheses about the etiology of autism is that cognitive deficits in ToM affect the understanding of the social world. ToM abilities refer to the awareness that human behaviors result from implicit mental states (i.e., thoughts, beliefs, memories, intents, and emotions) that are not always compatible with objective reality (Wellman, 1990). This awareness is required in social interactions as a guide to reciprocal behavior and all social interactions, from simple communication to more sophisticated behaviors such as deception, empathy, and humor. Many individuals with autism have difficulties in the ability to attribute mental states both to themselves and to others, as well as the ability to utilize these attributions in understanding and predicting behaviors. Indeed, difficulties in ToM are suggested to be core deficits in autism and may underlie the social and communicational impairments characteristic to the disorder.

ToM abilities are described as rich and complex mentalistic conceptions of people that begin to develop between the ages of 3 and 5 (Flavell, 2000; Gopnik, 1990), and thus require an aggregated operationalization. Task batteries and broader ranges of tasks are used to assess different components of ToM across different levels of complexity (Baron-Cohen, 2000; Hughes et al., 2000; Tager-Flusberg, 2001; Wellman, Cross, & Watson, 2001). The classic procedure for evaluating ToM abilities is the well-known, standard "false-belief task." A child is told a story about an object that is moved from its original location to a new location, without the knowledge of the main protagonist. Thus, the child must understand that a person's mental state may contradict reality—that is, a person may hold a false belief. Research has supported the notion that ToM abilities, as operationalized by the false-belief task, are associated with levels of skill in social behavior (Astington & Jenkins, 1995; Lalonde & Chandler, 1995; Watson, Nixon, Wilson, & Capage, 1999). However, this task has shown a ceiling effect for children with a mental age of 6 years—thus, some children with autism, especially those with high-functioning autism, pass these tasks even though they manifest mentalization difficulties in everyday life situations (Klin, 2000; Tager-Flusberg, 2001). Therefore, other tests and procedures must be employed for high-functioning individuals, to increase task sensitivity and detect more subtle difficulties in ToM abilities. For example, the Strange Stories test (Happé, 1994) is considered a more advanced ToM measure, in that it consists of everyday interpersonal situations where people say things they do not literally mean (e.g., ironic or sarcastic statements). At the end of each story, participants are asked a comprehension question and a justification question to test their understanding of the mental state described. Individuals with autism fail to provide context-appropriate mental state explanations for the story characters' nonliteral utterances (Happé, 1994; Happé et al., 1996; Jolliffe & Baron-Cohen, 1999; Vogeley et al., 2001).

Furthermore, individuals with Asperger syndrome or high-functioning autism have difficulties on measures requiring the integration of cross-modal information from faces, voices, and context to understand the mental states and complex emotions of others. For example, Golan and Baron-Cohen (2006) demonstrated that the performance of adults with Asperger syndrome or high-functioning autism was lower than that of adults with typical development on such measures as the Cambridge Mindreading Face–Voice Battery (Golan, Baron-Cohen, & Hill, 2006). This instrument uses short silent clips of adult actors expressing emotions facially, as well as voice recordings of short sentences expressing various emotional intonations, to measure complex emotion and mental state recognition via more naturalistic methods. In a meta-analysis of ToM abilities in individuals with ASD, Yirmiya, Erel, Shaked, and Solomonica-Levi (1998) concluded that deficits in ToM are not unique to such individuals, but that they are more severe than those experienced by individuals with diagnoses other than autism.

CONCLUSIONS

In this chapter, we described the assessment of social difficulties in individuals with ASD. We first presented the screening and diagnostic instruments that are used to assess social deficits as one of the three domains of behaviors constituting the core symptoms of ASD. Next, we discussed relationships that individuals with autism have with significant others—their attachment to their mothers, and their relationships with their agemates.

We would like to end this chapter by returning to the diathesis–stress model with which we opened the chapter, emphasizing both genetic vulnerability and environmental factors.

A dysfunction of mirror neurons, which may underlie the ability to imitate, has been proposed as the biological explanation or "cause" of the social and some other difficulties of individuals with autism. Meltzoff and Prinz (2002) have suggested that the ability to understand another person's feelings, intentions, and actions, which is crucial for relationships with others and for ToM, is associated with the ability to imitate, which develops during the very first weeks and months of life. Impairment in imitation ability is indeed one of the core symptoms included in the Social and Communicative Behaviors domain in DSM-5 criteria for autistic disorder (American Psychiatric Association, 2013). Thus, being able to imitate may be a key to our human understanding of what it means "for others to be like us and for us to be like others" (Meltzoff & Decety, 2003, p. 491). These authors have suggested that behavioral imitation is innate, that it precedes ToM in development and evolution, and that behavioral imitation and its neural substrate provide the mechanism by which ToM and empathy develop in humans. It is not surprising, therefore, that imitation skills have attracted attention in the search for underlying causes of the social difficulties that characterize autism.

A major step forward in understanding the brain mechanisms that may subserve imitation was the discovery of the mirror neuron system in the macaque monkey. Mirror neurons are a particular class of visual–motor neurons that discharge both when a monkey performs a particular action and when it observes another individual (monkey or human) performing a similar action (Di Pellegrino, Fadiga, Fogassi, Gallese, & Rizzolatti, 1992; Gallese, Fadiga, Fogassi, & Rizzolatti, 1996; Rizzolatti, Fadiga, Gallese, & Fogassi, 1996; see Rizzolatti & Craighero, 2004, for a review). Such neurons were originally discovered in area F5 of the monkey premotor cortex, and later in the areas around the intraparietal sulcus (Fogassi et al., 2005). Interestingly, the parietal mirror neurons discharge differently in response to identical motor actions when they are embedded in different action contexts, presumably enabling the observer to understand the intention of the agent. Although, relative to humans, monkeys are not very good imitators (Tomasello & Call, 1997; Iriki, 2006), these neurophysiological properties have led investigators to suggest a connection between the mirror neuron system and imitation, at least in monkeys (see Rizzolatti, Fogassi, & Gallese, 2001, for a review).

The neural circuits connecting regions populated by mirror neurons in monkeys are anatomically interconnected and also connected with the superior temporal sulcus, where higher-order visual neurons respond to seeing the action of others (Jellema, Baker, Wicker, & Perrett, 2000). These circuits seem optimal as precursors of neural mechanisms of imitation in humans as well (Iacoboni, 2005). Indeed, functional imaging studies of imitative behavior in humans have identified similar circuitry in the human brain (Iacoboni et al., 1999; Koski, Iacoboni, Dubeau, Woods, & Mazziotta, 2003). This circuitry comprises the human superior temporal sulcus and the human mirror neuron system—namely, the inferior frontal cortex, which seems particularly important for coding the goal of the imitated action (Koski et al., 2002), and the rostral part of the inferior parietal lobule (Chaminade, Meltzoff, & Decety, 2005; Decety, Chaminade, Grèzes, & Meltzoff, 2002).

There have been mixed findings concerning the association of this cortical network with imitative behavior and ToM (Hamilton, 2013; Sowden, Koehne, Catmur, Dziobek, & Bird, 2016). A functional magnetic resonance imaging study showed that during observation and imitation of facial expressions, children with ASD show less activity in mirror neuron areas (particularly the inferior frontal gyrus—the pars opercularis), as well as in the limbic system, than shown by typically developing children (Dapretto et al., 2006). Moreover, this reduction is correlated with the independently evaluated severity of ASD, which suggests that the malfunctioning of this circuit during a task involving social mirroring may indeed be part of the clinical picture of ASD. However, another study challenged the "broken mirror" hypothesis of autism by demonstrating impaired performance on an imitation task in the presence of normal mirror neuron system activation, assessed via electroencephalogram (Fan, Decety, Yang, Liu, & Cheng, 2010). So at the present time the jury is still out on whether mirror neurons may underlie the deficits in imitation and reciprocal social behavior that are inherent in ASD.

In summary, as reviewed in this chapter, our knowledge of the social deficits characterizing ASD is quite impressive. In addition, we now have more and more screening and diagnostic measures that are applicable across many developmental stages, from infancy to adulthood. Moreover, we are beginning to understand the neural circuitry that may be impaired in individuals with ASD. Based on these data, our next goal should be devising and empirically testing more intensive early intervention programs during the time that the brain shows a high degree of plasticity.

REFERENCES

Adrien, J. L., Lenoir, P., Martineau, J., Perrot, A., Hameury, L., Larmande, C., et al. (1993). Blind ratings of early symptoms of autism based upon family home movies. *Journal of the American Academy of Child and Adolescent Psychiatry, 32*(3), 617–626.

Adrien, J. L., Perrot, A., Hameury, L., Martineau, J., Roux, S., & Sauvage, D. (1991).

Family home movies: Identification of early autistic signs in infants later diagnosed as autistics. *Brain Dysfunction, 4*(6), 355–362.

Ainsworth, M. D. S. (1979). Infant–mother attachment. *American Psychologist, 34*(10), 932–937.

Ainsworth, M. D. S., Blehar, M. C., Waters, E., & Wall, S. (1978). *Patterns of attachment.* Hillsdale, NJ: Erlbaum.

Allison, C., Williams, J., Scott, F., Stott, C., Bolton, P., Baron-Cohen, S., et al. (2007). The Childhood Asperger Syndrome Test (CAST): Test–retest reliability in a high scoring sample. *Autism, 11*(2), 173–185.

American Psychiatric Association. (2013). *Diagnostic and statistical manual of mental disorders* (5th ed.). Arlington, VA: Author.

Astington, J., & Jenkins, J. (1995). Theory of mind development and social understanding. *Cognition and Emotion, 9*(2–3), 151–165.

Austin, E. J. (2005). Personality correlates of the broader autism phenotype as assessed by the Autism Spectrum Quotient (AQ). *Personality and Individual Differences, 38*(2), 451–460.

Baird, G., Charman, T., Baron-Cohen, S., Cox, A., Swettenham, J., Wheelwright, S., et al. (2000). A screening instrument for autism at 18 months of age: A 6-year follow-up study. *Journal of the American Academy of Child and Adolescent Psychiatry, 39*(6), 694–702.

Baird, G., Simonoff, E., Pickles, A., Chandler, S., Loucas, T., Meldrum, D., et al. (2006). Prevalence of disorders of the autism spectrum in a population cohort of children in South Thames: The Special Needs and Autism Project (SNAP). *Lancet, 368*(9531), 210–215.

Baranek, G. T. (1999). Autism during infancy: A retrospective video analysis of sensory–motor and social behaviors at 9–12 months of age. *Journal of Autism and Developmental Disorders, 29*(3), 213–224.

Barbaro, J., & Dissanaake, C. (2013). Early markers of autism spectrum disorders in infants and toddlers prospectively identified in the Social Attention and Communication Study. *Autism, 17*(1), 64–86.

Barnard-Brak, L., Brewer, A., Chesnut, S., Richman, D., & Schaeffer, A. M. (2016). The sensitivity and specificity of the Social Communication Questionnaire for autism spectrum with respect to age. *Autism Research, 9*(8), 838–845.

Baron-Cohen, S. (2000). Theory of mind and autism: A fifteen year review. In S. Baron-Cohen, H. Tager-Flusberg, & D. J. Cohen (Eds.), *Understanding other minds: Perspectives from developmental cognitive neuroscience* (pp. 3–20). Oxford, UK: Oxford University Press.

Baron-Cohen, S., Allen, J., & Gillberg, C. (1992). Can autism be detected at 18 months?: The needle, the haystack, and the CHAT. *British Journal of Psychiatry, 161*(6), 839–843.

Baron-Cohen, S., Cox, A., Baird, G., Swettenham, J., Nightingale, N., Morgan, K., et al. (1996). Psychological markers in the detection of autism in infancy in a large population. *British Journal of Psychiatry, 168*(2), 158–163.

Baron-Cohen, S., & Wheelwright, S. (2003). The Friendship Questionnaire: An investigation of adults with Asperger syndrome or high-functioning autism, and normal sex differences. *Journal of Autism and Developmental Disorders, 33*(5), 509–517.

Baron-Cohen, S., & Wheelwright, S. (2004). The Empathy Quotient: An investigation of adults with Asperger syndrome or high-functioning autism, and normal sex differences. *Journal of Autism and Developmental Disorders, 34*(2), 163–175.

Baron-Cohen, S., Wheelwright, S., Skinner, R., Martin, J., & Clubley, E. (2001).

The Autism-Spectrum Quotient (AQ): Evidence from Asperger syndrome/high-functioning autism, males and females, scientists and mathematicians. *Journal of Autism and Developmental Disorders, 31*(1), 5–17.

Barrera, M. E., & Maurer, D. (1981). Recognition of mother's photographed face by the three-month-old. *Child Development, 52*(2), 558–563.

Bauminger, N., & Kasari, C. (2000). Loneliness and friendship in high-functioning children with autism. *Child Development, 71*(2), 447–456.

Bauminger, N., Shulman, C., & Agam, G. (2003). Peer interaction and loneliness in high-functioning children with autism. *Journal of Autism and Developmental Disorders, 33*(5), 489–507.

Bauminger, N., Shulman, C., & Agam, G. (2004). The link between perceptions of self and of social relationships in high-functioning children with autism. *Journal of Developmental and Physical Disabilities, 16*(2), 193–214.

Bernier, R., Gerdts, J., Munson, J., Dawson, G., & Estes, A. (2012). Evidence for broader autism phenotype characteristics in parents from multiple-incidence autism families. *Autism Research, 5*(1), 13–20.

Berument, S. K., Rutter, M., Lord, C., Pickles, A., & Bailey, A. (1999). Autism Screening Questionnaire: Diagnostic validity. *British Journal of Psychiatry, 175*(5), 444–451.

Bowlby, J. (1969). *Attachment and loss: Vol. 1. Attachment*. New York: Basic Books.

Bryson, S. E., McDermott, C., Rombough, V., Brian, J., & Zwaigenbaum, L. (2000). *The Autism Observation Scale for Infants*. Unpublished manuscript.

Bryson, S. E., Zwaigenbaum, L., McDermott, C., Rombough, V., & Brian, J. (2008). The Autism Observation Scale for Infants: Scale development and reliability data. *Journal of Autism and Developmental Disorders, 38*(4), 731–738.

Chaminade, T., Meltzoff, A. N., & Decety, J. (2005). An fMRI study of imitation: Action representation and body schema. *Neuropsychologia, 43*(1), 115–127.

Channon, S., Charman, T., Heap, J., Crawford, S., & Rios, P. (2001). Real-life-type problem-solving in Asperger's syndrome. *Journal of Autism and Developmental Disorders, 31*(5), 461–469.

Clifford, S. M., & Dissanayake, C. (2008). The early development of joint attention in infants with autistic disorder using home video observations and parental interview. *Journal of Autism and Developmental Disorders, 38*(5), 791–805.

Constantino, J. N. (2012). *Social Responsiveness Scale, Second Edition (SRS-2)*. Torrance, CA: Western Psychological Services.

Clifford, S., Young, R., & Williamson, P. (2007). Assessing the early characteristics of autistic disorder using video analysis. *Journal of Autism and Developmental Disorders, 37*(2), 301–313.

Constantino, J. N., Gruber, C. P., Davis, S., Hayes, S., Passanante, N., & Przybeck, T. (2004). The factor structure of autistic traits. *Journal of Child Psychology and Psychiatry, 45*(4), 719–726.

Constantino, J. N., Lajonchere, C., Lutz, M., Gray, T., Abbacchi, A., McKenna, K., et al. (2006). Autistic social impairment in the siblings of children with pervasive developmental disorders. *American Journal of Psychiatry, 163*(2), 294–296.

Corsello, C., Hus, V., Pickles, A., Risi, S., Cook, E. H., Leventhal, B. L., et al. (2007). Between a ROC and a hard place: Decision making and making decisions about using the SCQ. *Journal of Child Psychology and Psychiatry, 48*(9), 932–940.

Dapretto, M., Davies, M. S., Pfeifer, J. H., Scott, A. A., Sigman, M., Bookheimer, S. Y., et al. (2006). Understanding emotions in others: Mirror neuron dysfunction in children with autism spectrum disorders. *Nature Neuroscience, 9*(1), 28–30.

Dawson, G., Estes, A., Munson, J., Schellenberg, G., Bernier, R., & Abbott, R. (2007). Quantitative assessment of autism symptom-related traits in probands and parents: Broader Phenotype Autism Symptom Scale. *Journal of Autism and Developmental Disorders, 37*(3), 523–536.

Decety, J., Chaminade, T., Grèzes, J., & Meltzoff, A. N. (2002). A PET exploration of the neural mechanisms involved in reciprocal imitation. *NeuroImage, 15*(1), 265–272.

Di Pellegrino, G., Fadiga, L., Fogassi, L., Gallese, V., & Rizzolatti, G. (1992). Understanding motor events: A neurophysiological study. *Experimental Brain Research, 91*(1), 176–180.

Dietz, C., Swinkels, S., van Daalen, E., van Engeland, H., & Buitelaar, J. K. (2006). Screening for autistic spectrum disorders in children aged 14–15 months: II. Population screening with the Early Screening of Autistic Traits Questionnaire (ESAT): Design and general findings. *Journal of Autism and Developmental Disorders, 36*(6), 713–722.

Dissanayake, C., & Crossley, S. A. (1996). Proximity and sociable behaviors in autism: Evidence for attachment. *Journal of Child Psychology and Psychiatry, 37*(2), 149–156.

Dissanayake, C., & Crossley, S. A. (1997). Autistic children's responses to separation and reunion with their mothers. *Journal of Autism and Developmental Disorders, 27*(3), 295–312.

Downs, A., & Smith, T. (2004). Emotional understanding, cooperation, and social behavior in high-functioning children with autism. *Journal of Autism and Developmental Disorders, 34*(6), 625–635.

Duvall, J. A., Lu, A., Cantor, R. M., Todd, R. D., Constantino, J. N., & Geschwind, D. H. (2007). A quantitative trait locus analysis of social responsiveness in multiplex autism families. *American Journal of Psychiatry, 164*(4), 656–662.

Dworzynski, K., Ronald, A., Hayiou-Thomas, M., Rijsdijk, F., Happé, F., Bolton, P. F., et al. (2007). Aetiological relationship between language performance and autistic-like traits in childhood: A twin study. *International Journal of Language and Communication Disorders, 42*(3), 273–292.

Eaves, L. C., Wingert, H., & Ho, H. H. (2006a). Screening for autism: Agreement with diagnosis. *Autism, 10*(3), 229–242.

Eaves, L. C., Wingert, H. D., Ho, H. H., & Mickelson, E. C. R. (2006b). Screening for autism spectrum disorders with the Social Communication Questionnaire. *Journal of Developmental and Behavioral Pediatrics, 27*(2), S95–S103.

Ehlers, S., Gillberg, C., & Wing, L. (1999). A screening questionnaire for Asperger syndrome and other high-functioning autism spectrum disorders in school age children. *Journal of Autism and Developmental Disorders, 29*(2), 129–141.

Ehlers, S., Nydén, A., Gillberg, C., Sandberg, A. D., Dahlgren, S., Hjelmquist, E., et al. (1997). Asperger syndrome, autism and attention disorders: A comparative study of the cognitive profiles of 120 children. *Journal of Child Psychology and Psychiatry, 38*(2), 207–217.

Fan, Y. T., Decety, J., Yang, C. Y., Liu, J. L., & Cheng, Y. (2010). Unbroken mirror neurons in autism spectrum disorders. *Journal of Child Psychology and Psychiatry, 51*(9), 981–988.

Feldman, R. (2007). Parent–infant synchrony and the construction of shared timing: Physiological precursors, developmental outcomes, and risk conditions. *Journal of Child Psychology and Psychiatry, 48*(3–4), 329–354.

Fine, S. E., Weissman, A., Gerdes, M., Pinto-Martin, J., Zackai, E. H.,

McDonald-McGinn, D. M., et al. (2005). Autism spectrum disorders and symptoms in children with molecularly confirmed 22q11.2 deletion syndrome. *Journal of Autism and Developmental Disorders, 35*(4), 461–470.

Flavell, J. H. (2000). Development of children's knowledge about the mental world. *International Journal of Behavioral Development, 24*(1), 15–23.

Fogassi, L., Ferrari, P. F., Gesierich, B., Rozzi, S., Chersi, F., & Rizzolatti, G. (2005). Parietal lobe: From action organization to intention understanding. *Science, 308*(5722), 662–667.

Freitag, C. M., Jensen, K., Elsuni, L., Sachse, M., Herpertz-Dahlmann, B., Schulte-Rüther, M., et al. (2016). Group-based cognitive behavioural psychotherapy for children and adolescents with ASD: The randomized, multicentre, controlled SOSTA-net trial. *Journal of Child Psychology and Psychiatry, 57*(5), 596–605.

Gallese, V., Fadiga, L., Fogassi, L., & Rizzolatti, G. (1996). Action recognition in the premotor cortex. *Brain, 119*(2), 593–609.

Gammer, I., Bedford, R., Elsabbagh, M., Garwood, H., Pasco, G., Tucker, L., et al. (2015). Behavioral markers for autism in infancy: Scores on the Autism Observational Scale for Infants in a prospective study of at-risk siblings. *Infant Behavior and Development, 38*, 107–115.

Goddard, L., Howlin, P., Dritschel, B., & Patel, T. (2007). Autobiographical memory and social problem-solving in Asperger syndrome. *Journal of Autism and Developmental Disorders, 37*(2), 291–300.

Golan, O., & Baron-Cohen, S. (2006). Systemizing empathy: Teaching adults with Asperger syndrome or high-functioning autism to recognize complex emotions using interactive multimedia. *Development and Psychopathology, 18*(2), 591–617.

Golan, O., Baron-Cohen, S., & Hill, J. (2006). The Cambridge Mindreading (CAM) Face–Voice Battery: Testing complex emotion recognition in adults with and without Asperger syndrome. *Journal of Autism and Developmental Disorders, 36*(2), 169–183.

Gopnik, A. (1990). Developing the idea of intentionality: Children's theories of mind. *Canadian Journal of Philosophy, 20*(1), 89–114.

Grzadzinski, R. L., Luyster, R., Spencer, A. G., & Lord, C. (2014). Attachment in young children with autism spectrum disorders: An examination of separation and reunion behaviors with both mothers and fathers. *Autism, 18*(2), 85–96.

Guo, Y. Q., Tang, Y., Rice, C., Lee, L. C., Wang, Y. F., & Cubells, J. F. (2011). Validation of the autism spectrum screening questionnaire, Mandarin Chinese version (CH-ASSQ) in Beijing, China. *Autism, 15*(6), 713–727.

Hamilton, A. F. D. C. (2013). Reflecting on the mirror neuron system in autism: A systematic review of current theories. *Developmental Cognitive Neuroscience, 3*, 91–105.

Hampton, J., & Strand, P. S. (2015). A review of level 2 parent-report instruments used to screen children aged 1.5–5 for autism: A meta-analytic update. *Journal of Autism and Developmental Disorders, 45*(8), 2519–2530.

Happé, F. (1994). Wechsler IQ profile and theory of mind in autism: A research note. *Journal of Child Psychology and Psychiatry, 35*(8), 1461–1471.

Happé, F., Ehlers, S., Fletcher, P., Frith, U., Johansson, M., Gillberg, C., et al. (1996). "Theory of mind" in the brain: Evidence from a PET scan study of Asperger syndrome. *NeuroReport, 8*(1), 197–201.

Hauck, M., Fein, D., Waterhouse, L., & Feinstein, C. (1995). Social initiations by autistic children to adults and other children. *Journal of Autism and Developmental Disorders, 25*(6), 579–595.

Howes, C. (1980). Peer Play Scale as an index of complexity of peer interaction. *Developmental Psychology, 16*(4), 371–372.

Hughes, C., Adlam, A., Happé, F., Jackson, J., Taylor, A., & Caspi, A. (2000). Good test–retest reliability for standard and advanced false-belief tasks across a wide range of abilities. *Journal of Child Psychology and Psychiatry, 41*(4), 483–490.

Iacoboni, M. (2005). Neural mechanisms of imitation. *Current Opinion in Neurobiology, 15*(6), 632–637.

Iacoboni, M., Woods, R. P., Brass, M., Bekkering, H., Mazziotta, J. C., & Rizzolatti, G. (1999). Cortical mechanisms of human imitation. *Science, 286*(5449), 2526–2528.

Iriki, A. (2006). The neural origins and implications of imitation, mirror neurons and tool use. *Current Opinion in Neurobiology, 16*(6), 660–667.

Jellema, T., Baker, C. I., Wicker, B., & Perrett, D. I. (2000). Neural representation for the perception of the intentionality of actions. *Brain and Cognition, 44*(2), 280–302.

Jolliffe, T., & Baron-Cohen, S. (1999). The Strange Stories Test: A replication with high-functioning adults with autism or Asperger syndrome. *Journal of Autism and Developmental Disorders, 29*(5), 395–406.

Jones, E. J. H., Gliga, T., Bedford, R., Charman, T., & Johnson, M. H. (2014). Developmental pathways to autism: A review of prospective studies of infants at risk. *Neuroscience and Biobehavioral Reviews, 39,* 1–33.

Kanner, L. (1943). Autistic disturbances of affective contact. *Nervous Child, 2*(3), 217–250.

Kanner, L. (1949). Nosology and psychodynamics in early childhood autism. *Journal of Orthopsychiatry, 19*(3), 416–426.

Ketelaars, C., Horwitz, E., Sytema, S., Bos, J., Wiersma, D., Minderaa, R., et al. (2008). Brief report: Adults with mild autism spectrum disorders (ASD): Scores on the Autism Spectrum Quotient (AQ) and comorbid psychopathology. *Journal of Autism and Developmental Disorders, 38*(1), 176–180.

Kleinman, J. M., Robins, D. L., Ventola, P. E., Pandey, J., Boorstein, H. C., Esser, E. L., et al. (2008). The Modified Checklist for Autism in Toddlers: A follow-up study investigating the early detection of autism spectrum disorders. *Journal of Autism and Developmental Disorders, 38*(5), 827–839.

Klin, A. (2000). Attributing social meaning to ambiguous visual stimuli in higher-functioning autism and Asperger syndrome: The Social Attribution Task. *Journal of Child Psychology and Psychiatry, 41*(7), 831–846.

Klin, A., Saulnier, C. A., Sparrow, S. S., Cicchetti, D. V., Volkmar, F. R., & Lord, C. (2007). Social and communication abilities and disabilities in higher functioning individuals with autism spectrum disorders: The Vineland and the ADOS. *Journal of Autism and Developmental Disorders, 37*(4), 748–759.

Kopp, S., & Gillberg, C. (2011). The Autism Spectrum Screening Questionnaire (ASSQ)—Revised Extended Version (ASSQ-REV): An instrument for better capturing the autism phenotype in girls?: A preliminary study involving 191 clinical cases and community controls. *Research in Developmental Disabilities, 32*(6), 2875–2888.

Koski, L., Iacoboni, M., Dubeau, M. C., Woods, R. P., & Mazziotta, J. C. (2003). Modulation of cortical activity during different imitative behaviors. *Journal of Neurophysiology, 89*(1), 460–471.

Koski, L., Wohlschläger, A., Bekkering, H., Woods, R. P., Dubeau, M. C., Mazziotta, J. C., et al. (2002). Modulation of motor and premotor activity during imitation of target-directed actions. *Cerebral Cortex, 12*(8), 847–855.

Kurita, H., Koyama, T., & Osada, H. (2005). Autism-Spectrum Quotient—Japanese version and its short forms for screening normally intelligent persons with pervasive developmental disorders. *Psychiatry and Clinical Neurosciences, 59*(4), 490–496.

Lalonde, C., & Chandler, M. (1995). False belief understanding goes to school: On the social–emotional consequences of coming early or late to a first theory of mind. *Cognition and Emotion, 9*(2–3), 167–185.

Landa, R. J., Holman, K. C., & Garrett-Mayer, E. (2007). Social and communication development in toddlers with early and later diagnosis of autism spectrum disorders. *Archives of General Psychiatry, 64*(7), 853–864.

Lawrence, E. J., Shaw, P., Baker, D., Baron-Cohen, S., & David, A. S. (2004). Measuring empathy: Reliability and validity of the Empathy Quotient. *Psychological Medicine, 34*(5), 911–924.

Lee, L., David, A. B., Rusyniak, J., Landa, R., & Newschaffer, C. J. (2007). Performance of the Social Communication Questionnaire in children receiving preschool special education services. *Research in Autism Spectrum Disorders, 1*(2), 126–138.

Li, G., Du, Y., Luan, F., Li, M., & Ousley, O. (2017). IQ profiles and clinical symptoms of Chinese school-aged boys with autism spectrum disorder. *European Journal of Psychiatry, 31*(2), 59–65.

Lord, C., Rutter, M., DiLavore, P. C., Risi, S., Gotham, K., & Bishop, S. L. (2012). *Autism Diagnostic Observation Schedule, 2nd edition (ADOS-2).* Los Angeles: Western Psychological Services.

Losche, G. (1990). Sensorimotor and action development in autistic children from infancy to early childhood. *Journal of Child Psychology and Psychiatry, 31*(5), 749–761.

Maestro, S., Muratori, F., Cavallaro, M. C., Pecini, C., Cesari, A., Paziente, A., et al. (2005). How young children treat objects and people: An empirical study of the first year of life in autism. *Child Psychiatry and Human Development, 35*(4), 383–396.

Maestro, S., Muratori, F., Cavallaro, M. C, Pei, F., Stern, D. D., Glose, B., et al. (2002). Attentional skills during the first 6 months of age in autism spectrum disorder. *Journal of the American Academy of Child and Adolescent Psychiatry, 41*(10), 1239–1245.

Main, M., & Solomon, J. (1990). Procedures for identifying infants as disorganized/disoriented during the Ainsworth Strange Situation. In M. T. Greenberg, D. Cicchetti, & E. M. Cummings (Eds.), *Attachment in the preschool years* (pp. 121–160). Chicago: University of Chicago Press.

Mattila, M. L., Jussila, K., Linna, S. L., Kielinen, M., Bloigu, R., Kuusikko-Gauffin, S., et al. (2012). Validation of the Finnish Autism Spectrum Screening Questionnaire (ASSQ) for clinical settings and total population screening. *Journal of Autism and Developmental Disorders, 42*(10), 2162–2180.

Mayes, S. D., & Calhoun, S. L. (2003). Analysis of WISC-III, Stanford–Binet:IV, and academic achievement test scores in children with autism. *Journal of Autism and Developmental Disorders, 33*(3), 329–341.

Mayes, S. D., & Calhoun, S. L. (2004). Similarities and differences in Wechsler Intelligence Scale for Children—Third Edition (WISC-III) profiles: Support for subtest analysis in clinical referrals. *Clinical Neurophysiology, 18*(4), 559–572.

McDuffie, A., Yoder, P., & Stone, W. (2005). Prelinguistic predictors of vocabulary in children with autism spectrum disorders. *Journal of Speech, Language, and Hearing Research, 48*(5), 1080–1097.

Meltzoff, A. N., & Decety, J. (2003). What imitation tells us about social cognition: A rapprochement between developmental psychology and cognitive neuroscience. *Philosophical Transactions of the Royal Society of London, Series B, 358*(1431), 491–500.

Meltzoff, A. N., & Moore, M. K. (1977). Imitation of facial and manual gestures by human neonates. *Science, 198*(4312), 75–78.

Meltzoff, A. N., & Moore, M. K. (1999). Persons and representations: Why infant imitation is important for theories of human development. In J. Nadel & G. Butterworth (Eds.), *Imitation in infancy* (pp. 9–35). Cambridge, UK: Cambridge University Press.

Meltzoff, A. N., & Prinz, W. (2002). *The imitative mind: Development, evolution and brain bases.* Cambridge, UK: Cambridge University Press.

Mundy, P., & Gomes, A. (1998). Individual differences in joint attention skill development in the second year. *Infant Behavior and Development, 21*(3), 469–482.

Mundy, P., Hogan, A., & Doehring, P. (1996). *A preliminary manual for the abridged Early Social-Communication Scales.* Coral Gables, FL: University of Miami. Available from *www.psy.miami.edu/faculty/pmundy.*

Mundy, P., Sigman, M., & Kasari, C. (1990). A longitudinal study of joint attention and language development in autistic children. *Journal of Autism and Developmental Disorders, 20*(1), 115–128.

Mundy, P., Sigman, M., Ungerer, J., & Sherman, T. (1986). Defining the social deficits of autism: The contribution of non-verbal communication measures. *Journal of Child Psychology and Psychiatry, 27*(5), 657–669.

Oppenheim, D., Koren-Karie, N., Dolev, S., & Yirmiya, N. (2009). Maternal insightfulness and resolution of the diagnosis are associated with secure attachment in preschoolers with autism spectrum disorders. *Child Development, 80*(2), 519–527.

Oppenheim, D., Koren-Karie, N., Dolev, S., & Yirmiya, N. (2012). Maternal sensitivity mediates the link between maternal insightfulness/resolution and child–mother attachment: The case of children with autism spectrum disorder. *Attachment and Human Development, 14*(6), 567–584.

Osterling, J. A., & Dawson, G. (1994). Early recognition of children with autism: A study of first birthday home videotapes. *Journal of Autism and Developmental Disorders, 24*(3), 247–257.

Osterling, J. A., Dawson, G., & Munson, J. A. (2002). Early recognition of 1-year-old infants with autism spectrum disorder versus mental retardation. *Development and Psychopathology, 14*(2), 239–251.

Ozonoff, S., Iosif, A. M., Young, G. S., Hepburn, S., Thompson, M., Colombi, C., et al. (2011). Onset patterns in autism: Correspondence between home video and parent report. *Journal of the American Academy of Child and Adolescent Psychiatry, 50*(8), 796–806.

Pascalis, O., de Schonen, S., Morton, J., Deruelle, C., & Fabre-Grenet, M. (1995). Mothers' face recognition by neonates: A replication and an extension. *Infant Behavior and Development, 18*(1), 79–86.

Ponnet, K., Buysse, A., Roeyers, H., & De Corte, K. (2005). Empathic accuracy in adults with a pervasive developmental disorder during an unstructured conversation with a typically developing stranger. *Journal of Autism and Developmental Disorders, 35*(5), 585–600.

Posserud, M. B., Lundervold, A. J., & Gillberg, C. (2006). Autistic features in a total population of 7–9-year-old children assessed by the ASSQ (Autism Spectrum

Screening Questionnaire). *Journal of Child Psychology and Psychiatry, 47*(2), 167–175.

Reiersen, A. M., Constantino, J. N., Volk, H. E., & Todd, R. D. (2007). Autistic traits in a population-based ADHD twin sample. *Journal of Child Psychology and Psychiatry, 48*(5), 464–472.

Reznick, J. S., Baranek, G. T., Reavis, S., Watson, L. R., & Crais, E. R. (2007). A parent-report instrument for identifying one-year-olds at risk for an eventual diagnosis of autism: The First Year Inventory. *Journal of Autism and Developmental Disorders, 37*(9), 1691–1710.

Rizzolatti, G., & Craighero, L. (2004). The mirror-neuron system. *Annual Review of Neuroscience, 27,* 169–192.

Rizzolatti, G., Fadiga, L., Gallese, V., & Fogassi, L. (1996). Premotor cortex and the recognition of motor actions. *Cognitive Brain Research, 3*(2), 131–141.

Rizzolatti, G., Fogassi, L., & Gallese, V. (2001). Neurophysiological mechanisms underlying the understanding and imitation of action. *Nature Reviews Neuroscience, 2*(9), 661–670.

Robins, D. L., Casagrande, K., Barton, M., Chen, C.-M. A., Dumont-Mathieu, T., & Fein, D. (2014). Validation of the Modified Checklist for Autism in Toddlers, revised with follow up (M-CHAT-R/F). *Pediatrics, 133*(1), 37–43.

Robins, D. L., & Dumont-Mathieu, T. M. (2006). Early screening for autism spectrum disorders: Update on the Modified Checklist for Autism in Toddlers and other measures. *Journal of Developmental and Behavioral Pediatrics, 27*(2), S111–S119.

Robins, D. L., Fein, D., Barton, M. L., & Green, J. A. (2001). The Modified Checklist for Autism in Toddlers: An initial study investigating the early detection of autism and pervasive developmental disorders. *Journal of Autism and Developmental Disorders, 31*(2), 131–144.

Rodrigue, J. R., Morgan, S. B., & Geffken, G. R. (1991). A comparative evaluation of adaptive behavior in children and adolescents with autism, Down syndrome, and normal development. *Journal of Autism and Developmental Disorders, 21*(2), 187–196.

Rogers, S. J., Ozonoff, S., & Maslin-Cole, C. (1991). A comparative study of attachment behavior in young children with autism and other psychiatric disorders. *Journal of the American Academy of Child and Adolescent Psychiatry, 30*(3), 483–488.

Rogers, S. J., Ozonoff, S., & Maslin-Cole, C. (1993). Developmental aspects of attachment behavior in young children with developmental disorders. *Journal of the American Academy of Child and Adolescent Psychiatry, 32*(6), 1274–1282.

Ronald, A., Happé, F., Bolton, P., Butcher, L. M., Price, T. S., Wheelwright, S., et al. (2006). Genetic heterogeneity between the three components of the autism spectrum: A twin study. *Journal of the American Academy of Child and Adolescent Psychiatry, 45*(6), 691–699.

Ronald, A., Happé, F., Price, T. S., Baron-Cohen, S., & Plomin, R. (2006). Phenotypic and genetic overlap between autistic traits at the extremes of the general population. *Journal of the American Academy of Child and Adolescent Psychiatry, 45*(10), 1206–1214.

Rutgers, A. H., Bakermans-Kranenburg, M. J., van IJzendoorn, M. H., & van Berckelaer-Onnes, I. A. (2004). Autism and attachment: A meta-analytic review. *Journal of Child Psychology and Psychiatry, 45*(6), 1123–1134.

Rutter, M., Bailey, A., & Lord, C. (2003). *Social Communication Questionnaire.* Los Angeles: Western Psychological Services.

Rutter, M., Le Couteur, A., & Lord, C. (2003). *Autism Diagnostic Interview—Revised (ADI-R)*. Los Angeles: Western Psychological Services.

Sally, D., & Hill, E. (2006). The development of interpersonal strategy: Autism, theory-of-mind, cooperation and fairness. *Journal of Economic Psychology, 27*(1), 73–97.

Sameroff, A. (2000). Developmental systems and psychopathology. In A. Sameroff, M. Lewis, & S. Miller (Eds.), *Handbook of developmental psychopathology* (2nd ed., pp. 23–40). New York: Kluwer Academic/Plenum.

Scheeren, A. M., & Stauder, J. E. A. (2008). Broader autism phenotype in parents of autistic children: Reality or myth? *Journal of Autism and Developmental Disorders, 38*(2), 276–287.

Scott, F., Baron-Cohen, S., Bolton, P., & Brayne, C. (2002). The CAST (Childhood Asperger Syndrome Test): Preliminary development of a UK screen for mainstream primary-school-age children. *Autism, 6*(1), 9–31.

Seibert, J. M., Hogan, A. E., & Mundy, P. C. (1982). Assessing interactional competencies: The Early Social-Communication Scales. *Infant Mental Health Journal, 3*(4), 244–245.

Seligman, M. E. P. (1970). On the generality of the laws of learning. *Psychological Review, 77*(5), 406–418.

Shapiro, T., Sherman, M., Calamari, G., & Koch, D. (1987). Attachment in autism and other developmental disorders. *Journal of the American Academy of Child and Adolescent Psychiatry, 26*(4), 480–484.

Siegel, D. J., Minshew, N. J., & Goldstein, G. (1996). Wechsler IQ profiles in diagnosing high-functioning autism. *Journal of Autism and Developmental Disorders, 26*(4), 389–406.

Sigman, M., & Mundy, P. (1989). Social attachment in autistic children. *Journal of the American Academy of Child and Adolescent Psychiatry, 28*(1), 74–81.

Sigman, M., & Ruskin, E. (1999). Continuity and change in the social competence of children with autism, Down syndrome, and developmental delays. *Monographs of the Society for Research in Child Development, 64*(1), 1–114.

Sigman, M., & Ungerer, J. A. (1984). Attachment behaviors in autistic children. *Journal of Autism and Developmental Disorders, 14*(3), 231–244.

Sowden, S., Koehne, S., Catmur, C., Dziobek, I., & Bird, G. (2016). Intact automatic imitation and typical spatial compatibility in autism spectrum disorder: Challenging the broken mirror theory. *Autism Research, 9*(2), 292–300.

Sparrow, S. S., Cicchetti, D. V., & Balla, D. A. (2005). *Vineland Adaptive Behavior Scales, Second Edition (Vineland–II)*. Circle Pines, MN: American Guidance Service.

Stone, W. L., & Caro-Martinez, L. (1990). Naturalistic observations of spontaneous communication in autistic children. *Journal of Autism and Developmental Disorders, 20*(4), 437–453.

Stone, W. L., Coonrod, E. E., Turner, L. M., & Pozdol, S. L. (2004). Psychometric properties of the STAT for early autism screening. *Journal of Autism and Developmental Disorders, 34*(6), 691–701.

Stone, W. L., & Ousley, O. Y. (1997). *STAT manual: Screening Tool for Autism in Two-Year-Olds*. Unpublished manuscript, Vanderbilt University, Nashville, TN.

Swinkels, S., Dietz, C., van Daalen, E., Kerkhof, I. H. G. M., van Engeland, H., & Buitelaar, J. K. (2006). Screening for autistic spectrum disorders in children aged 14 to 15 months: I. The development of the Early Screening of Autistic Traits Questionnaire (ESAT). *Journal of Autism and Developmental Disorders, 36*(6), 723–732.

Tager-Flusberg, H. (2001). A reexamination of the theory of mind hypothesis of autism. In J. A. Burack, T. Charman, N. Yirmiya, & P. R. Zelazo (Eds.), *The development of autism: Perspectives from theory and research* (pp. 173–193). Mahwah, NJ: Erlbaum.

Tomanik, S. S., Pearson, D. A., Loveland, K. A., Lane, D. M., & Shaw, J. B. (2007). Improving the reliability of autism diagnoses: Examining the utility of adaptive behavior. *Journal of Autism and Developmental Disorders, 37*(5), 921–928.

Tomasello, M., & Call, J. (1997). *Primate cognition.* Oxford, UK: Oxford University Press.

Travis, L. L., & Sigman, M. (1998). Social deficits and interpersonal relationships in autism. *Mental Retardation and Developmental Disabilities, 4*(2), 65–72.

Turner-Brown, L. M., Baranek, G. T., Reznick, J. S., Watson, L. R., & Crais, E. R. (2013). The First Year Inventory: A longitudinal follow-up of 12-month-old to 3-year-old children. *Autism, 17*(5), 527–540.

van IJzendoorn, M. H., Rutgers, A. H., Bakermans-Kranenburg, M. J., Swinkels, S. H. N., van Daalen, E., Dietz, C., et al. (2007). Parental sensitivity and attachment in children with autism spectrum disorder: Comparison with children with mental retardation, with language delays, and with typical development. *Child Development, 78*(2), 597–608.

Vogeley, K., Bussfeld, P., Newen, A., Herrmann, S., Happé, F., Falkai, P., et al. (2001). Mind reading: Neural mechanisms of theory of mind and self-perspective. *NeuroImage, 14*(1), 170–181.

Volkmar, E. R., Sparrow, S. S., Gourgreau, D., Cicchetti, D. V, Paul, R., & Cohen, D. J. (1987). Social deficits in autism: An operational approach using the Vineland Adaptive Behavior Scales. *Journal of the American Academy of Child and Adolescent Psychiatry, 26*(2), 156–161.

Wakabayashi, A., Baron-Cohen, S., Wheelwright, S., & Tojo, Y. (2006). The Autism-Spectrum Quotient (AQ) in Japan: A cross-cultural comparison. *Journal of Autism and Developmental Disorders, 36*(2), 263–270.

Watson, A. C., Nixon, C. L., Wilson, A., & Capage, L. (1999). Social interaction skills and the theory of mind in young children. *Developmental Psychology, 35*(2), 386–391.

Watson, L. R., Baranek, G. T., Crais, E. R., Reznick, J. S., Dykstra, J., & Perryman, T. (2007). The First Year Inventory: Retrospective parent responses to a questionnaire designed to identify one-year-olds at risk for autism. *Journal of Autism and Developmental Disorders, 37*(1), 49–61.

Wechsler, D. (2014). *Wechsler Intelligence Scale for Children—Fifth Edition (WISC-V).* San Antonio, TX: Psychological Corporation.

Weinfield, N. S., Sroufe, L. A., Egeland, B., & Carlson, E. (1999). The nature of individual differences in infant–caregiver attachment. In J. Cassidy & P. R. Shaver (Eds.), *Handbook of attachment: Theory, research, and clinical applications* (pp. 64–88). New York: Guilford Press.

Wellman, H. (1990). *The child's theory of mind.* Cambridge, MA: MIT Press.

Wellman, H., Cross, D., & Watson, J. (2001). Meta-analysis of theory-of-mind development: The truth about false belief. *Child Development, 72*(3), 655–684.

Werner, E., Dawson, G., Osterling, J., & Dinno, N. (2000). Brief report: Recognition of autism spectrum disorder before one year of age: A retrospective study based on home videotapes. *Journal of Autism and Developmental Disorders, 30*(2), 157–162.

Wetherby, A. M., Allen, L., Cleary, J., Kublin, K., & Goldstein, H. (2002). Validity and reliability of the Communication and Symbolic Behavior Scales Developmental Profile with very young children. *Journal of Speech, Language, and Hearing Research, 45*(6), 1202–1218.

Wetherby, A. M., Goldstein, H., Cleary, J., Allen, L., & Kublin, K. (2003). Early identification of children with communication disorders: Concurrent and predictive validity of the CSBS developmental profile. *Infants and Young Children, 16*(2), 161–174.

Wetherby, A. M., & Prizant, B. (1993). *Communication and Symbolic Behavior Scales—Normed Edition*. Baltimore: Brookes.

Wetherby, A. M., & Prizant, B. (2002). *Communication and Symbolic Behavior Scales Developmental Profile—First Normed Edition*. Baltimore: Brookes.

Wetherby, A. M., Watt, N., Morgan, L., & Shumway, S. (2007). Social communication profiles of children with autism spectrum disorders late in the second year of life. *Journal of Autism and Developmental Disorders, 37*(5), 960–975.

Wetherby, A. M., Woods, J., Allen, L., Cleary, J., Dickinson, H., & Lord, C. (2004). Early indicators of autism spectrum disorders in the second year of life. *Journal of Autism and Developmental Disorders, 34*(5), 473–493.

Williams, J., Allison, C., Scott, F., Stott, C., Bolton, P., Baron-Cohen, S., et al. (2006). The Childhood Asperger Syndrome Test (CAST): Test–retest reliability. *Autism, 10*(4), 415–427.

Williams, J., Scott, F., Stott, C., Allison, C., Bolton, P., Baron-Cohen, S., et al. (2005). The CAST (Childhood Asperger Syndrome Test): Test accuracy. *Autism, 9*(1), 45–68.

Woodbury-Smith, M. R., Robinson, J., Wheelwright, S., & Baron-Cohen, S. (2005). Screening adults for Asperger syndrome using the AQ: A preliminary study of its diagnostic validity in clinical practice. *Journal of Autism and Developmental Disorders, 35*(3), 331–335.

Yaari, M., Yitzhak, N., Harel, A., Friedlander, E., Bar-Oz, B., Eventov-Friedman, S., et al. (2016). Stability of early risk assessment for autism spectrum disorder in preterm infants. *Autism, 20*(7), 856–867.

Yang, S., Paynter, J. M., & Gilmore, L. (2016). Vineland Adaptive Behavior Scales: II. Profile of young children with ASD. *Journal of Autism and Developmental Disorders, 46*(1), 64–73.

Yirmiya, N., Erel, O., Shaked, M., & Solomonica-Levi, D. (1998). Meta-analyses comparing theory of mind abilities of individuals with autism, individuals with mental retardation, and normally developing individuals. *Psychological Bulletin, 124*(3), 283–307.

Yirmiya, N., & Ozonoff, S. (2007). The very early autism phenotype. *Journal of Autism and Developmental Disorders, 37*(1), 1–11.

Yirmiya, N., & Sigman, M. D. (2001). Attachment in autism. In J. Richter & S. Coates (Eds.), *Autism: Putting together the pieces* (pp. 53–63). London: Jessica Kingsley.

Yirmiya, N., Sigman, M. D., Kasari, C., & Mundy, P. (1992). Empathy and cognition in high-functioning children with autism. *Child Development, 63*(1), 150–160.

Zwaigenbaum, L., Bryson, S., Rogers, T., Roberts, W., Brian, J., & Szatmari, P. (2005). Behavioral manifestations of autism in the first year of life. *International Journal of Developmental Neuroscience, 23*(2), 143–152.

CHAPTER SEVEN

Assessing Speech, Language, and Communication in Autism Spectrum Disorder

Rhea Paul
Kaitlyn P. Wilson

In his initial descriptions of autism, Kanner (1943, 1946) highlighted atypical patterns of communication and they continue to be central to the DSM-5 (American Psychiatric Association, 2013) diagnosis of autism spectrum disorder (ASD). Whether verbal or nonverbal, communication deficits are a core symptom of ASD. Some people with ASD may begin talking at a later age than is typical, or they may remain nonverbal for life; others may gain minimally productive verbal skills, learning to produce words and sentences, but having difficulty using them effectively. This chapter explores how communication and its components (i.e., speech, language, pragmatics) are assessed for the dual purpose of establishing an ASD diagnosis and determining appropriate communication intervention goals for children with ASD. Before we begin this discussion, however, a group of key terms associated with this domain of functioning must be defined. These terms, and their relationships, are depicted graphically in Figure 7.1.

"Communication" is an overarching term that refers to all forms of sending and receiving messages, whether through use of spoken language, gestures, body language, written language, or sign language. "Language" represents a specific type of communication involving the formulation of ideas and messages through rule-based combinations of words. "Speech" is the expression of language through the use of sounds produced by oral gestures. It is important to remember that other modes besides speech are used

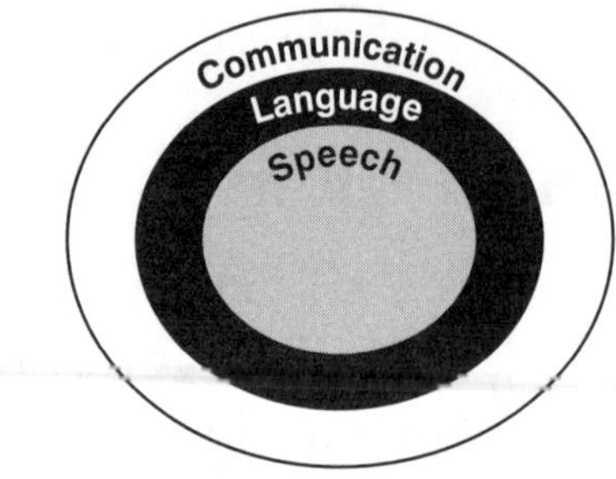

FIGURE 7.1. Domains of communication.

to express language-based ideas, such as writing or sign language. In the following discussion of communication and its assessment in children with ASD, these distinctions will be important to consider, as assessments of communication, language, and speech are distinct processes. In fact, ASD provides a useful model for understanding the difference between communication and language, as individuals with ASD may attain language skills but be unable to use language for the purpose of communicating (Kim, Paul, Tager-Flusberg, & Lord, 2014).

ASSESSING PRELINGUISTIC COMMUNICATION SKILLS

In the first years of life, children may show early signs of the communication deficits characteristic of ASD—however, ASD diagnoses are generally not made until the ages of 2–4 years (Centers for Disease Control and Prevention, 2016; Chawarska, Klin, Paul, & Volkmar, 2007; Woods & Wetherby, 2003). Thus, the assessment of communication skills in the first few years of life is based on the atypical development or presence of behaviors found in retrospective studies to be associated with a confirmed diagnosis of ASD later in early childhood (Klin, Volkmar, & Sparrow, 1992; Volkmar, Stier, & Cohen, 1985; Baranek, 1999; Maestro et al., 2002; Osterling, Dawson, & Munson, 2002), though few studies have relied on direct observations (e.g., Charman et al., 2003; Lord & Risi, 2000; Wetherby et al., 2004). Research has suggested that atypical development of certain early communication skills is highly correlated with ASD risk. These include deficits in attention to people, social smiling, and sharing of affect, as well as in preverbal forms of social communication, including use of gaze and gestures for sharing attention to objects (joint attention; e.g., Baron-Cohen et al., 1996; Charman et al., 1997; Lord, 1995; Mundy, Sigman, Ungerer, & Sherman, 1987; Swettenham et al., 1998; Wetherby et al., 2004). Communication impairments include limited responsiveness to speech, delayed development of language, and the use of others' bodies as tools (Lord, 1995; Wetherby et al., 2004). In one such study, Baron-Cohen et al. (1996) linked the absence of three key early communication skills (i.e., protodeclarative pointing, gaze monitoring, and pretend play) to a reliable risk of ASD at 18 months of age.

Assessing early communication skills can be difficult, as it requires analysis of many subtle behaviors and careful observation of the presence and nature (e.g., flexibility, appropriateness) of various aspects of communication. The communicative aspects assessed are typically considered within the following categories: the *frequency* of communicative attempts, the *functions* of these attempts, the *means* used to accomplish communicative goals, and the level of *responsiveness* to others' communicative attempts. These communicative aspects are discussed below, and within each discussion, the following considerations are outlined: signs of typical communication development, signs of possible ASD, and assessment methods.

Frequency of Communication

According to developmental benchmarks, typically developing children initiate communication at a rate of two acts/minute at 12 months, and seven acts/minute at 24 months (Chapman, 2000). As these data illustrate, the second year of life is typically accompanied by a large increase in the number of communicative acts, whether preverbal gestures, vocalizations, or words. In children with ASD, a depressed rate of preverbal communicative acts (Wetherby, Prizant, & Hutchinson, 1998) is exhibited during this early developmental period. In addition, children with ASD often fail to engage others in communication surrounding interests or enjoyment, which results in a lower frequency of communicative attempts than that of typically developing children.

Assessing the frequency of communication involves recording the number of intentional communicative acts made by a child within a certain time period or communicative context. For example, if a child and caregiver are engaged in a caregiving routine (e.g., dressing, bathing, feeding) for a specified amount of time (generally 10–15 minutes for the purpose of assessment), the number of intentional communicative acts initiated by the child is recorded by an observer. During this observation, the observer should count only those acts initiated by the child, and only those that meet the criteria for intentional communication—that is, they must:

- Consist of a gesture, vocalization, or verbal production.
- Be directed toward another person, with gaze, touch, gesture, or movement toward the person.
- Be interpretable as conveying a message or communicative function,

such as a request, protest, or direction of attention of a person to create joint attention or engage in social interaction.

Several measures have been developed that provide specific opportunities, or temptations, for a child to communicate. For example, the Communication and Symbolic Behavior Scales (CSBS; Wetherby & Prizant, 2002) tempts the child to communicate a request for help (e.g., gesture, vocalization, gaze) when he or she is unable to open a container with a desired object inside. The number of times the child responds to such communicative opportunities is then observed and recorded. Additional examples of scales that make use of this format include the Early Social Communication Scales (ESCS; Mundy, Hogan, & Doehring, 1996) and the Prelinguistic Communication Assessment (PCA; Stone, Ousley, Yoder, Hogan, & Hebpurn, 1997).

Recently, new methods for automated recording and analysis of child vocalizations have been developed (Oller et al., 2010; Warlaumont, Richards, Gilkerson, & Oller, 2014). These methods permit longer recordings, in more naturalistic settings (e.g., the home), and thus may afford new insights into speech development in early childhood. While these methods are much more efficient than detailed transcriptions of child vocalizations, their validity remains to be firmly established (e.g., how closely the number of communicative acts generated by the automated software corresponds with numbers transcribed by trained observers, how well the software parses child vocalizations from adult vocalizations and environmental sounds) and they do not measure communicative intentionality.

Functions of Communication

Both "protoimperative" (acts intended to regulate others' actions) and "protodeclarative" (acts intended to create social interaction or joint attention) communicative functions are seen in typically developing children by 18 months of age. Bruner (1977) groups these intentions into three general functions:

1. *Regulatory*: Requests and protests.
2. *Comments*: Calling attention to objects and activities of interest, for the purpose of creating joint attention.
3. *Social interaction*: Showing off, calling attention to oneself, or seeking comfort or attention from others.

In children ages 18–24 months, more advanced communicative functions typically emerge, and an understanding of conversational structure becomes apparent. During this stage, typically developing children begin to attend more to others' speech and to acknowledge the back-and-forth nature of discourse. As such, the communicative functions acquired at this time are what Chapman (1981, 2000) called "discourse functions." These discourse functions include the following:

1. *Requests for information*: Using language to gain information about the world. At the earliest stages, this function may consist of requests for the names of things (i.e., labels: "Whazzat?"). At a later stage, these requests may begin to include "wh-" words, rising intonation contours, or both.
2. *Acknowledgments*: Confirming that the previous utterance was received, through such behaviors as verbal imitation, nonverbal mimicking of intonation pattern, or head nods.
3. *Answers*: Responding to another person's request for information with a semantically appropriate remark.

Compared with typically developing children, children with ASD exhibit a limited range of communicative behaviors. Children with ASD primarily use regulatory functions (i.e., requests or protests), with limited use of communication for the purposes of social interaction, commenting, or establishing joint attention (Mundy & Stella, 2000). This finding reflects Woods and Wetherby's (2003) similar conclusion that most children with ASD have early deficits in the use of joint attention.

The methods suggested for assessing the frequency of communicative acts may be applied similarly to the assessment of communicative functions. The purpose of assessing communicative functions is to determine the range of such functions being utilized by the child. This can be accomplished through observation of the child in various communicative contexts, whether caregiving activities or play situations. Data can be recorded by marking the frequency of each of the functions listed above, or by using one of the communication scales cited earlier.

Means of Communication

Early means of communication include gaze, "babbling" (i.e., speech-like vocalizations), and conventional gestures (such as pointing, showing, and waving). Infants generally begin using gestures such as pointing between the ages of 6 and 10 months (Zinober & Martlew, 1985). Use of babbling and "protowords" (i.e., consistent patterns of vocalization used to express meaning) are also expected before the onset of speech.

Research suggests that children with ASD use nonconventional communicative means as infants and toddlers. Instead of using a conventional gesture, such as pointing, to show or ask for an object, a child with ASD may attempt to achieve the same communicative purpose through use of nonconventional gestures (Dawson, Meltzoff, Osterling, Rinaldi, & Brown, 1998; Stone et al., 1997). An example of this nonconventional means is a child who wants a pacifier and, instead of pointing to request the object, pulls the caregiver's hand to the pacifier. Children with ASD have also been found to have lower rates of babbling and other preverbal vocalizations, as well as atypical vocalizations (Esposito, Nakazawa, Venuti, & Bornstein, 2013; Patten et al., 2014; Sheinkopf, Mundy, Kimbrough-Oller, & Steffens, 2000).

Assessing a child's means of expressing communicative intent can be accomplished during structured observation of caregiver–child play, and can be evaluated concurrently with communicative frequency and function. Paul (2007) has provided a framework for structuring and compiling the observational data derived from this context (see Figure 7.2). This framework requires a record of each communicative act within the cell defined by its function and means. The frequency and range of both functions and means can be determined via this method when these data are compared to the frequency of communicative acts recorded. Measures such as the CSBS, ESCS, and PCA provide additional means for recording this type of observation, when structured communicative temptations are offered.

Responsiveness to Communication

By 12 months of age, typically developing children respond to their names by looking toward the speaker. By this time, children also have a receptive vocabulary of about 50 words (Chapman, 2000), and soon after, they produce their first word or approximation.

Nadig et al. (2007) found that a lack of response to hearing one's name is present in many but not all infants who are later diagnosed with ASD, and they suggest that a reduced response to one's name could also be a characteristic of the broader autism phenotype during infancy. Osterling and Dawson (1994) agree that infants and toddlers with ASD exhibit reduced responsiveness to their names and to speech in general. Parents of children with this reduced responsiveness may suspect deafness at first—therefore, a hearing evaluation is often the first step to an ASD diagnosis in young children.

Responsiveness can be assessed by observing a caregiver–child play session, by using the communicative temptations listed below (see the "Obtaining a Communication Profile" section), or by using the CSBS or ESCS. During these structured opportunities, the observer will count the number of times the child shows a reaction to communications directed to him or her. This method results in a record of the child's response to gestural and verbal bids for attention and interaction.

	Function of communication							
	Request	Protest	Sharing enjoyment	Comment/ joint attention	Initiating social interaction	Responding to gesture	Responding to name	Responding to speech
Gaze to person								
Three-point gaze*								
Conventional gesture								
Unconventional gesture								
Typical vocalization								
Unusual vocalization								
Echo								
Spontaneous speech								

*Child looks at object, at person, then back at object; or at person, at object, then back at person.

FIGURE 7.2. Summary of communication assessment for prelinguistic children. Adapted from Paul (2007). Copyright © 2007 C. V. Mosby, a division of Elsevier. Adapted by permission.

SPOKEN LANGUAGE ASSESSMENT IN CHILDREN WITH ASD

In 2001, the National Research Council reported that about 50% of children diagnosed with ASD would acquire functional speech. In 2005, Tager-Flusberg, Paul, and Lord estimated that more than 60% of children with ASD possessed spoken language. Recent emphasis on early communication intervention may contribute to current improvements in the percentage of these children who acquire speech. Wodka, Mathy, and Kalb (2013), for example, reported that over 70% of children with severe ASD acquired at least phrase speech by 8 years of age. In general, when children with ASD acquire spoken language, they do so by the age of 6 (Paul & Cohen, 1984; Tager-Flusberg et al., 2005), although there have been reported cases of nonverbal children acquiring language during adolescence (Mirenda, 2003; Windsor, Doyle, & Siegel, 1994). Children with ASD tend to show more severe receptive language difficulties than do children with other language disorders (Paul, Chawarska, Klin, & Volkmar, 2007) and their receptive skills may lag behind expressive language (Maljaars, Noens, Scholte, & van Berckelaer-Onnes, 2012). Receptive deficits are more difficult to target in an assessment than are expressive language deficits. A sampling of instruments that can be used at this level appears in Table 7.1 (see Dodd, Franke, Grzesik, & Stoskopf, 2014, for a helpful review of assessment instruments).

Children with ASD generally acquire expressive language, or begin to use words as the primary form of communication, between 2 and 6 years of age. Age of first words has been shown to be predictive of later cognitive and adaptive skills (Mayo, Chlebowski, Fein, & Eigsti, 2013). Below, we discuss communication assessment from this early stage of language use to the point at which a child produces more or less complete sentences. It is always important to remember that great variety exists in the language development of children with ASD. Some children may show delays in language development and be chronologically older than the typically expected age during this period of development. Others may show patterns of language acquisition similar to those seen in children with specific language disorders who are not on the autism spectrum (Tager-Flusberg & Joseph, 2003). Finally, some children with ASD may show normal or even precocious development of the forms of language (Landa, 2000; Tager-Flusberg et al., 2005)—that is, their deficits may be restricted to the pragmatic uses of communication.

Obtaining a Communication Profile

Following the identification of the presence or absence of basic language deficits through use of standardized tools, assessment efforts should focus on detailing a child's communication profile. The primary means for

TABLE 7.1. Standardized Instruments for Assessing Early Language Development

Instrument	Areas assessed
Clinical Evaluation of Language Fundamentals—Preschool (Wiig, Semel, & Secord, 2013)	Concepts, syntax, semantics, morphology
Peabody Picture Vocabulary Test—Fourth Edition (Dunn & Dunn, 2007)	Receptive vocabulary/expressive vocabulary
MacArthur–Bates Communicative Development Inventories (3rd ed.; Fenson et al., 2007)	Parent checklist that assesses receptive and expressive vocabulary, as well as use of play and gestures; later level assesses expressive vocabulary and early syntax
Preschool Language Scale, Fifth Edition (Zimmerman, Steiner, & Pond, 2012)	Receptive/expressive syntax, semantics, morphology
Reynell Developmental Language Scales—III (Edwards et al., 1999)	Receptive language/expressive language
Sequenced Inventory of Communicative Development—Revised (Hedrick, Prather, & Tobin, 1984)	Receptive language/expressive language
Test of Early Language Development—Third Edition (Hresko, Reid, & Hammill, 1999)	Receptive/expressive semantics and syntax
Test of Language Development—Primary: Fourth Edition (Newcomer & Hammill, 2008)	Receptive/expressive semantics and syntax
Vineland Adaptive Behavior Scales, Third Edition (Sparrow, Cicchetti, & Balla, 2016)	Receptive/expressive/written language

establishing a communication profile is collecting a sample of spontaneous speech during an interaction with the child. This interaction may consist of various play scenarios, a caregiving routine, or a shared book-reading activity. During these activities, language samples can be recorded on videotape or audiotape for later transcription and analysis. Increasingly, family members are being included in these processes, as they are asked to complete observation checklists, describe daily routines, interpret their child's actions, and/or validate assessment results (Crais, 1996).

As discussed above, young children with ASD often have a reduced frequency of communicative attempts—therefore, elicitation procedures may be necessary to gain an accurate picture of their communicative abilities. Communication elicitation generally involves tempting a child to communicate by setting up situations that produce desire for more or less of an action or object. Additional elicitation methods may strive to evoke confusion, surprise, or even disgust in the child. Here are some specific examples of temptations that can be used to elicit communication:

- Keeping toys to oneself, so the child needs to request them.
- Eating a snack without offering any to the child, to elicit requests.
- Offering the child the chance to pull objects out of opaque containers, to elicit comments.
- Engaging in a routine (such as rolling a ball back and forth), and then suddenly switching to another (such as pushing a truck).
- Engaging in social routines, such as tickle games or finger plays, and interrupting the routine to get the child to request its continuation.
- Offering the child an object or activity he or she does not like, to elicit a protest.
- Offering parts of toys or puzzles, but withholding some, so the child needs to request them.
- Pretending to misunderstand or not to hear a request or comment made by the child, in order to elicit a conversational repair.
- Suddenly doing something silly or unexpected, such as putting on a funny hat or "Groucho" glasses, to elicit a comment.

Assessment of Language Forms and Meanings

Certain communicative patterns are typical of children with ASD, whether they involve restricted use of typical communicative behaviors or overuse of atypical behaviors. The kinds of communicative behaviors that can be observed and recorded in children with ASD, and methods of analysis for each behavior, are outlined below.

1a. *Responsiveness*: Compared with typically developing children, children with ASD do not respond as consistently to hearing their names called, and may show minimal understanding of the conversational responsibility to respond when spoken to.

1b. *Analysis methods*: The number of times a child responds to his or her name can be examined as a proportion of the number of times the name was called. Likewise, the number of adult utterances to which the child responds with speech or meaningful gestures can be compared to the total number of adult utterances offered.

2a. *Echolalia*: This behavior is common in children with ASD in the early stages of spoken language acquisition. It includes immediate or delayed imitation of what is heard, or the repetition of strings of memorized language (i.e., scripts).

2b. *Analysis methods*: The proportion of echoed to spontaneous utterances can be analyzed. Echoed utterances can be further separated into immediate and delayed echolalia. The function of the echoed language should be recorded, in order to design intervention to replace the echoed language with more conventional means of communication to achieve the given functions.

3a. *Pronoun use*: Children with ASD often use the pronoun "you" in place of "I" or "me" when referring to themselves. This is thought to reflect their tendency to echo what they hear others say. For example, when a caregiver asks a child with ASD, "Are you hungry?" the child may respond with the phrase, "You hungry."

3b. *Analysis methods*: The number of inappropriate uses of pronouns in a speech sample can be calculated as a proportion of total pronoun use in the sample.

4a. *Vocabulary and syntax*: Children with ASD sometimes attach unusual or peculiar meanings to words or phrases. For example, a child with ASD may say, "Go on red riding," to mean "I want to go in the wagon." However, whereas association of semantic meaning to words is a relative deficit, syntax is generally a relative strength in children with ASD. Therefore, syntactic level, often determined by mean length of utterance (MLU), can be a baseline measure against which other areas of language skill may be measured.

4b. *Analysis methods*: Vocabulary diversity can be analyzed simply by recording the number of different words in the speech sample, or more formally by calculating the "type–token" ratio (i.e., number of different words divided by total number of words spoken). Language analysis programs such as Miller and Chapman's (2016) Systematic Analysis of Language Transcripts (SALT) automatically compute both vocabulary and MLU measures from transcripts entered into their data systems. These values can be compared with those in the SALT database of transcripts from typically developing children between the ages of 3 and 13 years. In addition, any idiosyncratic word use observed in children with ASD may be noted.

Assessing Pragmatics in Spoken Language

"Pragmatic" skills involve the *use* of language to communicate, as opposed to the content or form of language. Children with ASD may have above-average skills in language form (i.e., sound production, grammar) and/or content (i.e., vocabulary, semantic relations)—yet they may struggle with pragmatic skills such as taking turns, offering greetings, and maintaining or changing a conversational topic. Pragmatic language deficits are readily apparent to others and are potentially stigmatizing to children with ASD. By understanding the domains of pragmatic language clinicians, parents, and therapists of children with ASD can focus on goals that reflect the skills necessary for successful interaction with the social world.

1a. *Communicative functions*: The intended purposes for which communication is used.

1b. *Assessment*: Through observation, parent checklist, or a structured play method, the range of functions expressed can be noted. The functions seen in typically developing children between ages 5 and 7, as described by Tough (1977), appear in Figure 7.3. This form can be used as a recording device to assess the range of communicative functions expressed in free or structured play interactions between a child with ASD and an adult or peer.

2a. *Discourse management*: The organization of turns and topics in conversation.

Functions	Example from TD	Expressed by client: Frequency	Expressed by client: Example
Directing others	"You go there."		
Self-directing	"I'm gonna hide the ball."		
Reporting on past and ongoing events	"We played on the swings."		
Reasoning	"The gerbil ran away 'cause we forgot to lock the cage."		
Predicting	"Mom'll get mad if I play in the mud."		
Empathizing	"She's crying 'cause she fell down."		
Imagining	"I'm the mommy; I'll put the baby to bed."		
Negotiating	"If you give me the truck, I'll give you the ball."		

FIGURE 7.3. Chart for recording functions of communication expressed, with examples expressed by typically developing (TD) children at 4–7 years. Based on Chapman (1981) and Tough (1977).

2b. *Assessment*: During observations of interactions with a variety of conversational partners (e.g., peers, adults, familiar, unfamiliar), a clinician may focus on and record the child's ability to:

- Take a conversational turn at the appropriate time.
- Give partners speaking turns at the appropriate time.
- Reduce perseveration on preferred topics.
- Switch topics when cues (e.g., facial expressions, body language) are offered.
- Use appropriate transition phrases or cues (e.g., "On another topic," "I was also thinking") when initiating topic change.
- Initiate and maintain conversation on topics of interest to conversational partners.

3a. *Register variation*: Flexible use of language forms in accordance with the specific context of an interaction.

3b. *Assessment*: During interaction with the child and/or observation of the child interacting with a variety of other conversational partners, an evaluation is made of the child's ability to:

- Use polite forms.
- Speak appropriately to people of various ages and social status, using different language and speaking tones (i.e., informal language with peers, more formal language with teachers and other adults).
- Ask in different ways, depending on whether the request is a favor (e.g., to borrow something) or a right (e.g., to have a borrowed object returned).
- Use context-specific vocabulary according to the topic, conversational partner, and situation.

4a. *Presupposition*: Assuming what information a conversational partner needs to be given and what the partner already knows.

4b. *Assessment*: Observing the child in conversation with a variety of conversational partners, the clinician can note whether the child:

- Gives the appropriate amount of information—that is, avoids excessively discussing a topic or sounding pedantic on the one hand, and being too vague or causing confusion on the other.
- Uses pronouns appropriately (e.g., "he" if the subject is known or has been stated previously).
- Uses ellipsis appropriately (e.g., answering "Yes, I did" instead of "Yes, I went to the store" when asked, "Did you go to the store?").
- Creating cohesive conversational flow by appropriately relating statements to ideas introduced earlier in the conversation.

5a. *Conversational manner*: According to Grice (1996), contributions to conversation should be "clear, brief, and orderly."

5b. *Assessment*: Assessment of this domain should involve observation of the ability to speak succinctly and fluidly. For example, the clinician may note use of overly long, complex utterances; blatantly sparse conversational contributions; and/or disorganized, tangential, cluttered, or repetitive styles of speech.

The skills described above may be probed most efficiently in semistructured interactions, during which communication may be elicited in response to various situations, such as the following:

- Asking the child to pretend to be the "mommy" or "daddy" to a doll or toy.
- Having the child ask for an object, then (if the original request is blunt or abrupt) telling him or her to "ask more nicely."
- Providing an opportunity for the child to use contrastive stress—for example, by giving him or her a choice of two objects and presenting the wrong one.
- Asking for clarification of something the child said.
- Asking the child to describe a sequence, such as a set of pictures depicting a child dressing, and noting whether the child changes appropriately from noun at first mention ("the boy") to pronoun ("he") in later references; changes appropriately from full sentence in the first description ("The boy puts his sock on his foot") to elliptical sentence ("He puts his shoe on" ["his foot" is ellipted because it is redundant the second time]); and relates the sequence in a logical, organized manner.

An example of a simple assessment form that might be used for this semistructured assessment activity appears in Figure 7.4.

COMMUNICATION ASSESSMENT IN HIGH-FUNCTIONING SPEAKERS WITH ASD

Establishing Eligibility for Speech–Language Services

In the context of ASD, the label "high functioning" implies that an individual presents with a normal IQ (generally 70–80 or above) and can express ideas in a wide range of words and sentences. As a group, high-functioning children with ASD tend to exhibit advanced vocabulary and sentence structures, but poor pragmatic and social interaction skills. This discrepancy in abilities presents a challenge to the practitioner who needs to represent such

	Yes	No	No opportunity
Communicative functions	______	______	______
Directing others	______	______	______
Self-directing	______	______	______
Reporting	______	______	______
Reasoning	______	______	______
Predicting	______	______	______
Empathizing	______	______	______
Imagining	______	______	______
Negotiating	______	______	______
Discourse management	______	______	______
Waits turn to speak	______	______	______
Responds to speech with speech consistently	______	______	______
Responds to speech with relevant remark	______	______	______
Maintains other's topic for at least two turns	______	______	______
Shifts topics appropriately	______	______	______
Monitors interlocutor with gaze appropriately (looks at other when talking; looks at referents, then back at interlocutor)	______	______	______
Register variation	______	______	______
Talks appropriately to unfamiliar adult (clinician)	______	______	______
Demonstrates at least one register shift (e.g., in talk to baby doll or stuffed animal)	______	______	______
Uses politeness conventions in requests (e.g., "please")	______	______	______
Can increase politeness when told to "ask nicer"	______	______	______
Uses indirect requests spontaneously/ appropriately	______	______	______
Presupposition	______	______	______
Uses pronouns appropriately	______	______	______
Uses ellipsis appropriately	______	______	______
Uses stress appropriately for emphasis and contrast	______	______	______
Gives enough background information	______	______	______
Can provide additional information when requested ("A what?") for conversational repair	______	______	______
Manner of communication	______	______	______
Gives clear, relevant responses	______	______	______
Talks appropriate amount	______	______	______
Can relate sequence of actions clearly in organized fashion	______	______	______

FIGURE 7.4. Example form for assessing pragmatics in semistructured conversation: early language level. Adapted from Paul (2007). Copyright © 2007 C. V. Mosby, a division of Elsevier. Adapted by permission.

a child's complex communication needs and to provide justification for services for a child who presents with a relatively high verbal IQ and scores within or above the normal range on most standard language assessments. Despite these strengths in formal language, however, the high-functioning child with ASD will experience pragmatic and higher-level language deficits, which will become more obvious and problematic as social and educational demands increase with age.

In such cases, when traditional assessment materials are not adequate measures of communicative need, less traditional assessment methods may be considered. However, some standardized tests have shown potential for documenting the pragmatic weaknesses of higher-functioning individuals with ASD (Reichow, Salamack, Paul, Volkmar, & Klin, 2008; Swineford, Thurm, Baird, Wetherby, & Swedo, 2014), and may help to establish their eligibility for services from a speech–language pathologist to address their social communication deficits. Some of these tests are now described.

The Test of Pragmatic Language (TOPL-2; Phelps-Terasaki & Phelps-Gunn, 2007) was standardized with a sample of 1,016 students. The TOPL uses picture cues paired with verbal prompts to test social language skills in children ages 5–13 years. This test assesses six core components of pragmatic language (i.e., physical setting, abstraction, topic, purpose [speech acts], visual–gestural cues, and audience). Young, Diehl, Morris, Hyman, and Bennetto (2005) found the TOPL to be a viable tool in differentiating between children with and without ASD matched for verbal IQ and basic language skill, based on pragmatic language performance.

The Comprehensive Assessment of Spoken Language (CASL-2; Carrow-Woolfolk, 2017) has separate scales for both pragmatic judgment and supralinguistic forms (nonliteral uses of language, drawing inferences, and understanding of idiomatic language), which can be contrasted with lexical and syntactic skills. Reichow et al. (2008) showed that the Pragmatic and Inferences subtests of the CASL appeared to document the difficulties exhibited by speakers with ASD in adaptive use of language for communication.

The Test of Language Competence (TLC; Wiig & Secord, 1989) examines understanding of multiple meanings, figurative usage, and the ability to draw inferences and produce utterances appropriate for various contexts. Although the TLC and other tests aimed at assessing pragmatic skills can sometimes demonstrate significant discrepancies between language form and function in students with ASD at advanced language levels, even these measures occasionally fail to overcome the powerful cognitive strategies high-functioning individuals can marshal in the structured testing environment. For this reason, less formally structured, more naturalistic assessments are often necessary.

The Children's Communication Checklist–2 (CCC-2; Bishop, 2006) is a parent checklist that provides not only measures of basic language skills, but also a "communicative deviance" score that shows the discrepancy

TABLE 7.2. Topics of Discussion for PRS Interview

1. Greeting and small talk.
2. "Tell me about your school/job."
3. "Tell me about your friends."
4. "What makes you happy? Afraid? Angry? Annoyed? Proud?"
5. Ask individual to tell a story from a wordless picture book.
6. Ask individual to describe action in a comic strip; place strip out of reach to encourage use of gestures.
7. "What would you do if you won a million dollars?"

between language form and language use. The well-standardized CCC-2 can be used to document a significant discrepancy between semantic/syntactic and pragmatic skills that can be used to argue for the need for speech–language intervention, even in the presence of language test scores in the normal range.

The Autism Spectrum Screening Questionnaire (ASSQ; Ehlers, Gillberg, & Wing, 1999) is a checklist screener consisting of 27 items that can be completed by parents, teachers, or clinicians. Its aim is to identify symptoms characteristic of children and adolescents with high-functioning ASD. The ASQ may indicate areas of specific weakness, including pragmatic deficits and language use difficulties, that may be contrasted with language test scores.

The Pragmatic Rating Scale (PRS; Landa et al., 1992) was designed for evaluating conversational skills in parents of individuals with ASD, to determine whether weaknesses in pragmatics are common across family members. This scale identifies 30 pragmatic behaviors that reflect abnormalities thought to be typical of autism, based on reports of major pragmatic behaviors in the literature. The rating involves analysis of a 30-minute conversational interview sample with topics based on the Autism Diagnostic Observation Schedule, Second Edition (ADOS-2; Lord et al., 2012). See Table 7.2 for topics of discussion for a PRS interview.

Assessing Pragmatics and Prosody

High-functioning children with ASD demonstrate a range of social communication deficits:

- An impaired "theory of mind," or a limited ability to draw appropriate conclusions about others' thoughts and feelings. These deficits affect their presuppositional ability.
- Difficulties in feeling empathy, expressing emotion appropriately, or understanding the emotions of others.

- Obsessive interest in unusual topics, ranging from newts to plumbing equipment. They often have difficulty discussing nonpreferred topics.
- A tendency to make blunt comments that may offend others, such as pointing out a person's weight or appearance inappropriately.
- A tendency to be overly friendly in inappropriate ways; this may sometimes include inappropriate touching or asking explicitly for things (like sex) usually only hinted at in polite conversation.
- Use of incessant, repetitive questions that others may find annoying.
- Difficulties in understanding irony and humor in peer conversations.
- Inability to negotiate entry into peer activities.

All the while, these children may be showing age-appropriate or superior performance on basic tests of verbal skills. As high-functioning children with ASD progress in their education, they may encounter difficulty when asked to make inferences about characters' feelings, write essays on nonpreferred topics, or work in peer groups to complete tasks. As such, their pragmatic deficits will affect not only their success with social interactions but also their ability to achieve academic success and maintain self-confidence.

Another area of notable disability in high-functioning people with ASD is "prosody," or the musical aspects of speech (i.e., rate, volume, melody, and rhythm patterns) that accompany the linguistic signal and modulate its meaning. Research suggests that prosodic problems commonly seen in this population include inappropriate use of stress, hypernasal speech, and decreased speech fluency (Filipe, Frota, Castro, & Vicente, 2014; Lyons, Schoen Simmons, & Paul, 2014; Shriberg et al., 2001). Anecdotal reports also suggest trouble with modulating volume in speech and unusual intonation patterns (Pronovost, Wakstein, & Wakstein, 1966). The unique prosodic patterns of these children may render them odd, unapproachable, or unpleasant to others. In addition, teachers may interpret prosodic difficulties as defiant or passive–aggressive behavior. Some formal and informal measures that may be used to assess prosody are outlined below.

1a. *Formal assessment*: One formal screening instrument is the Prosody–Voice Screening Profile (PVSP; Shriberg, Kwiatkowski, & Rasmussen, 1990). The PVSP can be used to examine prosodic variables (i.e., stress, rate, fluency, loudness, pitch, voice quality) in free speech samples. As a screening measure, the PVSP has a suggested cutoff score of 80% for identifying a prosodic deficit—that is, if more than 80% of the subject's utterances are rated as inappropriate in one of the six areas above, according to the PVSP scoring procedures, the speech sample is considered to be demonstrating prosodic difficulties in that area.

1b. *Benefits*: The PVSP has been used to study prosody in a variety of communication disorders, and has a database of typical speakers for comparison. It has undergone extensive interjudge agreement studies and demonstrates adequate reliability at the level of summative prosody–voice codes.

1c. *Drawbacks*: The PVSP is highly labor-intensive, requiring transcription and utterance-by-utterance judgments to be made for each prosody–voice code. It also requires intensive training and practice before raters can attain adequate skill levels.

2a. *Informal assessment*: Speech samples may be gathered as part of the pragmatic assessment and evaluated informally for their prosodic characteristics. A clinician can make a judgment ("appropriate," "inappropriate," "no opportunity to observe") on each of the relevant domains of prosody, with special attention paid to stress, fluency, volume, intonation, and nasality. A recording sheet like that shown in Figure 7.5 can be used to summarize this assessment.

2b. *Benefits*: Informal assessment of a speech sample may allow for a more descriptive, qualitative analysis of prosody. This style of analysis and the impressions accompanying each judgment may be useful for describing prosodic traits in a school-based report, or for discussing these traits with a child's teacher or parent.

2c. *Drawbacks*: Although clinician judgments are often used to assess various aspects of communicative performance, prosody is an area in which few data exist to support the validity or reliability of these judgments. Clearly, the assessment of prosodic production is an area in which

	Appropriate	Inappropriate	No opportunity to observe
Loudness			
Syllable stress			
Sentence stress			
Pitch			
Intonation			
Nasality			
Intonation			
Rhythm			

FIGURE 7.5. A recording form for informal assessment of prosodic production in speech.

there is a great need for more research to establish boundaries of normality and develop more efficient methods of assessment.

Assessing Conversational and Narrative Skills

Speakers with high-functioning ASD are often most comfortable and successful when interacting with familiar, trusted adults (e.g., parents, teachers, therapists). The world of social interaction seems unregulated and unpredictable to these children, and responsive adults represent the safest, most predictable social partners. Interacting with peers, who are often unfamiliar and can seem fickle or intimidating, often evokes anxiety in these children, as peers generally will not understand or compensate for the interactive deficits these children display. During conversational interactions, children with ASD typically fail to take into account the interests of others, the need to share the conversational floor, and the necessity for reading nonverbal cues to gauge success of the conversation. Therefore, in order to assess their conversational skills and understand their difficulties in everyday social communication, it is important to observe them engaged in a variety of peer interactions.

Using a checklist or observational guide provides organization to a social communication observation. Larson and McKinley (2003) have provided several forms for guiding this type of assessment; a sample form appears in Figure 7.6. In the clinical setting, where it is usually not possible to observe a child in a natural interaction with a peer, social interaction skills may be assessed via a more structured method involving interaction with an adult. One such method is to use a seminaturalistic probe task, during which an adult conversational partner interjects specified questions into a conversation in order to assess the speaker's ability to provide appropriate responses. Examples of conversational probes useful for this purpose appear in Table 7.3.

An additional aspect of social communication that can be assessed in higher-functioning children with ASD is the ability to produce narratives. The pragmatic impairments that hinder these children during social interactions may affect their ability to create cohesive stories as well—that is, writing a narrative requires the ability to draw inferences and understand internal responses of characters, and these skills are often deficient in children with ASD. Asking a child to produce or interpret a narrative can be an efficient means of assessing his or her higher-level language abilities (e.g., use of inference, complex syntax, pronouns, sequential markers). Botting (2002) found narrative ability to have a direct correlation to pragmatic skill level. In another study, Norbury and Bishop (2003) reported on narratives from 8- to 10-year-old students with communication disorders, generated in response to the wordless picture book *Frog, Where Are You?* (Mayer, 1969). Their findings suggested a few key areas of higher-level language

	Appropriate	Inappropriate	No opportunity to observe	Comments
Listener role				
Vocabulary				
Syntax				
Main ideas				
Cooperative manner				
Gives feedback				
Speaker role: Language features				
Syntax				
Questions				
Figurative language				
Nonspecific language				
Precise vocabulary				
Word retrieval				
Mazes and dysfluencies				
Speaker role: Paralinguistic features				
Suprasegmental features				
Fluency				
Intelligibility				
Speaker role: Communicative functions				
Give information				
Receive information				
Describe				
Persuade				
Express opinion/belief				
Indicate readiness				
Solve problems verbally				
Entertain				

(continued)

FIGURE 7.6. A form for assessing peer conversation in speakers with ASD. From Larson and McKinley (2003). Copyright © 2003 Thinking Publications. Reprinted by permission.

	Appropriate	Inappropriate	No opportunity to observe	Comments
Conversational rules				
Verbal turns/topics				
Initiation				
Topic choice				
Topic maintenance				
Topic switch				
Turn taking				
Repair/revision				
Interruption				
Verbal politeness				
Quantity				
Sincerity				
Relevance				
Clarity				
Tact				
Nonverbal				
Gestures				
Facial expressions				
Eye contact				
Proxemics				

FIGURE 7.6. *(continued)*

deficit that are common to children with ASD, including incorrect use of pronouns and nouns to refer to story characters, and reduced syntactic complexity and accuracy (compared with that of typically developing peers).

Several tools are commercially available for assessing narrative, including:

The Bus Story language test (Renfrew, 1991)
Strong Narrative Assessment Procedure (SNAP: Strong, 1998)
Narrative rubrics (McFadden & Gillam, 1996)
Test of Narrative Language (Gillam & Pearson, 2004)

TABLE 7.3. Probes for Eliciting Conversational Behavior in Speakers with ASD

Behavior probed	Example	Target	Examples
Topic initiation	"By the way, I went camping over the weekend."	1. Responsiveness 2. Topic maintenance 3. Relevance	"I went canoeing." "My friend did that last month." "Weekends are the best!"
Questions	"So how was your vacation?"	1. Responsiveness 2. Topic maintenance 3. Relevance	"Not bad." "I met a guy from Canada." "I tried waterskiing." "Our hotel had dancing every night."
Requests for repair	"What kind of dancing?"	1. Responsiveness 2. Adjustment to listener 3. Repair strategy	"Samba." "Samba, it's a Latin dance." "Do you know any Latin dances?"
Sources of difficulty	"Can you get that pen for me?" [no pen in sight]	1. Assertiveness 2. Comprehension monitoring 3. Clarification requests	"I don't see any pen." "Did you say a pen?" "Do you mean a pencil?"

COMMUNICATION ASSESSMENT IN NONVERBAL CHILDREN WITH ASD

Despite current efforts to increase the number of children with ASD who acquire spoken language (National Research Council, 2001), a substantial portion of the population with ASD will remain nonverbal or minimally verbal (Tager-Flusberg & Kasari, 2013). Many of these individuals will rely on modes of augmentative and alternative communication (AAC), such as signs, pictures, and speech-generating devices. This section outlines the AAC assessment considerations unique to this population, as well as specific tools designed for assessment of nonverbal children in order to determine the most appropriate communication system for each individual.

AAC Assessment Considerations

AAC systems take many forms and, according to Light (1988), may be used to communicate wants and needs, transfer information, create social closeness, and express social etiquette. Although this range of typical communicative functions is ultimately attainable through use of AAC systems, children with ASD must use AAC methods that match their current level of communicative functioning. An AAC assessment aims to determine this functioning level by assessing all of the communicative attributes discussed previously, including communicative frequency, functions, means, and responsiveness. However, there are additional domains of assessment to consider in planning an AAC system. The domains described by Beukelman and Mirenda (2005) that are particularly relevant in planning such a system for a child with an ASD are cognitive/linguistic capabilities and language capabilities.

Cognitive/Linguistic Capabilities

In order to choose the most appropriate AAC method, it is important to determine the child's level of cognitive/linguistic functioning. A basic question involves determining into which of the following four broad stages a child's cognition falls:

1. The *preintentional stage,* when few goals can be held in mind to be pursued through actions. This corresponds to a level below 8 months in typical development and may be manifested by difficulty in demonstrating an understanding of permanence of objects and cause–effect relationships.
2. The *presymbolic stage,* when a child may be able to develop goals and intentions, but has difficulty creating mental representations or using symbolic play and behavior. This stage occurs from 8 to 18 months in typical development and may be manifested in an inability to use pretend play schemes.
3. The *preliterate stage,* when a child can use pretend play and symbols, but has no phonological awareness or knowledge of letter names and sounds. This stage occurs between 2 and 5 years of age in typical development, and can be seen in an unfamiliarity with letters and difficulty in detecting rhymes.
4. The *literate stage,* when a child demonstrates knowledge of or interest in letter names and sounds, and can detect rhymes.

The level of cognitive development as indexed by these general stages can be used, along with other information gathered in the assessment, to select the most appropriate means of AAC for each child.

Language Capabilities

Nonverbal children with ASD may not attain speech as a means of communication, but it is important to determine their receptive language skills as part of the AAC assessment. Within this domain, considerations include single-word comprehension and understanding of grammar and morphological rules. When it is developmentally appropriate to do so, literacy skills may also be assessed, as many AAC methods utilize letters or the written word. These often represent areas of relative strength for children with ASD (Chawarska et al., 2007). Miller and Paul (1995) suggest methods for assessing comprehension in nonverbal children.

Following a comprehensive assessment of a child's communicative capabilities, a decision is made regarding the most appropriate AAC method for the child. In general, AAC methods are considered to fall into one of two categories: *unaided* systems, which involve only the communicator's own body as the means of communication (e.g., sign language or gesture systems); and *aided* systems, which make use of other tools, such as picture boards or computers. However, a combination of these methods may be deemed appropriate for some children. In addition, once a device has been selected, the AAC assessment process should continue throughout the lifespan of the individual with ASD as his or her communication environments, needs, and capabilities change.

Assessment Tools for Nonverbal Children with ASD

Formal, norm-referenced assessment tools often require verbal responses, motor movements, and/or timed performance. For nonverbal children with ASD, this type of assessment, which compares them to their age-matched peers, may serve little purpose. Instead, Beukelman and Mirenda (2005) suggest the use of criterion-referenced assessment tools, which establish a child's ability to use certain communication strategies or tools. In addition, communication assessment may involve interviews of caregivers and other team members, as well as observation of natural interactions between the child and his or her typical communication partners. Several structured methods have been developed for use with these types of assessment. Some examples of such tools are now described.

The Augmentative Communication Assessment Profile (Goldman, 2002) is intended for children with ASD between 3 and 11 years of age, and identifies skills related to use of unaided systems, including signing, pointing, and picture exchange.

The Matching Assistive Technology and Child (Scherer, 1997) tool is intended for an infant or young child and is used by the entire team to identify the family's goals and preferences for the child, define the child's limitations, and determine the most appropriate technologies and training methods for the child and family.

The Developmental Assessment for Individuals with Severe Disabilities—Second Edition (DASH-2; Dykes & Erin, 1999) assesses children who are functioning at an age level from birth to 6 years, 11 months. The DASH-2 identifies the level of assistance (if any) required by the child in completion of various tasks, and assesses the child's skill level in language, sensory–motor, daily living, academics, and social–emotional domains.

The Communication Supports Checklist (McCarthy et al., 1998) is for use by programs serving individuals with severe disabilities, and is intended as a tool for determining programs' strengths and weaknesses as these relate to the communication needs of the populations they serve. Once completed, this tool offers program assistance in developing a communication supports action plan to better serve its clientele.

Checklists may be used to structure informal observations of the child's communication. During such observations, the clinician can note any maladaptive behaviors (such as head banging or rocking), record the situations during which these occur, and note the communicative functions they seem to serve. This information will be important during intervention planning, as self-injurious and maladaptive communication must be replaced by safer, more functional means. Overall, the purpose of an AAC assessment is to collect information within the child's natural environments—both through observation and input from parents, caretakers, and educators—to establish the most functional, comfortable, user-friendly, and versatile communication system possible for the child and family.

MULTICULTURAL CONSIDERATIONS IN ASD ASSESSMENT

The diagnostic criteria for ASD, as outlined by the American Psychiatric Association (2013) and the World Health Organization (1992), have been accepted throughout the world. Thus, we know that people with ASD are seen in every cultural, linguistic, and national group (Volkmar, 2005). However, because the core symptoms of ASD affect social and communicative skills, and because these skills are to some extent culturally determined, cultural sensitivity is necessary in assessing children with this condition. Within the United States, research has begun to explore the cultural differences, particularly those based on race and ethnicity, that affect diagnosis and treatment of ASD. For example, Mandell, Listerud, Levy, and Pinto-Martin (2002) studied Medicaid-eligible children to compare treatment time and age of diagnosis in African American and European American populations. They found that the European American children were typically diagnosed a year and a half earlier than their African American counterparts. In addition, it generally took more visits to the mental health office for African American children to receive a diagnosis of autism. The cultural differences that underlie this reality are important considerations for professionals interested in assessing, diagnosing, and treating ASD in the United States.

Differences between African American and European American parents in the management of their children with ASD may be affected by their previous clinical experiences, help-seeking behaviors, and support and advocacy networks. According to Diala et al. (2000), African Americans are less likely than their European American counterparts to seek mental health services, and are more likely to have negative experiences when they do seek help. Whaley (1998) explored the idea that attitudes of European American clinicians toward African American patients may be implicated in the observed racial differences in ASD treatment and outcomes. African Americans' negative experience of such attitudes may contribute to their reduced help-seeking behaviors. According to Kass, Weinick, and Monheit (1999), African Americans made 26% fewer visits to their regular medical care providers than did European Americans. Dyches, Wilder, Sudweeks, Obiakor, and Algozzine (2004) suggest that this relative reluctance to seek help from medical professionals may also be related to stronger support networks of families, friends, and churches in the African American culture. Whatever the underlying reason, it is increasingly clear that the cultural disparity regarding health care experiences in general is affecting the efficiency and quality of the ASD diagnostic process for people in the African American community.

Although the overall number of research studies on ASD is on the rise, racial and cultural differences as they relate to ASD in the United States have been generally overlooked in the literature. Even those studies that do investigate diagnosis and treatment of ASD in racially and culturally different groups often have limited validity, due to small sample sizes and other confounding factors (Dyches et al., 2004). Dyches et al. cited recruiting strategies as a major factor in limiting the pool of potential subjects for ASD research, as minority groups in the United States may prefer not to participate in research efforts due to language barriers, mistrust, or misunderstanding. The resulting paucity of research on American minority groups' use of health services and attitudes toward disorders such as ASD leaves clinicians ill equipped to address sociocultural issues in diagnosis and treatment. Beginning to consider the impact of cultural differences during assessment and treatment of ASD is a first step toward a more inclusive model. A few tools have already been developed to consider cultural differences in communication; these are now described.

The Diagnostic Evaluation of Language Variation (DELV; Seymour, Roeper, de Villiers, & de Villiers, 2005) comes in the form of a screening measure, a criterion-referenced test, and a norm-referenced test. The DELV is intended for children ages 4–12 years, and although it is sensitive to the linguistic and cultural characteristics of many African American children, it can be used for children of any race or ethnicity to identify the risk of a language disorder while considering the potential effects of variations from mainstream American English. It allows a culture-fair assessment of language form, and also contains a pragmatic section that can be useful for any client in documenting a discrepancy between skill levels in the formal and pragmatic domains of language.

Cultural Contexts for Early Intervention: Working with Families (Moore & Peréz-Méndez, 2003) is the title of both a video and a written manual designed for professionals who wish to become more skillful in assessment and intervention practices across cultures.

Multicultural Students with Special Language Needs: Practical Strategies for Assessment and Intervention (Roseberry-McKibbin, 2014) is a 364-page book that outlines key information about various cultural groups, including the groups' characteristics and traditions. In addition, this reference points out the variables that are most important to consider in assessing and planning intervention for children and families of various cultures.

In addition, the American Speech–Language–Hearing Association offers several manuals and compilations of articles to train clinicians to work with multicultural populations. These documents are available through its website (*www.asha.org*).

COMMUNICATION ASSESSMENT IN CONTEXT

The assessment of communication is, of course, part of the larger process of diagnostic evaluation and educational planning that goes into determining the strengths and needs of a child with ASD. In conducting this process, professionals from various disciplines collaborate with family members and other caregivers to determine a child's diagnostic classification and eligibility for publicly funded services, describe in detail the child's needs in all areas of functioning, identify the most appropriate goals for an intervention program, and monitor the program as it proceeds to ensure that it is efficient and effective.

Planning and Monitoring Communication Intervention

As we have seen, data from the communication assessment of a child with ASD will be gathered through a range of methods, including standard testing, structured observations, and parental interviews/questionnaires, as well as input from others with knowledge of the child's history and current presentation, who collectively form the child's treatment team. The assessment data will then be used to do the following:

- Identify the frequency, range, and means of communicative acts expressed. This involves determining the degree to which language or some other means (such as gesture) is used to express communicative functions.
- Establish the degree of reciprocity or responsiveness to communication the child shows.
- Describe the pattern of formal language acquisition—whether it is delayed, absent, similar to that seen in specific language disorder, or a relative strength.
- Compare the use of words and sentences with pragmatic abilities.
- Identify language patterns characteristic of ASD, such as pronoun reversals, echolalia, or prosodic abnormalities.
- Determine the most accessible form of AAC if the child is nonverbal.

This information will be shared with members of the child's treatment or educational team, including parents, other caregivers, teachers, and therapists—both to ensure its congruence with their understanding of the child, and to increase understanding of the child's current strengths and needs. The data are then used by the team to identify a set of goals for the child's communication intervention program. These goals will be based both on the portrait drawn of the child's strengths and needs by the assessment data, and also on the particular areas identified by the team as being most important to address, in order to improve the child's functioning in day-to-day settings.

Once individualized goals for the child's communication program have been established collaboratively in this way, one additional form of assessment may be introduced to assist in planning the intervention program. "Dynamic assessment" is designed to take a closer look at what factors, supports, or modifications enhance the child's communication performance. In dynamic assessment, the communicative context is manipulated through the use of prompts, cues, or various scaffolds to determine which of these best support positive changes in communication. Thus, dynamic assessment provides important initial information about what techniques or teaching styles may be appropriate to improve communication for a particular child. Dynamic assessment often takes place at the beginning of an intervention program, to identify the most effective ways to meet the aims identified by the assessment team.

SUMMARY

Communication assessment in individuals with ASD is a process that requires a broad understanding of both typical developmental patterns and those unique to ASD. Decisions regarding assessment methods will be made on the basis of each child's age, developmental level, verbal ability, and communication skills. Available and valid methods of assessing communication in children with ASD include formal evaluation of communication through standardized tools; informal evaluation through use of observations, checklists, and communication samples; and involvement of the family through interviews, questionnaires, and information sharing. A comprehensive assessment of communicative strengths and needs involves consideration of current performance, developmental history, cultural and linguistic factors, and the concerns expressed by caregivers and educators. It results in a family-centered plan to maximize the child's ability to communicate with the world.

Deficits in communication are core symptoms of ASD, and assessment of these skills is always a central part of the evaluation process. Children with ASD who are in the prelinguistic phase of communication may require assistance in establishing the communicative basis for a formal language system, while older nonverbal children may require assessment to identify the most appropriate AAC system. Assessment of communication for children in later stages of language use should consider the atypical communicative patterns that often accompany ASD, such as echolalia and pronoun errors, as well as the pragmatic and receptive language deficits that are common in this population. Although each communication assessment will be unique, due to the wide range of strengths and needs seen in this spectrum of disorders, the considerations discussed in this chapter offer a framework for thinking about the communication assessment process. A flexible, family-centered approach that includes everyone who cares for or provides treatment to a child will increase the validity of the information collected at each stage of the process, and will give the child the best possible chance to experience a communication intervention program that will open this vital channel between the child and his or her world.

REFERENCES

American Psychiatric Association. (2013). *Diagnostic and statistical manual of mental disorders* (5th ed.). Arlington, VA: Author.

Baranek, G. T. (1999). Autism during infancy: A retrospective video analysis of sensory–motor and social behaviors at 9–12 months of age. *Journal of Autism and Developmental Disorders, 29,* 213–224.

Baron-Cohen, S., Cox, A., Baird, G., Swettenham, J., Nightingale, N., Morgan, K., et al. (1996). Psychological markers in the detection of autism in infancy in a large population. *British Journal of Psychiatry, 168,* 158–163.

Beukelman, D. R., & Mirenda, P. (2005). *Augmentative and alternative communication: Supporting children and adults with complex communication needs* (3rd ed.). Baltimore: Brookes.

Bishop, D. (2006). *Children's Communication Checklist–2 (American Standardization Version).* London: Harcourt Assessment.

Botting, N. (2002). Narrative as a tool for the assessment of linguistic and pragmatic impairments. *Child Language Teaching and Therapy, 18,* 1–22.

Bruner, J. (1977). Early social interaction and language acquisition. In R. Schaffer (Ed.), *Studies in mother–infant interaction* (pp. 155–177). New York: Academic Press.

Carrow-Woolfolk, E. (2017). *Comprehensive Assessment of Spoken Language.* Austin, TX: Pearson Assessments.

Centers for Disease Control and Prevention. (2016). Prevalence and characteristics of autism spectrum disorder among children aged 8 years: Autism and Developmental Disabilities Monitoring Network, 11 Sites, United States, 2012. *Morbidity and Mortality Weekly Report Surveillance Summaries, 65,* 1–23.

Chapman, R. (1981). Analyzing communicative intents. In J. Miller (Ed.), *Assessing language production in children: Experimental procedures* (pp. 111–138). Boston: Allyn & Bacon.

Chapman, R. (2000). Children's language learning: An interactionist perspective. *Journal of Child Psychology and Psychiatry, 41,* 33–54.

Charman, T., Baron-Cohen, S., Swettenham, J., Baird, G., Drew, A., & Cox, A. (2003). Predicting language outcome in infants with autism and pervasive developmental disorder. *International Journal of Language and Communication Disorders, 38,* 265–285.

Charman, T., Swettenham, J., Baron-Cohen, S., Cox, A., Baird, G., & Drew, A. (1997). Infants with autism: An investigation of empathy, pretend play, joint attention, and imitation. *Developmental Psychology, 33,* 781–789.

Chawarska, K., Klin, A., Paul, R., & Volkmar, F. (2007). Autism spectrum disorder in the second year: Stability and change in syndrome expression. *Journal of Child Psychology and Psychiatry, 48,* 128–138.

Crais, E. (1996). Applying family-centered principles to child assessment. In P. McWilliam, P. Winton, & E. Crais (Eds.), *Practical strategies for family-centered early intervention* (pp. 69–96). San Diego, CA: Singular.

Dawson, G., Meltzoff, A., Osterling, J., Rinaldi, J., & Brown, E. (1998). Children with autism fail to orient to naturally occurring social stimuli. *Journal of Autism and Developmental Disorders, 28,* 479–485.

Diala, C., Muntaner, C., Walrath, C., Nickerson, K., LaVest, T., & Leaf, P. (2000). Racial differences in attitudes toward professional mental health care in the use of services. *American Journal of Orthopsychiatry, 70,* 455–464.

Dodd, J. L., Franke, L. K., Grzesik, J. K., & Stoskopf, J. (2014). Comprehensive multidisciplinary assessment protocol for autism spectrum disorder. *Journal of Intellectual Disability, 2,* 68–82.

Dunn, L., & Dunn, L. (2007). *Peabody Picture Vocabulary Test—Fourth Edition.* Bloomington, MN: Pearson Assesssments.

Dyches, T. T., Wilder, L. K., Sudweeks, R. R., Obiakor, F. E., & Algozzine, B. (2004). Multicultural issues in autism. *Journal of Autism and Developmental Disorders, 34,* 211–221.

Dykes, M., & Erin, J. (1999). *A Developmental Assessment for Students with Severe Disabilities—Second Edition.* Austin, TX: PRO-ED.

Edwards, S., Fletcher, P., Garman, M., Highes, A., Letts, C., & Sinka, I. (1999). *Reynell Developmental Language Scales–III.* Windsor, UK: NFER-Nelson.

Ehlers, S., Gillberg, C., & Wing, L. (1999). A screening questionnaire for Asperger syndrome and other high-functioning autism spectrum disorders in school age. *Journal of Autism and Developmental Disorders, 29,* 129–141.

Esposito, G., Nakazawa, J., Venuti, P., & Bornstein, M. H. (2013). Componential deconstruction of infant distress vocalizations via tree-based models: A study of cry in autism spectrum disorder and typical development. *Research in Developmental Disabilities, 34,* 2717–2724.

Fenson, L., Dale, P., Reznick, S., Thal, D., Bates, E., Hartung, J., et al. (2007). *MacArthur–Bates Communicative Developmental Inventories* (3rd ed.). Baltimore: Brookes.

Filipe, M. G., Frota, S., Castro, S. L., & Vicente, S. G. (2014). Atypical prosody in Asperger syndrome: Perceptual and acoustic measurements. *Journal of Autism and Developmental Disorders, 44,* 1972–1981.

Gillam, R., & Pearson, N. (2004). *Test of Narrative Language.* Greenville, SC: Super-Duper.

Goldman, H. (2002). *Augmentative Communication Assessment Profile.* London: Speechmark.

Grice, P. (1996). Logic and conversation. In H. Deirsson & M. Losonsky (Eds.), *Readings in language and mind* (pp. 121–133). New York: Wiley.

Hedrick, D., Prather, E., & Tobin, A. (1984). *Sequenced Inventory of Communication Development—Revised.* Austin, TX: PRO-ED.

Hresko, W., Reid, K., & Hamill, D. (1999). *Test of Early Language Development—Third Edition.* Austin, TX: PRO-ED.

Kanner, L. (1943). Autistic disturbances of affective contact. *Nervous Child, 2,* 217–250.

Kanner, L. (1946). Irrelevant and metaphorical language in early infantile autism. *American Journal of Psychiatry, 103,* 242–246.

Kass, B., Weinick, R., & Monheit, A. (1999). *Racial and ethnic differences in health* (MEPS Chartbook No. 2). Rockville, MD: U.S. Department of Health and Human Services.

Kim, S. Paul, R. Tager-Flusberg, H., & Lord, C. (2014). Language and communication in ASD. In F. Volkmar, S. Rogers, R. Paul, & K. Pelphrey (Eds.), *Handbook of autism spectrum disorders: Vol. 1* (4th ed., pp. 176–190). New York: Wiley.

Klin, A., Volkmar, F., & Sparrow, S. (1992). Autistic social dysfunction: Some limitations of the theory of mind hypothesis. *Journal of Child Pschology and Psychiatry, 33,* 861–876.

Landa, R. (2000). Social language use in Asperger syndrome and high-functioning autism. In A. Klin, F. R. Volkmar, & S. S. Sparrow (Eds.), *Asperger syndrome* (pp. 125–155). New York: Guilford Press.

Landa, R., Piven, J., Wzorek, M., Gayle, J., Cloud, D., Chase, G., et al. (1992). Social language use in parents of autistic individuals. *Psychological Medicine, 22,* 245–254.

Larson, V., & McKinley, N. (2003). *Communication solutions for older students: Assessment and intervention strategies.* Eau Claire, WI: Thinking.

Light, J. (1988). Interaction involving individuals using augmentative and alternative communication systems: State of the art and future directions. *Augmentative and Alternative Communication, 4,* 66–82.

Lord, C. (1995). Follow-up of two-year-olds referred for possible autism. *Journal of Child Psychology and Psychiatry, 36,* 1365–1382.

Lord, C., & Risi, S. (2000). Diagnosis of autism spectrum disorders in young children.

In A. M. Wetherby & B. M. Prizant (Eds.), *Autism spectrum disorders: A transactional developmental perspective* (pp. 11–30). Baltimore: Brookes.

Lord, C., Rutter, M., DiLavore, P. C., Risi, S., Gotham, K., & Bishop, S. L. (2012). *Autism Diagnostic Observation Schedule, Second Edition (ADOS-2)*. Torrance, CA: Western Psychological Services.

Lyons, M., Schoen-Simmons, E., & Paul, R. (2014). Prosodic development in middle childhood and adolescence in high-functioning autism. *Autism Research, 7*(2), 181–196.

Maestro, S., Muratori, F., Cavallaro, M. C., Pei, F., Stern, D., Golse, B., et al. (2002). Attentional skills during the first 6 months of age in autism spectrum disorder. *Journal of the American Academy of Child and Adolescent Psychiatry, 41*, 1239–1245.

Maljaars, J., Noens, I., Scholte, E., & van Berckelaer-Onnes, I. (2012). Language in low-functioning children with autistic disorder: Differences between receptive and expressive skills and concurrent predictors of language. *Journal of Autism and Developmental Disorders, 42*, 2181–2191.

Mandell, D. S., Listerud, J., Levy, S. E., & Pinto-Martin, J. A. (2002). Race differences in the age at diagnosis among Medicaid-eligible children with autism. *Journal of the American Academy of Child and Adolescent Psychiatry, 41*, 1447–1453.

Mayer, M. (1969). *Frog, where are you?* New York: Dial Books.

Mayo, J., Chlebowski, C., Fein, D. A., & Eigsti, I. M. (2013). Age of first words predicts cognitive ability and adaptive skills in children with ASD. *Journal of Autism and Developmental Disorders, 43*, 253–264.

McCarthy, C. F., Mclean, L. K., Miller, J. F., Brown, D. P., Romski, M. A., Rourk, J. D., et al. (1998). *Communication Supports Checklist for programs serving individuals with severe disabilities*. Baltimore: Brookes.

McFadden, T., & Gillam, R. (1996). An examination of the quality of narrative produced by children with language disorders. *Language, Speech and Hearing Services in Schools, 27*, 48–56.

Miller, J., & Chapman, R. (2016). *Systematic Analysis of Language Transcripts*. Madison: University of Wisconsin.

Miller, J., & Paul, R. (1995). *The clinical assessment of language comprehension*. Baltimore: Brookes.

Mirenda, P. (2003). "He's not really a reader": Perspectives on supporting literacy development in individuals with autism. *Topics in Language Disorders, 23*, 271–282.

Moore, S. M., & Peréz-Méndez, C. (2003). *Cultural contexts for early intervention: Working with families*. Rockville, MD: American Speech–Language–Hearing Association.

Mundy, P., Hogan, A., & Doehring, P. (1996). *Preliminary manual for the Abridged Early Social Communication Scales*. Available from *www.psy.miami.edu/faculty/pmundy*.

Mundy, P., Sigman, M., Ungerer, J., & Sherman, T. (1987). Nonverbal communication and play correlates of language development in autistic children. *Journal of Autism and Developmental Disorders, 17*, 349–364.

Mundy, P., & Stella, J. (2000). Joint attention, social orienting, and nonverbal communication in autism. In A. M. Wetherby & B. M. Prizant (Eds.), *Autism spectrum disorders: A transactional developmental perspective* (pp. 55–77). Baltimore: Brookes.

Nadig, A. S., Ozonoff, S., Young, G. S., Rozga, A., Sigman, M., & Rogers, S. J. (2007). A prospective study of response to name in infants at risk for autism. *Archives of Pediatrics and Adolescent Medicine, 161,* 378–383.

National Research Council. (2001). *Educating children with autism.* Washington, DC: National Academy Press.

Newcomer, P. L., & Hammill, D. D. (2008). *Test of Language Development—Primary: Fourth Edition* (TOLD-P:4). Austin, TX: PRO-ED.

Norbury, C., & Bishop, D. V. M. (2003). Narrative skills of children with communication impairments. *International Journal of Language and Communication Disorders, 38,* 287–314.

Oller, D. K., Niyogi, P., Gray, S., Richards, J. A., Gilkerson, J., Xu, D., et al. (2010). Automated vocal analysis of naturalistic recordings from children with autism, language delay, and typical development. *Proceedings of the National Academy of Sciences, 107,* 13354–13359.

Osterling, J., & Dawson, G. (1994). Early recognition of children with autism: A study of first birthday home videos. *Journal of Autism and Developmental Disorders, 24,* 247–258.

Osterling, J., Dawson, G., & Munson, J. A. (2002). Early recognition of 1-year-old infants with autism spectrum disorder versus mental retardation. *Developmental and Psychopathology, 14,* 239–251.

Patten, E., Belardi, K., Baranek, G. T., Watson, L. R., Labban, J. D., & Oller, D. K. (2014). Vocal patterns in infants with autism spectrum disorder: Canonical babbling status and vocalization frequency. *Journal of Autism and Developmental Disorders, 44,* 2413–2428.

Paul, R. (2005). Assessing communication. In F. R. Volkmar, R. Paul, A. Klin, & D. Cohen (Eds.), *Handbook of autism and pervasive developmental disorders: Vol. 2* (3rd ed., pp. 799–816). Hoboken, NJ: Wiley.

Paul, R. (2007). *Language disorders from infancy through adolescence: Assessment and intervention* (3rd ed.). St. Louis, MO: Mosby.

Paul, R., Chawarska, K., Klin, A., & Volkmar, F. (2007). Dissociations in development of early communication in ASD. In R. Paul (Ed.), *Language disorders from a developmental perspective: Essays in honor of Robin Chapman* (pp. 163–194). Hillsdale, NJ: Erlbaum.

Paul, R., & Cohen, D. (1984). Outcomes of severe disorders of language acquisition. *Journal of Autism and Developmental Disorders, 14,* 405–421.

Phelps-Terasaki, D., & Phelps-Gunn, T. (2007). *The Test of Pragmatic Language–2.* Austin, TX: PRO-ED.

Pronovost, W., Wakstein, M., & Wakstein, D. (1966). A longitudinal study of speech behavior and language comprehension in fourteen children diagnosed as atypical or autistic. *Exceptional Children, 33,* 19–26.

Reichow, B., Salamack, S., Paul, R., Volkmar, F. R., & Klin, A. (2008). Pragmatic assessment in speakers with autism spectrum disorders: A comparison of a standard measure with parent report. *Communication Disorders Quarterly, 29,* 169–176.

Renfrew, C. (1991). *The Bus Story: A test of continuous speech* (22nd ed.). Oxford, UK: Author.

Roseberry-McKibbin, C. (2014). *Multicultural students with special language needs: Practical strategies for assessment and intervention* (4th ed.). Oceanside, CA: Academic Communication Associates.

Scherer, M. (1997). *Matching assistive technology and child*. Webster, NY: Institute for Matching Person and Technology.

Seymour, H. N., Roeper, T. W., de Villiers, J., & de Villiers, P. A. (2005). *Diagnostic Evaluation of Language Variation*. San Antonio, TX: Harcourt Assessment.

Sheinkopf, S. J., Mundy, P., Kimbrough-Oller, D., & Steffens, M. (2000). Vocal atypicalities of preverbal autistic children. *Journal of Autism and Developmental Disorders, 30*(4), 345–354.

Shriberg, L. D., Kwiatkowski, J., & Rasmussen, C. (1990). *The Prosody–Voice Screening Profile*. Tucson, AZ: Communication Skill Builders.

Shriberg, L. D., Paul, R., McSweeney, J., Klin, A., Cohen, D., & Volkmar, F. R. (2001). Speech and prosody characteristics of adolescents and adults with high-functioning autism and Asperger syndrome. *Journal of Speech, Language, and Hearing Research, 44*(5), 1097–1115.

Sparrow, S. S., Cicchetti, D., & Balla, D. (2016). *Vineland Adaptive Behavioral Scales, Third Edition (Vineland–III)*. Austin, TX: Pearson Assessments.

Stone, W. L., Ousley, O. Y., Yoder, P. J., Hogan, K. L., & Hepburn, S. L. (1997). Nonverbal communication in two- and three-year-old children with autism. *Journal of Autism and Developmental Disorders, 27,* 677–696.

Strong, C. (1998). *Strong Narrative Assessment Procedure (SNAP)*. Eau Claire, WI: Thinking.

Swettenham, J., Baron-Cohen, S., Charman, T., Cox, A., Baird, G., Drew, A., et al. (1998). The frequency and distribution of spontaneous attention shifts between social and nonsocial stimuli in autistic, typically developing, and nonautistic developmentally delayed infants. *Journal of Child Psychology and Psychiatry, 39,* 747–753.

Swineford, L. B., Thurm, A., Baird, G., Wetherby, A. M., & Swedo, S. (2014). Social (pragmatic) communication disorder: A research review of this new DSM-5 diagnostic category. *Journal of Neurodevelopmental Disorders, 6,* 41–48.

Tager-Flusberg, H., & Joseph, R. (2003). Identifying neurocognitive phenotypes in autism. *Philosophical Transactions of the Royal Society of London, Series B, 358,* 303–314.

Tager-Flusberg, H., & Kasari, C. (2013). Minimally verbal school-aged children with autism spectrum disorder: The neglected end of the spectrum. *Autism Research, 6,* 468–478.

Tager-Flusberg, H., Paul, R., & Lord, C. (2005). Language and communication in autism. In F. R. Volkmar, R. Paul, A. Klin, & D. Cohen (Eds.), *Handbook of autism and pervasive developmental disorders: Vol. 2* (3rd ed., pp. 335–364). Hoboken, NJ: Wiley.

Tough, J. (1977). *The development of meaning*. New York: Halsted Press.

Volkmar, F. R. (2005). International perspectives. In F. R. Volkmar, R. Paul, A. Klin, & D. Cohen (Eds.), *Handbook of autism and pervasive developmental disorders: Vol. 2* (3rd ed., pp. 1193–1252). Hoboken, NJ: Wiley.

Volkmar, F. R., Stier, D. M., & Cohen, D. J. (1985). Age of recognition of pervasive developmental disorder. *American Journal of Psychiatry, 142,* 1450–1452.

Warlaumont, A. S., Richards, J. A., Gilkerson, J., & Oller, D. K. (2014). A social feedback loop for speech development and its reduction in autism. *Psychological Science, 25,* 1314–1324.

Wetherby, A. M., & Prizant, B. M. (2002). *Communication and Symbolic Behavior Scales*. Baltimore: Brookes.

Wetherby, A. M., Prizant, B. M., & Hutchinson, T. (1998). Communicative, social–affective, and symbolic profiles of young children with autism and pervasive developmental disorder. *American Journal of Speech–Language Pathology, 7,* 79–91.

Wetherby, A. M., Woods, J., Allen, L., Cleary, J., Dickinson, H., & Lord, C. (2004). Early indicators of autism spectrum disorders in the second year of life. *Journal of Autism and Developmental Disorders, 34,* 473–493.

Whaley, A. L. (1998). Racism in the provision of mental health services: A social-cognitive analysis. *American Journal of Orthopsychiatry, 68*(1), 47–57.

Wiig, E. H., & Secord, W. (1989). *Test of Language Competence.* New York: Psychological Corporation.

Wiig, E. H., Semel, E., & Secord, W. (2013). *Clinical Evaluation of Language Fundamentals—Preschool, Third Edition (CELF-Preschool 3).* San Antonio, TX: Harcourt Assessment.

Windsor, J., Doyle, S., & Siegel, G. (1994). Language acquisition after mutism: A longitudinal case study of autism. *Journal of Speech and Hearing Research, 37,* 96–105.

Wodka, E., Mathy, P., & Kalb, L. (2013). Predictors of phrase and fluent speech in children with autism and severe language delay. *Pediatrics, 131,* 1128–1135.

Woods, J., & Wetherby, A. M. (2003). Early identification of and intervention for infants and toddlers who are at risk for autism spectrum disorder. *Language, Speech and Hearing Services in Schools, 34,* 180–193.

World Health Organization. (1992). *International classification of diseases* (10th rev.). Geneva, Switzerland: Author.

Young, E. C., Diehl, J. J., Morris, D., Hyman, S. L., & Bennetto, L. (2005). The use of two language tests to identify pragmatic language problems in children with autism spectrum disorders. *Language, Speech, and Hearing Services in Schools, 36,* 62–72.

Zimmerman, I., Steiner, V., & Pond, R. (2012). *Preschool Language Scale, Fifth Edition (PLS-5).* San Antonio, TX: Psychological Corporation.

Zinober, B., & Martlew, M. (1985). Developmental changes in four types of gesture in relation to acts and vocalization from 10 to 21 months. *British Journal of Developmental Psychology, 3,* 293–306.

CHAPTER EIGHT

Assessment of Intellectual Functioning in Autism Spectrum Disorder

Laura Grofer Klinger
Joanna L. Mussey
Sarah O'Kelley

> Even though most of these children were at one time or another looked upon as feebleminded, they are all unquestionably endowed with good *cognitive potentialities*. . . . The astounding vocabulary of the speaking children, the excellent rote memory for events of several years before, the phenomenal rote memory for poems and names, and the precise recollection of complex patterns and sequences, bespeak good intelligence. . . .
>
> —KANNER (1943, p. 217; emphasis in original)

Kanner's (1943) original description of the intellectual abilities of children with autism spectrum disorder (ASD) highlights the juxtaposition of cognitive delays and cognitive strengths that characterize this disorder. Even when an intellectual evaluation suggests that a child with ASD is developmentally delayed, children with ASD often have some peaks in their abilities. This combination of strengths and weaknesses creates an uneven profile of cognitive abilities in individuals with ASD (see Figure 8.1). This uneven cognitive profile presents a conundrum for psychologists trying to decide which IQ test to administer.

Consider the case example of Jason, an 8-year-old boy with a diagnosis of ASD. Jason had an extensive vocabulary, although the majority of his speech consisted of delayed echolalia, and he was unable to participate in a lengthy reciprocal conversation. He loved puzzles and spent hours every day arranging objects into geometric patterns. Jason's mother referred him to our clinic for a psychological evaluation to assist in academic placement and accommodations for the third grade. If Jason were evaluated with

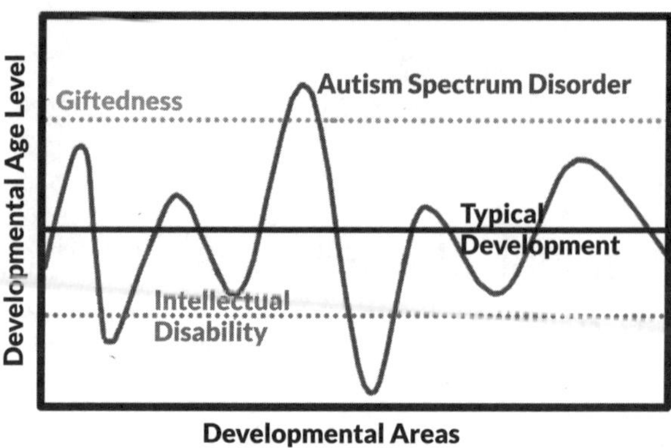

FIGURE 8.1. Uneven cognitive profile in ASD.

an IQ test that required him to formulate answers to complex questions (e.g., the Wechsler Intelligence Scale for Children—Fifth Edition [WISC-V]; Wechsler, 2014), he would be likely to show significant impairments and receive a score in the range of mild intellectual disability. However, in contrast, if Jason were administered a nonverbal test of intelligence measuring visual sequencing and pattern perception skills (e.g., the Leiter International Performance Scale—Third Edition [Leiter–3]; Roid, Miller, Pomplun, & Koch, 2013), he would be likely to show average or above-average performance. Hence the conundrum faced by the psychologist: Which test would be most appropriate for Jason? Which test would be the best measure of Jason's true abilities? Which test is the best measure of the "cognitive potentialities" that Kanner described?

The purpose of this chapter is to provide a set of guidelines for deciding which intelligence test may be the most appropriate when evaluating a person with ASD.[1] There is no "best test" for measuring intellectual functioning in persons with ASD. Instead, the psychologist must consider the reasons that an intellectual evaluation is being requested for this particular individual; the literature on intellectual strengths and weaknesses in ASD; the unique social, communication, and behavioral symptoms of ASD that may interfere with intellectual testing; and the specific properties of the intellectual tests that are being considered. Thus, before we can provide

---

[1]As previous research that is cited in this chapter may have separated their ASD group into DSM-IV-TR (American Psychiatric Association, 2000) subtypes, such as autistic disorder or Asperger's disorder, in our discussions of this literature, we maintain these groupings as reported in the research publication. Otherwise, to reflect current nomenclature, the term "ASD" is generally used in discussions.

a set of guidelines for choosing an intellectual assessment battery, each of these issues is discussed in detail.

OVERLAP BETWEEN ASD AND INTELLECTUAL DISABILITY

Historically, it was believed that the majority of children with ASD have a dual diagnosis of intellectual disability, although there was little empirical evidence to support these claims (Edelson, 2006). In his review of 36 epidemiological studies published between 1966 and 2003, Fombonne (2005) reported that the median rate of intellectual disability in individuals diagnosed with autistic disorder was 70.4% (range = 40–100%). More recent studies, however, suggest that the rate of intellectual disability is considerably lower. The Autism and Developmental Disabilities Monitoring (ADDM) Network (Christensen et al., 2016) surveillance data from nine sites in the United States reported that 31.6% (range = 20–50%) of 8-year-old children with ASD were classified as having IQ scores in the range of intellectual disability (IQ ≤ 70). Across sites, 24.5% of children scored in the borderline range (IQ = 71–85) and 43.9% in the average or above-average range of intellectual ability (IQ > 85). A total population study of children and young adults in Sweden indicated that 25.6% of individuals with ASD had an intellectual disability with younger birth cohorts showing a consistent increase of ASD without comorbid intellectual disability (Idring et al., 2015). These decreasing rates could be the result of a broadening of the ASD diagnostic criteria, improved identification of more mildly affected individuals, and/or more available and effective early intervention. Regardless of why the rates of comorbid diagnoses of ASD and intellectual disability are decreasing, there is a growing need for intellectual assessments that are appropriate for individuals with ASD who have a wide range of intellectual abilities.

Lower IQ scores have been associated with gender, race/ethnicity, and the presence of comorbid medical conditions. Females with autism tend to receive lower scores on both verbal and nonverbal measures of intelligence with a more equivalent sex ratio in persons with ASD who have comorbid intellectual disability (Rubenstein, Wiggins, & Lee, 2015; Volkmar, Szamari, & Sparrow, 1993). Data from the 2016 ADDM study estimated that 37% of females with ASD had IQ scores indicating intellectual disability compared with 30% of males (Christensen et al., 2016). However, some research has suggested that females affected with ASD without comorbid intellectual disability may be undiagnosed or misdiagnosed, which may result in this uneven distribution of intellectual abilities across gender (see Kirkovski, Enticott, & Fitzgerald, 2013, for a review). With regard to race/ethnicity, the estimated prevalence of ASD with intellectual disability in European American children was significantly lower (3.3 per 1,000) than African American children (5.8 per 1,000; Christensen et al., 2016). Additional research is needed on the etiology of these differences, but this variation might be attributable to a variety of factors, including regional and socioeconomic disparities in access to services, underrecognition of symptoms of ASD in some groups, or cultural differences influencing the decision to seek services, among others. Individuals with ASD and a comorbid seizure disorder are more likely to have intellectual disability. Specifically, a meta-analysis of studies found the pooled prevalence of epilepsy was 21.5% in individuals with ASD with intellectual disability and 8% in those with ASD without intellectual disability (Amiet et al., 2008).

REFERRAL QUESTIONS FOR INTELLECTUAL TESTING IN ASD

When a clinician is choosing an appropriate instrument to assess developmental or intellectual functioning, it is important to consider the reason(s) why the testing is being conducted. There are several different reasons for evaluating developmental and intellectual abilities in individuals with ASD: (1) as part of a diagnostic battery to determine whether an ASD is present, (2) as part of an educational battery to evaluate the strengths and weaknesses that should be targeted by a child's individualized education program or transition support plan, (3) as a measure of treatment effectiveness, and (4) as an aid in estimating long-term prognosis.

Diagnostic Assessment

Intellectual testing is a recommended part of an interdisciplinary diagnostic evaluation (Johnson, Myers, & the Council on Children with Disabilities, 2007; Volkmar et al., 2014). Intellectual assessment results can be used to facilitate comorbid diagnosis of ASD and intellectual disability. Klin, Saulnier, Tsatsanis, and Volkmar (2005) described intellectual assessment as a frame for interpreting the results of diagnostic testing. This "frame" can be used to evaluate whether a child's social and communication delays are greater than expected from the child's developmental level, or whether they are equivalent to the child's developmental level. In a child who receives an ASD diagnosis, social and communicative skills are delayed below developmental level. For example, if a developmental evaluation indicates that a 4-year-old child has the cognitive development of a 2-year-old, then his or her social and communication skills (e.g., eye contact, pointing, symbolic play, reciprocal interactions, affect) should be compared with the skills expected of a 2-year-old. If a discrepancy between developmental level and social communication skills is not present, then diagnoses of other developmental delays or language disorder should be considered.

Intellectual assessment results can also be used to determine whether comorbid ASD and intellectual disability is present. While DSM-5 (American Psychiatric Association, 2013) diagnostic criteria do not rely on cognitive development to diagnose ASD, the presence or absence of accompanying intellectual impairment should be documented and specified. Separate estimates of verbal and nonverbal skills are necessary in light of the characteristically uneven cognitive profile in ASD.

Assessment of Current Strengths and Weaknesses

Intellectual testing is often helpful in clarifying the specific strengths and weaknesses present in an individual child or adult and highlighting the areas that need to be addressed by intervention. Klin et al. (2005) recommended that intellectual assessment should

> describe patterns of both verbal and nonverbal functioning across several domains: (1) problem solving (e.g., can the child generate strategies and integrate information?), (2) concept formation (e.g., can the child abstract rules from specific instances or understand principles of categorization, order, time, number, and causation, and generalize knowledge from one context to another?), (3) reasoning (e.g., can the child transform information to solve visual–perceptual and verbal problems?), (4) style of learning (e.g., can the child learn from modeling, imitation, using visual cues, or verbal prompts?), and (5) memory skills (e.g., how many items of information can the child retain; . . . are the child's memory skills in one modality better than in another such as visual or verbal?). (p. 777)

This assessment of strengths and weaknesses is especially important given the uneven profile of cognitive skills that typically characterizes individuals with ASD. IQ profiles may provide additional information for clinicians regarding the individual with ASD with whom they are working (Chiang, Tsai, Cheung, Brown, & Li, 2014). This information can give insight into difficulties they are experiencing related to areas of cognitive weakness as well as ideas for interventions and strategies that capitalize upon strengths to compensate for or address weaknesses.

Assessment of Intervention Effectiveness

Although IQ scores are commonly used as a measure of treatment effectiveness, there are several cautions involved in using IQ testing for this purpose. Importantly, the use of the same IQ test on multiple occasions raises concerns about possible practice effects and concerns about whether the testing is developmentally appropriate at both testing points. For example, a developmental test such as the Bayley Scales of Infant and Toddler Development, Third Edition (Bayley–III; Bayley, 2005) may be appropriate for a 2-year-old beginning intervention, but is no longer appropriate for a 4-year-old at the conclusion of intervention. However, if a different test is administered at pre- and posttreatment, it is unclear whether gains are due to testing error, the different social and communication requirements of the test, or whether a true increase in developmental level or IQ has occurred. For example, while two commonly used measures for assessing developmental level in young children with ASD—the Mullen Scales of Early Learning and the Differential Ability Scales—may be highly correlated, large mean differences in cognitive ability across tests occur (Farmer, Golden, & Thurm, 2016). Even when the same test is administered at both time points, there are concerns that the items may measure different skills at different ages. For example, instruments may include measures of social skills (e.g., playing peek-a-boo, reading a book with the examiner) for infants and toddlers that may not be components of the same test at older ages. In this example, earlier scores could partially be attributed to the child's social rather than intellectual delays.

Despite these cautions, changes in cognitive abilities are considered a hallmark of effective interventions—especially early interventions (e.g., Eikeseth, Smith, Jahr, & Eldevik, 2007; Estes et al., 2015). The National Research Council (2001) recommends that while intellectual testing provides useful information in measuring treatment effectiveness, this type of testing is not sufficient and should not be used as the sole measure of treatment outcome. Indeed, the assessment of specific skills targeted by an intervention (e.g., social skills, communication skills, play skills) may be better measures of treatment mediators and moderators than IQ (see Vivanti, Prior, Williams, & Dissanayake, 2014, for a review).

Predictions of Long-Term Outcome

IQ testing is often used as a prognostic indicator of long-term outcome for children and adolescents with ASD. A review of 23 longitudinal studies of preschool and school-age children points to stability of IQ in the majority of studies evaluated (Begovac, Begovac, Majic, & Vidovic, 2009). Anderson, Liang, and Lord (2014) conducted a long-term follow-up study on 85 children initially seen between 2 and 3 years of age and followed until the age of 19 years. Verbal IQ at age 3 was a strong predictor of intellectual ability at age 19. Each standard deviation increase in age 3 verbal IQ increased the odds of being in the cognitively able group of youth 21-fold. For cognitively able youth, large gains in verbal IQ were observed between ages 2 and 3. These findings point to the importance of assessing intellectual ability when diagnosing ASD.

However, this does not mean that IQ scores are always stable across the lifespan. Mayes and Calhoun (2003) found a significant correlation between age and full scale IQ (FSIQ) in their sample of 164 children (ages 3–15 years) with autism. The average IQ score increased from 53 for children 3 years of age to 91 for children 8 years of age and older. For children with IQ scores below 80, both verbal and nonverbal IQ scores increased. For children with IQ scores greater than or equal to 80, only verbal IQ increased significantly with age. After 8 years of age, both verbal and nonverbal IQ was relatively stable. Because this was a cross-sectional study, it is possible that the increase in IQ can be attributed to the fact that children who are more severely disordered are generally evaluated at a younger age, while more high-functioning children are not seen until school age. Nevertheless, this research suggests that it is important to reevaluate intellectual functioning in middle childhood or early adolescence to better predict long-term outcome.

In addition to predicting adult intellectual abilities, childhood IQ is a strong predictor of adult independent living skills. Indeed, in discussing adult outcomes for their 40-year follow-up study, Howlin, Goode, Hutton, and Rutter (2004) concluded that "only individuals with an IQ in the normal range (70+) have a real chance of living independently as they reach adulthood" (p. 225). Other follow-up studies from middle childhood to adulthood (Beadle-Brown, Murphy, & Wing, 2006; Smith, Maenner, & Seltzer, 2012; Taylor & Seltzer, 2011) have reported similar findings indicating that IQ is a good predictor of long-term educational attainment, communication skills, independent living skills, and competitive employment.

Taken together, these studies suggest that IQ scores may be an important predictor of long-term outcome in terms of cognitive functioning and independent living skills once a child reaches middle childhood. Thus, an IQ test is an important component of an assessment battery designed to estimate long-term prognosis.

PROFILE OF STRENGTHS AND WEAKNESSES IN ASD

It has historically been believed that individuals with ASD have a specific profile of intellectual ability characterized by a higher nonverbal IQ than verbal IQ (see Lincoln, Hansel, & Quirmbach, 2007, for a review). For example, individuals with ASD have frequently shown relative and absolute strengths on nonverbal visual–spatial tasks involving puzzles and arranging patterns or blocks into designs (e.g., Ghaziuddin & Mountain-Kimchi, 2004; Ozonoff, South, & Miller, 2000). Recently, however, this general belief has been called into question. Ankenman, Elgin, Sullivan, Vincent, and Bernier (2014) examined 1,954 children with ASD between the ages of 4 and 17 years—the children had a wide range of cognitive abilities (verbal IQ range = 30–167 and nonverbal IQ range = 33–161). Overall, the majority of individuals (58.8%) showed no cognitive split between verbal and nonverbal abilities. Those children with higher nonverbal than verbal abilities tended to be younger, male, and have more significant impairments in social communication skills.

Indeed, a variety of cognitive profiles have been described in children with ASD. In a sample of 456 young children with ASD (ages 24–66 months), Munson and colleagues (2008) identified four different profiles of intellectual functioning: very low verbal and low nonverbal scores, with an average difference of 22 points (59% of the sample); very low verbal abilities, with nonverbal scores higher by approximately 42 points (12.5%); commensurate verbal and nonverbal abilities, yet mild to moderate impairments in cognitive functioning (21.7%); and commensurate verbal and nonverbal performance, with overall functioning in the low average range (7%). Children with the largest discrepancy between verbal and nonverbal abilities (Group 2) were younger, suggesting that age may play a factor in cognitive profiles. Additionally, there has been some evidence that individuals with less severe symptoms of ASD without intellectual disability (what under DSM-IV would have been called Asperger syndrome or high-functioning autism) tend to display an intellectual profile characterized by higher verbal IQ than nonverbal IQ, although this profile is not ubiquitous (Ehlers et al., 1997; Ghaziuddin & Mountain-Kimchi, 2004; Joseph, Tager-Flusberg, & Lord, 2002; Ozonoff et al., 2000). Thus, cognitive profiles may vary by age, IQ, and ASD symptom severity such that, contrary to prevailing beliefs, no single pattern appears indicative of an ASD diagnosis.

Rather than focusing on specific strengths and weaknesses across broad categories of verbal and nonverbal abilities assessed by IQ tests, investigators have begun to identify specific cognitive strengths and weaknesses in persons with ASD. In a large sample of individuals with ASD, caregivers reported that 62.5% demonstrated unusual islets of ability or "splinter skills" that represented relative strengths in comparison with other skills and absolute strengths in comparison with same-age peers (Meilleur, Jelenic, & Mottron, 2015). These splinter skills were reported in memory, visuospatial skills, reading, drawing, music, and mathematical calculations. Individuals with special isolated skills tended to be older and have higher intelligence levels. Depending on the specific tasks, these splinter skills could skew scores during IQ testing.

In addition to these isolated strengths, individuals with ASD have been reported to show specific weaknesses in a variety of cognitive areas. Cognitive impairments are thought to have a significant impact on daily life, particularly with regard to their social interactions. There are several theories regarding early-developing cognitive impairments—specifically, researchers have proposed that ASD is characterized by atypical perception, attention, intuitive learning, flexible thinking, and perspective taking. Perceptual theories suggest that individuals with ASD have a cognitive style in which they tend to focus on the details rather than the bigger picture, which may account for their success on nonverbal perceptual tasks such as block designs (i.e., weak central coherence; Happé & Booth, 2008; Happé & Frith, 2006). Furthermore, Mottron, Dawson, Soulieres, Hubert, and Burack (2006) have suggested that this type of enhanced perceptual processing is present not only in visual perception but across a wide range of perceptual domains. Attention theories have highlighted difficulties in disengaging and shifting attention, with sustained attention relatively intact in persons with ASD (Courchesne et al., 1994; Keehn, Muller, & Townsend, 2013; Renner, Klinger, & Klinger, 2006). Difficulties in shifting focus have been described as part of an overall impaired learning style characterized by rigid, inflexible thinking (i.e., impaired executive functioning; Geurts, Corbett, & Solomon, 2009; Ozonoff & Jenson, 1999; Russo et al., 2007). Difficulties in taking into account both one's own perspective and the perspective of another person (i.e., impaired theory of mind; Baron-Cohen, 2001) are considered hallmark cognitive problems experienced by individuals with ASD. Other learning theories have highlighted difficulties in integration of information due to impaired complex information processing (Minshew, Goldstein, & Siegel, 1997; Williams, Goldstein, & Minshew, 2006) and impaired implicit or intuitive learning (Klinger, Klinger, & Pohlig, 2007). Across this research, a pattern of strengths (i.e., perceptual processing, sustained attention, and simple information processing) and weaknesses (i.e., central coherence, shifting attention, flexible thinking, perspective taking, implicit learning, and complex information processing) has emerged to describe the learning styles of individuals with ASD. However, these learning differences have rarely been examined within the same group of individuals. In a recent study examining executive function, central coherence, and theory-of-mind skills within the same individuals with ASD, the majority of individuals with ASD demonstrated a weakness in one of these cognitive domains—however, only 32% show multiple cognitive atypicalities across all three domains (Brunsdon et al., 2015). Those with difficulties in multiple cognitive domains showed higher levels of autism symptomatology.

Taken together, research on cognitive strengths and weaknesses suggests that there is no single underlying cognitive deficit in those with ASD.

Instead, ASD is characterized by an atypical pattern of cognitive strengths and weaknesses, although the pattern may differ across individuals with ASD. Because of this characteristically uneven cognitive profile, a child's overall IQ scores may be an average of widely discrepant scores (see Figure 8.1) and thus may not meaningfully describe the child's true ability (Klin et al., 2005). An average IQ score may overestimate ability in a child's weakest skills and underestimate ability in a child's strongest skills. Isolated peaks in performance on some tasks are not necessarily indicative of skills in other areas, or even in related areas. For example, an 8-year-old child may be able to decode written material at the level of a 10-year-old, but may have the reading comprehension ability of a 6-year-old. Thus, it is critical for the evaluator to have knowledge of the varying learning differences that have been associated with ASD in order to avoid erroneous conclusions by focusing on islets of strengths or specific weaknesses when interpreting testing results.

DEVELOPMENTAL AND BEHAVIORAL ISSUES IN ASSESSING PERSONS WITH ASD

Successful performance on an IQ test requires the ability to sit and attend to another person's instructions. However, as discussed above, the characteristics of ASD include difficulties with attention, social interaction, and language understanding. Thus, the traditional standardized assessment paradigm is often a challenge for children with ASD (and for the examiners trying to administer the tests). At a minimum, an examiner should have experience administering intellectual assessments, as well as some knowledge about how the symptoms of ASD may interfere with test administration and performance. Ideally, the examiner will have experience interacting with individuals with ASD. An understanding of the symptoms and treatment approaches for ASD will assist the examiner in choosing an appropriate test and structuring the testing session to ensure that an individual's performance is representative of his or her true abilities.

Developmental Issues in IQ Assessment

It is important for an examiner to consider an individual's chronological and mental ages when choosing and administering an IQ test. This is particularly important in testing children with significant developmental delays, who demonstrate a wide discrepancy between chronological and mental age. Such a child is likely to receive the lowest standard score provided by an assessment instrument. When this happens, it is difficult to translate the score into a meaningful description of the child's current ability. For example, if an IQ score of 50 is the lowest standard score provided by the assessment instrument, it is impossible to know whether the child's IQ is truly in this moderate range of intellectual disability, or whether a test with a wider range of standard scores would indicate severe or profound intellectual disability.

For older individuals with significant developmental delays, it would be more appropriate to administer a test with a wider age range that will accommodate their level of delay. For example, a 12-year-old who is functioning at a 4-year-old level will probably be unable to complete any items on a test designed for elementary school-age children, but may be able to perform some of the simpler tasks on a test designed for ages that span the preschool and elementary school years. For a young child, it may be more useful to consider the child's mental age (by calculating age equivalent scores) rather than to focus on a standard score (Akshoomoff, 2006). A focus on mental age equivalent scores in young children has several advantages. First, it highlights a focus on current developmental level rather than IQ. This is particularly important for young children with ASD, as the research discussed above on the stability of IQ in children with ASD suggests that children can show large improvements in IQ scores from the preschool to elementary school years. Thus, the use of a mental age score provides information about current ability without implying permanent intellectual disability. Second, the use of mental age equivalents may be more meaningful to caregivers or teachers, as they provide estimates of developmentally appropriate academic, behavioral, and adaptive expectations. For example, it would be developmentally inappropriate to expect a 3½-year-old child who is functioning at the 15-month level to learn to write his or her name, be toilet trained, or understand the link between his or her actions and time out as a discipline technique.

Finally, when an examiner is testing a child with significant developmental delay, Akshoomoff (2006) recommends allowing parents to observe developmental testing and asking the parents for feedback about whether the child seemed to be performing to the best of his or her abilities. Indeed, this is the approach we use in our ASD clinics. We have found that this extra information is useful in helping the examiner consider how to interpret the current results. For example, when an examiner is trying to decide whether a child's refusal behavior occurred because the task demands were too complicated for the child or because the child was simply not interested in trying the task, a parent's view is often helpful, particularly when the parent indicates that the child has never been able to complete similar tasks at home or school. Allowing parents to observe and provide their opinions is also helpful in preparing parents for the feedback meeting. Parents who feel that their child showed his or her best skills during tests are more likely to accept estimates of developmental level or IQ as accurate representations of their child's current abilities.

Interference of ASD Symptoms

Individuals with ASD have the most difficulty on tests involving the use of social and language skills that are specifically impaired in ASD—including attending to social information (Dawson et al., 2004), imitation (Rogers, Hepburn, Stackhouse, & Wehner, 2003), joint attention (Sigman, Mundy, Sherman, & Ungerer, 1986), and understanding of personal pronouns. These types of tasks are likely to produce lower scores than tasks requiring skills that are often strengths in individuals with ASD (e.g., perception, rote memory). This is particularly evident when testing very young children with ASD (e.g., 2- to 4-year-old children). For example, such children with ASD may have difficulty completing tasks that assess the ability to play reciprocal social games (e.g., peek-a-boo), the ability to use an index finger to point to objects (e.g., joint attention), the ability to imitate the examiner's actions, and the ability to understand directions that use the pronouns "I" and "you." These types of tasks are frequently found on assessments designed to measure cognitive abilities in infants and toddlers. Thus, low scores on these cognitive measures may be associated with decreased attention, social engagement, and emotion regulation rather than true cognitive delays (Akshoomoff, 2006). Although it may be impossible to find a test that does not involve these social and communication skills, an examiner should be aware of which tasks are likely to be particularly difficult for a child with ASD.

Ideas for Structuring the Testing Session

In order for an assessment to be considered valid, it must be administered in a standardized fashion, involving correct object placement and verbal and nonverbal directions. However, an experienced clinician can combine standardized administration with behavior management techniques that increase cooperation and motivation, and thus lead to a more valid estimate of the individual's ability. If a child spends the entire testing session screaming or running in circles in the testing room, the results are unlikely to be a true estimate of the child's abilities, no matter how standardized the administration of materials may be.

Lincoln et al. (2007) offer several ideas for how to encourage cooperation and reduce a child's attempt to leave the testing situation. For example, they suggest that it is often helpful for the examiner to position the side of the testing table against a wall, to have an assistant or parent sit next to the child, to position him- or herself behind the child (although this requires the examiner to be flexible enough to administer items from a different perspective than is typically used), or to conduct the testing while sitting on the floor. In our clinical experiences, we have successfully used each of these strategies. For graduate students learning test administration, it is often helpful to have an assistant in the room who can manage the child's behavior (e.g., by providing rewards, encouraging the child to stay seated) while the examiner focuses on administering test items. This not only provides the examiner an opportunity to display testing materials correctly but reduces the overall test-taking time.

Individuals with ASD often become quite anxious when aspects of their routine are changed. For instance, parents of very young children with ASD frequently report that their children become upset when they take a different route to school or home. IQ testing is clearly not part of a regular daily routine—thus, being brought to a new place, meeting a new person, and being asked to do new tasks can be extremely stressful for a child with ASD. The use of a visual schedule can significantly reduce the child's anxiety about the testing session. Pictures depicting the various subtests (e.g., blocks, puzzles, book, and a question mark) can be put in vertical order on a piece of paper, with a check box next to each picture. As the child moves through each task, he or she can check each box (or put a sticker in each box) as a task is completed. Ideally, the examiner will know that this type of structure is needed ahead of time. However, if necessary, a quickly written column of numbers with boxes associated with each number will work. With higher-functioning children and adolescents, a written list will suffice (e.g., a simple list of words associated with each task—"Blocks," "Questions," "Find the same").

Typically, we vary our social interaction style with young children by using facial expressions, eye contact, and different words of praise throughout the testing session. However, given that difficulties with social skills are the hallmark deficits of ASD, it is often helpful to minimize the social component of the testing by developing a social routine. This is particularly important for young children with ASD, who may not understand a visual schedule (unless they are in an intervention program that uses this technique). For example, the examiner can establish a routine of saying, "Time to work. Look," presenting the test item, waiting for a response, and then saying "Good working." This type of routine not only minimizes the child's anxiety about being in a new place but also makes the examiner more predictable.

Individuals with ASD often have intense interests that interfere with their performance on standardized testing. For example, a young boy obsessed with trains may bring trains to the testing room, insist on holding a train during testing, and talk repetitively about the train that he saw on the way to the clinic. In this example, IQ scores will certainly be affected by his obsession—timed motor tasks will be hindered by the fact that the child is clutching a train, and verbal items will be hindered by the fact that he answers every question by talking about the train he saw. Koegel, Koegel, and Smith (1997) have suggested children with ASD can be motivated to complete assessment tasks if they are rewarded with breaks to play with objects related to their interests or to talk about their interests. Thus, in this example, the child may be given the opportunity to play with trains as a reward for completing a task. For example, the examiner can build a train station (e.g., a tissue box) and tell the child that the trains need to stay in the station until the puzzles are done: "After we finish the puzzles, we can play with the trains. The trains need to stay in the station until the puzzles are finished." The examiner can further structure the environment by adding train play to the schedule (i.e., a picture of a train or the word "train" after every subtest) and by using a timer to tell the child how long he has to play with the train before returning to the IQ test. This level of structure helps to improve the child's understanding of when he will be allowed to play with the trains, and thus to improve the child's motivation to complete the IQ subtests. As a result, the child is eminently more "testable" and is likely to receive higher IQ scores than would have been obtained by allowing the child to clutch a train and talk about it incessantly during testing.

Overall, if an examiner has experience and an understanding of ASD symptoms and intervention approaches, few children with ASD should truly be "untestable" (Ozonoff, Goodlin-Jones, & Solomon, 2007). Koegel et al. (1997) found significant improvements in IQ when the testing session was modified to increase attention and motivation (e.g., by providing predictable breaks contingent upon on-task performance, allowing a child's mother to be present in the testing room, permitting the child to sit on the floor). However, unless the structure of the assessment session is adapted to fit the specific needs of the child with ASD, the "test session becomes one of assessing motivation, attention, or compliance more than of assessing language or intelligence" (Koegel et al., 1997, p. 241).

MEASURES OF INTELLECTUAL FUNCTIONING

Clinicians and researchers have a number of tools available to them for assessing developmental level and intellectual ability of individuals with ASD. Some of these measures were standardized on individuals with ASD, although inclusion criteria for each measure may have differed. However, other measures did not specifically include individuals with ASD during standardization, although individuals with ASD were not explicitly excluded according to the norming criteria provided in the technical manuals. Table 8.1 briefly summarizes the characteristics of the instruments reviewed below.

TABLE 8.1. Cognitive and Adaptive Measures for Individuals with ASD

Measure	Age range	Administration time (minutes)	Individuals with ASD included in standardization
		Cognitive measures	
Preschool age			
Bayley–III	1–42 m	30–90	DSM-IV AD, AS, and PDD
DAS-II (Early Years battery)	2 y, 6 m to 3 y, 5 m	20	None
WPPSI-IV (young level)	2 y, 6 m to 3 y, 11 m	30–45	DSM-IV AD and AS
Mullen	Birth–5 y, 8 m	15–60	None
School age			
DAS-II (School-Age battery)	3 y, 6 m to 17 y, 11 m	30	None
WPPSI-IV (older level)	4 y, 0 m to 7 y, 7 m	45–60	DSM-IV AD and AS
WISC-V	6 y, 0 m to 16 y, 11 m	48–65	DSM-5 ASD with and without language delay
Adult			
WAIS-IV	16–90 y	65–90	None
Lifespan			
SB5	2–85 y	45–75	DSM-IV AD
Leiter–3	3– >75 y	25–40	None
WASI-II	6–90 y	15–30	None
KBIT-2	4–90 y	15–30	None
		Adaptive measures	
Vineland–II	Birth–90 y	20–60	DSM-IV AD
ABAS-3	Birth–89 y	20	DSM-IV AD and AS

Note. Bayley–III, Bayley Scales of Infant and Toddler Development, Third Edition; DAS-II, Differential Ability Scales—Second Edition; WPPSI-IV, Wechsler Preschool and Primary Scale of Intelligence—Fourth Edition; Mullen, Mullen Scales of Early Learning; WISC-V, Wechsler Intelligence Scale for Children—Fifth Edition; Leiter–3, Leiter International Performance Scale—Third Edition; WAIS-IV, Wechsler Adult Intelligence Scale—Fourth Edition; SB5, Stanford–Binet Intelligence Scales, Fifth Edition; WASI-II, Wechsler Abbreviated Scale of Intelligence—Second Edition; KBIT-2, Kaufman Brief Intelligence Test, Second Edition; Vineland–II, Vineland Adaptive Behavior Scales, Second Edition; ABAS-3, Adaptive Behavior Assessment System—Third Edition; AD, autistic disorder; AS, Asperger syndrome; PDD, pervasive developmental disorder; m, months; y, years.

Bayley Scales of Infant and Toddler Development, Third Edition

The Bayley–III (Bayley, 2005) measures the strengths and abilities of children from 1 to 42 months of age in the areas of cognitive, motor, language, social–emotional, and adaptive behaviors. Composite scores are available for each area assessed. Depending on a child's age, the Bayley–III can be administered in approximately 30–90 minutes. Administration time for the entire battery is approximately 50 minutes for children ages 12 months and younger, and approximately 90 minutes for children ages 13 months and older.

During standardization, data were collected on a group of 70 children between the ages of 16 and 42 months who met DSM-IV criteria for a pervasive developmental disorder (PDD). On the Bayley–III, these children obtained significantly lower scores on all subtest scales (Cognitive, Receptive Communication, Expressive Communication, Fine Motor, Gross Motor, and Social–Emotional) and composite measures (Language and Motor) than did children in the matched control group. Similarly, Ray-Subramanian, Huai, and Weismer (2011) examined the early development of 23- to 39-month-old children with DSM-IV diagnoses of autistic disorder and pervasive developmental disorder not otherwise specified (PDD-NOS) using the Bayley–III. Only 9% of children had standard scores of 100 or greater (mean cognitive composite = 85) and the mean developmental age (in months) on the cognitive scale was approximately 7 months lower than the mean chronological age of the sample.

The Bayley–III is one of the few standardized instruments that are available to evaluate young children with significant developmental delays who would not meet basal requirements on most preschool instruments, resulting in an inability to calculate meaningful standard scores. The most recent version of the Bayley was extended upward to include 3½-year-old children—thus, the Bayley–III is a good choice when testing a 2- or 3-year-old who is functioning below the 24-month level of development. However, a standard score of 50 is the lowest score provided by the Bayley–III, making it impossible to get a specific standard score for children who are extremely delayed and necessitating the use of age equivalent scores. The Bayley–III can also be administered to children older than 42 months to estimate the child's developmental level, if other measures are inappropriate due to a low mental age. However, these results must be interpreted cautiously, as a standard score cannot be computed.

Mullen Scales of Early Learning

The Mullen is designed to measure cognitive functioning in children from birth through 68 months of age (Mullen, 1995). This instrument assesses a child's gross motor, fine motor, visual reception, receptive language, and expressive language abilities. Each of the individual scales yields *T*-scores (mean = 50) and age equivalents. The Mullen also provides an overall Early Learning Composite standard score, which is based on the standardized *T*-scores from the four cognitive scales (Visual Reception, Fine Motor, Receptive Language, and Expressive Language). The amount of time necessary to administer the Mullen varies between approximately 15 and 60 minutes, depending on a child's age, with older children requiring more time.

During standardization of the Mullen, children with known physical or developmental disabilities (including ASD) were not included in the sample. However, a recent study of 399 children (half with ASD) suggests that the Mullen has good convergent and divergent validity in measuring development in young children with ASD (Swineford, Guthrie, & Thurm, 2015). Several studies have used the Mullen to examine cognitive profiles in infants and toddlers who are at risk for developing ASD because of an older sibling with an ASD diagnosis (e.g., Landa & Garrett-Mayer, 2006; Ozonoff et al., 2010). Overall, these studies suggest that children who later receive a diagnosis of ASD show typical cognitive profiles at 6 months of age with developmental delays becoming evident by 12–14 months of age. Further, studies using the Mullen in young children with ASD have found a similar profile of personal strengths in nonverbal cognitive skills and weaknesses in verbal skills, with receptive language more impaired than expressive language (Barbaro & Dissanayake, 2012; Carter et al., 2007; Chawarska, Klin, Paul, Macari, & Volkmar, 2009; Hartley & Sikora, 2009).

Thus, the Mullen appears to capture early emerging developmental delays in toddlers who are at risk for ASD. Further, like the Bayley–III, the Mullen is one of the few standardized instruments available to evaluate young children with significant developmental delays who would not meet basal requirements on most preschool assessment instruments. The Mullen is appropriate for children up to 5½ years of age, and thus, is a good choice when testing preschool-age children with significant delays. Because the Mullen covers the entire preschool age range, it is also a good choice for early intervention studies examining change across the preschool years. However, even with this range, 73% of children with ASD in Akshoomoff's (2006) study received the lowest standard score (a *T*-score of 20) provided by the Mullen on one or more scales. A *T*-score of 20 is more than 3 standard deviations below average and represents an overall standard score of 55 or below. In this situation, age equivalent scores may be a more appropriate way to interpret test performance (Akshoomoff, 2006).

Differential Ability Scales—Second Edition

The Differential Ability Scales—Second Edition (DAS-II; Elliot, 2007) is a brief but comprehensive measure of ability, which makes it attractive for use with individuals with ASD. The DAS-II is designed to measure cognitive strengths and weaknesses in individuals between the ages of 2 years, 6 months, and 17 years, 11 months. The Early Years battery consists of a lower level (ages 2 years, 6 months, to 3 years, 5 months) and an upper level (ages 3 years, 6 months, to 6 years, 11 months), each taking approximately 30 minutes to administer. The School-Age battery consists of six subtests for individuals ages 7 years, 0 months, to 17 years, 11 months. The entire battery takes approximately 40 minutes to administer. Testing at each level of the DAS-II yields a General Conceptual Ability (GCA) composite score. For the lower-level Early Years battery, cluster scores for Verbal Ability and Nonverbal Ability are also calculated. For both the upper-level Early Years and the School-Age batteries, cluster scores for Verbal Ability, Nonverbal Reasoning Ability, and Spatial Ability are calculated. In addition, for children 3 years, 6 months, of age or older, a Special Nonverbal Composite may be derived from the appropriate nonverbal core subtests from each battery, which may be a useful measure of cognitive ability for nonverbal individuals with ASD. For individuals between the ages of 5 years, 0 months, and 8 years, 11 months, examiners have the option of administering either the Early Years battery or the School-Age battery "out of level" to either lower- or higher-functioning individuals. The DAS-II provides norms for this full age range across the tasks contributing to these batteries—this is particularly useful for assessing an individual with ASD, as it allows for more accurate assessment based on the individual's mental rather than chronological age. Additional diagnostic subtests that measure working memory, processing speed, and school readiness are also available for individuals of different ages for the DAS-II.

Unlike most other cognitive assessment instruments, the DAS-II does not require a strict administration order for its subtests, which allows the testing session to be individualized for each examinee. For example, it may be beneficial to begin with a nonverbal task for an individual with ASD, to build rapport and familiarity with the testing environment. An examiner may also choose to begin with a subtest that overlaps batteries, such as the Pattern Construction subtest, in order to observe and estimate informally the examinee's level of functioning (e.g., receptive and expressive language, cognitive flexibility) as a guide in selecting the most appropriate test battery (i.e., choosing either the Early Years or School-Age level, or only administering tasks that yield the Special Nonverbal Composite).

Individuals with ASD were not included in the standardization sample although several studies are available regarding its utility with individuals with ASD. Kuriakose (2014) administered the DAS-II School-Age battery to 23 children with a DSM-IV-TR diagnosis of autistic disorder or Asperger's disorder between the ages of 7 and 16 years. Average GCA score in this sample was 88.0 and a profile of higher nonverbal (Nonverbal

Reasoning Ability and Spatial Ability) than verbal (Verbal Ability) abilities was observed. Specifically, the lowest average subtest score was obtained on Word Definitions, while the highest average subtest scores were on Pattern Construction and Matrices.

Overall, the DAS-II offers the opportunity to identify a child's specific strengths and weaknesses; is appropriate across a wide chronological and mental age range; and has some flexibility in test administration, which is helpful when testing children with ASD. Because of the large age range, the DAS-II may be a good choice for intervention studies that will use IQ testing as one measure of outcome across an extended period of time. However, the DAS-II is less useful in testing young children with ASD who are performing below the 2½-year level, as they are unlikely to meet basal requirements on most subtests, resulting in an inability to calculate meaningful standard scores.

Stanford–Binet Intelligence Scales, Fifth Edition

The Stanford–Binet Intelligence Scales, Fifth Edition (SB5; Roid, 2003) assesses intelligence and cognitive abilities in individuals from 2 to 85+ years of age. To obtain an FSIQ, the SB5 requires an average 45–75 minutes of testing time. In addition, the SB5 contains separate sections for Nonverbal IQ (based on five nonverbal subtests) and Verbal IQ (based on five verbal subtests), which can be useful for testing individuals with ASD who are nonverbal or have limited language abilities. Each of these sections requires approximately 30 minutes. In addition, five factor scores can be computed (Fluid Reasoning, Knowledge, Quantitative Reasoning, Visual–Spatial Processing, and Working Memory)—these can be used to identify a pattern of strengths and weaknesses in performance. Each factor score includes a verbal and a nonverbal subtest. Moreover, an Abbreviated Battery IQ can be calculated from two subtests if necessary. This is often helpful when the child is displaying difficulty attending to task demands and the examiner is concerned about being able to complete the lengthier full battery of tests. The SB5 revision was designed to make the test more sensitive to assessing younger children with developmental delays than the previous version.

The SB5 standardization sample included 83 children and adolescents with diagnoses of autistic disorder between the ages of 2 and 17 years. This sample included 79% males and was predominately European American. Individuals with autistic disorder performed similarly to those in the developmental delay group, but had slightly lower means on all subtest and composite scales. Studies examining cognitive profiles of children and adolescents with ASD on the SB5 have found remarkably consistent results (Coolican, Bryson, & Zwaigenbaum, 2008; Matthews et al., 2015), including significantly higher Nonverbal IQ compared to Verbal IQ scores

(37–50% across studies). Specifically, children with ASD demonstrated relative strengths on several nonverbal subtests including Fluid Reasoning, Quantitative Reasoning, and Visual–Spatial Processing skills and strengths on one verbal subtest (Quantitative Reasoning). This profile of higher Nonverbal than Verbal IQ was found only in children older than 6 years of age. Further, both studies found that the Abbreviated Battery IQ was not statistically different from the FSIQ for the majority of children (i.e., 73% of the Coolican et al., 2008, sample). However, when the scores differed, the Abbreviated Battery IQ was typically higher than the FSIQ. Thus, Coolican et al. (2008) recommended being cautious when using the Abbreviated Battery IQ as it may overestimate overall ability in some individuals with ASD.

Because of its wide age range, the SB5 may be an appropriate measure for testing a child with significant developmental delays (e.g., a 10-year-old child with the mental age of a preschool child) who might not meet basal requirements on tests that are solely developed for school-age children. In addition, the SB5 may be a good choice for intervention studies that will use IQ testing as one measure of outcome across an extended period of time. Although the SB5 provides a Nonverbal IQ score that may be appropriate for children with limited language, some of the nonverbal tasks require imitation and receptive language skills, which are both areas of weakness in children with ASD. For example, the Nonverbal Working Memory task requires the child to imitate the examiner's motor movements by tapping a series of blocks. At a more sophisticated level, children are asked to imitate the examiner's movements in reverse order, requiring that the child understand the verbal directions to do so. Thus, the nonverbal measures on the SB5 are not completely independent of language understanding and can be negatively impacted by symptoms of ASD.

Wechsler Preschool and Primary Scale of Intelligence—Fourth Edition

The Wechsler Preschool and Primary Scale of Intelligence—Fourth Edition (WPPSI-IV; Wechsler, 2012) assesses cognitive functioning in young children across two age bands: ages 2 years, 6 months, to 3 years, 11 months; and ages 4 years, 0 months, to 7 years, 7 months. For both age bands, the WPPSI-IV yields an FSIQ, a Primary Index scale, and the Ancillary Index scale. For younger children, the WPPSI-IV FSIQ and Primary Index scales comprise three composite scores: Verbal Comprehension, Visual Spatial, and Working Memory. For the older children, two additional composites, Fluid Reasoning and Processing Speed, are included. The Ancillary scales include the Vocabulary Acquisition Index, the Nonverbal Index, the General Ability Index (GAI), and for older children, the Cognitive Proficiency Index (CPI). It is estimated that the average administration time to obtain an FSIQ is 30–60 minutes, with less time for younger children. The standardization sample included a group of 38 children with DSM-IV-TR autistic disorder (ages 2 years, 10 months, to 7 years, 6 months; 79% male) and 38 children with Asperger's disorder (ages 3 years, 10 months, to 7 years, 6 months; 79% male). For both groups, the lowest performance was noted on the Comprehension subtest along with poor scores on the Processing Speed Index. In both groups, the highest scores were obtained on the Visual Spatial Index. Because the WPPSI-IV provides a Verbal Comprehension Index, a Visual Spatial Index, a Working Memory Index, and a Nonverbal Index, it offers an opportunity to identify a pattern of strengths and weaknesses in children with ASD. However, some of the nonverbal tasks require language understanding—thus, they are not completely independent of a child's language delays. The WPPSI-IV is designed to include both younger preschool-age children and older children entering elementary school, making it appropriate for beginning school-age children who have significant developmental delays. However, the WPPSI-IV is less useful when testing 2- and 3-year-old children with ASD who are performing below the 2½-year level, as they are unlikely to meet basal requirements on most subtests, resulting in an inability to calculate meaningful standard scores.

Wechsler Intelligence Scale for Children—Fifth Edition

The WISC-V (Wechsler, 2014) is designed to assess intelligence in children ages 6 years, 0 months, to 16 years, 11 months. There are five primary index scales with two subtests in each scale: Verbal Comprehension (Similarities, Comprehension), Visual Spatial (Block Design, Visual Puzzles), Fluid Reasoning (Matrix Reasoning, Figure Weights), Working Memory (Digit Span, Picture Span), and Processing Speed (Coding, Symbol Search). The FSIQ is composed of seven of these subtests. Administration of the seven FSIQ subtests can be completed within approximately 50 minutes and the 10 primary subtests can be completed in approximately 65 minutes. Additional subtests are available to compute ancillary index scales that may be helpful in identifying a profile of strengths and weaknesses for children with ASD: Quantitative Reasoning, Auditory Working Memory, Nonverbal, General Ability, and Cognitive Proficiency.

A sample of 27 children between the ages of 6 and 16 years who had a diagnosis of ASD with language impairment were included as a special group during clinical validity testing. The average FSIQ for this group was 75.2. Within the primary index scales, highest performance was on the Fluid Reasoning Index (mean = 84.4) and Visual Spatial Index (mean = 82.2), while the indices with lowest scores were Working Memory (mean = 76.9) and Processing Speed (mean = 76.1). The Verbal Comprehension

Index fell in the middle with a mean score of 78.2. Additionally, a sample of 30 children between the ages of 7 and 15 years who had a diagnosis of ASD without accompanying language impairment were administered the WISC-V. The average FSIQ for this group was 96.3. Within the five primary index scales, highest performance was on the Verbal Comprehension Index (mean = 100. 9) and Visual Spatial Index (mean = 100.1), while the indices with lowest scores were Working Memory (mean = 93.6) and Processing Speed (mean = 87.6). The Fluid Reasoning Index in this sample fell between the other scores with a mean score of 98.6.

Although the WISC-V is too recent to have been widely studied for individuals with ASD, a wealth of literature is available regarding the performance of individuals with ASD on the previous edition (Wechsler Intelligence Scale for Children, Fourth Edition [WISC-IV]; Wechsler, 2003). Studies examining the performance of children with ASD on the WISC-IV consistently documented both relative and normative weaknesses on the Comprehension, Coding, Symbol Search, Letter–Number Sequencing, and Digit Span subtests, and the Processing Speed Index (Lincoln et al., 2007; Mayes & Calhoun, 2008; Oliveras-Rentas, Kenworthy, Roberson, Martin, & Wallace, 2012). Further, literature on the WISC-IV supports the use of two of the ancillary index scores: the GAI, which measures cognitive reasoning skills (Verbal Comprehension, Perceptual Reasoning) and the CPI, which measures cognitive efficiency (Working Memory, Processing Speed). The GAI is often higher than the FSIQ because it examines cognitive reasoning in the absences of working memory and processing speed demands that have been shown to be impaired in those with ASD (Kuriakose, 2014; Mayes & Calhoun, 2008; Oliveras-Rentas et al., 2012). In a study of children with ASD without intellectual disability (i.e., IQ > 70), Mayes and Calhoun (2008) reported that both Working Memory and Processing Speed Index scores were lower than Verbal Comprehension and Perceptual Reasoning Index scores in 74% of their sample of 54 children. In studies of children with ASD, including a wider range of intellectual ability, the lowest average subtest score has been consistently obtained on Comprehension, while the highest average subtest score has been consistently obtained on Block Design (Kuriakose, 2014; Lincoln et al., 2007). In the Kuriakose (2014) study, almost half of the children with ASD received a greater Perceptual Reasoning Index score compared to their Verbal Comprehension Index score. Further, 40% showed significantly lower Processing Speed Index scores compared to Verbal Comprehension Index scores.

Because the WISC-V provides separate measures of verbal and nonverbal reasoning, working memory, and processing speed, it provides an opportunity to identify a pattern of strengths and weaknesses in children with ASD. The WISC-V replaces the previous Perceptual Reasoning Index with two primary indices: Visual Spatial and Fluid Reasoning. This allows for visual perceptual abilities to be assessed separately from abstract thinking and inductive and deductive reasoning. The Working Memory Index and Processing Speed Index provide measurement of the poor motor skills and attention difficulties experienced by individuals with ASD. However, the use of timed tests and the need for verbal understanding even on measures of perceptual reasoning may lead examiners to underestimate the nonverbal abilities of some individuals with ASD (Carothers & Taylor, 2013; Klin et al., 2005), which is where the GAI and the CPI may provide useful information. When comparing performance on the WISC-V to other tests, it may be appropriate to use the GAI rather than the FSIQ. For example, in the Kuriakose (2014) study of the WISC-IV, the GAI was most similar to the DAS-II GCA, while the FSIQ was an average of 8 points lower. Although not completely language-free, the Nonverbal Index may also provide additional information on general intellectual ability that minimizes expressive language demands. Younger school-age children with significant delays are unlikely to meet basal requirements on most subtests, resulting in an inability to calculate meaningful standard scores.

Wechsler Adult Intelligence Scale—Fourth Edition

The Wechsler Adult Intelligence Scale—Fourth Edition (WAIS-IV; Wechsler, 2008) is designed to assess intelligence in individuals between the ages of 16 years, 0 months, and 90 years, 11 months. Based on 10 core subtests, the Verbal Comprehension Index, Perceptual Reasoning Index, Working Memory Index, Processing Speed Index, and FSIQ scores are computed, and like the WISC-V, a GAI and CPI can also be calculated. The standardization data indicate that administration of the 10 subtests required to calculate FSIQ can be completed in approximately 65–90 minutes.

During the standardization process, 40 individuals with DSM-IV-TR Asperger's disorder (ages 16–40 years; 78% male) and 16 individuals with autistic disorder (ages 16–28 years; 94% male) were administered the WAIS-IV. Mean FSIQ for the group with Asperger's disorder was 97, while the mean FSIQ for the group with autistic disorder was 79. The Processing Speed Index was an area of weakness for individuals in both groups. For the group with Asperger's disorder, their highest mean score was obtained on the Verbal Comprehension Index with the Information and Vocabulary subtests being two of their three highest subtests. For the group with autistic disorder their highest mean score was obtained on the Perceptual Reasoning Index with their three highest scores on nonverbal tasks and their lowest scores on the Comprehension subtest of the Verbal Comprehension Index. Similar to other Wechsler measures, the GAI was 5 or more points greater than FSIQ for more than 55% of the group with Asperger's disorder and 38% of the group with autistic disorder.

To examine WAIS-IV cognitive profiles, Holdnack, Goldstein, and Drozdick (2011) compared individuals with typical development, those with DSM-IV-TR autistic disorder, and those with DSM-IV-TR Asperger's disorder. Overall, there were no significant differences between the control group and the group with Asperger's disorder. Both of these groups had higher scores than the group of participants with autistic disorder. Individuals with autistic disorder scored lower on the Verbal Comprehension Index and the Processing Speed Index with the Comprehension subtest being the lowest. Holdnack et al. (2011) concluded that the cognitive profile of individuals with autistic disorder on the WAIS-IV includes difficulties in language, particularly when social judgment is required, and speed of information processing.

Few publications have examined the WAIS-IV in ASD. More research is needed to examine the profile associated with ASD on the WAIS-IV. The fact that the WAIS-IV provides specific index scores measuring Verbal Comprehension, Perceptual Reasoning, Working Memory, and Processing Speed suggests that the WAIS-IV may be a good choice for identifying a profile of strengths and weaknesses in adults with ASD. However, as with the WISC-V, the use of timed tests and the need for verbal understanding even on measures included in the Perceptual Reasoning Index score may lead examiners to underestimate the nonverbal abilities of some individuals with ASD. During standardization of the WISC-V, 112 individuals were given both the WISC-V and the WAIS-IV and the uncorrected correlation between the FSIQ obtained on each measure was high (.84; Canivez & Watkins, 2016). Thus, the WAIS-IV may be a good choice for reevaluating an older adolescent or young adult who had previously been given the WISC-V.

Leiter International Performance Scale—Third Edition

The Leiter–3 (Roid et al., 2013) is designed to assess nonverbal intellectual ability, memory, and attention in children, adolescents, and adults between the ages of 3 years and more than 75 years. Administration requires no verbal instructions from the examiner or verbal responses from the individual. The Leiter–3 contains two groupings of subtests: a Cognitive Battery and an Attention/Memory Battery. The Cognitive Battery consists of five subtests of nonverbal intellectual ability related to visualization and reasoning with four subtests required to obtain a Nonverbal IQ—this battery can be administered in approximately 45 minutes. The Attention/Memory Battery has five subscales including two nonverbal attention subtests, one interference (Stroop) subtest, and two memory subtests and composite scores for Nonverbal Memory and Processing Speed can be obtained—these five subtests can be administered in approximately 30 minutes. The Leiter–3 includes a return to the original Leiter "block-and-frame" format that involves the examinee placing blocks into "slots" in the "frame." This format has been associated with increased ability to maintain attention and obtain valid scores for children with ASD, communication difficulties, or children who benefit from "hands-on" materials (Tsatsanis et al., 2003).

A total of 64 individuals with ASD ages 3–22 years (mean age 9 years) who met DSM-IV criteria were among the special groups included in the Leiter–3 standardization sample. On the Cognitive Battery, individuals with ASD had lower means on the Nonverbal IQ, Nonverbal Memory Composite, and Processing Speed Composite than the majority of other special populations evaluated with the exception of individuals with an intellectual disability. A similar pattern of lower mean performance for individuals with ASD compared with the other special groups was also evident on the individual subtests of the Attention/Memory Battery.

As the Leiter–3 was recently published, few research studies have examined profiles scores for individuals with ASD. Kuschner, Bennetto, and Yost (2007) used the Leiter–R Brief IQ to examine the cognitive profile of preschool-age children with high-functioning ASD (average Leiter–R Brief IQ of 80). They found that, compared with children of similar chronological and nonverbal mental age with developmental delays, the children with ASD showed specific strengths in tasks measuring the ability to focus on specific visual details (Figure Ground subtest) and to mentally manipulate and synthesize visual information (Form Completion subtest). The children with ASD were specifically impaired on a subtest measuring abstract reasoning and concept formation (Repeated Patterns subtest). These results suggest that children with ASD may not have overall strengths in all areas of nonverbal processing, and instead have strengths in visual perception. This is consistent with cognitive theories of ASD, including the theories of weak central coherence (Happé & Frith, 2006) and enhanced perceptual processing (Mottron et al., 2006).

The Leiter–3 is an excellent choice for testing either a nonverbal/minimally verbal child with ASD or a child with significantly impaired receptive and expressive language. This is one of the few tests that would be appropriate for an older child with a very small vocabulary (e.g., a 15-year-old who is able to speak in single words only). An additional strength of the Leiter–3 is the presence of teaching trials to ensure that the examinee understands task demands, including demonstrating and even taking the child's hand to teach. However, a great many instructions are provided via descriptive gestures and facial expressions—both social stimuli that are very difficult for children with ASD to understand. Tager-Flusberg et al. (2016) suggested modifications of the Leiter–3 when testing minimally verbal children with ASD including the addition of simple language (e.g., "just one" or "match") and an increased reliance on modeling and hand-over-hand guidance rather than social gestures. Further, for examinees with fine motor difficulties that prevented them from putting cards into the appropriate slots, they recommend allowing examinees to place cards in front of the slots. Using these modifications, Nonverbal IQ scores were successfully obtained for 30 out of 32 minimally verbal children and adolescents with ASD who typically pose a challenge for valid assessments. Additionally, for individuals who function at a low level of ability and are expected to be retested using the Leiter–3, Growth Scores designed using item response theory are available to measure small increments of growth. However, this test is not appropriate for young children with delays. As on other tests that begin at the 3-year range, preschool children with ASD who have significant developmental delays are unlikely to understand task demands and achieve a basal score on the Leiter–3.

Brief IQ Measures

Brief IQ measures are frequently used when time constraints do not allow administration of an entire battery. When a full battery of tests is desired but the examiner is unsure whether a child will be able to maintain attention and motivation, it is often helpful to administer a measure with a short form that allows IQ to be calculated from performance on a few subtests. Both the SB5 and the Leiter–3 have these types of brief IQ measures, which provide standardized scores based on their respective standardization samples. However, when the original purpose is to use a brief IQ measure—as is often the case when a lengthy research battery is being administered—the examiner could instead choose a stand-alone brief measure of intelligence.

Wechsler Abbreviated Scale of Intelligence—Second Edition

The Wechsler Abbreviated Scale of Intelligence—Second Edition (WASI-II; Wechsler, 2011) was developed to be a short measure of intelligence that can be used in clinical, psychoeducational, and research settings for individuals between the ages of 6 and 90 years. The two-subtest form of the WASI-II FSIQ requires approximately 15 minutes to complete and the four-subtest form can be completed in approximately 30 minutes. The profile of scores available from the WASI-II includes the Verbal Comprehension Index, Perceptual Reasoning Index, and FSIQ (two- or four-subtest forms). WASI-II subtests and items were revised to closely parallel those of the WISC-IV and WAIS-IV. The WASI-II does not include an evaluation of working memory or processing speed, which may be important aspects of cognitive functioning to assess depending on the purpose of the assessment, but may be a good choice when time is limited. Although individuals with ASD were not excluded from the WASI-II standardization sample, they were also not included as a special group while the clinical validity of this measure was being established.

Kaufman Brief Intelligence Test, Second Edition

The Kaufman Brief Intelligence Test, Second Edition (KBIT-2; Kaufman & Kaufman, 2004) is designed to be a brief measure of verbal and nonverbal intelligence for individuals ages 4–90 years. The KBIT-2 requires approximately 15–30 minutes to administer and yields a Verbal domain score, a Nonverbal domain score, and an IQ Composite score. During the standardization process, ASD was not included as an exclusionary condition and was also not included within the sample of conditions or diagnoses for validity purposes. The special populations included in the standardization sample were individuals with learning disability, speech–language disorders, attention-deficit/hyperactivity disorder (ADHD), intellectual disability, traumatic brain injury, and dementia.

MEASURES OF ADAPTIVE BEHAVIOR

Assessments of individuals with any suspected developmental disability, including ASD, should include a measure of adaptive functioning in addition to cognitive functioning. This is necessary for classification and diagnostic purposes (e.g., ascertaining whether an individual meets criteria for intellectual disability), as well as in determining an individual's personal strengths and weaknesses beyond cognitive ability. Measures of adaptive functioning are also useful in planning interventions and for measuring response to intervention, as they do not necessarily involve the risk of practice effects from repeated administration. Recently, findings that adaptive behavior measures were closely correlated with adult outcome has implications for intervention programs that foster independence in adulthood for individuals with ASD (Farley et al., 2009) and adds to the importance of measuring these skills across the lifespan.

The two most commonly used measures of adaptive behavior in individuals with ASD are the Vineland Adaptive Behavior Scales, Second Edition (Vineland–II; Sparrow, Cicchetti, & Balla, 2005) and the Adaptive Behavior Assessment System—Third Edition (ABAS-3; Harrison & Oakland, 2015). Both measures offer potential benefits for clinicians and researchers working with individuals with ASD that warrant discussion. Each of these measures is reviewed below and is also summarized in Table 8.1.

Vineland Adaptive Behavior Scales, Second Edition

The Vineland–II (Sparrow et al., 2005) is a revision of the widely popular Vineland Adaptive Behavior Scales (Sparrow, Balla, & Cicchetti,, 1984). A survey by Luiselli et al. (2001) of assessment practices of national service centers for individuals with autism in 30 states in the United States reported that 60.6% of centers use the original version of the Vineland as their primary measure of adaptive behavior, and a review of available research in the area of ASD would certainly support similar popularity in research protocols as well. There are several versions of administration: two survey forms (a 383-item Survey Interview Form, which is administered by an examiner, and a Parent/Caregiver Rating Form, which is a checklist); an Expanded Interview Form, which permits more comprehensive assessment for use in planning interventions; and a Teacher Rating Form, which is based on classroom observation and focuses on academic functioning. The Survey Interview Form may be completed in 20–60 minutes, and the Parent/Caregiver Rating Form generally takes between 30 and 60 minutes to complete. The Vineland–II may be used with individuals from birth to age 90 to assess functioning in four domains and 11 subdomains. Individuals 7 years of age and older are assessed in the domains of Communication (Receptive, Expressive, and Written); Daily Living Skills (Personal, Domestic, and Community); and Socialization (Interpersonal Relationships, Play and Leisure Time, and Coping Skills). Children 6 years, 11 months, of age and younger are assessed on an additional Motor Skills domain (Gross and Fine). An optional Maladaptive Behavior Index consisting of three subscales (Internalizing, Externalizing, and Other) and a group of Maladaptive Critical Items are available for individuals older than 3 years and provide additional measures of how an individual's adaptive functioning may be limited by difficult behaviors. Standard scores with a mean of 100 (standard deviation = 15) are calculated for each of the four domains and for an overall Adaptive Behavior Composite. Age equivalents are available for subdomains, but not for summary domains.

The Vineland–II manual provides data regarding 77 individuals with autism that were obtained during standardization. This sample included 31 children between the ages of 2 and 10 who were considered nonverbal (i.e., using five or fewer words) and 46 individuals between the ages of 3 and 19 who were considered verbal. Significant differences ($p < .01$) were obtained for both groups in comparison to an age-matched nonclinical reference group for the domain, subdomain, and Adaptive Behavior Composite scores. Adaptive Behavior Composite means were 50.7 for the nonverbal group and 65.7 for the verbal group. For the verbal group, the lowest domain score was found in Socialization. In both groups, the largest adaptive functioning deficits were found in the Interpersonal Relationships, Play and Leisure Time, and Expressive Language subdomains. Within the Maladaptive domain, both groups obtained significantly higher mean scores on the Internalizing subscale than the nonclinical sample did, but their Externalizing subscale scores were within the average range. The nonverbal group was rated overall as having more maladaptive behaviors than the verbal group, with scores in the elevated range.

Studies using the Vineland–II in toddlers with ASD demonstrate significant weaknesses in the Communication and Socialization domains (Paul, Loomis, & Chawarska, 2014; Ray-Subramanian et al., 2011). In school-age children and adolescents with ASD, Vineland scores have been reported to be below expectations based on IQ, even in individuals with average or higher intellectual skills (Doobay, Foley-Nicpon, Ali, & Assouline, 2014; Duncan & Bishop, 2015). In Duncan and Bishop's study of 417 adolescents with average IQ (mean of 105.7), delays were reported in the Socialization (71.1), Communication (78.7), and Daily Living Skills (79.9) domains.

Significant impairments in the Daily Living Skills domain have been consistently reported in adolescents and young adults with ASD (Bal, Kim, Cheong, & Lord, 2015; Matthews et al., 2015). In a study examining daily living skills from 2 to 21 years of age (Bal et al., 2015), two trajectories were identified. In the first group, although daily living skills were delayed, approximately 12 years in daily living skills were gained from 2 to 21 years of age. In contrast, in the second group, only 3–4 years of daily living skills were gained across the same time span. This widening gap in daily living skills was associated with both poor language skills and poor nonverbal mental age during early childhood. Notably, both groups showed evidence of a decline in domestic skills during later adolescence. In the Duncan and Bishop (2015) study, half of the adolescents were significantly below chronological age and IQ expectations, and a quarter had daily living skills in the low range of adaptive functioning (i.e., below 70).

Adaptive Behavior Assessment System—Third Edition

The ABAS-3 (Harrison & Oakland, 2015) provides five different forms to be used across the age range of birth–89 years, each of which takes about 20 minutes to complete. Each form is completed by the relevant rater. A Parent/Primary Caregiver Form and a Teacher/Day Care Form are available for children. The Adult Form can be self-rated or completed by a family member, or by a supervisor or other respondent familiar with the individual. In addition to rating the frequency of behaviors, raters are asked to check a box for each item indicating whether they guessed about the individual's performance for that item, which allows for interpreting whether the respondent is an appropriate rater for the individual being assessed. The ABAS-3 describes the level of an individual's functional skills that are required for daily living (i.e., self-care and interactions with others) without the assistance of others. Specific skill areas assessed by the ABAS-3 include Communication, Community Use (depending on the individual's age), Functional (Pre-)Academics, Home/School Living (depending on the rater), Motor (depending on the individual's age), Health and Safety, Leisure, Self-Care, Self-Direction, Social, and Work (depending on whether the individual is employed). Scores for each skill area are combined into three separate Adaptive Domain composite scores: Conceptual (communication and academic skills), Social (interpersonal and social competence skills), and Practical (independent living and daily living skills). The sum of scaled scores for each skill area is also used to calculate a General Adaptive Composite (GAC). Each composite score has a mean of 100 and standard deviation of 15.

While no research has been published on the use of the ABAS-3 in individuals with ASD, several studies have used the Adaptive Behavior Assessment System—Second Edition (ABAS-II; Harrison & Oakland, 2003) in children and young adults with ASD (Kenworthy, Case, Harms, Martin, & Wallace, 2010; Lopata et al., 2012). Kenworthy et al. (2010) compared adaptive behaviors of 12- to 22-year-olds with ASD to matched controls using the ABAS-II Parent Form. The group of individuals with ASD with IQs above 80 demonstrated significant deficits in overall adaptive behavior (GAC), on the three adaptive domain composite scales (Conceptual, Social, and Practical), and on all nine subscale skill areas. Specifically, the composite scores for this group were generally ≥ 1.5 standard deviations below the population mean and far below the group's IQ level. Lopata et al. (2012) used the ABAS-II Parent Form to examine adaptive functioning of children ages 7–12 years with ASD who had IQs above 70 on the WISC-IV. Compared with normative expectations (as well the group's average IQ), the group with ASD displayed lowest scores in the skill areas of Social (more than 2 standard deviations below), Home Living (nearly 2 standard deviations below), and Self-Direction (more than 1.5 standard deviations below), yet scored in the average range in the areas of Functional Academics, Health and Safety, and Community Use. Kenworthy et al. (2010) found a correlation between IQ and ABAS-II Conceptual domain score for individuals with ASD. Across both studies, a similar adaptive behavior profile on the ABAS-II emerges with significant difficulties in the Social area and personal strengths in Functional Academics for individuals with ASD without intellectual disability—yet, consistent with research on the Vineland, the overall ASD adaptive behavior profile reveals more impairment than might be expected given the IQ of these samples.

GUIDELINES FOR CHOOSING A MEASURE OF INTELLECTUAL FUNCTIONING

As is clear from this review, there are multiple options for assessment of cognitive and adaptive functioning in individuals with ASD. Unlike some other aspects of assessment, such as determining an appropriate diagnosis, there is no clear "gold standard" for assessing either area of functioning in children, adolescents, or adults with ASD. Instead, the flexibility of available instruments allows researchers and clinicians to adopt an *individualized* assessment approach rather than a static ASD cognitive and adaptive battery. Examiners should take the following considerations into account when choosing the appropriate tools for a cognitive and/or adaptive assessment.

Considerations in Choosing a Measure of Cognitive Ability

Language Ability

One of the most limiting factors in cognitive assessment of an individual with ASD is often the verbal ability of the examinee. Some of the available measures permit separate assessment of nonverbal and verbal ability in producing qualitatively and quantitatively useful scores. However, some assessments, including the Wechsler intelligence tests and the SB5, require some level of receptive language to understand nonverbal task directions. As a result, determining both the individual's level of language use and his or her level of understanding of verbal directions is essential in choosing an appropriate measure. Even when the nonverbal tasks are appropriate, individuals with limited language may not receive any credit on the language measures, resulting in an invalid assessment.

For older children who have no or limited language, the Leiter–3 is an appropriate choice, as no language use on the part of the examiner or examinee is required. Kasari, Brady, Lord, and Tager-Flusberg (2013) argued that the Leiter is the only measure of nonverbal cognitive abilities well suited for use with minimally verbal school-age children with ASD. However, the Leiter–3 may not be as appropriate for preschool children with ASD. Although the Leiter–3 is normed for children from 3 years of age onward, young nonverbal children with ASD may not understand task directions and may not be able to complete enough items to obtain a valid score. For these children, instruments that are appropriate from birth onward (i.e., the Bayley–III or the Mullen) may be the most beneficial.

Chronological Age and Developmental Level

With measures available spanning the age range from birth to 90 years, there is no age level at which an individual's ability may not be assessed. In measuring cognitive skills, it is best to choose a measure for which population norms are available for the individual's chronological age. Choosing an age-appropriate measure will add to the reliability and validity of the scores yielded by a cognitive measure, and will aid in greater understanding regarding the individual's abilities compared with same-age peers. When several measures are appropriate, the examiner should consider choosing an instrument that is appropriate for children several years younger than the examinee. For example, when deciding which developmental test to administer to a 3-year-old with ASD, the examiner has a wide range of tests that are appropriate for the child's chronological age, including the Bayley–III, Mullen, DAS-II, SB5, and WPPSI-IV. However, if the child is delayed, he or she may have difficulty completing tests that are designed for children 2½ years of age or older, and floor effects are likely. Thus, the examiner might consider a developmental test that is appropriate for children several years younger, such as the Bayley–III or the Mullen. In the case that the age-appropriate measure is too difficult (e.g., requires too much receptive or expressive language) and no other instruments are available, it is reasonable to choose an alternative measure that may provide age equivalents rather than standard scores. For example, if an individual is older than 5½ years in chronological age, but below 2½ years in mental age, there is no instrument that fits both the child's chronological and mental age. In this case, either the Bayley–III or Mullen may be administered, and age equivalent scores should be calculated.

Behavioral Difficulties

Even when the testing session is structured as described earlier in this chapter, some examinees may exhibit behavioral difficulties that make it difficult to complete a lengthy evaluation or raise concerns about the validity of the results. Behavioral difficulties are often a sign of frustration and fatigue in individuals with ASD. Examiners are therefore encouraged to choose the most succinct measure that will yield informative data for the purpose of the assessment when individuals have short attention spans or low tolerance of seated, formalized testing. This approach will prove more satisfying for both the examiners and examinees than relying on a single measure without considering the examinee's attention span in choosing an appropriate measure. The DAS-II was designed to be a relatively quick assessment instrument and is a good choice when time is a concern—in addition, for children older than 2½ years of age, a brief IQ can be obtained after the first few subtests are completed. The KBIT-2 is also appropriate for children at least 4 years of age, and the WASI-II is appropriate for children at least 6 years of age.

Modality of Administration

Recently, technological advances have moved assessment into the digital era. One example of this movement is illustrated through Pearson's Q-interactive system, which uses two connected tablets for administration (one for the examiner to use for administration and one for the examinee to use to view and respond to stimuli). While some of the measures mentioned above are currently available in this Q-interactive format, including the WISC-V and WAIS-IV, these measures are also still offered in the traditional paper-and-pencil format. In a technical report on the WISC-V, Pearson examined a group of 30 school-age children with ASD and co-occurring language disorder. The same pattern of strengths and weaknesses was found using the Q-interactive version as has been found by other researchers using the paper version (Raiford, Drozdick, & Zhang, 2015). However, to date no research has directly examined the comparability of scores across the two versions in the same sample of children with ASD.

As this is a relatively new and unstudied format, some concerns regarding the use of a tablet during administration for individuals with ASD exist regarding potential behavioral complications beyond the statistical equivalencies of this format. This requires an examiner to make a decision to use a format that fits the individual being assessed. For example, administration using a tablet may not be the best fit for an individual with behavioral difficulties that may result in the tablet being thrown. Sometimes individuals have very specific ways in which they are used to using familiar items, such as tablets, and not being able to play a favorite game or use the tablet in the desired way might result in frustration for some individuals. Technology, such as tablets, may also be very exciting for some individuals and they may have a tendency to try to touch everything on the screen, making administration and accuracy of responding more difficult. Alternatively, computer administration may yield higher scores than the standard format as has been found with the Wisconsin Card Sorting Task (Ozonoff, 1995). Thus, an experienced examiner needs to carefully assess whether the paper- or technology-based format is the best fit for the examinee in order to obtain the most accurate information possible. Additional use and research on this new administration modality is needed to help resolve some of these questions for use with individuals with ASD.

The Purpose of the Assessment

Determining the need for an assessment and the value of its results for the individual with ASD is of ultimate importance in choosing a measure of cognitive ability for individuals with ASD. The underlying need for the assessment is typically for a comprehensive measure of a range of cognitive abilities, but in other situations a screener of general cognitive ability will suffice. Examiners should keep in mind what will happen to the scores after the assessment is completed as well. For example, certain agencies (e.g., school systems) may only accept comprehensive measures and FSIQ or composite scores when making eligibility decisions. While a brief IQ measure may fit with a child's attention span, if an insurance company requires an FSIQ to qualify for autism-related services, then the examiner must choose the best measure that provides an FSIQ. If an assessment is intended to be part of a series of administrations to track an individual's development over time, one of the instruments that covers a wider age range may be of preference (e.g., the SB5 for the entire lifespan, the Mullen for measurements across the preschool years, or the Leiter–3 or DAS-II for multiple assessments throughout childhood and adolescence).

Because of the uneven profile of strengths and weaknesses characterizing individuals with ASD, an examiner is often faced with the decision to choose an instrument that highlights an examinee's strengths or weaknesses. For example, a child with limited language but good nonverbal perception abilities may receive higher scores on a nonverbal IQ test such as the Leiter–3, but perform much more poorly on a test with receptive and expressive language demands such as the WISC-V. The choice between measures depends on the purpose of the evaluation. If the goal of the evaluation is to highlight the fact that the child is not developmentally delayed in all areas and, in fact, has some age-level skills, the Leiter–3 may be a good choice. However, if the purpose of the assessment is to identify strengths and weaknesses that may have an impact on school performance, a test that includes verbal ability is important for providing a good predictor of the child's performance in a classroom that requires verbal comprehension and expression. Identifying the child's verbal weaknesses is likely to result in additional school accommodations—this may not occur if only a nonverbal IQ test is administered.

Considerations in Choosing an Adaptive Behavior Measure

With several available measures of adaptive functioning that are generally similar in underlying concepts, type of information obtained, and age ranges of the standardization, the main decision for an examiner lies in whether detailed, qualitative information or simply a quick measure of an individual's adaptive level is needed. Test format is another consideration. The Vineland–II is available in both interview and checklist forms, while the ABAS-3 is exclusively a checklist. Still another aspect to consider in choosing an adaptive measure is the desired respondent (i.e., parent/caregiver, teacher, employer, or the examinee him- or herself). The ABAS-3 provides forms for the largest range of respondents, including a self-report, but the Vineland–II allows for data from caregivers and teachers to be obtained. Examiners are encouraged to obtain data regarding adaptive functioning from multiple respondents when possible, particularly in clinical assessments, because research has found that parents and other raters tend to provide qualitatively different data from their perspectives on an individual. For example, Szatmari, Archer, Fisman, and Streiner (1994) reported that while overall correlations of parent and teacher reports were good, teachers rated individuals with PDD as having higher adaptive skills on the Vineland than their parents did. Furthermore, parental reports on the Vineland yielded greater distinction at the subdomain level between individuals with high-functioning autism and Asperger syndrome than were apparent from teacher reports (Szatmari et al., 1994). There have also been some discrepancies reported between individuals' self-report and that of other respondents, such as individuals not perceiving themselves to have significant difficulties when other respondents may report concerns or difficulties (Barnhill et al., 2000). Clinically, discrepancy between self- and caregiver report of independent behavior is a concern when evaluations are being conducted to qualify an adolescent or adult for services (e.g., employment supports through Vocational Rehabilitation). If an adult with ASD does not perceive the level of supports that are being provided for him or her to live or work independently, he or she may not qualify for services based on a self-report questionnaire. In our clinical work, this is a significant issue with regard to adult psychological assessments conducted to determine whether an adult qualifies for services. We strongly recommend that clinicians and researchers carefully consider the feasibility of multiple respondents and carefully interpret the discrepancies that may arise.

Given that the newest versions of the available adaptive measures have taken efforts to expand the available variability of scores for very young children with ASD, it may also be possible to choose any of these measures to assess response to intervention. For example, a screener form of the Vineland showed promise in detecting progress in preschool-age children over an 11-month period, with gains in the Vineland domain scores reported after a year of schooling was received (Charman, Howlin, Berry, & Prince, 2004).

SUMMARY

In this chapter, we have asserted that there is no "best test" for measuring intellectual functioning in persons with ASD. Because of the uneven profiles that characterize individuals with ASD and the behavioral difficulties that often occur during standardized testing, the examiner needs to have experience administering and interpreting standardized assessments and an understanding of how the symptoms of ASD may interfere with test performance. The examiner is encouraged to provide additional structure to increase the examinee's attention and motivation to complete the assessment, while still maintaining a standardized test administration. In addition, it is important to choose the right instrument in order to ensure that an accurate estimate of developmental ability is obtained and that the resulting scores will meet the purpose of the evaluation. The examiner is encouraged to consider the following sequence of questions when deciding which test is most appropriate:

1. Which instruments are appropriate for the examinee's chronological age?
2. Is the child nonverbal, necessitating a nonverbal IQ test?
3. Given the examinee's estimated mental age, is it appropriate to choose a test that extends several years below the examinee's chronological age?
4. If there are no appropriate measures that include both the examinee's chronological age and expected mental age, is a test that provides age equivalents available?
5. Is a full scale or brief IQ score more appropriate? The answer to this question depends on whether the referral agency would prefer one type of measure and whether behavioral difficulties may interfere with testing success.
6. If the assessment is being conducted to measure whether the examinee is showing an increase or decrease in skills across time, which measure is most appropriate, given the proposed range of assessments? For example, if the child was previously evaluated with a Wechsler scale, it may be most appropriate to administer another Wechsler scale. If the child is participating in a longitudinal research project, which measure is most appropriate, given the proposed age range of the study?
7. Is the assessment being conducted to highlight the individual's strengths or to highlight areas of weakness that may need additional intervention? This is particularly important if the examinee has discrepant verbal and nonverbal abilities.

CASE EXAMPLE

At the beginning of this chapter, we introduced Jason, a young boy with a diagnosis of ASD, and raised a question about which IQ test would be the most appropriate for him. After interviewing his mother to obtain his developmental and social history, we used the questions above to choose an appropriate test. Below is a summary of the developmental history that we obtained, a discussion of our decision-making process in choosing IQ and adaptive behavior instruments, a condensed version of the test results, and a discussion of the appropriateness of these results in addressing the referral questions.

Developmental and Social History

Jason, age 8 years, 6 months, was referred to a university-based autism clinic by his school system. An updated evaluation was requested to provide additional recommendations for school accommodations. Jason was currently in the third grade. He received resource room services daily for reading and math, and spent the remainder of his day in a regular education classroom. He also received speech therapy services two times per week for 30 minutes each time.

Jason's mother reported that she first became concerned about Jason's development when he was 12 months old, because he was not responding to his name and had not yet begun to speak. Although his motor milestones developed within normal limits (e.g., he walked at 11 months), Jason's language was delayed. He spoke his first words at 2½ years and did not combine words into short sentences until he was 3½ years old. His mother reported that Jason did not use gestures, eye contact, or facial expressions to help compensate for his language difficulties. He was diagnosed with ASD at the age of 3 years.

In the area of language and communication skills, Jason's mother reported that he had an extensive vocabulary, although the majority of his speech consisted of delayed echolalia, in which he repeats lines from his favorite movies. She noted that it was difficult to hold a conversation with Jason because he did not comment on remarks made by others, responded only when asked a direct question, and tended to initiate only conversations that are related to his own interests. He occasionally mixed up his pronouns, referring to himself as "you" and other people as "I," although this is much improved from when he was a preschooler. He has learned to use gestures such as nodding his head "yes" or "no," but does not use descriptive gestures.

In the area of social development, Jason's mother reported that he referred to his classmates as his "friends," but that these friendships were not reciprocated and he did not see these children outside of school. His mother commented that Jason often watched other children and seemed to want to join in their games. However, he rarely approached other children and she thought that he didn't know how to join their activities. When other children approached Jason, he was beginning to respond to them, but typically insisted that they play games according to his own rules. His eye contact had improved from his preschool years, especially with familiar people, although it was mostly fleeting.

In the area of repetitive behavior and play, Jason's mother reported that he was "obsessed" with stuffed animals (Beanie Babies) and had collected hundreds of them. She noted that he has memorized the names and "birth dates" of every animal in his collection. He spent his free time either reading the guide that described the characteristics of each of the stuffed animals in his collection or arranging his animals into geometric shapes and patterns. His mother noted that Jason was excellent at completing puzzles and could even complete them "upside down" (i.e., when he was only looking at the blank cardboard on the back of the pieces).

Choosing an Appropriate IQ Test and Structuring the Environment

We used the sequence of questions recommended earlier to identify the appropriate IQ test for Jason. Because his mother wanted a comprehensive evaluation to identify his strengths and weaknesses, including appropriate academic accommodations, we chose to administer a full scale IQ battery. Jason's mother was concerned about how his IQ might change across time—thus, we wanted to choose an instrument that could be given again in the future to track any changes. Although we considered the Leiter–3 because of Jason's poor use of language for communicative purposes, we decided that a measure of his verbal skills was necessary to provide a realistic estimate of the difficulties he was likely to encounter in the third grade. However, we wanted to choose an instrument that would show the discrepancy between his verbal and nonverbal skills, so that his strengths would also be identified. Given his chronological age and these other considerations, we identified the WISC-V, SB5, and DAS-II as being appropriate measures for Jason's evaluation. We chose the WISC-V because we suspected that Jason's symptoms of autism might interfere with some of the imitation demands on the Nonverbal Working Memory subtest of the SB5, and we were concerned that he might perform at the floor level of the DAS-II School-Age battery because it begins at 7 years. Further, we chose the WISC-V as we wanted to examine Jason's processing speed and CPI because both skills are important to performance in a general education third-grade classroom. Finally, we chose to use the paper-and-pencil traditional administration of the WISC-V as little data are available on the validity of the electronic administration version with school-age children with ASD. Jason was given a schedule showing a picture denoting each of the 10 subtests on the WISC-V that would be administered to obtain an FSIQ and all of the Primary Index scales. For every subtest that he completed, he earned a sticker of an animal. In addition, Jason brought several of his stuffed animals with him to the testing session and was allowed several minutes to play with the animals after he completed every set of two subtests. Following the WISC-V, Jason's mother was interviewed with the Vineland–II to assess Jason's adaptive behavior. We chose the interview form as a method of gathering additional information about Jason's mother's concerns about his development and the supports that she provides at home.

WISC-V Results

Jason obtained a Verbal Comprehension Index of 76 (5th percentile), a Visual Spatial Index of 92 (30th percentile), a Fluid Reasoning Index of 76 (5th percentile), a Working Memory Index of 72 (3rd percentile), and a Processing Speed Index of 49 (below the 1st percentile). Jason's FSIQ was 82 and was at the 12th percentile compared with other children his age. This score was classified by the WISC-V as Low Average. There was a 95% chance that his true IQ score was within the range of 77–88. The FSIQ is an aggregate of the five index scores and is usually considered the best measure of global intellectual functioning. However, Jason showed significant differences across index scores, suggesting that the FSIQ might not be an accurate representation of his overall ability. Specifically, Jason's Visual Spatial Index was significantly higher than all of his other index scores. It was 16 points higher than his Verbal Comprehension Index—this discrepancy is seen only in 13% of children Jason's age. Furthermore, Jason's Processing Speed Index was significantly lower than all of his other index scores. It was 43 points lower than his Visual Spatial Index—this discrepancy is seen in less than 1% of children Jason's age.

The Verbal Comprehension Index is a measure of verbal concept formation, verbal reasoning, and knowledge acquired from one's environment. Jason's Verbal Comprehension Index was classified as Very Low; his subtest scores ranged from 5 to 6 (8–12 is average). Jason's Verbal Comprehension Index scores were consistent across subtests. Notably, he often echoed the examiner's words and provided little additional information to answer the examiner's questions.

The Visual Spatial Index assesses skills such as the ability to integrate and synthesize part–whole relationships, attentiveness to visual detail, visual–motor integration, and visual–spatial reasoning. Jason's Visual Spatial Reasoning Index was in the Average range; his subtests scores ranged from 6 to 11 (8–12 is average). His highest score was on a task requiring him to use objects to re-create visual patterns (Block Design). The Fluid Reasoning Index assesses skills such as inductive and quantitative reasoning, broad visual intelligence, simultaneous processing, and abstract thinking. Jason's Fluid Reasoning Index was classified as Very Low; his subtest scores ranged from 5 to 7 (8–12 is average). He obtained his highest score on a task requiring him to indicate which response option completes a matrix or series of images (Matrix Reasoning), but struggled more on a task involving quantitative fluid reasoning (Figure Weights).

The Working Memory Index is a measure of an individual's ability to attend to verbally or visually presented information, to process information in memory, and then to formulate a response. Jason's Working Memory Index was classified as Very Low—his subtest scores ranged from 4 to 6

(8–12 is average). Jason could remember small amounts of information, but seemed to have more difficulty as the subtests increased the amount of information he had to remember and manipulate.

The Processing Speed Index is a measure of an individual's ability to scan visual information, process simple or routine visual information efficiently, and to perform tasks quickly based on that information. Jason's Processing Speed Index was in the Extremely Low range—his subtest scores ranged from 1 to 2 (8–12 is average). It should be noted that Jason had particular difficulty with these subtests as he became anxious and upset when he made a mistake and could not correct his work. He began to repeat lines from a movie rather than complete the task. His level of anxiety and frustration probably interfered with his ability to complete this task within the time constraints, resulting in a Processing Speed Index that might be an underestimate of his true abilities in this area.

As Jason's lowest scores were obtained on three of the four subtests comprising the Working Memory Index and Processing Speed Index, and the large amounts of discrepancy among his Visual Spatial Index and his Processing Speed Index and the other three Primary Index scales, it may be more meaningful to consider the Ancillary Index Scales of the GAI and CPI. Jason obtained a GAI of 78 (7th percentile), which is classified in the Very Low range of functioning when the influence of working memory and processing speed difficulties are minimized. This is not a clinically significant difference from his FSIQ. Jason obtained a CPI of 54 (less than the 1st percentile), which is classified in the Extremely Low range of functioning. It was 24 points lower than his GAI—this discrepancy is seen in less than 5% of children Jason's age. Thus, while his general cognitive ability or cognitive "horsepower" is within the Low Average range, his ability to efficiently process information is much lower and may be negatively impacting him.

Vineland–II Results

Jason's mother was the respondent for the Vineland–II. Based on the information gathered from the interview, Jason obtained an Adaptive Behavior Composite of 71, which falls in the Moderately Low range of adaptive functioning. Jason's mother reported moderately low levels of skills in all areas assessed. In the area of Communication, Jason obtained a score of 79 (8th percentile). His mother reported that he could follow simple and complex instructions, speak in full sentences, and print simple words from memory. However, he has not yet learned to follow three-step commands or engage in back-and-forth conversation. In the area of Daily Living Skills, Jason obtained a score of 74 (4th percentile). His mother reported that he could brush his teeth and dress independently, but had not yet learned to use simple appliances. In the Socialization domain, Jason obtained a score of 64 (1st percentile). His mother described him as showing interest in same-age peers and answering questions when familiar adults made small talk—however, he has not yet learned to talk about shared interests with others, play with other children his own age, or share his toys. In the Motor Scales domain, Jason obtained a score of 78 (7th percentile) and was described as being able to draw shapes and run easily. He has difficulty using a keyboard to type short words, catching a ball, tying knots, and using a bicycle without training wheels.

Discussion of the Case Example Information

Jason's performance on the WISC-V was consistent with previous research reviewed in this chapter, indicating that individuals with ASD often display an uneven profile of performance. Jason's WISC-V profile was characterized by some skills that were significantly below his chronological age and other skills that were equivalent to his chronological age. He also showed the commonly observed pattern of significantly greater visual–spatial perception skills than verbal reasoning skills. Fitting this pattern, his highest subtest score was on the Block Design subtest (which measures visual–spatial perception). The WISC-V highlighted Jason's strengths and weaknesses, providing an opportunity to recommend additional school assistance when receptive or expressive language was required by building on his strengths (e.g., increased use of written or picture directions rather than verbal directions, and use of manipulatives when solving math problems). Also, by examining his CPI indicating that Jason processes information less efficiently, we were able to recommend that he receive accommodations to allow for extra processing time (e.g., fewer items on a worksheet, extended test-taking time) while continuing to allow him to participate in the traditional academic curriculum for third grade.

Similarly, the Vineland–II provided a profile that was consistent with previous research showing overall delays with specific deficits in social skills. Given Jason's WISC-V Visual Spatial Index score of 92, specific ideas for increasing adaptive behavior goals using visual supports were recommended. For example, the use of visual work systems (Hume, Loftin, & Lantz, 2009; Hume, Plavnick, & Odom, 2012) could be used to teach the steps involved in daily living skills such as using a microwave. We believe that by considering the recommended questions for choosing an appropriate IQ and adaptive behavior assessment, we were able to provide a comprehensive set of recommendations for school and home accommodations to help Jason reach his full potential.

REFERENCES

Akshoomoff, N. (2006). Use of the Mullen Scales of Early Learning for the assessment of young children with autism spectrum disorders. *Child Neuropsychology, 12,* 269–277.

American Psychiatric Association. (2000). *Diagnostic and statistical manual of mental disorders* (4th ed., text rev.). Washington, DC: Author.

American Psychiatric Association. (2013). *Diagnostic and statistical manual of mental disorders* (5th ed.). Arlington, VA: Author.

Amiet, C., Gourfinkel-An, I., Bouzamondo, A., Tordjman, S., Baulac, M., Lechat, P., et al. (2008). Epilepsy in autism is associated with intellectual disability and gender: Evidence from a meta-analysis. *Biological Psychiatry, 64,* 577–582.

Anderson, D. K., Liang, J. W., & Lord, C. (2014). Predicting young adult outcome among more and less cognitively able individuals with autism spectrum disorders. *Journal of Child Psychology and Psychiatry, 55,* 485–494.

Ankenman, K., Elgin, J., Sullivan, K., Vincent, L., & Bernier, R. (2014). Nonverbal and verbal cognitive discrepancy profiles in autism spectrum disorders: Influence of age and gender. *American Journal on Intellectual and Developmental Disabilities, 139,* 84–99.

Bal, V. H., Kim, S.-H., Cheong, D., & Lord, C. (2015). Daily living skills in individuals with autism spectrum disorder from 2 to 21-years of age. *Autism, 19*(7), 774–784.

Barbaro, J., & Dissanayake, C. (2012). Developmental profiles of infants and toddlers with autism spectrum disorders identified prospectively in a community-based setting. *Journal of Autism and Developmental Disorders, 42,* 1939–1948.

Barnhill, G. P., Hagiwara, R., Myles, B. S., Simpson, R. L., Brick, M. L., & Griswold, D. E. (2000). Parent, teacher, and self-report of problem and adaptive behaviors in children and adolescents with Asperger syndrome. *Diagnostique, 25,* 147–167.

Baron-Cohen, S. (2001). Theory of mind and autism: A review. *International Review of Research in Mental Retardation, 23,* 169–184.

Bayley, N. (2005). *Manual for the Bayley Scales of Infant and Toddler Development, Third Edition (Bayley–III).* San Antonio, TX: Harcourt Assessment.

Beadle-Brown, J., Murphy, G., & Wing, L. (2006). The Camberwell cohort 25 years on: Characteristics and changes in skills over time. *Journal of Applied Research in Intellectual Disabilities, 19,* 317–329.

Begovac, I., Begovac, B., Majic, G., & Vidovic, V. (2009). Longitudinal studies of IQ stability in children with childhood autism—literature study. *Psychiatria Danubina, 21,* 310–319.

Brunsdon, V. E., Colvert, E., Ames, C., Garnett, T., Gillan, N., Hallett, V., et al. (2015). Exploring the cognitive features in children with autism spectrum disorder, their co-twins, and typically developing children within a population-based sample. *Journal of Child Psychology and Psychiatry, 56*(8), 893–902.

Canivez, G. L., & Watkins, M. W. (2016). Review of the Wechsler Intelligence Scale for Children—Fifth Edition: Critique, commentary, and independent analyses. In A. S. Kaufman, S. E. Raiford, & D. L. Coalson (Eds.), *Intelligent testing with the WISC-V* (pp. 683–702). Hoboken, NJ: Wiley.

Carothers, D. E., & Taylor, R. L. (2013). Differential effect of features of autism on IQs reported using Wechsler scales. *Focus on Autism and Other Developmental Disabilities, 28,* 54–59.

Carter, A. A., Black, D. O., Tewani, S., Connolly, C. E., Kadlec, M. B., & Tager-Flusberg, H. (2007). Sex differences in toddlers with autism spectrum disorders. *Journal of Autism and Developmental Disorders, 37,* 86–97.

Charman, T., Howlin, P., Berry, B., & Prince, E. (2004). Measuring developmental progress of children with autism spectrum disorder on school entry using parent report. *Autism, 8,* 89–100.

Chawarska, K., Klin, A., Paul, R., Macari, S., & Volkmar, F. (2009). A prospective study of toddlers with ASD: Short-term diagnostic and cognitive outcomes. *Journal of Child Psychology and Psychiatry, 50,* 1235–1245.

Chiang, H., Tsai, L. Y., Cheung, Y. K., Brown, A., & Li, H. (2014). A meta-analysis of differences in IQ profiles between individuals with Asperger's disorder and high-functioning autism. *Journal of Autism and Developmental Disorders, 44,* 1577–1596.

Christensen, D. L., Baio, J., Van Naarden Braun, K., Bilder, D., Charles, J., Constantino, J. N., et al. (2016). Prevalence and characteristics of autism spectrum disorder among children aged 8 years—autism and developmental disabilities monitoring network, 11 sites, United States, 2012. *Morbidity and Mortality Weekly Report Surveillance Summaries, 65*(3), 1–23.

Coolican, J., Bryson, S. E., & Zwaigenbaum, L. (2008). Brief report: Data on the Stanford–Binet Intelligence Scales (5th ed.) in children with autism spectrum disorder. *Journal of Autism and Developmental Disorders, 38,* 190–197.

Courchesne, E., Townsend, J. P., Akshoomoff, N. A., Yeung-Courchesne, R., Press, G. A., Murakami, J. W., et al. (1994). A new finding: Impairment in shifting attention in autistic and cerebellar patients. In H. Broman & J. Grafman (Eds.), *Atypical cognitive deficits in developmental disorders: Implications for brain function* (pp. 101–137). Hillsdale, NJ: Erlbaum.

Dawson, G., Toth, K., Abbott, R., Osterling, J., Munson, J., Estes, A., et al. (2004). Early social attention impairments in autism: Social orienting, joint attention, and attention to distress. *Developmental Psychology, 40,* 271–283.

Doobay, A. F., Foley-Nicpon, M., Ali, S. R., & Assouline, S. G. (2014). Cognitive, adaptive, and psychosocial differences between high ability youth with and without autism spectrum disorder. *Journal of Autism and Developmental Disorders, 44,* 2026–2040.

Duncan, A. W., & Bishop, S. L. (2015). Understanding the gap between cognitive abilities and daily living skills in adolescents with autism spectrum disorders with average intelligence. *Autism, 19*(1), 64–72.

Edelson, M. G. (2006). Are the majority of children with autism mentally retarded? *Focus on Autism and Other Developmental Disabilities, 21,* 66–83.

Ehlers, S., Nyden, A., Gillberg, C., Sandberg, A. D., Dahlgren, S., Hjelmquist, E., et al. (1997). Asperger syndrome, autism, and attention disorders: A comparative study of the cognitive profiles of 120 children. *Journal of Child Psychology and Psychiatry, 38,* 207–217.

Eikeseth, S., Smith, T., Jahr, E., & Eldevik, S. (2007). Outcomes for children with autism who began intensive behavioral treatment between ages 4 and 7: A comparison controlled study. *Behavior Modifications, 31,* 264–278.

Elliot, C. D. (2007). *Differential Ability Scales—Second Edition.* San Antonio, TX: Harcourt Assessment.

Estes, A., Munson, J., Rogers, S. J., Greenson, J., Winter, J., & Dawson G. (2015).

Long-term outcomes of early intervention in 6-year-old children with autism spectrum disorder. *Journal of the American Academy of Child and Adolescent Psychiatry, 54*, 580–587.

Farley, M. A., McMahon, W. M., Fombonne, E., Jenson, W. R., Miller, J., Gardner, M., et al. (2009). Twenty-year outcome for individuals with autism and average or near-average cognitive abilities. *Autism Research, 2*, 109–118.

Farmer, C., Golden, C. & Thurm, A. (2016). Concurrent validity of the Differential Ability Scales, Second Edition with the Mullen Scales of Early Learning in young children with and without neurodevelopmental disorders. *Child Neuropsychology, 22*(5), 556–569.

Fombonne, E. (2005). Epidemiological studies of pervasive developmental disorders. In F. R. Volkmar, R. Paul, A. Klin, & D. Cohen (Eds.), *Handbook of autism and pervasive developmental disorders: Vol. 1. Diagnosis, development, neurobiology, and behavior* (3rd ed., pp. 42–69). Hoboken, NJ: Wiley.

Geurts, H. M., Corbett, B., & Solomon, M. (2009). The paradox of cognitive flexibility in autism. *Trends in Cognitive Sciences, 13*, 74–82.

Ghaziuddin, M., & Mountain-Kimchi, K. (2004). Defining the intellectual profile of Asperger syndrome: Comparison with high-functioning autism. *Journal of Autism and Developmental Disorders, 34*, 279–284.

Happé, F. G. E., & Booth, R. D. L. (2008). The power of the positive: Revisiting weak coherence in autism spectrum disorders. *Quarterly Journal of Experimental Psychology, 61*, 50–63.

Happé, F., & Frith, U. (2006). The weak coherence account: Detail-focused cognitive style in autism spectrum disorders. *Journal of Autism and Developmental Disorders, 36*, 5–25.

Harrison, P. L., & Oakland, T. (2003). *Adaptive Behavior Assessment System—Second Edition*. San Antonio, TX: Psychological Corporation.

Harrison, P., & Oakland, T. (2015). *Adaptive Behavior Assessment System—Third Edition*. Torrance, CA: Western Psychological Services.

Hartley, S. L., & Sikora, D. M. (2009). Sex differences in autism spectrum disorder: An examination of developmental functioning, autistic symptoms, and coexisting behavior problems in toddlers. *Journal of Autism and Developmental Disorders, 39*, 1715–1722.

Holdnack, J., Goldstein, G., & Drozdick, L. (2011). Social perception and WAIS-IV performance in adolescents and adults diagnosed with Asperger's syndrome and autism. *Assessment, 18*, 192–200.

Howlin, P., Goode, S., Hutton, J., & Rutter, M. (2004). Adult outcomes for children with autism. *Journal of Child Psychology and Psychiatry, 45*, 212–229.

Hume, K., Loftin, R., & Lantz, J. (2009). Increasing independence in autism spectrum disorders: A review of three focused interventions. *Journal of Autism and Developmental Disorders, 39*(9), 1329–1338.

Hume, K., Plavnick, J., & Odom, S. L. (2012). Promoting task accuracy and independence in students with autism across educational setting through the use of individual work systems. *Journal of Autism and Developmental Disorders, 42*(10), 2084–2099.

Idring, S., Lundberg, M., Sturm, H., Dalman, C., Gumpert, C., Rai, D., et al. (2015). Changes in prevalence of autism spectrum disorders in 2001–2011: Findings from the Stockholm youth cohort. *Journal of Autism and Developmental Disorders, 45*(6), 1766–1773.

Johnson, C. P., Myers, S. M., & the Council on Children with Disabilities. (2007). Identification of and evaluation of children with autism spectrum disorders. *Pediatrics, 120,* 1183–1215.

Joseph, R. M., Tager-Flusberg, H., & Lord, C. (2002). Cognitive profiles and social-communicative functioning in children with autism spectrum disorder. *Journal of Child Psychology and Psychiatry, 43,* 807–821.

Kanner, L. (1943). Autistic disturbances of affective contact. *Nervous Child, 2,* 217–250.

Kasari, C., Brady, N., Lord, C., & Tager-Flusberg, H. (2013). Assessing the minimally verbal school-aged child with autism spectrum disorder. *Autism Research, 6,* 479–493.

Kaufman, A. S., & Kaufman, N. L. (2004). *Kaufman Brief Intelligence Test, Second Edition (KBIT-2).* Circle Pines, MN: American Guidance Service.

Keehn, B., Muller, R. A., & Townsend, J. (2013). Atypical attentional networks and the Avwwvemergence of autism. *Neuroscience and Biobehavioral Reviews, 37,* 164–183.

Kenworthy, L., Case, L., Harms, M. B., Martin, A., & Wallace, G. L. (2010). Adaptive behavior ratings correlate with symptomatology and IQ among individuals with high-functioning autism spectrum disorders. *Journal of Autism and Developmental Disorders, 40*(4), 416–423.

Kirkovski, M., Enticott, P. G., & Fitzgerald, P. B. (2013). A review of the role of female gender in autism spectrum disorders. *Journal of Autism and Developmental Disorders, 43,* 2584–2603.

Klin, A., Saulnier, C., Tsatsanis, K., & Volkmar, F. R. (2005). Clinical evaluation in autism spectrum disorders: Psychological assessment within a transdisciplinary framework. In F. R. Volkmar, R. Paul, A. Klin, & D. J. Cohen (Eds.), *Handbook of autism and pervasive developmental disorders: Vol. 2. Assessment, interventions, and policy* (3rd ed., p. 772–798). Hoboken, NJ: Wiley.

Klinger, L. G., Klinger, M. R., & Pohlig, R. L. (2007). Implicit learning impairments in autism spectrum disorders: Implications for treatment. In J. M. Perez, P. M. Gonzalez, M. L. Comi, & C. Nieto (Eds.), *New developments in autism: The future is today* (pp. 76–103). London: Jessica Kingsley.

Koegel, L. K., Koegel, R. L., & Smith, A. (1997). Variables related to differences in standardized test outcome for children with autism. *Journal of Autism and Developmental Disorders, 27,* 233–243.

Kuriakose, S. (2014). Concurrent validity of the WISC-IV and the DAS-II in children with autism spectrum disorder. *Journal of Psychoeducational Assessment, 32,* 283–294.

Kuschner, E. S., Bennetto, L., & Yost, K. (2007). Patterns of nonverbal cognitive functioning in young children with autism spectrum disorders. *Journal of Autism and Developmental Disorders, 37,* 795–807.

Landa, R., & Garrett-Mayer, E. (2006). Development in infants with autism spectrum disorders: A prospective study. *Journal of Child Psychology and Psychiatry, 47,* 629–638.

Lincoln, A. J., Hansel, E., & Quirmbach, L. (2007). Assessing intellectual abilities of children and adolescents with autism and related disorders. In S. R. Smith & L. Handler (Eds.), *The clinical assessment of children and adolescents: A practitioner's handbook* (pp. 527–544). Mahwah, NJ: Erlbaum.

Lopata, C., Fox, J. D., Thomeer, M. L., Smith, R. A., Volker, M. A., Kessel, C. M., et al. (2012). ABAS-II ratings and correlates of adaptive behavior in children with HFASDs. *Journal of Developmental and Physical Disabilities, 24,* 391–402.

Luiselli, J. K., Campbell, S., Cannon, B., DiPietro, E., Ellis, J. T., Taras, M., et al. (2001). Assessment instruments used in the education and treatment of persons with autism: Brief report of a survey of national service centers. *Research in Developmental Disabilities, 22,* 389–398.

Matthews, N. L., Pollard, E., Ober-Reynolds, S., Kirwan, J., Malligo, A., & Smith, C. J. (2015). Revisiting cognitive and adaptive functioning in children and adolescents with autism spectrum disorder. *Journal of Autism and Developmental Disorders, 45*(1), 138–156.

Mayes, S. D., & Calhoun, S. L. (2003). Ability profiles in children with autism: Influence of age and IQ. *Autism, 6,* 65–80.

Mayes, S. D., & Calhoun, S. L. (2008). WISC-IV and WIAT-II profiles in children with high-functioning autism. *Journal of Autism and Developmental Disorders, 38,* 428–439.

Meilleur, A. A. S., Jelenic, P., & Mottron, L. (2015). Prevalence of clinically and empirically defined talents and strengths in autism. *Journal of Autism and Developmental Disorders, 45*(5), 1354–1367.

Minshew, N. J., Goldstein, G., & Siegel, D. J. (1997). Neuropsychologic functioning in autism: Profile of a complex information processing disorder. *Journal of the International Neuropsychological Society, 3,* 303–316.

Mottron, L., Dawson, M., Soulieres, I., Hubert, B., & Burack J. (2006). Enhanced perceptual functioning in autism: An update, and eight principles of autistic perception. *Journal of Autism and Developmental Disorders, 36,* 27–43.

Mullen, E. M. (1995). *Mullen Scales of Early Learning.* Circle Pines, MN: American Guidance Service.

Munson, J., Dawson, G., Sterling, L., Beauchaine, T., Zhou, A., Koehler, E., et al. (2008). Evidence for latent classes of IQ in young children with autism spectrum disorder. *American Journal on Mental Retardation, 113,* 439–452.

National Research Council. (2001). *Educating children with autism.* Washington, DC: National Academy Press.

Oliveras-Rentas, R. E., Kenworthy, L., Roberson, R. B., III, Martin, A., & Wallace, G. L. (2012). WISC-IV profile in high-functioning autism spectrum disorders: Impaired processing speed is associated with increased autism communication symptoms and decreased adaptive communication abilities. *Journal of Autism and Developmental Disorders, 42,* 655–664.

Ozonoff, S. (1995). Reliability and validity of the Wisconsin Card Sorting Test in studies of autism. *Neuropsychology, 9*(4), 491–500.

Ozonoff, S., Goodlin-Jones, B. L., & Solomon, M. (2007). Autism spectrum disorders. In E. J. Mash & R. A. Barkley (Eds.), *Assessment of childhood disorders* (4th ed., pp. 487–525). New York: Guilford Press.

Ozonoff, S., Iosif, A., Baguio, F., Cook, I. C., Hill, M. M., Hutman, T., et al. (2010). A prospective study of the emergence of early behavioral signs of autism. *Journal of the American Academy of Child and Adolescent Psychiatry, 49,* 256–266.

Ozonoff, S., & Jensen, J. (1999). Brief report: Specific executive function profiles in three neurodevelopmental disorders. *Journal of Autism and Developmental Disorders, 29,* 171–177.

Ozonoff, S., South, M., & Miller, J. N. (2000). DSM-IV defined Asperger syndrome:

Cognitive, behavioral and early history differentiation from high-functioning autism. *Autism, 4,* 29–46.

Paul, R., Loomis, R., & Chawarska, K. (2014). Adaptive behavior in toddlers under two with autism spectrum disorders. *Journal of Autism and Developmental Disorders, 44,* 264–270.

Raiford, S. E., Drozdick, L., & Zhang, O. (2015). Q-interactive special group studies?: The WISC-V and children with autism spectrum disorder and accompanying language impairment or attention-deficit/hyperactivity disorder. *Q-Intereactive Technical Report 11,* 1–19.

Ray-Subramanian, C. E., Huai, N., & Weismer, S. E. (2011). Brief report: Adaptive behavior and cognitive skills for toddlers on the autism spectrum. *Journal of Autism and Developmental Disorders, 41,* 679–684.

Renner, P., Klinger, L. G., & Klinger, M. R. (2006). Exogenous and endogenous attention orienting in autism spectrum disorders. *Child Neuropsychology, 12,* 361–382.

Rogers, S. J., Hepburn, S., Stackhouse, T., & Wehner, E. (2003). Imitation performance in toddlers with autism and those with other developmental disorders. *Journal of Child Psychology and Psychiatry, 44,* 763–781.

Roid, G. H. (2003). *Stanford–Binet Intelligence Scales, Fifth Edition.* Itasca, IL: Riverside.

Roid, G. H., Miller, L. J. Pomplun, M., & Koch, C. (2013). *Leiter International Performance Scale—Third Edition (Leiter–3).* Wood Dale, IL: Stoelting.

Rubenstein, E., Wiggins, L. D., & Lee, L. C. (2015). A review of the differences in developmental, psychiatric, and medical endophenotypes between males and females with autism spectrum disorder. *Journal of Developmental and Physical Disabilities, 27,* 119–139.

Russo, N., Flanagan, T., Iarocci, G., Berringer, D., Zelazo, P. D., & Burack, J. A. (2007). Deconstructing executive deficits among persons with autism: Implications for cognitive neuroscience. *Brain and Cognition, 65,* 77–86.

Sigman, M., Mundy, P., Sherman, T., & Ungerer, J. (1986). Social interactions of autistic, mentally retarded, and normal children with their caregivers. *Journal of Child Psychology and Psychiatry, 27,* 647–656.

Smith, L. E., Maenner, M. J., & Seltzer, M. M. (2012). Developmental trajectories in adolescents and adults with autism: The case of daily living skills. *Journal of the American Academy of Child and Adolescent Psychiatry, 51,* 622–631.

Sparrow, S. S., Balla, D. A., & Cicchetti, D. V. (1984). *Vineland Adaptive Behavior Scales.* Circle Pines, MN: American Guidance Service.

Sparrow, S. S., Cicchetti, D. V., & Balla, D. A. (2005). *Vineland Adaptive Behavior Scales, Second Edition.* Circle Pines, MN: American Guidance Service.

Swineford, L., Guthrie, W., & Thurm, A. (2015). Convergent and divergent validity of the Mullen Scales of Early Learning in young children with and without autism spectrum disorder. *Psychological Assessment, 27*(4), 1364–1378.

Szatmari, P., Archer, L., Fisman, S., & Streiner, D. L. (1994). Parent and teacher agreement in the assessment of pervasive developmental disorders. *Journal of Autism and Developmental Disorders, 24,* 703–717.

Tager-Flusberg, H., Plesa Skwerer, D., Joseph, R. M., Brukilacchio, B., Decker, J., Eggleston, B., et al. (2016). Conducting research with minimally verbal participants with autism spectrum disorder. *Autism.* {Epub ahead of print]

Taylor, J. L., & Seltzer, M. M. (2011). Employment and post-secondary educational activities for young adults with autism spectrum disorders during the transition to adulthood. *Journal of Autism and Developmental Disorders, 41*, 566–574.

Tsatsanis, K. D., Dartnall, N., Cicchetti, D., Sparrow, S. S., Klin, A., & Volkmar, F. R. (2003). Concurrent validity and classification accuracy of the Leiter and Leiter–R in low-functioning children with autism. *Journal of Autism and Developmental Disorders, 33*(1), 23–30.

Vivanti, G., Prior, M., Williams, K., & Dissanayake, C. (2014). Predictors of outcomes in autism early intervention: Why don't we know more? *Frontiers in Pediatrics, 2*, 1–10.

Volkmar, F., Siegel, M., Woodbury-Smith, M., King, B., McCracken, J., State, M., et al. (2014). Practice parameter for the assessment and treatment of children and adolescents with autism spectrum disorder. *Journal of the American Academy of Child and Adolescent Psychiatry, 53*, 237–257.

Volkmar, F. R., Szatmari, P., & Sparrow, S. S. (1993). Sex differences in pervasive developmental disorders. *Journal of Autism and Developmental Disorders, 23*, 579–591.

Wechsler, D. (2003). *Wechsler Intelligence Scale for Children, Fourth Edition* (WISC-IV). San Antonio, TX: Psychological Corporation.

Wechsler, D. (2008). *Wechsler Adult Intelligence Scale—Fourth Edition* (WAIS-IV). San Antonio, TX: Pearson.

Wechsler, D. (2011). *Wechsler Abbreviated Scale of Intelligence—Second Edition* (WASI-II). San Antonio, TX: NCS Pearson.

Wechsler, D. (2012). *Wechsler Preschool and Primary Scale of Intelligence—Fourth Edition* (WPPSI-IV). San Antonio, TX: Psychological Corporation.

Wechsler, D. (2014). *Wechsler Intelligence Scale for Children—Fifth Edition* (WISC-V). Bloomington, MN: Pearson.

Williams, D. L., Goldstein, G., & Minshew, N. J. (2006). Neuropsychologic functioning in children with autism: Further evidence for disordered complex information processing. *Child Neuropsychology, 12*, 279–298.

CHAPTER NINE

Clinical Assessment of Neuropsychological Functioning in Autism Spectrum Disorder

Blythe A. Corbett
Yasmeen S. Iqbal

Neuropsychology may be conceptualized as a bridge between neurology and psychology, which looks at the relationship between the brain and behavior—it has emerged as a clinical and research discipline in the last 50 years. Over this period of time, the field has progressed from the administration of basic paper-and-pencil-type tasks to elaborate, comprehensive batteries evaluating many domains of functioning. In the last decade, structural and functional neuroimaging has corroborated and extended many of the contributions advanced by clinical neuropsychology. The goals of neuropsychological assessment include integrating the factors of development, brain function, behavior, and social context to inform clinical judgments and research.

The purpose of a neuropsychological evaluation can be to identify cognitive strengths and weaknesses, establish a baseline of functioning, determine premorbid functioning, document performance status and changes in performance, and guide treatment. In addition, it can assist with differential diagnosis and the identification of individual differences among and within groups. In research, the use of neuropsychological instruments permits the exploration of theoretical frameworks and provides useful objective measures for comparison across groups or conditions. The field of pediatric neuropsychology has evolved as a specialized division within neuropsychology to emphasize child development and how factors such as learning and behavior are related to the development of brain systems and structures. In addition, pediatric neuropsychology provides a model for the understanding of neuroplasticity in development.

A comprehensive neuropsychological assessment includes information from a variety of sources in addition to standardized tests, described below. These sources can include medical and educational records, clinical observation, parent and teacher reports and ratings, and diagnostic interviews. This chapter is intended to provide an overview of the neuropsychological assessment process in relation to autism spectrum disorder (ASD; American Psychiatric Association, 2013) as well as briefly review relevant research findings. However, it is not intended to provide the necessary training and extensive knowledge required of a pediatric neuropsychologist that includes a deep appreciation of child development, the central nervous system, and the emergence of cognitive processes across the lifespan (Batchelor & Dean, 1995; Yeates, Ris, & Taylor, 2000). In addition, it is not possible within the scope of this chapter to present an exhaustive list of measures that could be used within each domain of functioning. Rather, the ones described below are examples of tools developed with the sensitivity to provide information on the functioning of each domain, and we have tried to include those that we have found helpful and that have good reported reliability and validity.

Neuropsychological assessment utilizes quantitative approaches that involve standardized behavior ratings and norm-referenced test data. Qualitative data, such as patient history; observations of behavior during testing; observations of social interaction, play, and communication; and neurological signs are also very important, but the interpretation of these data ultimately relies on the expertise of the examiner (Turkheimer, 1989).

Neuropsychological measures provide standardized scores based on normative data ideally from a large sample of children derived from the population of interest. Although various scores may be generated, the majority provide metrics that are derived by subtracting the population mean from an individual's raw score and then dividing by the population standard deviation. The standardized score allows us to determine how close the child's performance is to a comparison group. Psychological measures usually provide normative data in the form of standardized scores with a mean of 100 and a standard deviation of 15, or scaled scores with a mean of 10 and a standard deviation of 3, or *T*-scores with a mean of 50 and a standard deviation of 10.

DOMAINS OF FUNCTIONING

A comprehensive neuropsychological assessment typically involves the assessment of many areas of functioning, including overarching cognitive or intellectual ability, adaptive skills, attention, sensory processing, motor ability, language, executive functioning, visual–spatial and visual–motor ability, memory, academic skills, and social–emotional functioning. The neuropsychological assessment can assist in corroborating diagnostic procedures, contribute to a unique profile of ability and deficit, and assist in formulating appropriate treatments and interventions (Lezak, 1995; Lezak & Bigler, 2012).

In the following section, we address the primary areas of cognitive functioning, focusing on descriptions of standardized measures that assess these various areas of ability. Several neuropathological models have been proposed over the years in an attempt to explain the core or related symptoms in autism or using the current nosology—ASD. These terms will be used interchangeably, especially when discussing previous research that occurred prior to the common use of ASD. When applicable, we present summaries of these core or "primacy" models within the relevant domain.

Cognitive Functioning

At the foundation of a neuropsychological assessment is intellectual testing, which provides the framework for the interpretation of other quantitative and qualitative measures and observations. In ASD, the child's level of measured intelligence is affected by some factors that are either not relevant or not as important in typical development—these include the severity of symptoms, level of adaptive functioning, motivation to participate in testing, and treatment provided (Filipek et al., 1999). According to the latest estimates, the prevalence rate for ASD is one in 68 children in the United States (Centers for Disease Control and Prevention, 2016). It is estimated that 31% of children with ASD are classified as having an intellectual disability (IQ ≤ 70), 25% in the borderline range (IQ = 71–85), and 44% in the average or above-average range of intellectual ability (IQ > 85; Centers for Disease Control and Prevention, 2016). Since intellectual ability is dependent on many factors (and influences many cognitive skills in turn), cognitive impairment may be due to difficulties in a number of contributing areas including language, processing speed, broad knowledge, and social comprehension. It is important to note that although impairments in social behavior are usually considered the hallmark deficit in autism, it is cognitive ability that serves as a better predictor of outcome (Filipek et al., 1999; Stevens et al., 2000). In addition, cognitive level influences the expression of autism symptoms, including social behavior and repetitive interests. For example, for children with low IQ, social disability may manifest as lack of interest in peers, while for children (and those who are older) with higher IQ, social disability may manifest in wanting to have friends, accompanied by social awkwardness, immaturity, and rigidity, thus preventing actual mutual friendships from developing. In the

Repetitive Behavior domain, the child with low IQ may present with multiple motor stereotypes and unusual visual behaviors, while the child with higher IQ may manifest this characteristic more in resistance to changes in routines and preoccupations with unusual topics. As with any child, when the profile of cognitive subtests is uneven (as is the rule rather than the exception in autism), the overall IQ score must be interpreted with caution, and used more as a rough index of overall current functioning than as a real measure of cognitive ability.

A brief overview of several of the overall cognitive measures is provided.

Measures

The Wechsler Intelligence Scale for Children—Fifth Edition (WISC-V; Wechsler, 2014) is considered one of the gold standards for measuring intellectual functioning. The Wechsler scales provide separate scores based on verbal and nonverbal problem-solving skills, short-term memory, and processing speed. The WISC-V is used to measure cognitive functioning in children 6 years, 0 months, to 16 years, 11 months, of age. The primary use of IQ testing in this population is to differentiate between high- and low-functioning ASD. However, it has been helpful in the support of differential diagnosis (Williams, Goldstein, Kojkowski, & Minshew, 2008) and has been utilized as a predictor for functional outcome (e.g., Billstedt, Gillberg, & Gillberg, 2005). While research on the intellectual profile testing on the WISC-V is mixed, individuals with high-functioning ASD often show strengths in Matrix Reasoning and Similarities subtests and weaknesses on the Comprehension subtest (Oliveras-Rentas, Kenworthy, Roberson, Martin, & Wallace, 2012). Nevertheless, though it is an improvement from previous Wechsler scales, the instrument is not a stand-alone neuropsychological test (see Baron, 2005, for a review). The normative sample for the WISC-V consisted of 2,200 English-speaking U.S children, ages 6 years, 0 months to 16 years, 11 months, stratified according to the 2012 U.S. census. The standardization also included specialized populations, such as autism, making it a good tool in ASD research and practice. Additionally, the WISC-V and Wechsler Individual Achievement Test—Third Edition (WIAT-III; Wechsler, 2009) are conormed, making the WISC-V useful in assessing learning disability.

The Wechsler Preschool and Primary Scale of Intelligence—Fourth Edition (WPPSI-IV; Wechsler, 2012) is a measure of general intellectual abilities that provides separate scores based on verbal and nonverbal problem-solving skills. It is intended for use with young children from 2 years, 6 months, to 7 years, 7 months, of age. Although the measure was developed for assessment of cognitive abilities in preschoolers and young children, some of the task demands may be challenging for children with neurodevelopmental disorders, such as ASD. It represents a downward extension of the WISC tests. This measure was normed on 1,700 children ages 2 years, 2 months, to 7 years, 7 months.

The Wechsler Abbreviated Scale of Intelligence—Second Edition (WASI-II; Wechsler, 2011) is an abbreviated measure of general intelligence, which is used to obtain an estimated IQ across much of the lifespan, from 6 to 90 years of age. This instrument was developed to fill the need for a shorter, yet reliable assessment of full scale intelligence (FSIQ). As such, this measure provides prediction intervals from WASI-II FSIQ to the comprehensive WISC-V FSIQ. Since the administration of this measure takes only about 30 minutes to complete, it is frequently used in research, and can be useful for the lower-functioning individual, as long as his or her mental age is close to 6 years or above. Four subtests (Vocabulary, Block Design, Similarities, and Matrix Reasoning) are used to calculate Verbal IQ, Performance IQ, and FSIQ. The standardization of the WASI-II was conducted on a nationally representative sample consisting of approximately 2,300 individuals.

The Stanford–Binet Intelligence Scales, Fifth Edition (SB5; Roid, 2003), is a standardized measure of general intelligence that follows a theoretical model, or a general intelligence factor (*g*), as well as additional secondary factors including crystallized ability, fluid ability, and short-term memory (Cattell, 1971). The SB5 is unique in that it covers a wide age span by assessing cognitive functioning from 2 years through adulthood. This makes it advantageous for following children over time—however, one should use caution in interpreting changes in some of the subtests (e.g., Comprehension) because as the child progresses, the task demands change considerably. Normative data is based on 4,800 individuals ages 2 to over 80. The sample is representative of the 2000 U.S. census.

The Bayley Scales of Infant and Toddler Development—Third Edition (Bayley–III; Bayley, 2005) is used to assess the mental, motor, and behavioral functioning of children from the age of 1 to 42 months. The Mental scale provides assessment of early sensory–perceptual abilities, vocalization, early verbal communication, problem solving, memory, habituation, learning, generalization, and classification. The Motor Development scale assesses body control, gross motor coordination, fine motor manipulation, posture, and mobility. The Infant Behavior Rating scale provides ratings of the child's attention, arousal, emotion regulation, orientation, engagement, and quality of motor control. The five subtests include measures of Adaptive Behavior, Cognitive Functioning, Language, Motor, and Social–Emotional Skills. The Language domain measures both expressive and receptive communication, and both preverbal and vocabulary abilities. Specifically, behaviors such as babbling and gesturing, turn taking, and object identification are assessed. Normative data is derived from 1,700 children ages 1–42 months, and is reflective of the 2000 U.S. census.

The Kaufman Assessment Battery for Children, Second Edition (KABC-II; Kaufman & Kaufman, 2004), is grounded in two models known as the Cattell–Horn–Carroll (CHC) psychometric model of broad and narrow abilities, and Luria's processing model (Kaufman & Kaufman, 2004). Some of the subtests on the Kaufman are very appealing to children with ASD and can keep their attention relatively well. The KABC-II also includes six achievement tests and covers the age range from 3 to 18 years of age. Normative data is based on 3,025 individuals ranging in age from 3 years, 0 months, to 18 years, 11 months. The sample is representative of the 2001 U.S. census.

The Cognitive Assessment System, Second Edition (CAS2; Naglieri & Das, 2014), is a test developed to measure planning, attention, simultaneous, and successive (PASS) processing, which are the four areas of the PASS theoretical framework. It is intended for children 5 years, 0 months, to 18 years, 11 months. The CAS2 has been used in studies including children with intellectual disability, learning disabilities, attention-deficit/hyperactivity disorder (ADHD), and special populations (see Naglieri & Das, 2005). This test was normed on a large sample of children and adolescents (including those with autism) ages 5–18 (N = 1,342), who closely represented the U.S. population on a number of important demographic variables (Naglieri & Das, 1997).

The Differential Ability Scales—Second Edition (DAS-II; Elliott, 2006) includes both Verbal and Nonverbal measures of intelligence for children ranging in age from 2 years, 6 months, to 17 years, 11 months, of age. Many subtests are included in this measure, with several specifically developed for preschool-age children, others designed for school-age children, and still others that can be used for both age groups. Individual subtests on this measure are less multifactorial than subtests on some other widely used measures, and thus easier to interpret. For this reason, the DAS-II is often used in research studies—it can also be used to measure performance changes over time. The DAS-II has a normative sample of 3,475 children and adolescents, representative of the general U.S. population.

The Mullen Scales of Early Learning (MSEL; Mullen, 1995) is a measure of verbal and nonverbal abilities that utilizes five different scales (Gross Motor, Visual Reception, Fine Motor, Receptive Language, and Expressive Language) for children ages 1–68 months. Verbal versus nonverbal ability has been studied widely in ASD research, making the MSEL a measure that is reliably used. Recently, good convergent reliability was established for the MSEL compared with the DAS-II (Elliott, 1990, 2006) for Verbal IQ, Performance IQ, and Nonverbal IQ–Verbal IQ profiles (Bishop, Guthrie, Coffing, & Lord, 2011). A large study utilizing a sample of 456 children with ASD revealed evidence for multiple IQ-based subgroups on intelligence level, patterns of strengths and weakness, and level of severity (Munson et al., 2008). Since the MSEL provides separate estimates of functioning in nonverbal problem solving (Visual Reception) and receptive and expressive language for children in infancy and toddlerhood, it is also widely used in research studies of young children with ASD. The MSEL has a total normative sample of 1,849 children ranging from 2 to 69 months. It should be noted that the norms were acquired in the 1980s, with demographics similar to the 1990 U.S. census but with a slightly different geographic distribution than the U.S. population (Bradley-Johnson, 1997).

Adaptive Functioning

Adaptive functioning involves skills and behaviors necessary for age-appropriate day-to-day functioning that encompass communication, socialization, self-care, community use, and independent living skills. In order for an individual to receive a diagnosis of intellectual impairment, both IQ and adaptive functioning must fall into the impaired range (usually a standard score < 70 on most standardized tests). Adaptive skills are often measured clinically as perhaps more ecologically valid measurements of everyday functioning (Volkmar, 2003). In children with ASD, adaptive functioning is often significantly impaired despite demonstration of clear cognitive potential (Klin et al., 2007). Adaptive functioning is often used as a dependent measure in treatment studies to determine whether targeted skills generalize to adaptive skills in the home or school settings. For example, improvement in social functioning has been shown to increase self-care and home living skills (Corbett et al., 2014).

Measures

The Vineland Adaptive Behavior Scales, Second Edition (Vineland–II; Sparrow, Cicchetti, & Balla, 2005), is a semistructured parent interview designed to assess a child's ability to perform daily activities required for personal and social sufficiency. The main areas covered include communicative, daily living skills, socialization, and motor skills. Additionally, maladaptive behavior is an optional subject that may be assessed. The Vineland–II assesses adaptive behaviors of individuals from birth to 90 years, 11 months, and has norms of 3,695 participants based on the 2000 U.S. census. An expanded interview form is also available to obtain additional information after the initial interview. This instrument is one of the most common measures utilized in the assessment of adaptive functioning and is widely used in current autism research (e.g., Klin et al., 2007). For example, the adaptive behavior profiles of children with high-functioning

ASD were examined by one group of researchers using the Vineland–II who reported weaknesses in the Interpersonal, Play and Leisure, and Receptive subdomains compared with significantly higher areas of functioning in the Written, Community, and Personal subdomains (Lopata, Smith, Volker, Thomeer, & McDonald, 2013). More expansively, the same study found that functioning in the Socialization domain was significantly lower than in the Communication and Daily Living domains, indicating characteristic social impairments in high-functioning ASD (Lopata et al., 2013). Another recent study using the Vineland–II examined correlates of functioning for toddlers (under age 2) with ASD and found Daily Living scores to be significantly correlated with nonverbal ability and total Autism Diagnostic Observation Schedule (ADOS) scores, while scores on Receptive Communication were significantly correlated with ADOS total algorithm (Paul, Loomis, & Chawarska, 2014).

The Adaptive Behavior Assessment System—Second Edition (ABAS-II; Harrison & Oakland, 2003) is another adaptive measure for ages 0–89 years that is also widely used. The ABAS-II can be administered as an interview or questionnaire. The domains assessed are similar to those in the Vineland–II, but broken down somewhat differently to include assessment of Communication, Community Use, Functional Academics, Health and Safety, Leisure, Self-Care, Self-Direction, Social Functioning, and Work Aptitude. The forms for children ages 0–5 years has a standardized group of 3,100 children, and the teacher, parent, and adult forms for those over 5 years of age are normed on 5,270 individuals. All standardization samples are representative of the 2000 U.S. census. Of particular relevance, the ABAS-II has also been widely referenced in the ASD literature within the context of functional ability. A study conducted by Kenworthy, Case, Harms, Martin, and Wallace (2009) reported findings on the association among functional ability, intelligence, and symptom severity in children with high-functioning ASD. Specifically, their findings revealed significant positive associations between communication skills on the ABAS-II and intelligence, and a significant negative correlation between global adaptive functioning and severity of ASD symptoms (Kenworthy et al., 2009). As noted, improvement in Self-Care and Home Living Skills on the ABAS-II has been reported in youth with ASD in response to peer-mediated, theare-based treatment (Corbett et al., 2014).

Attention

Attention is a fundamental cognitive domain that is multifaceted and pertains to many different skills, including the ability to sustain attention, the ability to switch from one focus of attention to another or from one task to another (often referred to as "mental flexibility"), and "selective attention," or the ability to focus on one stimulus and inhibit attention to distractions.

Individuals with ASD display a variety of strengths and weaknesses across the various components of attention (see Allen & Courchesne, 2001, for a review). It has been previously reported that sustained attention is usually intact for preferred activities, while sustained attention for nonpreferred activities is usually impaired (Garretson, Fein, & Waterhouse, 1990). In other words, motivational contingencies impact the level of performance, making the provision of adequate incentives crucial for good performance (Garretson et al., 1990). Children with ASD who have comorbid symptoms of ADHD, which is quite common, also exhibit impaired ability in both visual and auditory attention as well as behavioral inhibition (Corbett & Constantine, 2006). Individuals with ASD often orient to a new stimulus much more slowly (Townsend, Harris, & Courchesne, 1996) and show impairment in their ability to shift attention (Courchesne et al., 1994). However, other studies have shown specific rather than general attention-shifting deficits, again underscoring that the level of impairment is often dependent on the specific task stimuli as well as conditions such as distraction and motivation (Pascualvaca, Fantie, Papageorgiou, & Mirsky, 1998).

There are a number of fundamental or primacy theories of autism that consider attention and arousal to be central to the disorder and to involve dysfunction of the attentional systems of the frontal lobes, parietal cortex, and cerebellum. It has been reported that children with autism exhibit deficits in selective attention (Ciesielski, Courchesne, & Elmasian, 1990) that include difficulty with rapid shifts in attention. In fact, Courchesne et al. (1994) proposed that difficulty in shifting attention might underlie the social and cognitive deficits in autism (Courchesne et al., 1994; Lewy & Dawson, 1992; Pierce, Glad, & Schreibman, 1997). Kinsbourne (1991) suggests that perseverative attentional focus is a fundamental feature of autism, perhaps resulting from an attempt to defend against an unstable arousal system. Dawson, Meltzoff, Osterling, Rinaldi, and Brown (1998) showed that orienting to external stimuli is reduced in children with autism, and that orienting to social stimuli (e.g., someone clapping, someone calling the child's name) is especially impaired.

The following measures may be considered in a comprehensive neuropsychological assessment, especially when aspects of attention are impaired or comorbid symptoms of ADHD (inattention and poor inhibition) are suspected. As in studies of ADHD, when multiple measures are used together, prediction of ADHD status improves even if overall diagnosis is limited (Doyle, Biederman, Seidman, Weber, & Faraone, 2000).

Measures

The Integrated Visual and Auditory (IVA) Continuous Performance Test (CPT) (Sandford & Turner, 2000) was designed to help in the diagnosis and quantification of the symptoms of ADHD, but it has also been used to measure attention and self-control across a variety of neurodevelopmental and psychiatric conditions. The IVA combines measures of inattention and impulsivity in a counterbalanced design across both visual and auditory modalities. It is similar to the Test of Variables of Attention (TOVA; Greenberg, Leark, Dupuy, Corman, & Kindschi, 1991; Greenberg & Waldman, 1993), which is also a computerized test of attention. For these tasks, the child is required to press a button when a specific target stimulus is flashed on a computer screen and to refrain from pressing the button when an alternate stimulus is presented. These tasks assess vigilance (sustained attention over time), response inhibition and impulsivity, speed of information processing, and the consistency in attentional focus over time. On this measure children with autism have shown significant deficits in visual and auditory attention, vigilance, and poorer visual response inhibition when compared with children with ADHD and typical development (Corbett & Constantine, 2006; Corbett, Constantine, Hendren, Rocke, & Ozonoff, 2009). The authors suggest that many children with ASD present with symptoms of ADHD and these measures can help identify impairment in sustained attention and inhibition. The normative sample on the IVA consists of 1,700 individuals, and is age grouped and divided by gender.

The Test of Everyday Attention for Children (TEA-Ch; Manly et al., 2001) comprises a series of tasks that measure selective, focused, sustained, and divided attention (the ability to share attention between two tasks). As the name implies, the TEA-Ch was designed to have better ecological validity (Manly et al., 2001) and facilitates motivation by using stimuli that are inherently dynamic and interesting to children. It is designed for ages 6–16, and norms were developed with a group of 293 male and female participants from Australia between the ages of 6 and 16.

The Test of Auditory Discrimination (TOAD; Goldman, Fristoe, & Woodcock, 1970) is a measure of auditory attention, discrimination, and distractibility. The TOAD assesses auditory factors of attention by requiring the individual to identify speech sounds under ideal listening conditions (quiet) and under controlled background noise (distraction). The instrument has been shown to be discriminating in individuals with ADHD (Corbett & Stanczak, 1999) and may have utility for assessing auditory distractibility in individuals with autism. This assessment can be used in persons from the age of 3 years, 8 months, through 70+ years—however, the norm sample is quite old.

The child's attention in everyday situations (such as a classroom) may not be adequately captured by tests of sustained, focused, or divided attention given in a lab, on a computer, and with one-on-one adult attention. Furthermore, the child's attention may vary considerably from one time to another (Barkley, 1991). For these reasons, it is important to gather information from teachers and parents, either informally, or, preferably, using validated rating scales, such as the measures listed below.

The Conners' Parent Rating Scale—Revised (CPRS-R; Conners, 2001) is a parent-rating scale that provides a narrow range of information about behaviors associated with attention and/or hyperactivity as well as oppositional behavior. The CPRS-R is often considered a standard and valid measure frequently used in the assessment of ADHD (Goldstein & Goldstein, 1998). Different versions are available that vary in terms of the respondent (parent, teacher, self), scope of questions, and length of the questionnaire. It is important to note that there is limited correlation between the CPRS-R and other cognitive measures (e.g., see Naglieri, Goldstein, Delauder, & Schwebach, 2005). Nevertheless, the parent, and especially the teacher, versions can assist in a comprehensive clinical evaluation to clarify the expression of symptoms across settings. The CPRS-R norms are derived from over 2,000 parents of children and adolescents ages 3–17 for the teacher and parent forms, and from individuals ages 12–17 for the self-forms, all from the United States and Canada.

Sensory Functioning

Differences and deficits in sensory processing have been widely reported in children with autism (Watling, Deitz, & White, 2001). Dunn and colleagues presented a subtype model based on thresholds of sensory responsiveness and the self-regulatory strategies employed (Dunn, 1999; Dunn & Brown, 1997). Liss, Saulnier, Fein, and Kinsbourne (2006) proposed an overarousal hypothesis to help explain the atypical sensory (overreactivity) and attention (overfocusing) abnormalities. More recently, based on a large sample of children with ASD between 2 and 10 years of age, four distinct sensory subtypes were identified: (1) sensory adaptive, (2) taste–smell sensitive, (3) postural inattentive, and (4) generalized sensory difference (Lane, Molloy, & Bishop, 2014).

Regarding specific domains, many children and adults with autism show unusual patterns in visual processing. For example, when searching for targets individuals with autism usually are faster and more accurate, suggesting enhanced visual discrimination (O'Riordan, 2004; O'Riordan, Plaisted, Driver, & Baron-Cohen, 2001). It has been reported that children with autism show superior auditory discrimination and comparable tactile ability when compared with control subjects (O'Riordan & Passetti, 2006). Taken together with previous findings in visual processing, these studies suggest enhanced perceptual discrimination ability in autism. Behaviorally, one often observes that children with ASD evidence visual fascinations, often spending their free time in staring at absorbing visual stimuli, such as spinning wheels, lights, mirrors, and shadows; or lining up toys and sighting along the lines; or squinting or looking at things out of the corner of their eye (Liss et al., 2006). Conversely, they often seem to have difficulty tolerating tactile stimuli (e.g., being touched, haircuts, certain clothing, and certain foods) and auditory stimuli, and may cover their ears as protection from discomfort (Liss et al., 2006).

Measures

The Sensory Profile (SP; Dunn, 1999) is a parent questionnaire related to sensory sensitivity across several domains, including Auditory, Visual, Vestibular, Tactile, Oral, and Multisensory Processing. Differences on this measure have been reported in autism for sensory-seeking behavior, emotional reactivity, low endurance and tone, oral sensitivity, inattention and distractibility, and more (Watling et al., 2001). The SP is designed for ages 3–10 years—however, an infant/toddler measure is available for those under 3 years, and an adolescent/adult form is available for those over the age of 11. A shorter questionnaire, the Short Sensory Profile (SSP), is also available. (See Liss et al., 2006, for a description of additional, autism-specific questions.) Normative data is based on more than 1,200 children nationwide ages 3–10. Norms for adolescents and adults is based on a sample of 950 individuals ages 11–97 with and without disabilities from the midwestern United States. The SP is often used in research in children with ASD. For example, patterns of hyper- and hyposensitivity have been associated with diurnal regulation of cortisol (Corbett, Schupp, Levine, & Mendoza, 2009) and sensory challenges have been associated with behavioral problems, but not cognitive or adaptive functioning (O'Donnell, Deitz, Kartin, Nalty, & Dawson, 2012). Recently, the SP was used to classify young children with ASD into four distinct sensory subtypes (Adaptive, Taste/Smell, Postural/Inattentive, and Generalized Difference) that were further distinguished based on the focus and severity of the sensory dimension (Lane et al., 2014).

Motor Functioning

Motor functioning is an often overlooked area in the assessment of individuals with autism. While fine and gross motor disturbances were once characterized as an associated feature of ASD, the current general consensus attributes deficits in motor coordination as a more pervasive and cardinal feature (Fournier, Hass, Naik, Lodha, & Carraugh, 2010). Early motor functioning may predict diagnostic and cognitive outcome (Sutera et al., 2007), as well as daily living and adaptive skills (MacDonald, Lord, & Ulrich, 2013). Studies on motor abilities in children with autism have found differences in gait (Vilensky, Damasio, & Maurer, 1981), as well as with running speed, agility, balance, and bilateral coordination (Ghaziuddin, Butler, Tsai, & Ghaziuddin, 1994). Additionally, other studies have shown significant motor delays compared with normative data (Berkeley,

Zittel, Pitney, & Nichols, 2001; Manjiviona & Prior, 1995; Mari, Castiello, Marks, Marraffa, & Prior, 2003; Mayes & Calhoun, 2003). In infants, subtle motor differences have been identified, including excessive mouthing of objects (Baranek, 1999). Other studies looking at infants have found hypotonia, hypoactivity, unusual postures (Adrien et al., 1993), and movements such as delays in head-righting reactions and atypical motor patterns (Teitelbaum et al., 2004; Teitelbaum, Teitelbaum, Nye, Fryman, & Maurer, 1998). It is important to point out that some reports of intact motor skills in young children with ASD are based on parent report of developmental milestones, such as independent walking (Gillberg et al., 1990), but this is disregarded by other researchers (Provost, Lopez, & Heimerl, 2007) who argue that other motor skills learned later are more complex, and thus learning to walk at a typical age does not ensure other motor skills will be acquired normally. Although a neurologist may be required to do a thorough motor exam, including examination of reflexes, postural abnormalities, and abnormal movements, there are excellent instruments available for neuropsychologists to use in examining motor skill.

Measures

The Purdue Pegboard Test—Revised Edition (Lafayette Instruments, 1999; Tiffin & Asher, 1948) assesses fine motor speed, coordination, and finger and hand dexterity. The measure requires the individual to place pegs in holes on a fixed board using the dominant, nondominant, and then both hands. The norms for this measure are old and are based on children ages 5–16 years. Norms are also available for adults.

The Nine-Hole Peg Test of Finger Dexterity (Mathiowetz, Volland, Kashman, & Weber, 1992) is a measure of fine motor dexterity with current normative data on samples of 826 elementary students (Smith, Hong, & Presson, 2000) and 406 children (Poole et al., 2005). It is highly correlated with the Purdue Pegboard Test and assesses skills for both the dominant and nondominant hands.

The Beery–Buktenica Developmental Test of Visual–Motor Integration—Sixth Edition (Beery, Buktenica, & Beery, 2010) is used to assess an individual's ability to integrate visuoperceptual skills with motor functioning. It is available in a short and long format, and is used for children between the ages of 1 and 18 years, and adults. The short form is commonly used for those between the ages of 2 and 8. There are also supplemental tests available to address visual perception and motor coordination abilities. Normative data was standardized on 1,737 individuals and is representative of the 2006 U.S. census.

Since there is a lack of stand-alone measures of functioning in various domains, including Motor Skills, select subtests from comprehensive batteries can by utilized to screen for strength or impairment in specific skill areas.

The Fingertip Tapping subtest from the NEPSY—Second Edition (NEPSY-II: Korkman, Kirk, & Kemp, 2007) is a test of motor speed and finger dexterity using the index finger and thumb of each hand. The task involves repetitive and sequential tapping. It is developed for ages 3–16. Normative data for the NEPSY-II was developed based on a sample of 1,000 children ages 3–12, and is representative of children from the 1995 U.S. census.

The Imitating Hand Positions subtest from the NEPSY-II (Korkman et al., 2007) measures performance in imitating finger and hand positions in both hands within a time limit and is intended for ages 3–16. Norms come from 1,000 children ages 3–12.

Language

Impairments in communication, especially receptive and expressive language, are part of the diagnostic criteria for ASD (American Psychiatric Association, 2013). Children with ASD exhibit a variety of early deficits in communication, including delays in comprehension, reduced attention to language, limited nonverbal communication and gesture, immediate and delayed echolalia (repetition of meaningless sounds, words, or phrases), and atypical prosody (emotional intonation in speech; e.g., Eigsti, Bennetto, & Dadlani, 2007; Howlin, 2003; Lyons, Schoen-Simmons, & Paul, 2014; Narzisi, Muratori, Calderoni, Fabbro, & Urgesi, 2013; Tager-Flusberg, 1981, 1996; Tager-Flusberg & Joseph, 2003).

There are a number of components of language that include phonology (understanding and producing speech sounds), semantics (meaning of words), pragmatics (social aspects of communication), prosody (speech rhythm, tempo, and pitch), and grammar (includes both use of word order and grammatical parts of speech, such as "ing"). Individuals with ASD can exhibit problems in any of these areas, all of which are essential for understanding and using language. In general, though grammar and phonology tend to be relatively spared, prosody and pragmatics are almost always impaired, and semantics is variable (Kelley, Paul, Fein, & Naigles, 2006).

Typical brain development is generally manifested by left hemispheric specialization for spoken language and gesture, findings which have been widely reported by neuroimaging, lesion, and animal studies. There are theories (Prior, 1979; Prior & Bradshaw, 1979; Rutter, 1974, 1979; Rutter, Bartak, & Newman, 1971) that view ASD as primarily a disorder of language, but other views hold that it is caused by language deficits along with social impairment and repetitive behavior (Bishop, 1989, 2000a, 2000b; Bishop & Norbury, 2002; Hollander, 1997; Hollander et al., 1999; Hollander,

Dolgoff-Kaspar, Cartwright, Rawitt, & Novotny, 2001; Hollander, Phillips, & Yeh, 2003), while still others document the presence of language disorders in some children with ASD (Kjelgaard & Tager-Flusberg, 2001). Changes to the diagnostic criteria (American Psychiatric Association, 2013) now require primary deficits in Social Communication—thereby emphasizing how once-separate domains clearly overlap in the ASD profile. Moreover, children with ASD typically exhibit significant delays in various communication and language areas, but especially pragmatics (Tager-Flusberg, Paul, & Lord, 2005). In general, years of language study in ASD suggests that although many individual children will be found with deficits in any given area of language, children with ASD, as a group, tend to have spared phonology and syntax, with impaired prosody and pragmatics. Children with ASD present a complex semantic picture in which basic word meanings may be a strength, but connotations are ignored and certain classes of words with social content are limited. (For an expanded review of language in ASD see Chapter 7.)

A working group of leading experts in the study of language development and disorders including ASD provides a developmental framework (Tager-Flusberg et al., 2009) in which to conceptualize and measure language to include gathering multiple sources of objective information (e.g., natural language samples, standardized measures, parent report) on phases of speech from preverbal communication and first words to complex language.

Measures

The Peabody Picture Vocabulary Test—Fourth Edition (PPVT-IV; Dunn & Dunn, 2007) is a single-word receptive vocabulary task that can be administered from 2½ to over 90 years of age. As such, it is a frequently used measure in clinical settings and research. A companion Expressive Vocabulary Test (conormed with the PPVT-IV) has also been published—the early items are useful, but the later ones require the child to produce a synonym for a common word, which can be difficult for children with ASD. Norms are based on a sample of 4,000 individuals representative of the U.S. population.

The Expressive One-Word Picture Vocabulary Test, 4th Edition (EOWPVT-4; Martin & Brownell, 2011a), is an individually administered measure that assesses for single-word expressive English vocabulary, and may be administered to those 2–80+ years. The EOWPVT-4 is a norm-referenced test that provides items for young children, and this updated version also provides norms for geriatric ages over 80 years. The EOWPVT-4 requires the identification of objects, actions, or concepts presented in full-color pictures. The 190 items (vocabulary words) are presented in a developmental sequence with more basic concepts presented from age-based starting points, and then proceed to more advanced stimuli to establish a ceiling. Normative data is based on a large sample that is representative of the national population collected in 2010. A companion receptive version, the Receptive One-Word Picture Vocabulary Test, 4th Edition (ROWPVT-4; Martin & Brownell, 2011b), has been written by the same authors and has been conormed with the EOWPVT-4.

The ROWPVT-4 is an individually administered measure examining the ability of persons to match spoken English words to objects, actions, or concepts that are presented in a multiple-choice format using full-color pictures. The ROWPVT-4 is norm referenced for persons 2–90+ years, containing items for young children as well as for older adults. The test includes 190 items presented in a developmental sequence (based on a 2010 normative sample). As noted above, the ROWPVT-4 has been conormed with the EOWPVT-4, which allows a thorough assessment of single-word receptive and expressive vocabulary. The ROWPVT-4 and EOWPVT-4 and similar measures are often used in clinical practice and research. Even so, it is essential to highlight that single-word vocabulary tests alone can overestimate language skills in the child with autism (Pellicano, Maybery, Durkin, & Maley, 2006). As such, we present the following more comprehensive measures that include tests of complex language, to be used in a neuropsychological assessment when possible.

The Clinical Evaluation of Language Fundamentals—Fourth Edition (CELF-4; Semel, Wiig, & Secord, 2003) is a battery of three receptive and three expressive language measures. The subtests include tasks measuring auditory attention, classification, concept formation, syntax, word structure, and grammar. The test has been developed for ages 5–21. Normative data comes from a sample of 2,650 individuals that is representative of the 2000 U.S. census, and includes children with diagnosed language disorders and other conditions. Recently, lower performance on the CELF-4 in children with ASD was associated with reduced functional connectivity in the cortical language network—namely, between the inferior frontal and superior temporal brain regions (Verly et al., 2014). Performance on the CELF-4 has also been highly predictive of other aspects of functioning, such as prosodic development (Lyons et al., 2014).

The Test of Language Competence—Expanded Edition (TLC-E; Wiig & Secord, 1989) assesses metalinguistic higher-level language functioning, which includes a child's ability to understand and use the abstract, figurative, ambiguous, and inferential aspects of language. As such, this is a good measure for children with higher-functioning ASD with good basic word knowledge but demonstrate difficulty with more abstract and complex language formation. It is designed for ages 5–18 years. The TLC-E can be used to identify delays in linguistic competence as well as in the child's use of semantic, syntactic, and pragmatic strategies. In addition to measuring basic syntactic and semantic abilities, an important feature of the TLC-E is the assessment of situational and contextual aspects of conversation abilities. The test is divided into two levels, based on developmental content and context: Level 1 is intended for ages 5–8, and Level 2 is intended for 9–18 years. The normative data were based on a large representative national sample for Level 1 (2,188 students) and Level 2 (1,796 students).

The Preschool Language Scales—Fifth Edition (PLS-5; Zimmerman, Steiner, & Pond, 2011) is a comprehensive language measure designed for children from birth to 7 years, 11 months. The PLS-5 evaluates receptive and expressive language through parent interviews and direct assessment of the child. The standardization normative sample consisted of 1,400 children collected across the United States, including children with disabilities. Case samples and clinical studies are provided for children with ASD and language disorders, respectively. Moreover, significant care was given to examine bias in the selection of test items and art. According to the manual, split-half reliabilities range from .80 to .97; sensitivity for the Total Language score is .83 and specificity is .80.

The Reynell Development Language Scales (Reynell & Gruber, 1990) has been used to assess language delay in young children 3 years, 0 months, to 7 years, 6 months, of age and provides data on typically developing children from 2 years, 0 months, to 7 years, 6 months. Specifically, it provides a measure of expressive language including vocabulary and word combinations, as well as grammatical items using a combination of play-based activities and stimulus materials. The new version was standardized in the United Kingdom on 1,200 children. A unique feature of the Reynell is that it comes with a multilingual toolkit for interpretation of results from children who are not monolingual.

The Comprehensive Assessment of Spoken Language (CASL; Carrow-Woolfolk, 1999) measures different aspects of spoken and written language, including the identification of antonyms and syntax, as well figurative and pragmatic language. It is for use with ages 3–21. Normative data were developed from a nationwide sample of 1,700 individuals.

Since social communication is a core area of impairment in ASD, the utilization of select subtests from test batteries can be meaningful. For example, the NEPSY-II (Korkman et al., 2007) includes six subtests in the Language domain and previous research has shown significantly lower performance for children with ASD for Comprehension of Instructions, Speeded Naming, Phonological Processing, and Repetition of Nonsense Words (only measures of Oromotor Sequences and Phonological Word Generation were relatively spared) compared with typically developing control subjects (Narzisi et al., 2013).

Additionally, examination of narrative functioning and storytelling may be meaningful to assess. For example, from the NEPSY-II Memory and Learning Core (Korkman et al., 2007) the narrative memory subtest, Bus Story, examines information, sentence length, and subordinate clauses. In a study of 21 children with high-functioning ASD between 7 and 8 years of age, notable impairment in narrative functioning was observed in many children with ASD, even in those with average verbal speech and language comprehension (Miniscalco, Hagberg, Kacsjö, Westerlug, & Gillberg, 2007).

Memory

Memory, like attention, is complex and encompasses many domains including visual, verbal, auditory, rote, short-term, nonverbal, episodic (events), and face memory. Different aspects of memory have been studied in children and adults with autism (e.g., Bennetto, Pennington, & Rogers, 1996; Bowler, Gardiner, & Berthollier, 2004; Rogers, Bennetto, McEvoy, & Pennington, 1996) but the research findings are equivocal in regard to consistently identifying specific areas of deficit (O'Shea, Fein, Cillessen, Klin, & Schultz, 2005). Not surprisingly, verbal memory is often impaired (Kamio & Toichi, 1998), while visuospatial memory is usually intact, with the exception of social stimuli such as faces and social situations (Williams, Goldstein, & Minshew, 2005). While spatial working memory tends to be impaired (Luna et al., 2002; Williams, Goldstein, Carpenter, & Minshew, 2005), the findings regarding working memory are varied and may depend on the type of task performed (Ozonoff & Strayer, 2001). Although it has been reported that episodic memory is often deficient in individuals with autism (Millward, Powell, Messer, & Jordan, 2000), there are many reports in the clinical literature of individuals who show exceptional, detailed memory pertaining to events to which they were motivated to attend. It has been postulated that episodic memory deficits may be more representative of an inefficient cognitive processing style rather than a difficulty with storage and retrieval (Southwick, Bigler, Froehlich, Lange, & Lainhart, 2011). Finally, source memory has been found to be impaired, yet it appears that it may be influenced by the type of context information to be remembered, and may be especially impaired when it involves social information (O'Shea et al., 2005).

Measures

The California Verbal Learning Test—Children's Version (CVLT-C; Delis, Kramer, Kaplen, & Ober, 1994) requires the child to learn two lengthy "shopping lists," each of which contains several categories of items. This test assesses the strategies the child uses to learn the lists and is useful in identifying problems with encoding, retention, and retrieval of verbal information. The computerized version of the test provides additional variables, including the efficiency of new learning, measures of proactive and retroactive interference, consistency of learning over trials, the difference between recall and recognition (an indicator of retrieval problems), retention of learning over a delay period, and the degree to which the child clusters the words by meaning (an indicator of depth and automaticity of semantic processing). Since this test is relatively brief compared with more comprehensive measures of memory assessment, the CVLT-C is used widely in clinical practice and research. More specifically, it has been used to study memory functioning in ASD populations. For example, one study utilizing the CVLT-C demonstrated that children with high-functioning ASD performed comparably to typically developing peers in overall memory performance but benefited significantly more when provided with external support for retrieval of information (Phelan, Filliter, & Johnson, 2011). Findings such as those aforementioned are particularly valuable when determining test selection in research and clinical settings. The CVLT-C is intended for children ages 5–16, and has a standardization sample of 920 children based on the 1988 U.S. census (Strauss, Sherman, & Spreen, 2006).

The NEPSY-II Memory for Faces subtest (Korkman et al., 2007) is a measure of face recognition and memory. It requires the child to identify a series of faces after a brief exposure and following a 30-minute delay. It is developed for children 3–16 years. Norms are based on 1,000 children, and is representative of the 1995 U.S. census. There is significant evidence that children with ASD often show impairment in face processing ability (e.g., Adolphs, Sears, & Piven, 2001; Corbett, Carmean, et al., 2009; Critchley et al., 2000; Pierce, Muller, Ambrose, Allen, & Courchesene, 2001; Schultz et al., 2003). Importantly, it is amenable to treatment as shown by significant improvement on the NEPSY-II Memory for Faces task following participation in a peer-mediated theater intervention program (Corbett et al., 2011, 2014).

The Wide Range Assessment of Memory and Learning, Second Edition (WRAML2; Sheslow & Adams, 2003), is a comprehensive battery of different aspects of visual and verbal memory. The subtests can be administered individually and cover the following domains: Verbal, Visual, and Attention and Concentration. From these subtests, scores of General Memory, Working Memory, Visual Memory, and Attention and Concentration are derived. In addition, there are recognition subtests of Verbal, Visual, Design, and Story Memory. The WRAML2 is designed for ages 5–90 years, and norms were developed for this group from a national sample.

The Children's Memory Scale (CMS; Cohen, 1997) is a well-developed battery of visual and verbal learning and immediate and delayed memory. It includes tasks dependent on recall, recognition, and attentional processes, and parallels the widely used Wechsler Memory Scale (WMS; Wechsler, 2009b) for adults. Specifically, the CMS looks at working memory and learning characteristics in addition to both short and long delay, as well as verbal and visual memory. It is designed for children and adolescents 5–16 years, and has normative data based on a sample of 1,000 typically developing children ages 5–16, and is representative of the 1995 U.S. census.

The Test of Memory and Learning—Second Edition (TOMAL-2; Reynolds & Voress, 2007) consists of 14 subtests to assess verbal and nonverbal memory functions. The TOMAL-2 includes eight core subtests that are aggregated for a Verbal Memory Composite Index and a Nonverbal Memory Composite Index. A Supplemental Composite Index comprises subtests that provide scores for Verbal Delayed Recall, Attention/Concentration, Sequential Recall, Free Recall, Associative Recall, and Learning. Research utilizing the previous edition of the TOMAL has demonstrated broad differences between individuals with ASD and typically developing controls across many aspects of memory functioning, including verbal and nonverbal, immediate and delayed, attention and concentration, sequential recall, free recall, associative recall, and multiple-trial learning (Southwick et al., 2011). In an effort to explain the theoretical foundation for the TOMAL-2, a conceptual model of the behavioral correlates of memory functioning is provided in the test manual for examiners to reference when testing clinical populations. The normative sample for the TOMAL-2 included 1,900 individuals between 5 and 59 years of age in 31 states and is representative of gender, age, ethnicity, geographic distribution, and urban and rural populations.

Executive Functioning

"Executive functioning" (EF) is an umbrella term that refers to mental control processes that enable physical, cognitive, and emotional self-control (Denckla, 1996; Lezak, 1995; Pennington & Ozonoff, 1996), and are necessary to maintain effective goal-directed behavior (Welsh & Pennington, 1988). Executive functions generally include response inhibition, working memory, cognitive flexibility (set shifting), planning, and fluency (Ozonoff & Strayer, 1997; Pennington & Ozonoff, 1996).

A variety of investigations have shown deficits among individuals with ASD in various executive functions, especially set shifting and planning (Ozonoff & Jensen, 1999). More recent reports comparing children with ASD to populations with identified EF deficits, such as ADHD, and typically developing children demonstrate deficits on tasks of EF. For example, Corbett, Constantine, et al. (2009) found that children with ASD performed significantly worse on tasks assessing vigilance compared with normal controls, and demonstrated deficits in response inhibition and working memory compared with children with ADHD. Some theorists have suggested that problematic EF is a central cognitive feature of autism (Ozonoff, Pennington, & Rogers, 1991; Pennington & Ozonoff, 1996; Russell, 1997), which implicates the prefrontal cortex in the pathophysiology of ASD. Although deficits in EF may be present in several neurodevelopmental disorders when compared with other populations, such as ADHD or Tourette syndrome, children with autism typically demonstrate broader and more impaired EF skills (Geurts, Verte, Oosterlaan, Roeyers, & Sergeant, 2004; Goldberg et al., 2005). Difficulty in shifting set (and consequently, perseveration) has been noted in autism for many years; this especially holds true for shifting attention away from preferred activities, but may also apply to shifting cognitive set away from any ongoing activity. While EF may be often associated with autism, others would argue that it is by no means universal or directly associated with other domains of functioning such as adaptive or language ability (Landa & Goldberg, 2005; Liss et al., 2001). Since EF is associated with deficits in social behavior, communication, and adaptive skills in children with autism (Gilotty, Kenworthy, Sirian, Black, & Wagner, 2002), it is valuable to assess EF in determining the child's neuropsychological profile.

Measures

The Delis–Kaplan Executive Function System (D-KEFS; Delis, Kaplan, & Kramer, 2001) consists of nine tests that measure a variety of verbal and nonverbal executive functions. It includes tasks assessing many aspects of EF, including initiating problem-solving behavior and assessment of verbal and nonverbal problem-solving abilities, inhibition and flexibility (switching), word generation, rule learning, verbal abstraction skills, and design fluency. The subtests include Verbal and Design Fluency, Card Sorting, Trail-Making Test, Color–Word Interference Test, Word Context Test, 20 Questions, Proverbs Test, and a Tower Test. Given the heterogeneity in the expression of EF deficits in individuals with ASD, this can be a particularly useful test in evaluation because of the selection of subtests designed to assess specific functions. For example, findings from a recent study comparing performance on the D-KEFS for individuals with ASD, individuals with nonverbal learning disabilities (NLD), and typically developing peers revealed variability among D-KEFS subtests (Semrud-Clikeman, Fine, & Bledsoe, 2014). Specifically, significant group differences were found between ASD and NLD for Sort Recognition and Contrast scores, and Sort Recognition and Free Sorts but not for performance on Trail Making or Verbal Fluency subtests (Semrud-Clikeman et al., 2014). The test is designed for individuals between the ages of 8 and 89, and the normative sample includes 1,750 nonclinical individuals. The sample was based on the 2000 U.S. census (Homack, Lee, & Riccio, 2005).

The Controlled Oral Word Association ("F–A–S"; Spreen & Benton, 1977) is an often used measure of speed and efficiency in producing words according to specified constraints. The letters *F, A,* and *S* are the most commonly used letters for this test. The individual is required to produce orally as many words as possible beginning with a certain letter in a limited period of time (usually 60 seconds). There are norms for ages 6–95 years—however, it should be noted that the norms are old.

The D-KEFS Verbal Fluency Test (Delis et al., 2001) is a more comprehensive verbal fluency test in that it consists of three testing conditions: Letter Fluency (producing words beginning with a certain letter), Category Fluency (producing words from specified categories), and Category Switching (switching between different conditions). Together these three conditions provide information regarding the individual's vocabulary knowledge, ability to fluently retrieve words beginning with the same letter, and the ability to retrieve lexical items from a designated category. It is developed for ages 8–89, and has normative data for this age range that comes from a sample of 1,750 participants and is based on the 2000 U.S. census (Homack et al., 2005).

The Wisconsin Card Sorting Task (WCST; Heaton, Chelune, Talley, Kay, & Curtis, 1993; Heaton & Psychological Assessment Resources Staff, 2000) is a measure of inhibition and cognitive flexibility. There are different versions but most have conditions consisting of color naming (word finding), word reading (reading speed), and inhibition (verbal inhibition). There is versatility in administration of this task such that it can be administered by hand or by computer. A study examining performance on the computerized version of the WCST among individuals with ASD, ADHD, and normal controls determined impairment in the ASD group on total errors, number of categories achieved, and perseverative and nonperseverative errors compared with typically developing peers (Tsuchiya, Oki, Yahara, & Fujieda, 2005). The WCST is intended for ages 6 years, 5 months, to 89 years, 0 months, and has normative data for 899 individuals in this age range. The newer versions of the WCST can be performed on a computer (e.g., Heaton & Psychological Assessment Resources Staff, 2000).

The Children's Color Trails Test I and II (CCTT-I & CCTT-II; Llorente, Williams, Satz, & D'Elia, 2003) are analogous to trail-making tests administered to adults that measure alternating and sustained visual attention, sequencing ability, psychomotor speed, cognitive flexibility, and inhibition. The CCTT-I requires the individual to rapidly connect different-colored circles in the correct numerical order (1, 2, 3, . . .). The CCTT-II requires connecting the circles in numerical order while switching between colored numbers. Normative data is available for ages 8–16.

The Stroop Color and Word Test: Children's Version (e.g., Golden, Freshwater, & Golden, 2004) is a measure of inhibition and flexibility that exposes the child to different reading conditions. Although there are different versions, it typically consists of color naming (word finding), word reading (reading speed), inhibition (verbal inhibition), and inhibition switching (cognitive flexibility). The children's version has normative data from 182 children ages 5–14.

As noted above in the "Attention" section, neuropsychological measures may not correlate with rating scales, especially across settings (Naglieri et al., 2005). As such, practitioners must interpret their findings cautiously and resist the temptation to generalize the findings too broadly. Nevertheless, the inclusion of questionnaires and rating scales can still provide additional valuable information regarding the child's functioning across constructs and settings.

The Behavior Rating Inventory of Executive Function (BRIEF; Gioia, Isquith, Guy, & Kenworthy, 2000) is a parent-report instrument that yields separate scores for various areas of EF, including initiation, working memory, planning/organizing, inhibition, emotional control, behavior regulation, and shifting. While a group of children with ASD showed impairments on most scales, initiation and working memory were found to have particular relationships with adaptive functioning in this group (Gilotty, Kenworthy, Sirian, Black, & Wagner, 2002). The BRIEF is designed for ages 5–18. Normative data samples were based on protocols from 1,419 parents and 720 teachers that were acquired from public and private school settings in the state of Maryland.

Academic Functioning

Academic achievement in children with ASD is a relatively understudied area with findings that indicate a wide range of associated factors. In the recent literature, academic achievement for children with ASD has been associated with social and communication skills (Estes, Rivera, & Bryan, 2011; Jones et al., 2009) and attention (e.g., May, Rinehart, & Wilding 2013). In general, children with autism, when compared with control subjects, tend to perform poorly on achievement measures that involve a comprehension component, but perform well and consistently with level of cognitive ability on mechanical reading, spelling, and computational tasks (Minshew, Goldstein, Taylor, & Siegel, 1994).

Reading has been examined in several studies of children with ASD (Frith & Snowling, 1983; Goldberg, 1987; Loveland & Tunali-Kotoski, 1997; Minshew, Goldstein, & Siegel, 1995; Minshew et al., 1994; Myles et al., 2002; O'Connor & Hermelin, 1994; Patti & Lupinetti, 1993; Venter, Lord, & Schopler, 1992; Whitehouse & Harris, 1984). In general, decoding or basic word identification is an area of strength (commensurate with overall cognitive development, or more advanced cognitive ability) for many children with ASD with poor reading comprehension (Goldberg, 1987; O'Connor & Hermelin, 1994; Patti & Lupinetti, 1993). On the other hand, comprehension of written material can be quite impaired, especially when any nonliteral meaning must be inferred (Minshew et al., 1994). In addition, children with ASD may rely more on syntactic structure rather than semantics combined with real-world knowledge (e.g., they will be unbothered by the sentence "The elephant was chased by the mouse"). Similarly, comprehension may be relatively good at the single-word level but impaired for material of sentence length and beyond; therefore, assessments of single-word comprehension may overestimate reading ability (Newman et al., 2007).

A small number of children with ASD show advanced decoding at an early age (Newman et al., 2007). These "hyperlexic" children have not been well studied, and it is likely that their advanced reading skills may not be functionally useful in most cases. However, it appears that their reading skills may level off at around 10 years of age and become comparable to age-matched typically developing peers (Newman et al., 2007).

Fewer studies have examined the component processes of writing in children with ASD. In general, writing is an area of weakness (Gross, 1994; Mayes & Calhoun, 2003). For many children, this includes all aspects of writing affecting graphomotor skills, word retrieval, spelling, word spacing, alignment, formulation of sentences, and organization of longer works. Our collective clinical experience suggests that writing tends to be an area disliked by children with ASD, and their efforts may be minimal and compositions short.

There is limited research on mathematics and autism. It does appear, however, that a child's performance on math is closely associated with their level of IQ (Mayes & Calhoun, 2003). Additionally, it has been reported that children with autism perform equally well on computation tasks (Minshew et al., 1994).

Although a clear distinction can be made between measures of achievement and ability level (Naglieri & Bornstein, 2003), for the purpose of this section, we include both tests of academic achievement (acquired skills) and ability (capacity) in determining the individual's level of current and potential functioning.

Measures

The Wechsler Individual Achievement Test—Third Edition (WIAT-III; Wechsler, 2009a) is a measure of basic academic skills, designed for children 5–19 years of age. It consists of fourteen subtests that produce six composite scores for basic reading, mathematics, oral language, reading comprehension and fluency, total achievement, and written expression. The assessments elicit written or oral responses. One of the advantages of the WIAT-III is that it has been used in convergent studies with the WISC-V, WPPSI-IV, and DAS-II across 3,000 nationally represented children, adolescents, and adults.

The Woodcock–Johnson III Tests of Achievement (WJ-III; Woodcock, McGrew, & Mather, 2001) consists of an Achievement and a Cognitive battery, assessing reading, math, and writing skills and is intended for ages 2–90+. The WJ-III can be used to measure general academic performance. Updated norms reflecting the 2005 U.S. census are available, and come from a sample of 8,782 individuals.

The Phonological Processing subtest from the NEPSY-II (Korkman et al., 2007) is a measure of phonological processing skill assessing the capacity to perceive and manipulate the phonemic elements (i.e., individual sound elements) of words, which is an important skill for lexical reading. This measure is for ages 3–16. Norms are based on a sample of 1,000 children ages 3–12.

The Tests of Written Language—Fourth Edition (TOWL-4; Hammill & Larsen, 2009) is a comprehensive assessment of written language designed for ages 9–17. The TOWL-4 consists of an essay format and a traditional test format to measure both spontaneous and contrived language. It provides an assessment of many areas of language, including syntax, spelling, vocabulary, and style. Additionally, through story construction, plot and character development can be assessed. Normative data for the TOWL-4 is derived from an age-stratified sample of individuals across 18 states whose demographic characteristics approximate the 2005 U.S. census.

Social–Emotional/Perceptual Skills

By definition, social perception and expression are areas of significant weakness in autism and many consider social functioning to be the single most important core deficit. As part of their difficulty interpreting the social world, individuals with autism often demonstrate impaired processing of emotions (Fein, Lucci, Braverman, & Waterhouse, 1992; Gepner, Deruelle, & Grynfeltt, 2001; Hobson, 1986a, 1986b; Hobson, Ouston, & Lee, 1988; Humphreys, Minshew, Leonard, & Behrmann, 2007), abnormal processing of faces (e.g., Adolphs, Baron-Cohen, & Tranel, 2002; Adolphs et al., 2001; Baron-Cohen et al., 1999, 2000; Critchley et al., 2000; Schultz et al., 2003), impaired judgment of mental state (Baron-Cohen et al., 1999), and deficits in theory of mind (e.g., Baron-Cohen, Leslie, & Frith, 1985; Boucher, 1989).

These and other findings from pathology studies have implicated regions involved in social processing to include structures in the medial temporal lobe, such as the amygdala, superior temporal gyrus, superior temporal sulcus, and the orbital frontal gyrus. Social and emotional primacy theories have been proposed emphasizing various aspects of perceptual abilities (Adolphs et al., 2001, 2002; Baron-Cohen et al., 1985, 1999, 2000; Critchley et al., 2000; Hobson, 1986a, 1986b; Hobson et al., 1988; Schultz et al., 2003). Children with ASD have been found to be slightly impaired on tasks of emotion perception where emotion was matched to context (Fein et al., 1992). In addition, difficulty in imitating actions, theory of mind, and the presence of language impairments, such as echolalia, has led some researchers to believe that an abnormality in the development of mirror neurons, found in the frontal cortex, may exist in children with autism (Williams, Whiten, Suddendorf, & Perrett, 2001).

Measures

There is an absence of measures to assess emotion perception—however, a few tests do address this ability.

The Autism Diagnostic Observation Schedule, Second Edition (ADOS-2; Lord et al., 2012), is a diagnostic measure of current behaviors indicative of autism including the Social, Communication, and Behavioral domains—however, it can be used to assess social–emotional functioning. Specifically, the measure contains specific tasks that elicit social and play interactions that can be coded on a behaviorally anchored scale. The ADOS-2 has moderate to high internal consistency on all domains across five modules (.47–.90). For the total score, the overall test–retest correlations range from .64 to .88 within an average of 10 months. The instrument shows good content and construct validity following a confirmatory factor analysis of a two-domain solution (Social Affect and Restrictive and Repetitive Behaviors). As for the predictive validity, Modules 1–3 show high sensitivity and specificity.

Face Recognition (Benton, Sivan, Hamsher, Varney, & Spreen, 1994) is used as a measure of the individual's capacity to identify and discriminate photographs of unfamiliar human faces. The test requires the child to choose a target face among different distracters. The stimuli are presented in black and white with different profiles and contrasts. This is a challenging task for many individuals and the norms are quite old—as a result, Face Recognition may not be as useful for some individuals other than to document impairment. It is intended for persons over the age of 8 years. Normative data comes from 286 typical adults and 266 children with normal intelligence ages 6–14.

The Social Perception domain from the NEPSY-II (Korkman et al., 2007) was released in spring 2007, which includes subtests of Theory of Mind and Affect Recognition. It is intended for ages 3–16. The NEPSY-II has normative data from a sample of 1,000 children ages 3–12. Since ASD is characterized by impairment in social functioning, these tasks are useful in a neuropsychological battery to identify potential challenges in these areas. Additionally, Memory for Faces, summarized above, is also a useful subtest to examine the child's ability to identify and remember faces.

Affect Recognition (Korkman et al., 2007) examines the ability to recognize emotions from a series of photographs of children's faces, which has been shown to be an area of difficulty for some but not all children with ASD (e.g., Corbett, Carmean, et al., 2009; Corbett et al., 2011; Loukusa, Mäkinen, Kuusikko-Gauffin, Ebeling, & Moilanen, 2014). The stimuli include happy, sad, neutral, fear, angry, and disgust. The tasks require the child to identify children showing similar affect as a model picture. There is also an Affect Memory component that requires identifying children showing similar expressions after viewing one exemplar for 5 seconds. The NEPSY-II has been used to examine affect recognition in ASD with mixed findings (Corbett et al., 2011, 2014; Narzisi et al., 2013).

Theory of Mind (Korkman et al., 2007) examines perspective taking, abstract social communication (e.g., idioms), and contextual processing, such as how a character's emotional expressions match given social situations. Children with ASD tend to perform more poorly on this measure, especially on the verbal items rather than the pictorial contextual part of the task (Narzisi, et al., 2013). However, following treatment, significant improvements have been demonstrated using this Theory-of-Mind measure in children with ASD (Corbett et al., 2011, 2014).

Visual–Spatial Skills

Visual–spatial skills are typically thought of as an area of strength in children with autism (Bertone, Mottron, Jelenic, & Faubert, 2005; Caron, Mottron, Rainville, & Chouinard, 2004; O'Riordan, 2004; O'Riordan & Passetti, 2006; O'Riordan et al., 2001; Shah & Frith, 1993). Individuals with high-functioning autism have demonstrated superior accuracy in a map-learning task related to cued recall and shorter latency (Caron et al., 2004). It has been proposed that the enhanced discrimination, detection, and memory for simple visual stimuli may explain the superior performance often observed on visual–spatial tasks in individuals with autism. As noted, persons with autism tend to show greater aptitude with feature detection and perform well on measures of visual–spatial construction ability (Shah & Frith, 1993). Frith (1989) was the first to put forth the theory of weak central coherence, proposing that individuals with autism show impairment in the ability to integrate information in a meaningful, coherent whole. Thus, this impairment results in a bias toward local processing rather than global processing. The weak central coherence deficit may be observed on tasks that require more global processing, such as categorization tasks and enhanced performance on other tasks such as block design. As a theory, the weak central hypothesis has received equivocal support and so should not serve as the basis of interpretation in neuropsychological testing (Jolliffe & Baron-Cohen, 2001; Mottron, Burack, Iarocci, Belleville, & Enns, 2003).

It has been suggested that the symptoms of autism are the result of a complex information processing deficit (Minshew, Goldstein, & Siegel, 1997). Similarly, Rimland (1964) conceptualized autism as the primary result of poor integration of information. Additionally, less functional connectivity has been reported in children with autism compared with typically developing children (Just, Cherkassky, Keller, & Minshew, 2004), supporting the notion of a fundamental deficit in integrating information at neural and cognitive levels.

Measures

The Arrows subtest (similar to Judgment of Line Orientation) from the NEPSY-II (Korkman et al., 2007) assesses the child's ability to judge the direction, angularity, and orientation of lines. This task requires the child to select arrows pointing to a center target. It is important to note that this test does not require a motor response. It is intended for ages 3–16. Normative data is derived from 1,000 children across this age range.

The Gestalt Closure subtest from the KABC-II (Kaufman & Kaufman, 2004) assesses the ability to "mentally fill in the gaps" on degraded pictures of familiar objects and figures. This subtest is similar to the Gestalt Completion Task (Street, 1931). The KABC-II was normed on a sample of 3,025 individuals ages 3 years, 0 months, to 18 years, 11 months, and is representative of the 2001 U.S. census.

The Motor-Free Visual Perception Test, Third Edition (MVPT-3; Colarusso & Hammill, 2003), is a measure of visual perception for children and adults ages 4–85. The tasks include Matching, Form Discrimination, Figure Ground, Closure, and Visual Memory, and, as the name suggests, are completed without depending on motor skills. Standardization scores are based on a sample of 1,856 individuals from 36 states and is representative of the U.S. population. It should be noted that age groups are not evenly distributed across the sample (McCane, 2006).

The Rey–Osterrieth Complex Figure Test (ROCFT; Osterrieth, 1944; Rey, 1944) provides a comprehensive evaluation of a wide range of visual–spatial abilities designed to assess for visuospatial recall memory, visuospatial recognition memory, response bias, processing speed, and visuospatial constructional ability. There are several versions of this test and it may sometimes be referred to as the Rey Complex Figure Test (RCFT), the Complex Figure Test (CFT), and the Rey Figure (RF). This measure is one of the most commonly used tests in neuropsychological evaluation (Camara, Nathan, & Puente, 2000), in part due to its utility in assessing many cognitive processes. It also has particular applicability in obtaining qualitative information on approach to figure copy. For example, the examiner may wish to record a patient's strategy in copying elements of the design by providing colored pencils and noting the order of their use, or utilizing a flowchart method that notes the ordering by numbers and directionality by arrows (Strauss et al., 2006). Such qualitative aspects of this measure can be particularly useful when assessing individuals with ASD as there is some indication that they may display a local processing (as opposed to global processing) bias (Rinehart, Bradshaw, Moss, Brereton, & Tonge, 2000). The RCFT is intended for individuals 6–93 years of age and there are several sets of normative data that provided the wide variability in administration (Strauss et al., 2006).

COMPREHENSIVE ASSESSMENT

Although clinicians may choose to select many instruments, the NEPSY-II offers comprehensive assessment using a single measure. The NEPSY-II (Korkman et al., 2007) includes six domains, comprising Executive Functioning and Attention, Language, Memory and Learning, Sensorimotor Functioning, Visuospatial Processing, and Social Perception. Recently, the battery was administered to 22 children with high-functioning ASD matched to 44 healthy control children on age, gender, race, and education. The findings showed that the NEPSY-II is a useful and valid neuropsychological measure for identifying strengths and weaknesses for children with high-functioning ASD (Narzisi et al., 2013). As noted by the authors, this instrument is able to carefully capture the neuropsychological profile, thereby identifying primary and secondary deficits (Luria, 1962) to guide educational and intervention services.

WORKING FROM A NEUROPSYCHOLOGICAL MODEL

As can be seen from the aforementioned review of neuropsychological assessment, research findings, and overarching theories, there is no clear neuropsychological profile for ASD. Instead, the heterogeneity and complexity of the disorder are marked by variability, which further supports the need for more comprehensive testing. It is also plausible that many measures may not be sensitive to the cognitive problems inherent in children with ASD or specific enough to be helpful for an individual child. Even so, the advantage of working from a neuropsychological model allows a framework in which to structure the assessment by evaluating ability and deficit across many areas of functioning. Furthermore, by conceptualizing the disorder in terms of many facets of function allows for a different and potentially more meaningful interpretation of the disorder. In other words, if one only assesses cognitive or language functioning in the assessment of ASD, it is unlikely that a theoretical framework related to other domains of functioning will emerge. In contrast, it is likely that by expanding the measures used in clinical practice and research, more useful information may contribute to our understanding of the behavioral endophenotypes of autism.

TREATMENT RECOMMENDATIONS

Perhaps a more important reason for providing a thorough neuropsychological assessment is that by identifying specific deficits and areas of strength to compensate, the results can better guide treatment. The findings can help identify the target behaviors to address and signal what strategies to use for comprehensive and individualized treatment planning (Batchelor & Dean, 1995; Yeates et al., 2000). Table 9.1 is intended to be merely a guide as to how neuropsychological findings in cognitive functioning, adaptive skills, attention, and so on may guide specific recommendations across the various domains of functioning.

ACKNOWLEDGMENTS

We would like to dedicate the chapter to the late David King, PhD (1950–2005), for his clinical insights in neuropsychological assessment, passion for neuroscience, commitment to his patients, and his unwavering dedication to mentorship, all of which helped inspire this chapter.

REFERENCES

Adolphs, R., Baron-Cohen, S., & Tranel, D. (2002). Impaired recognition of social emotions following amygdala damage. *Journal of Cognitive Neuroscience, 14*(8), 1264–1274.

Adolphs, R., Sears, L., & Piven, J. (2001). Abnormal processing of social information from faces in autism. *Journal of Cognitive Neuroscience, 13*(2), 232–240.

TABLE 9.1. A Guide to Treatment Recommendations

Domain	Home recommendations	Educational recommendations
Cognitive functioning	• Provide a stimulating environment • Expose child to variety of activities	• Full inclusion when possible with aide • Individualized curriculum
Adaptive functioning	• Include child in day-to-day activities • Provide opportunities to learn with supervision • Teach individual adaptive skills broken down into small steps and reinforced	• Provide an aide when needed • Teach independent self-care skills • Teach functional academics • Home and community skills
Attention	• Structure activities • Provide visual cues and reminders • Use repetition and clarification	• Seating near teacher • Limit extraneous visual and auditory stimuli • Provide breaks • Take apart tasks and show how information ties together • Use repetition • Provide teacher outlines • Increased time for tasks
Sensory functioning	• Limit extraneous stimuli, especially in child's room • Be cognizant of child's sensory issues • Prepare for stressful situations	• Use headphones • Computer-based teaching • Individualized work environment for study • Give gross motor breaks and intersperse preferred activities • Cubicle work • Reinforce increasing tolerance of stimulation
Motor functioning	• Physical exercise • Trampoline and swings • Craft activities that require fine motor skills	• Physical education • Teach typing skills • Have another student take notes
Language	• Talk frequently to your child regardless of level of his or her language • Reinforce attempts at communication • Carry over behavioral or language therapy lessons at home for increased practice and generalization	• Speech and language therapy as needed • Augmented communication devices when necessary

(continued)

TABLE 9.1. *(continued)*

Domain	Home recommendations	Educational recommendations
Memory	• Shorter assignments • Chunk information into groups • Shape new information by gradually introducing more information • Link new information to old • Use visual schedules	• Provide repetition as needed • Teach how things are associated, especially new knowledge • Organize information visually
Executive functioning	• Establish and maintain an organized room • Provide a structured home environment • Engage in activities, like cooking, that require planning and organization • Chart chores and daily behavior • Play family concentration and word-finding games	• Provide structure • Teach basic organizational strategies • Different color binders and folders • Use checklists • Highlight important information • Present information more clearly, slowly
Academic functioning	• Have good communication with teacher • Be available during homework • Find real-life examples of school lessons	• Individualized curriculum • Ensure that it is stimulating • Utilize areas of strength • Visual materials • Graph paper for math
Social–emotional/ perceptual skills	• Exposure to peers for brief playdates with supervision • Video modeling • When watching TV label emotions and social situations with child • Use social stories and comic strip conversations	• Buddy system at school • Social skills • Structured activities • Group learning projects • After-school activities with children with shared interest
Visual–spatial skills	• Provide blocks, puzzles, and construction tasks for play	• If any area of strength, utilize it in teaching • Use visually cued instruction
General functioning	• Consistent behavior plan across environments	• Notebook between school and home

Adrien, J. L., Lenoir, P., Martineau, J., Perrot, A., Hameury, L., Larmande, C., et al. (1993). Blind ratings of early symptoms of autism based upon family home movies. *Journal of the American Academy of Child and Adolescent Psychiatry, 32*(3), 617–626.

Allen, G., & Courchesne, E. (2001). Attention function and dysfunction in autism. *Frontiers in Bioscience, 6,* D105–D119.

American Psychiatric Association. (2013). *Diagnostic and statistical manual of mental disorders* (5th ed.). Arlington, VA: Author.

Baranek, G. T. (1999). Autism during infancy: A retrospective video analysis of sensory–motor and social behaviors at 9–12 months of age. *Journal of Autism and Developmental Disorders, 29*(3), 213–224.

Barkley, R. A. (1991). The ecological validity of laboratory and analogue assessment methods of ADHD symptoms. *Journal of Abnormal Child Psychology, 19*(2), 149–178.

Baron, I. S. (2005). Test review: Wechsler Intellligence Scale for Children—Fourth Edition (WISC-IV). *Child Neuropsychology, 11*(5), 471–475.

Baron-Cohen, S., Leslie, A. M., & Frith, U. (1985). Does the autistic child have a "theory of mind"? *Cognition, 21*(1), 37–46.

Baron-Cohen, S., Ring, H. A., Bullmore, E. T., Wheelwright, S., Ashwin, C., & Williams, S. C. (2000). The amygdala theory of autism. *Neuroscience and Biobehavioral Reviews, 24*(3), 355–364.

Baron-Cohen, S., Ring, H. A., Wheelwright, S., Bullmore, E. T., Brammer, M. J., Simmons, A., et al. (1999). Social intelligence in the normal and autistic brain: An fMRI study. *European Journal of Neuroscience, 11*(6), 1891–1898.

Batchelor, E. S., Jr., & Dean, R. S. (1995). *Pediatric neuropsychology.* Boston: Allyn & Bacon.

Bayley, N. (2005). *Bayley Scales of Infant Development, Third Edition.* San Antonio, TX: Harcourt Assessment.

Beery, K. E., Buktenica, N. A., & Beery, N. A. (2010). *Beery–Buktenica Developmental Test of Visual–Motor Integration, Sixth Edition.* San Antonio, TX: Pearson Assessment.

Bennetto, L., Pennington, B. F., & Rogers, S. J. (1996). Intact and impaired memory functions in autism. *Child Development, 67*(4), 1816–1835.

Benton, A. L., Sivan, A. B., Hamsher, K. deS., Varney, N. R., & Spreen, O. (1994). *Contributions to neuropsychological assessment: A clinical manual* (2nd ed.). New York: Oxford University Press.

Berkeley, S. L., Zittel, L. L., Pitney, L. V., & Nichols, S. E. (2001). Locomotor and object control skills of children diagnosed with autism. *Adapted Physical Activity Quarterly, 18,* 405–416.

Bertone, A., Mottron, L., Jelenic, P., & Faubert, J. (2005). Enhanced and diminished visuo–spatial information processing in autism depends on stimulus complexity. *Brain, 128*(Pt. 10), 2430–2441.

Billstedt, E., Gillberg, I., & Gillberg, C. (2005). Autism after adolescence: Population-based 13- to 22-year follow-up study of 120 individuals with autism diagnosed in childhood. *Journal of Autism and Developmental Disorders, 35*(3), 351–360.

Bishop, D. V. M. (1989). Autism, Asperger's syndrome and semantic–pragmatic disorder: Where are the boundaries? *British Journal of Disorders of Communication, 24*(2), 107–121.

Bishop, D. V. M. (2000a). Development of the Children's Communication Checklist (CCC): A method for assessing qualitative aspects of communicative impairment in children. *Journal of Child Psychology and Psychiatry and Allied Disciplines, 39*(6), 879–891.

Bishop, D. V. M. (2000b). What's so special about Asperger syndrome?: The need for further exploration of the borderlands of autism. In A. Klin, F. R. Volkmar, & S. S. Sparrow (Eds.), *Asperger syndrome* (pp. 254–277). New York: Guilford Press.

Bishop, D. V. M., & Norbury, C. F. (2002). Exploring the borderlands of autistic disorder and specific language impairment: A study using standardised diagnostic instruments. *Journal of Child Psychology and Psychiatry, 43*(7), 917–929.

Bishop, S. L., Guthrie, W., Coffing, M., & Lord, C. (2011). Convergent validity of the Mullen Scales of Early Learning and the Differential Ability Scales in children with autism spectrum disorders. *American Journal on Intellectual and Developmental Disabilities, 116*(5), 331–343.

Boucher, J. (1989). The theory of mind hypothesis of autism: Explanation, evidence and assessment. *British Journal of Disorders of Communication, 24*(2), 181–198.

Bowler, D. M., Gardiner, J. M., & Berthollier, N. (2004). Source memory in adolescents and adults with Asperger's syndrome. *Journal of Autism and Developmental Disorders, 34*(5), 533–542.

Bradley-Johnson, S. (1997). Mullen Scales of Early Learning. *Psychology in the Schools, 34*(4), 379–382.

Camara, W. J., Nathan, J. S., & Puente, A. E. (2000). Psychological test usage: Implications in professional psychology. *Professional Psychology: Research and Practice, 31,* 141–154.

Caron, M. J., Mottron, L., Rainville, C., & Chouinard, S. (2004). Do high functioning persons with autism present superior spatial abilities? *Neuropsychologia, 42*(4), 467–481.

Carrow-Woolfolk, E. (1999). *Comprehensive assessment of spoken language.* Bloomington, MN: Pearson Assessments.

Cattell, R. B. (1971). *Abilities: Their structure, growth and action.* New York: Harcourt, Brace Janovich.

Centers for Disease Control and Prevention. (2016). Prevalence and characteristics of autism spectrum disorder among children aged 8 years—Autism and Developmental Disabilities Monitoring Network, 11 Sites, United States, 2012. *Morbidity and Mortality Weekly Report Surveillance Summaries, 65,* 1–23.

Ciesielski, K. T., Courchesne, E., & Elmasian, R. (1990). Effects of focused selective attention tasks on event-related potentials in autistic and normal individuals. *Electroencephalography and Clinical Neurophysiology, 75*(3), 207–220.

Cohen, M. (1997). *Children's Memory Scale.* San Antonio, TX: Psychological Corporation.

Colarusso, R. P., & Hammill, D. D. (2003). *Motor-Free Visual Perception Test, Third Edition (MVPT-3).* Novato, CA: Academic Therapy.

Conners, K. C. (2001). *Conners' Rating Scales—Revised: Manual.* Tonawanda, NY: Multi-Health Systems.

Corbett, B. A., Carmean, V., Ravizza, S., Wendelken, C., Henry, M. L., Carter, C., et al. (2009). A functional and structural study of emotion and face processing in children with autism. *Psychiatry Research, 173*(3), 196–205.

Corbett, B. A., & Constantine, L. J. (2006). Autism and attention deficit hyperactivity disorder: Assessing attention and response control with the integrated visual and auditory continuous performance test. *Child Neuropsychology, 12*(4–5), 335–348.

Corbett, B. A., Constantine, L. J., Hendren, R., Rocke, D., & Ozonoff, S. (2009). Examining executive functioning in children with autism spectrum disorder, attention deficit hyperactivity disorder and typical development. *Psychiatry Research, 166*(2–3), 210–222.

Corbett, B. A., Gunther, J., Comins, D., Price, J., Ryan, N., Simon, D., et al. (2011). Theatre as therapy for children with autism. *Journal of Autism and Developmental Disorders, 41*(4), 505–511.

Corbett, B. A., Schupp, C. W., Levine, S., & Mendoza, S. (2009). Comparing cortisol, stress and sensory sensitivity in children with autism. *Autism Research, 2*, 39–49.

Corbett, B., & Stanczak, D. E. (1999). Neuropsychological performance of adults evidencing attention-deficit hyperactivity disorder. *Archives of Clinical Neuropsychology, 14*(4), 373–387.

Corbett, B. A., Swain, D. M., Coke, C., Simon, D., Newsom, C., Houchins-Juarez, N., et al. (2014). Improvement in social deficits in autism spectrum disorders using a theatre-based peer mediated intervention. *Autism Research, 7*(1), 4–16.

Courchesne, E., Townsend, J., Akshoomoff, N. A., Saitoh, O., Yeung-Courchesne, R., Lincoln, A. J., et al. (1994). Impairment in shifting attention in autistic and cerebellar patients. *Behavioral Neuroscience, 108*(5), 848–865.

Critchley, H. D., Daly, E. M., Bullmore, E. T., Williams, S. C., Van Amelsvoort, T., Robertson, D. M., et al. (2000). The functional neuroanatomy of social behaviour: Changes in cerebral blood flow when people with autistic disorder process facial expressions. *Brain, 123*(Pt. 11), 2203–2212.

Dawson, G., Meltzoff, A. N., Osterling, J., Rinaldi, J., & Brown, E. (1998). Children with autism fail to orient to naturally occurring social stimuli. *Journal of Autism and Developmental Disorders, 28*(6), 479–485.

Delis, D. C., Kaplan, E., & Kramer, J. H. (2001). *Delis–Kaplan Executive Function System*. San Antonio, TX: Psychological Corporation.

Delis, D. C., Kramer, J. H., Kaplen, E., & Ober, B. A. (1994). *California Verbal Learning Test—Children's Version: Manual*. San Antonio, TX: Psychological Corporation.

Denckla, M. B. (1996). Biological correlates of learning and attention: What is relevant to learning disability and attention-deficit hyperactivity disorder? *Journal of Developmental and Behavioral Pediatrics, 17*(2), 114–119.

Doyle, A. E., Biederman, J., Seidman, L. J., Weber, W., & Faraone, S. V. (2000). Diagnostic efficiency of neuropsychological test scores for discriminating boys with and without attention deficit-hyperactivity disorder. *Journal of Consulting and Clinical Psychology, 68*(3), 477–488.

Dunn, L. M., & Dunn, D. M. (2007). *The Peabody Picture Vocabulary Test—Fourth Edition*. Circle Pines, MN: American Guidance Service.

Dunn, W. (1999). *Short Sensory Profile*. San Antonio, TX: Psychological Corporation.

Dunn, W., & Brown, C. (1997). Factor analysis on the sensory profile from a national sample of children without disabilities. *American Journal of Occupational Therapy, 51*(7), 490–495.

Eigsti, I. M., Bennetto, L., & Dadlani, M. B. (2007). Beyond pragmatics: Morphosyntactic development in autism. *Journal of Autism and Developmental Disorders, 37*(6), 1007–1023.

Elliott, C. D. (1990). *Differential Ability Scales.* San Antonio, TX: Psychological Corporation.

Elliott, C. (2006). *Differential Abilities Scale–II.* San Antonio, TX: Harcourt Assessment.

Estes, A., Rivera, V., & Bryan, M. (2011). Discrepancies between academic achievement and intellectual ability in higher functioning school-aged children with autism spectrum disorder. *Journal of Autism and Developmental Disorders, 41,* 1044–1052.

Fein, D., Lucci, D., Braverman, M., & Waterhouse, L. (1992). Comprehension of affect in context in children with pervasive developmental disorders. *Journal of Child Psychology and Psychiatry, 33*(7), 1157–1167.

Filipek, P. A., Accardo, P. J., Baranek, G. T., Cook, E. H., Jr., Dawson, G., Gordon, B., et al. (1999). The screening and diagnosis of autistic spectrum disorders. *Journal of Autism and Developmental Disorders, 29*(6), 439–484.

Fournier, K. A., Hass, C. J., Naik, S. A., Lodha, N., & Carraugh, J. H. (2010). Motor coordination in autism spectrum disorders: A synthesis and meta-analysis. *Journal of Autism and Developmental Disorders, 40,* 1227–1240.

Frith, U. (1989). A new look at language and communication in autism. *British Journal of Disorders of Communication, 24*(2), 123–150.

Frith, U., & Snowling, M. (1983). Reading for meaning and reading for sound in autistic and dyslexic children. *British Journal of Developmental Psychology, 1*(4), 329–342.

Garretson, H. B., Fein, D., & Waterhouse, L. (1990). Sustained attention in children with autism. *Journal of Autism and Developmental Disorders, 20*(1), 101–114.

Gepner, B., Deruelle, C., & Grynfeltt, S. (2001). Motion and emotion: A novel approach to the study of face processing by young autistic children. *Journal of Autism and Developmental Disorders, 31*(1), 37–45.

Geurts, H. M., Verte, S., Oosterlaan, J., Roeyers, H., & Sergeant, J. A. (2004). How specific are executive functioning deficits in attention deficit hyperactivity disorder and autism? *Journal of Child Psychology and Psychiatry, 45*(4), 836–854.

Ghaziuddin, M., Butler, E., Tsai, L., & Ghaziuddin, N. (1994). Is clumsiness a marker for Asperger syndrome? *Journal of Intellectual Disability Research, 38*(Pt. 5), 519–527.

Gillberg, C., Ehlers, S., Schaumann, H., Jakobsson, G., Dahlgren, S. O., Lindblom, R., et al. (1990). Autism under age 3 years: A clinical study of 28 cases referred for autistic symptoms in infancy. *Journal of Child Psychology and Psychiatry, 31*(6), 921–934.

Gilotty, L., Kenworthy, L., Sirian, L., Black, D. O., & Wagner, A. E. (2002). Adaptive skills and executive function in autism spectrum disorders. *Child Neuropsychology, 8*(4), 241–248.

Gioia, G., Isquith, P., Guy, S., & Kenworthy, L. E. (2000). *Behavior Rating Inventory for Executive Function.* Odessa, FL: Psychological Assessment Resources.

Goldberg, M. C., Mostofsky, S. H., Cutting, L. E., Mahone, E. M., Astor, B. C., Denckla, M. B., et al. (2005). Subtle executive impairment in children with autism and children with ADHD. *Journal of Autism and Developmental Disorders, 35*(3), 279–293.

Goldberg, T. E. (1987). On hermetic reading abilities. *Journal of Autism and Developmental Disorders, 17*(1), 29–44.

Golden, C. J., Freshwater, S. M., & Golden, Z. (2004). *Stroop Color and Word Test: Children's Version*. Wood Dale, IL: Stoelting.

Goldman, R., Fristoe, M., & Woodcock, R. W. (1970). *Test of Auditory Discrimination*. Circle Pines, MN: American Guidance Service.

Goldstein, S., & Goldstein, M. (1998). *Managing attention deficit hyperactivity disorder in children: A guide for practitioners*. New York: Wiley.

Greenberg, L., Leark, R. A., Dupuy, T. R., Corman, C. L., & Kindschi, C. L. (1991). *Test of Variables of Attention (TOVA)*. Los Alamitos, CA: WPS.

Greenberg, L., & Waldman, I. (1993). Developmental normative data on the Test of Variables of Attention (TOVA). *Journal of Child and Adolescent Psychiatry, 34*, 1019–1030.

Gross, J. (1994). Asperger's syndrome: A label worth having? *Educational Psychology, 10*(2), 104–110.

Hammill, D. D., & Larsen, S. C. (2009). *Test of Written Language—Fourth Edition*. Austin, TX: PRO-ED.

Harrison, P. L., & Oakland, T. (2003). *Adaptive Behavior Assessment System, Second Edition (ABAS-II)*. San Antonio, TX: Psychological Corporation.

Heaton, R. K., Chelune, G. J., Talley, J. L., Kay, G. G., & Curtis, G. (1993). *Wisconsin Card Sorting Test (WCST) manual: Revised and expanded*. Lutz, FL: Psychological Assessment Resources.

Heaton, R. K., & Psychological Assessment Resources Staff. (2000). *WCST–64: Computer Version 2 Research Edition (WCST-64:CV2)*. Lutz, FL: Psychological Assessment Resources.

Hobson, R. P. (1986a). The autistic child's appraisal of expressions of emotion. *Journal of Child Psychology and Psychiatry, 27*(3), 321–342.

Hobson, R. P. (1986b). The autistic child's appraisal of expressions of emotion: A further study. *Journal of Child Psychology and Psychiatry, 27*(5), 671–680.

Hobson, R. P., Ouston, J., & Lee, A. (1988). Emotion recognition in autism: Coordinating faces and voices. *Psychological Medicine, 18*(4), 911–923.

Hollander, E. (1997). The obsessive-compulsive spectrum disorders. *International Review of Psychiatry, 9*(1), 99–110.

Hollander, E., DelGiudice-Asch, G., Simon, L., Schmeidler, J., Cartwright, C., DeCaria, C. M., et al. (1999). B lymphocyte antigen D8/17 and repetitive behaviors in autism. *American Journal of Psychiatry, 156*(2), 317–320.

Hollander, E., Dolgoff-Kaspar, R., Cartwright, C., Rawitt, R., & Novotny, S. (2001). An open trial of divalproex sodium in autism spectrum disorders. *Journal of Clinical Psychology, 62*(7), 530–534.

Hollander, E., Phillips, A. T., & Yeh, C. C. (2003). Targeted treatments for symptom domains in child and adolescent autism. *The Lancet, 362*(9385), 732–734.

Homack, S., Lee, D., & Riccio, C. A. (2005). Test review: Delis–Kaplan Executive Function System. *Journal of Clinical and Experimental Neuropsychology, 27*(5), 599–609.

Howlin, P. (2003). Outcome in high-functioning adults with autism with and without early language delays: Implications for the differentiation between autism and Asperger syndrome. *Journal of Autism and Developmental Disorders, 33*(1), 3–13.

Humphreys, K., Minshew, N., Leonard, G. L., & Behrmann, M. (2007). A fine-grained analysis of facial expression processing in high-functioning adults with autism. *Neuropsychologia, 45*(4), 685–695.

Jolliffe, T., & Baron-Cohen, S. (2001). A test of central coherence theory: Can adults with high-functioning autism or Asperger syndrome integrate fragments of an object? *Cognitive Neuropsychiatry, 6*(3), 193–216.

Jones, C. R., Happe, F., Golden, H., Marsden, A. J., Tregay, J., Simonoff, E., et al. (2009). Reading and arithmetic in adolescents with autism spectrum disorders: Peaks and dips in attainment. *Neuropsychology, 23*(6), 718–728.

Just, M. A., Cherkassky, V. L., Keller, T. A., & Minshew, N. J. (2004). Cortical activation and synchronization during sentence comprehension in high-functioning autism: Evidence of underconnectivity. *Brain, 127*(8), 1811–1821.

Kamio, Y., & Toichi, M. (1998). Affective understanding in high-functioning autistic adolescents. *Japanese Journal of Child and Adolescent Psychiatry, 39*, 340–351.

Kaufman, A. S., & Kaufman, N. L. (2004). *Kaufman Assessment Battery for Children, Second Edition*. Circle Pines, MN: American Guidance Service.

Kelley, E., Paul, J. J., Fein, D., & Naigles, L. R. (2006). Residual language deficits in optimal outcome children with a history of autism. *Journal of Autism and Developmental Disorders, 36*(6), 807–828.

Kenworthy, L., Case, L., Harms, M. B., Martin, A., & Wallace, G. L. (2009). Adaptive behavior ratings correlate with symptomatology and IQ among individuals with high-functioning autism spectrum disorders. *Journal of Autism and Developmental Disorders, 40*, 416–423.

Kinsbourne, M. (1991). Overfocusing: An apparent subtype of attention deficit hyperactivity disorder. In N. Amir, I. Rapin, & D. Branski (Eds.), *Pediatric neurology: Vol. 1. Behavior and cognition of the child with brain dysfunction* (pp. 18–35). Basel, Switzerland: Karger.

Kjelgaard, M. M., & Tager-Flusberg, H. (2001). An investigation of language impairment in autism: Implications for genetic subgroups. *Language and Cognitive Processes, 16*(2–3), 287–308.

Klin, A., Saulnier, C. A., Sparrow, S. S., Cicchetti, D. V., Volkmar, F. R., & Lord, C. (2007). Social and communication abilities and disabilities in higher functioning individuals with autism spectrum disorders: The Vineland and the ADOS. *Journal of Autism and Developmental Disorders, 37*(4), 748–759.

Korkman, M., Kirk, U., & Kemp, S. (2007). *NEPSY—Second Edition*. San Antonio, TX: Harcourt Assessment.

Lafayette Instruments. (1999). *Purdue Pegboard Test—Revised Edition*. Lafayette, IN: Author.

Landa, R. J., & Goldberg, M. C. (2005). Language, social, and executive functions in high functioning autism: A continuum of performance. *Journal of Autism and Developmental Disorders, 35*(5), 557–573.

Lane, A. E., Molloy, C. A., & Bishop, S. L. (2014). Classification of children with autism spectrum disorder by sensory subtype: A case for sensory-based phenotypes. *Autism Research, 7*(3), 322–333.

Lewy, A. L., & Dawson, G. (1992). Social stimulation and joint attention in young autistic children. *Journal of Abnormal Child Psychology, 20*(6), 555–566.

Lezak, M. (1995). *Neuropsychological assessment* (3rd ed.). New York: Oxford University Press.

Lezak, M., & Bigler, E. (2012). *Neuropsychological assessment* (5th ed.). New York: Oxford University Press.

Liss, M., Fein, D., Allen, D., Dunn, M., Feinstein, C., Morris, R., et al. (2001). Executive functioning in high-functioning children with autism. *Journal of Child Psychology and Psychiatry, 42*(2), 261–270.

Liss, M., Saulnier, C., Fein, D., & Kinsbourne, M. (2006). Sensory and attention abnormalities in autistic spectrum disorders. *Autism, 10*(2), 155–172.

Llorente, A. M., Williams, J., Satz, P., & D'Elia, L. F. (2003). *Children's Color Trails Test.* Lutz, FL: Psychological Assessment Resources.

Lopata, C., Smith, R. A., Volker, M. A., Thomeer, M. L., & McDonald, C. A. (2013). Comparison of adaptive behavior measures for children with HFASDs. *Autism Research and Treatment, 2013,* Article 415989.

Lord, C., Rutter, M., DiLavore, P. C., Risi, S., Gotham, K., & Bishop, S. (2012). *Autism Diagnostic Observation Schedule, Second Edition.* Torrance, CA: Western Psychological Services.

Loukusa, S., Mäkinen, L., Kuusikko-Gauffin, S., Ebeling, H., & Moilanen, I. (2014). Theory of Mind and emotion recognition skills in children with specific language impairment, autism spectrum disorder and typical development: Group differences and connection to knowledge of grammatical morphology, word-finding abilities and verbal working memory. *International Journal of Langauge and Communication Disorders, 49*(4), 498–507.

Loveland, K. A., & Tunali-Kotoski, B. (1997). The school age child with autism. In D. J. Cohen & F. R. Volkmar (Eds.), *Handbook of autism and pervasive developmental disorders* (2nd ed., pp. 283–308). New York: Wiley.

Luna, B., Minshew, N. J., Garver, K. E., Lazar, N. A., Thulborn, K. R., Eddy, W. F., et al. (2002). Neocortical system abnormalities in autism: An fMRI study of spatial working memory. *Neurology, 59*(6), 834–840.

Luria, A. R. (1962). *Higher cortical functions in man.* Moscow: Moscow University Press.

Lyons, M., Schoen-Simmons, E., & Paul, R. (2014). Prosodic development in middle childhood and adolescence in high-functioning autism. *Autism Research, 7*(2), 181–196.

MacDonald, M., Lord, C., & Ulrich, D. (2013). The relationship of motor skills and adaptive behavior skills in young children with autism spectrum disorders. *Research in Autism Spectrum Disorders, 7*(11), 1383–1390.

Manjiviona, J., & Prior, M. (1995). Comparison of Asperger syndrome and high-functioning autistic children on a test of motor impairment. *Journal of Autism and Developmental Disorders, 25*(1), 23–39.

Manly, T., Anderson, V., Nimmo-Smith, I., Turner, A., Watson, P., & Robertson, I. H. (2001). The differential assessment of children's attention: The Test of Everyday Attention for Children (TEA-Ch), normative sample and ADHD performance. *Journal of Child Psychology and Psychiatry, 42*(8), 1065–1081.

Mari, M., Castiello, U., Marks, D., Marraffa, C., & Prior, M. (2003). The reach-to-grasp movement in children with autism spectrum disorder. *Philosophical Transactions of the Royal Society of London, Series B: Biological Sciences, 358*(1430), 393–403.

Martin, N. A., & Brownell, R. (2011a). *Expressive One-Word Picture Vocabulary Test, 4th Edition.* North Tonawanda, NY: Multi-Health System.

Martin, N. A., & Brownell, R. (2011b). *Receptive One-Word Picture Vocabulary Test, 4th Edition.* North Tonawanda, NY: Multi-Health System.

Mathiowetz, V., Volland, G., Kashman, N., & Weber, K. (1992). Nine Hole Peg

Test (NHPT). In D. T. Wade (Ed.), *Measurement in neurological rehabilitation* (p. 171). New York: Oxford University Press.

May, T., Rinehart, N., & Wilding, J. (2013). The role of attention in the academic attainment of children with autism spectrum disorder. *Journal of Autism and Developmental Disorders, 43,* 2147–2158.

Mayes, S. D., & Calhoun, S. L. (2003). Ability profiles in children with autism: Influence of age and IQ. *Autism, 7*(1), 65–80.

McCane, S. J. (2006). Test review: Motor-Free Visual Perception Test. *Journal of Psychoeducational Assessment, 24*(3), 265.

Millward, C., Powell, S., Messer, D., & Jordan, R. (2000). Recall for self and other in autism: Children's memory for events experienced by themselves and their peers. *Journal of Autism and Developmental Disorders, 30*(1), 15–28.

Miniscalco, C. Hagberg, B., Kaesjö, B., Westerlug, M., & Gillberg, C. (2007). Narrative skills, cognitive profiles and neuropsychisatric disorders in 7–8-year-old children with late developing language. *International Journal of Language and Communication Disorders, 42*(6), 665–681.

Minshew, N. J., Goldstein, G., & Siegel, D. J. (1995). Speech and language in high functioning autistic individuals. *Neuropsychology, 9,* 255–261.

Minshew, N. J., Goldstein, G., & Siegel, D. J. (1997). Neuropsychologic functioning in autism: Profile of a complex information processing disorder. *Journal of International Neuropsychological Society, 3*(4), 303–316.

Minshew, N. J., Goldstein, G., Taylor, H. G., & Siegel, D. J. (1994). Academic achievement in high functioning autistic individuals. *Journal of Clinical Experimental Neuropsychology, 16*(2), 261–270.

Mottron, L., Burack, J. A., Iarocci, G., Belleville, S., & Enns, J. T. (2003). Locally oriented perception with intact global processing among adolescents with high-functioning autism: Evidence from multiple paradigms. *Journal of Child Psychology and Psychiatry, 44*(6), 904–913.

Mullen, E. M. (1995). *Mullen Scales of Early Learning.* Circle Pines, MN: American Guidance Service.

Munson, J., Dawson, G., Sterling, L., Beauchaine, T., Zhou, A., Koehler, E., et al. (2008). Evidence for latent classes of IQ in young children with autism spectrum disorder. *American Journal of Mental Retardation, 113*(6), 439–452.

Myles, B. S., Hilgenfeld, T. D., Barnhill, G. P., Griswold, D. E., Hagiwara, T., & Simpson, R. L. (2002). Analysis of reading skills in individuals with Asperger syndrome. *Focus on Autism and Other Developmental Disabilitites, 17*(1), 44–47.

Naglieri, J. A., & Bornstein, B. T. (2003). Intelligence and achievement: Just how correlated are they? *Journal of Psychoeducational Assessment, 21*(3), 244.

Naglieri, J. A., & Das, J. P. (1997). *Cognitive Assessment System.* Itasca, IL: Riverside.

Naglieri, J. A., & Das, J. P. (2005). Planning, attention, simultaneous, successive (PASS) theory: A revision of the concept of intelligence. In D. P. Flanagan & P. L. Harrison (Eds.), *Contemporary intellectual assessment* (2nd ed., pp. 136–182). New York: Guilford Press.

Naglieri, J. A., & Das, J. P. (2014). *Cognitive Assessment System, Second Edition.* Itasca, IL: Riverside.

Naglieri, J. A., Goldstein, S., Delauder, B. Y., & Schwebach, A. (2005). Relationships between the WISC-III and the Cognitive Assessment System with Conners' rating scales and continuous performance tests. *Archives of Clinical Neuropsychology, 20*(3), 385–401.

Narzisi, A., Muratori, F., Caldersoni, S., Fabbro, F., & Urgesi, C. (2013). Neuropsychological profile in high functioning autism spectrum disorder. *Journal of Autism and Developmental Disorders, 43*(8), 1895–1909.

Newman, T. M., Macomber, D., Naples, A. J., Babitz, T., Volkmar, F., & Grigorenko, E. L. (2007). Hyperlexia in children with autism spectrum disorders. *Journal of Autism and Developmental Disorders, 37*(4), 760–774.

O'Connor, N., & Hermelin, B. (1994). Two autistic savant readers. *Journal of Autism and Developmental Disorders, 24*(4), 501–515.

O'Donnell, S., Deitz, J., Kartin, D., Nalty, T., & Dawson, G. (2012). Sensory processing, problem behavior, adaptive behavior, and cognition in preschool children with autism spectrum disorders. *American Journal of Occupational Therapy, 66*(5), 586–594.

Oliveras-Rentas, R. E., Kenworthy, L., Roberson, R. B., III, Martin, A., & Wallace, G. L. (2012). WISC-IV profile in high functioning autism spectrum disorders: Impaired processing speed is associated with increased autism communication symptoms and decreased adaptive communication abilities. *Journal of Autism and Developmental Disorders, 42*(5), 655–664.

O'Riordan, M. A. (2004). Superior visual search in adults with autism. *Autism, 8*(3), 229–248.

O'Riordan, M. A., & Passetti, F. (2006). Discrimination in autism within different sensory modalities. *Journal of Autism and Developmental Disorders, 36*(5), 665–675.

O'Riordan, M. A., Plaisted, K. C., Driver, J., & Baron-Cohen, S. (2001). Superior visual search in autism. *Journal of Experimental Psychology: Human Perception and Performance, 27*(3), 719–730.

O'Shea, A. G., Fein, D. A., Cillessen, A. H., Klin, A., & Schultz, R. T. (2005). Source memory in children with autism spectrum disorders. *Developmental Neuropsychology, 27*(3), 337–360.

Osterrieth, P. A. (1944). Le test de copie d'une figure complexe. *Archives of Psychology, 30*, 206–356.

Ozonoff, S., & Jensen, J. (1999). Brief report: Specific executive function profiles in three neurodevelopmental disorders. *Journal of Autism and Developmental Disorders, 29*(2), 171–177.

Ozonoff, S., Pennington, B. F., & Rogers, S. J. (1991). Executive function deficits in high-functioning autistic individuals: Relationship to theory of mind. *Journal of Child Psychology and Psychiatry, 32*(7), 1081–1105.

Ozonoff, S., & Strayer, D. L. (1997). Inhibitory function in nonretarded children with autism. *Journal of Autism and Developmental Disorders, 27*(1), 59–77.

Ozonoff, S., & Strayer, D. L. (2001). Further evidence of intact working memory in autism. *Journal of Autism and Developmental Disorders, 31*(3), 257–263.

Pascualvaca, D. M., Fantie, B. D., Papageorgiou, M., & Mirsky, A. F. (1998). Attentional capacities in children with autism: Is there a general deficit in shifting focus? *Journal of Autism and Developmental Disorders, 28*(6), 467–478.

Patti, P. J., & Lupinetti, L. (1993). Brief report: Implications of hyperlexia in an autistic savant. *Journal of Autism and Developmental Disorders, 23*(2), 397–405.

Paul, R., Loomis, R., & Chawarska, K. (2014). Adaptive behavior in toddlers under two with autism spectrum disorders. *Journal of Autism and Developmental Disorders, 44*, 264–270.

Pellicano, E., Maybery, M., Durkin, K., & Maley, A. (2006). Multiple cognitive capabilities/deficits in children with an autism spectrum disorder: "Weak" central coherence and its relationship to theory of mind and executive control. *Development and Psychopathology, 18*(1), 77–98.

Pennington, B. F., & Ozonoff, S. (1996). Executive functions and developmental psychopathology. *Journal of Child Psychology and Psychiatry, 37*(1), 51–87.

Phelan, H. L., Filliter, J. H., & Johnson, S. A. (2011). Brief report: Memory performance on the California Verbal Learning Test—Children's Version in autism spectrum disorder. *Journal of Autism and Developmental Disorders, 41*(4), 518–523.

Pierce, K., Glad, K. S., & Schreibman, L. (1997). Social perception in children with autism: An attentional deficit? *Journal of Autism and Developmental Disorders, 27*(3), 265–282.

Pierce, K., Muller, R. A., Ambrose, J., Allen, G., & Courchesene, E. (2001). Face processing occurs outside the fusiform "face area" in autism: Evidence from functional MRI. *Journal of Neurology, 124*(10), 2059–2073.

Poole, J. L., Burtner, P. A., Torres, T. A., McMullen, C. K., Markham, A., Marcum, M. L., et al. (2005). Measuring dexterity in children using the Nine-Hole Peg Test. *Journal of Hand Therapy, 18*(3), 348–351.

Prior, M. R. (1979). Cognitive abilities and disabilities in infantile autism: A review. *Journal of Abnormal Child Psychology, 7*(4), 357–380.

Prior, M. R., & Bradshaw, J. L. (1979). Hemisphere functioning in autistic children. *Cortex, 15*(1), 73–81.

Provost, B., Lopez, B. R., & Heimerl, S. (2007). A comparison of motor delays in young children: Autism spectrum disorder, developmental delay, and developmental concerns. *Journal of Autism and Developmental Disorders, 37*(2), 321–328.

Rey, A. (1944). L'examen psychologique dans les cas d'encephalopathie traumatique. *Archives of. Psychology, 30,* 206–356.

Reynell, J. K., & Gruber, C. P. (1990). *Reynell Developmental Language Scales—U.S. Edition.* Los Angeles: Western Psychological Services.

Reynolds, C., & Voress, J. K. (2007). *Test of Memory and Learning—Second Edition.* Austin, TX: PRO-ED.

Rimland, B. (1964). *Infantile autism: The syndrome and its implications for a neural theory of behavior.* New York: Appleton-Century-Crofts.

Rinehart, N. J., Bradshaw, J. L., Moss, S. A., Brereton. A. V., & Tonge, B. J. (2000). Atypical interference of local detail on global processing in high-functioning autism and Asperger's disorder . *Journal of Child Psychology and Psychiatry, 41*(6), 769–778.

Rogers, S. J., Bennetto, L., McEvoy, R., & Pennington, B. F. (1996). Imitation and pantomime in high-functioning adolescents with autism spectrum disorders. *Child Development, 67*(5), 2060–2073.

Roid, G. H. (2003). *Stanford–Binet Intelligence Scales, Fifth Edition.* Itasca, IL: Riverside.

Russell, J. (1997). *Autism as an executive disorder.* New York: Oxford University Press.

Rutter, M. (1974). The development of infantile autism. *Psychological Medicine, 4,* 147–163.

Rutter, M. (1979). Language, cognition and autism. *Annals of the Academy of Medicine, Singapore, 8*(3), 301–311.

Rutter, M., Bartak, L., & Newman, S. (1971). Autism—A central disorder of cognition and language. In M. Rutter (Ed.), *Infantile autism: Concepts, characteristics and treatment* (pp. 148–171). London: Churchill-Livingstone.

Sandford, J. A., & Turner, A. (2000). *Integrated Visual and Auditory Continuous Performance Test manual.* Richmond, VA: Brain Train.

Schultz, R. T., Grelotti, D. J., Klin, A., Kleinman, J., Van der Gaag, C., Marois, R., et al. (2003). The role of the fusiform face area in social cognition: Implications for the pathobiology of autism. *Philosophical Transactions of the Royal Society of London, Series B: Biological Sciences, 358*(1430), 415–427.

Semel, E., Wiig, E. H., & Secord, W. A. (2003). *Clinical Evaluation of Language Fundamentals—Fourth Edition.* San Antonio, TX: Harcourt Assessment.

Semrud-Clikeman, M., Fine, J. G., & Bledsoe, J. (2014). Comparison among children with autism spectrum disorder, nonverbal learning disorder and typically developing children on measures of executive functioning. *Journal of Autism and Developmental Disorders, 44*(2), 331–342.

Shah, A., & Frith, U. (1993). Why do autistic individuals show superior performance on the Block Design task? *Journal of Child Psychology and Psychiatry, 34*(8), 1351–1364.

Sheslow, D., & Adams, W. (2003). *Wide Range Assessment of Memory and Learning, Second Edition (WRAML2).* San Antonio, TX: Harcourt Assessment.

Smith, Y. A., Hong, E., & Presson, C. (2000). Normative and validation studies of the Nine-Hole Peg Test with children. *Perceptual and Motor Skills, 90*(3, Pt. 1), 823–843.

Southwick, J. S., Bigler, E. D., Froehlich, A., Lange, N., & Lainhart, J. E. (2011). Memory functioning in children and adolescents with autism. *Neuropsychology, 25*(6), 702–710.

Sparrow, S. S., Cicchetti, D. V., & Balla, D. A. (2005). *Vineland Adaptive Behavior Scales: Second Edition (Vineland–II).* Livonia, MN: Pearson Assessments.

Spreen, O., & Benton, A. L. (1977). *Neurosensory Center Comprehensive Examination for Aphasia (NCCEA).* Victoria, BC, Canada: University of Victoria Neuropsychology Laboratory.

Stevens, M. C., Fein, D. A., Dunn, M., Allen, D., Waterhouse, L. H., Feinstein, C., et al. (2000). Subgroups of children with autism by cluster analysis: A longitudinal examination. *Journal of the American Academy of Child and Adolescent Psychiatry, 39*(3), 346–352.

Strauss, E., Sherman, E. M., & Spreen, O. (2006). *A compendium of neuropsychological tests: Administration, norms and commentary* (3rd ed.). New York: Oxford University Press.

Street, R. F. (1931). A Gestalt Completion Test. *Teachers College Contributions to Education, 481,* vii, 65.

Sutera, S., Pandey, J., Esser, E. L., Rosenthal, M. A., Wilson, L. B., Barton, M., et al. (2007). Predictors of optimal outcome in toddlers diagnosed with autism spectrum disorders. *Journal of Autism and Developmental Disorders, 37*(1), 98–107.

Tager-Flusberg, H. (1981). On the nature of linguistic functioning in early infantile autism. *Journal of Autism and Developmental Disorders, 11*(1), 45–56.

Tager-Flusberg, H. (1996). Brief report: Current theory and research on language and communication in autism. *Journal of Autism and Developmental Disorders, 26*(2), 169–172.

Tager-Flusberg, H., & Joseph, R. M. (2003). Identifying neurocognitive phenotypes in autism. *Philosophical Transactions of the Royal Society of London, Series B: Biological Sciences, 358*(1430), 303–314.

Tager-Flusberg, H., Paul, R., & Lord, C. E. (2005). Language and communication in autism. In F. Volkmar, R. Paul, A. Klin, & D. J. Cohen (Eds.), *Handbook of autism and pervasive developmental disorder* (3rd ed., pp. 335–364.) New York: Wiley.

Tager-Flusberg, H., Rogers, S., Cooper, R. S., Landa, R., Lord, C., Paul, R., et al. (2009). Defining spoken language benchmarks and selecting measures of expressive language development for young children with autism spectrum disorders. *Journal of Speech, Language and Hearing, 52*(3), 643–652.

Teitelbaum, O., Benton, T., Shah, P. K., Prince, A., Kelly, J. L., & Teitelbaum, P. (2004). Eshkol–Wachman movement notation in diagnosis: The early detection of Asperger's syndrome. *Proceedings of the National Academy of Sciences USA, 101*(32), 11909–11914.

Teitelbaum, P., Teitelbaum, O., Nye, J., Fryman, J., & Maurer, R. G. (1998). Movement analysis in infancy may be useful for early diagnosis of autism. *Proceedings of the National Academy of Sciences USA, 95*(23), 13982–13987.

Tiffin, J., & Asher, E. J. (1948). The Purdue Pegboard: Norms and studies of reliability and validity. *Journal of Applied Psychology, 32*, 234–247.

Townsend, J., Harris, N. S., & Courchesne, E. (1996). Visual attention abnormalities in autism: Delayed orienting to location. *Journal of International Neuropsychological Society, 2*(6), 541–550.

Tsuchiya, E., Oki, J., Yahara, N., & Fujieda, K. (2005). Computerized version of the Wisconsin Card Sorting Test in children with high-functioning autistic disorder or attention-deficit/hyperactivity disorder. *Brain and Development, 27*, 233–236.

Turkheimer, E. (1989). Techniques of quantitative measurement of morphological structures of the central nervous system. In R. A. Yeo, E. D. Bigler, & E. Turkheimer (Eds.), *Neuropsychological functioning and brain imaging* (pp. 47–64). New York: Plenum Press.

Venter, A., Lord, C., & Schopler, E. (1992). A follow-up study of high-functioning autistic children. *Journal of Child Psychology and Psychiatry, 33*(3), 489–507.

Verly, M., Verhoeven, J., Zink, I., Mantini, D., Oudenhove, L. V., Lagae, L., et al. (2014). Structural and functional underconnectivity as a negative predictor for language in autism. *Human Brain Mapping, 35*(8), 3602–3615.

Vilensky, J. A., Damasio, A. R., & Maurer, R. G. (1981). Gait disturbances in patients with autistic behavior: A preliminary study. *Archives of Neurology, 38*(10), 646–649.

Volkmar, F. (2003). Adaptive skills. *Journal of Autism and Developmental Disorders, 33*(1), 109–110.

Watling, R. L., Deitz, J., & White, O. (2001). Comparison of Sensory Profile scores of young children with and without autism spectrum disorders. *American Journal of Occupational Therapy, 55*(4), 416–423.

Wechsler, D. (2009a). *Wechsler Individual Achievement Test—Third Edition*. San Antonio, TX: Harcourt Assessment.

Wechsler, D. (2009b). *Wechsler Memory Scale—Fourth Edition*. San Antonio, TX: Psychological Corporation.

Wechsler, D. (2011). *Wechsler Abbreviated Scale of Intelligence—Second Edition*. San Antonio, TX: Psychological Corporation.

Wechsler, D. (2012). *Wechsler Preschool and Primary Scale of Intelligence—Fourth Edition*. New York: Psychological Corporation.

Wechsler, D. (2014). *Wechsler Intelligence Scale for Children—Fifth Edition*. New York: Psychological Corporation.

Welsh, M. C., & Pennington, B. F. (1988). Assessing frontal lobe functioning in children: View from developmental psychology. *Developmental Neuropsychology, 4*, 199–230.

Whitehouse, D., & Harris, J. C. (1984). Hyperlexia in infantile autism. *Journal of Autism and Developmental Disorders, 14*(3), 281–289.

Wiig, E. H., & Secord, W. (1989). *Test of Language Competence—Expanded Edition.* San Antonio, TX: Psychological Corporation.

Williams, D. L., Goldstein, G., Carpenter, P. A., & Minshew, N. J. (2005). Verbal and spatial working memory in autism. *Journal of Autism and Developmental Disorders, 35*(6), 747–756.

Williams, D. L., Goldstein, G., Kojkowski, N., & Minshew, N. J. (2008). Do individuals with high functioning autism have the IQ profile associated with nonverbal learning disability? *Research in Autism Spectrum Disorders,* 2(2), 353–361.

Williams, D. L., Goldstein, G., & Minshew, N. J. (2005). Impaired memory for faces and social scenes in autism: Clinical implications of memory dysfunction. *Archives of Clinical Neuropsychology, 20*(1), 1–15.

Williams, J. H., Whiten, A., Suddendorf, T., & Perrett, D. I. (2001). Imitation, mirror neurons and autism. *Neuroscience and Biobehavioral Reviews, 25*(4), 287–295.

Woodcock, R. W., McGrew, K. S., & Mather, N. (2001). *Woodcock–Johnson III.* Itasca, IL: Riverside.

Yeates, K. O., Ris., M. D., & Taylor, H. G. (2000). *Pediatric neuropsychology: Research, theory and practice.* New York: Guilford Press.

Zimmerman, I. L., Steiner, V. G., & Pond, R. E. (2011). *Preschool Language Scale—Fifth Edition.* San Antonio, TX: Harcourt Assessment.

CHAPTER TEN

Assessment of Comorbid Psychiatric Conditions in Autism Spectrum Disorder

Lesley Deprey
Sally Ozonoff

The occurrence of two or more clinical diagnoses, known as "comorbidity," has received much attention in the child psychopathology literature in recent years (Matson & Cervantes, 2014). Co-occurrence of disorders within the same time interval can be defined narrowly, more broadly, or even with reference to the entire lifetime (e.g., "concurrent" vs. "successive" comorbidity; Angold, Erkanli, Costello, & Rutter, 1996; Costello, Foley, & Angold, 2006). The issue of comorbidity and autism spectrum disorder (ASD) has become increasingly important, as DSM-5 (American Psychiatric Association, 2013) no longer excludes most additional diagnoses in children with ASD. This is in accordance with what has long been recognized—that ASD can co-occur with a number of other conditions and that these additional problems have a substantial negative impact on functioning (Lecavalier, 2006). Several large studies, most based on clinically referred samples, have reported that over 70% of children with ASD were above diagnostic thresholds for another emotional or behavioral disorder and that over 40% may have two or more comorbid mental health conditions (Gjevik, Eldevik, Fjæran-Granum, & Sponheim, 2011; Joshi et al., 2010; Kaat, Gadow, & Lecavalier, 2013; Simonoff et al., 2008). Children with ASD have been found to have more psychiatric comorbidity than children with intellectual disability (Brereton, Tonge, & Einfeld, 2006). In contrast to typical development, males and females with ASD are reported to experience similar rates of co-occurring psychiatric conditions (Worley

& Matson, 2011). Thus, this is an area that must be addressed in any comprehensive evaluation of a child with ASD. Comorbidity should be considered whenever there are signs of psychiatric problems that are not part of ASD; when there are marked changes in functioning from baseline, or an existing problem is markedly exacerbated; or when an individual with ASD does not respond as expected to interventions that are traditionally effective (Lainhart, 1999).

Assessment of comorbidity is inherently complex and has presented a persistent puzzle for both research and clinical work (Krueger & Markon, 2006). Children may demonstrate mixed symptoms that stem from a single disorder with unusual presentation or from the simultaneous occurrence of multiple disorders (Caron & Rutter, 1991). Although students and clinicians are often taught to make a single diagnosis whenever possible, comorbidity is common in epidemiological studies of many child psychiatric disorders. A person who meets criteria for a mental health disorder is more likely to meet criteria for another disorder than expected by chance, given that mental disorder constructs are correlated and dimensional (Krueger & Markon, 2006; Regier, Narrow, Kuhl, & Kupfer, 2009). In general, individuals diagnosed with more than one disorder present with greater symptom severity and impairment than those meeting criteria for a single condition (Gadow, Guttmann-Steinmetz, Rieffe, & DeVincent, 2012).

It is important to understand, however, that there are also a variety of ways in which an apparent picture of comorbidity can be falsely created. In a seminal paper, Caron and Rutter (1991) reminded us that detection artifacts, such as referral biases, can distort impressions of the frequency of comorbidity. It is also possible that a disorder has been misconceived, so that overlapping diagnostic criteria, artificial subdivisions of syndromes, or one disorder representing an early manifestation of another disorder may present a false picture of comorbidity. Beyond such artifactual comorbidities, these authors describe the mechanisms that may underlie true comorbidity, such as shared risk factors or one disorder creating a risk for another disorder. Changes from DSM-IV-TR to DSM-5 now allow for a range of comorbid clinical presentations to be identified along with ASD, when historically such additional diagnoses (e.g., attention-deficit/hyperactivity disorder [ADHD], psychosis) were considered exclusionary (American Psychiatric Association, 2000, 2013).

Developmental specialists involved in both clinical and research endeavors must be knowledgeable about the interplay between neurodevelopment and mental health issues, as the presentation of comorbid conditions results in more challenging assessments. The complexity of diagnosing ASD, with its broad range of symptom severity and intellectual functioning, is already a difficult task. Differences in clinical presentation associated with comorbidity add to the complexities of diagnostic assessment.

Although differential diagnosis is challenging, it is essential, as treatment of the ASD symptoms alone will usually not result in improvement in the other behavioral or emotional problems that coexist. Undertreatment or partial treatment can result in significant functional impairment.

This chapter begins with a discussion of theoretical and methodological issues associated with comorbidity in ASD. We then discuss specific psychiatric conditions known to co-occur with ASD, including mood disorders, anxiety disorders, ADHD, tic disorders, and psychotic disorders. Each section reviews the literature on prevalence rates, differential diagnosis, and differences in symptom expression when the disorder or disorders co-occur with ASD. After this, we discuss different instruments that can be helpful in the assessment of possible comorbidities and the differential diagnostic process. We end the chapter with directions for future research.

CHALLENGES IN ASSESSING COMORBID CONDITIONS

Clinicians encounter several difficulties when assessing children with ASD whose functioning may also be affected by other forms of psychopathology.

Standardization and Norming Issues

Standardized assessment instruments should be utilized to evaluate impairment and range of possible diagnosable disorders (Kazdin, 1993). Unfortunately, most behavior checklists and diagnostic interview tools were standardized without children with ASD, making interpretation of scores challenging. It is not clear that norms developed for children without developmental disorders and with average cognitive functioning are relevant for children with ASD, with or without intellectual disability. Thus, it is sometimes hard to know whether a child is scoring in the clinical range on an instrument because he or she has ASD, or because he or she is experiencing the particular difficulties that the tool measures.

Insight and Self-Report Problems

A second set of difficulties in assessing potential psychiatric problems in children with ASD and/or intellectual disability is limitations in the ability to process and talk about emotions and internal experiences (Sovner, 1996). In the assessment of psychopathology, the gold standard method is self-report, which captures "the experiencing self"—the individual centered in the phenomenon (Derogatis, 1983). Unfortunately, limitations in insight and mentalizing pose considerable challenges to obtaining accurate, clinically useful information when self-report is utilized in individuals with ASD (Mazefsky, Kao, & Oswald, 2011). Many studies have demonstrated the difficulties individuals with ASD experience in attributing mental and emotional states to others (Baron-Cohen, O'Riordan, Stone, Jones, & Plaisted, 1999; Jolliffe & Baron-Cohen, 1999; Sicotte & Stemberger, 1999). Such difficulties are also proposed to cause these individuals impairments in recognizing and describing their own emotional and mental states (Baron-Cohen, Tager-Flusberg, & Cohen, 2000; Ben Shalom et al., 2006; Berthoz & Hill, 2005). Individuals with ASD tend to focus on physical, concrete characteristics rather than on inner abstract experiences (Hill, Berthoz, & Frith, 2004). It has been suggested that children with ASD lack an "inner language" to describe their socioemotional difficulties (Walters, Barrett, & Feinstein, 1990). Functional communication and pragmatic language skills may be limited. Response perseveration can also have an impact on self-report ratings (Ben Shalom et al., 2006). For all these reasons, self-reporting of internal phenomena—essential to most assessments of psychopathology—may be less useful with children with ASD, especially those who are younger or lower functioning (Mazefsky et al., 2011).

It is possible, however, that some higher-functioning adolescents and adults may be able to provide useful self-reports. One study found that adolescents and adults with ASD did not differ from comparison subjects on a measure of "private self-consciousness," defined as attention to the private aspects of the self, such as feelings and motives (Blackshaw, Kinderman, Hare, & Hatton, 2001). Autobiographical writings of adults with ASD reveal awareness of their interpersonal and socioemotional difficulties (Happé, 1991; Spicer, 1998). A previous study found that self-report using the Minnesota Multiphasic Personality Inventory–2 yielded profiles consistent with the ASD phenotype, with elevations on scales measuring social isolation, introversion, and rigidity; these findings indicated that the adult participants were able to describe their difficulties validly (Ozonoff, Garcia, Clark, & Lainhart, 2005). A case study of a young adult with high-functioning autism suggested that he had "accurate knowledge of his traits" (Klein, Chan, & Loftus, 1999, p. 413). Although such evidence is indirect, this collective body of work suggests that there may be some capacity for introspection, and therefore for accurate self-reporting on dimensions of psychopathology, in older and higher-functioning individuals on the autism spectrum. Nevertheless, we believe that self-report measures should still be used cautiously with the ASD population.

Differences in Symptom Manifestation

A third complication in the assessment of comorbidities in ASD is that differences in clinical expression can influence the range and quality of symptoms displayed. Symptoms of another condition may look different in the context of ASD and symptom expression may be influenced by lowered cognitive capacity (Sovner, 1996). Individuals with ASD may not demonstrate certain symptoms, such as the feelings of guilt often seen in depression or the grandiosity and inflated self-esteem typical of mania, due to cognitive limitations, lack of understanding of certain concepts, or reduced social and peer comparison. Anxiety may be manifested as obsessive questioning or insistence on sameness, rather than as rumination or somatic complaints. Emotional problems and oppositionality may present when minor changes are made to routines. ASD alone involves differences in socioemotional expression (such as reductions in reciprocity, joint attention, and coordination of gaze and gesture) that will affect social responsiveness during an assessment, as well as overall clinical impressions. Changes in sleep and/or eating behaviors may be less obvious because of the motivation of individuals with ASD to follow routines (Lainhart, 1999). In the sections on specific comorbid conditions below, we review what is known for each disorder about potential differences between typical symptom manifestation and manifestation within the context of ASD.

Principal and Secondary Diagnoses

Another challenge in the assessment of comorbid mental health conditions is the relative rankings of diagnoses in accounting for functional impairment. DSM-5 permits the assignment of one diagnosis as principal when it is chiefly responsible for referral and/or more impairing at the time of evaluation. So, for example, an adolescent with ASD who is also displaying feelings of sadness, hopelessness, and worthlessness, insomnia, and thoughts of suicide might receive a principal DSM-5 diagnosis of major depressive disorder (severe) and a secondary diagnosis of ASD.

Solutions to Assessment Challenges

One of the best ways to evaluate the presence of comorbidities in ASD is to focus on changes in behavior from baseline. Significant changes in behavior from how the individual was described in the past—such as increases in social withdrawal, repetitive motor movements, aggression/outbursts, resistance to change, irritability, and avoidance of novelty, or decreases in activities that once brought pleasure—can be crucial to making an accurate diagnosis (Lainhart, 1999). For example, a decrease in the amount of time spent discussing a special interest (e.g., the solar system or Canadian prime ministers) may be helpful in evaluating anhedonia and the onset of a mood disorder. In addition, the appearance of new challenging behaviors that have not been part of the clinical picture in the past, such as self-injury or aggression, will indicate the need for further evaluation. Unexplained decreases in self-care and other everyday living skills may also present diagnostic clues related to comorbidities in ASD. Comorbidity should be suspected when such changes from baseline are accompanied by significant clinical impairment in functioning and decreased adaptive behavior. Evaluations of risk factors (especially family history of comorbid conditions) and of environmental factors (e.g., appropriate access to services and support) are other key elements to making an accurate differential diagnosis.

Differential Diagnosis versus Comorbidity

So far, we have discussed psychiatric problems that may coexist with ASD. However, it is of course also possible that a child has another disorder alone, and that in fact the diagnosis of ASD is inaccurate. Thus, another important part of the process of case formulation is differential diagnosis: Does the child have both ASD and another disorder, or just another disorder? The rest of this chapter will help clinicians address the first half of this question, but how can an evaluator tell whether it would be more parsimonious to ascribe difficulties to just one condition? For example, poor eye contact and low social initiative may be indicative of ASD, but also of depression. How does a clinician go about deciding whether the difficulties are due to one or the other of these explanations, rather than comorbidity? The answer is deceptively simple. Examining the developmental history for the consistency of symptoms over time and pervasiveness across situations will help the clinician immensely in the process of differential diagnosis. Children with depression alone, for example, do not exhibit the widespread and long-term difficulties in social interaction, communication, and behavior that are characteristic of ASD. Children who present with a restricted range of facial expressions, poor eye contact, and low social initiative, and who also display limited empathy, few gestures, pedantic speech, or unusual interests, are likely to have both ASD and a mood disorder. The package of social and communication limitations, combined with odd or repetitive behaviors, expressed consistently throughout the lifetime, should alert the clinician that ASD must be part of the differential diagnosis. No other condition includes all of these difficulties. Then, if additional problems not encompassed by the ASD criteria are present, if there are changes from baseline indicating onset of new difficulties, or if the individual is not responding as expected to treatment, comorbidity should be considered (Lainhart, 1999). If, however, the social and communication difficulties are limited to behaviors that might plausibly stem from depression and do not extend to pragmatic communication, symbolic activities, empathy, or stereotyped behaviors, or have not been part of the developmental history but are of recent onset, then the differential diagnosis is more likely to include just the mood disorder. See also Mazefsky et al. (2012) for a helpful discussion of this topic.

In the next section, we consider specific disorders that commonly co-occur with ASD.

ASD AND SPECIFIC COMORBIDITIES

ASD and Depression

Prevalence

A large epidemiological investigation, the National Health and Nutrition Examination Survey (NHANES), estimated that the prevalence of mood disorders in U.S. children ages 8–15 years is 3.7% (Merikangas et al., 2010). Prevalence rates are somewhat lower in preschoolers (2%; Wichstrøm et al., 2012) and substantially higher in adolescents (10.0%; Kessler, Petukhova, Sampson, Zaslavsky, & Wittchen, 2012). Depression and other mood disorders have long been among the most commonly reported mental health problems in individuals with ASD, with rates between 19 and 56% reported in recent large clinically ascertained samples of youth and adults with ASD (Hofvander et al., 2009; Joshi et al., 2010; Kaat et al., 2013). Until recently, there were few population-based studies of the prevalence of psychiatric disorders within ASD, making it difficult to know whether comorbidity rates were truly higher than average or were artifacts of referral biases. In the past several years, however, a number of epidemiological studies have been conducted that shed light on this issue, including the Danish National Birth Cohort study (Abdallah et al., 2011) and the National Survey of Children's Health (NSCH) study (Close, Lee, Kaufmann, & Zimmerman, 2012). The NSCH study found rates of comorbid depression that were well above general population rates for both children (12.5%) and adolescents (31.3%) with ASD (Close et al., 2012). A lower prevalence of 6.8%, but still higher than the general population risk, was reported in the Danish study (Abdallah et al., 2011). Among close relatives of individuals with ASD, rates of depression have also been found to be increased (Piven & Palmer, 1999). As in the general population, children with ASD who suffer from depression are more likely to have a family history of depression (Ghaziuddin & Greden, 1998).

Diagnostic Criteria and Symptom Expression

Criteria in the fifth edition of the *Diagnostic and Statistical Manual of Mental Disorders* (DSM-5) for a major depressive episode include depressed and/or irritable mood or loss of interests for at least 2 weeks, accompanied by at least four additional symptoms; these may include changes in weight, sleep patterns, activity level, psychomotor agitation or retardation, suicidal ideation, self-injurious behavior, feelings of worthlessness, and unwarranted feelings of guilt (American Psychiatric Association, 2013).

Several studies have examined the phenomenology of depression in individuals with ASD and differences in symptom expression are often found (Magnuson & Constantino, 2011). Lainhart (1999; Lainhart & Folstein,

1994) has remarked that the presenting complaint is often not mood related, but rather new or worsened aggression, agitation, self-injurious behavior, increased compulsive behaviors, hypoactivity, or an overall deterioration in everyday functioning across environments. Similarly, Ghaziuddin, Ghaziuddin, and Greden (2002) have noted that although some individuals with ASD can communicate some of their feelings to others, the expression of sadness is one of the most difficult. In a summary of published case studies of ASD and depression, depressed mood was a frequently cited symptom, but in only one case was the affected individual able to report the change in mood directly (Stewart, Barnard, Pearson, Hasan, & O'Brien, 2006). However, increases in irritability (Mayes, Calhoun, Murray, Ahuja, & Smith, 2011) and sleep disturbances are frequently reported and may be alternate expressions of sadness. Symptoms that may be specific to depression when it is comorbid with ASD and that were also common in this case series included losing interest in a special topic, evidencing a decrease in adaptive functioning, a loss of bowel control, and an increase in maladaptive behaviors (particularly aggression and self-injury; Stewart et al., 2006).

ASD and Bipolar Disorder

Prevalence

Approximately 2% of adolescents in the general population meet criteria for bipolar I disorder (Kessler et al., 2012), hereafter referred to as simply bipolar disorder. The prevalence of bipolar disorder in ASD remains unknown, with no epidemiological studies yet performed to estimate rates of comorbidity. Reported rates of mania in selected clinical samples of children and adolescents with ASD span a wide range, from 2 to 31% (Joshi et al., 2010, 2012; Kaat et al., 2013; Leyfer et al., 2006), with highest rates described in samples derived from psychiatric clinic referrals (Joshi et al., 2010). A recent systematic review of the literature on adults with ASD reported similar rates, from 6 to 21% (Vannucchi et al., 2014).

Diagnostic Criteria and Symptom Expression

A manic episode is characterized by elevated or irritable mood, grandiosity, decreased need for sleep, pressured speech, flight of ideas, distractibility, increases in goal-directed activity or psychomotor agitation, and involvement in activities that have a high potential for negative consequences (American Psychiatric Association, 2013). Symptoms of hypomania present with a shorter duration (lasting 4 days or less) than those associated with a full manic episode (i.e., 1-week duration). Mania and hypomania can be difficult to diagnose in ASD, due to superficial similarities in presentation or overlap of symptoms. Nonspecific behaviors that often occur in children with ASD, such as irritability, overactivity, lack of fear, and overtalkativeness (Lainhart, 1999; Stahlberg, Soderstrom, Rastam, & Gillberg, 2004), may be quite difficult to differentiate from bipolar symptoms. Sleep disturbance, particularly decreased need for sleep, is already common among children with ASD (Oyane & Bjorvatn, 2005; Polimeni, Richdale, & Francis, 2005; Wiggs & Stores, 2004). Only when clear changes from an individual's typical pattern are evident might sleep disturbances be indicative of mania, so obtaining a detailed sleep history and examining it for clear changes is critical. Leyfer et al. (2006) have commented that children with ASD (without bipolar disorder) often demonstrate poorly modulated, fluctuating mood and overreactive emotions. They may speak at an abnormal rate, describe preoccupations or ideas in an excited manner, or laugh for no apparent reason, all of which could be confused with symptoms of mania. Children with ASD may engage in dangerous activities, as do individuals experiencing mania, but for very different reasons. Depending on a child's mental age, he or she may not comprehend that particular activities are unsafe or may not link cause and effect, resulting in participation in potentially dangerous experiences. According to Leyfer et al. (2006), both their empirical results and clinical experience suggest that the comorbidity of ASD and bipolar disorder is relatively rare. Thus, in most cases, care must be taken to differentiate core symptoms of ASD from comorbid symptoms of mania (e.g., flight of ideas, pressured speech). As with depression, the key to identifying bipolar disorder in individuals with ASD is to evaluate mood relative to baseline behavior—that is, did these persons generally display positive affect before, but at present do they seem grouchy, cranky, or angry most of the time? Did they typically have a mild reaction to interruptions in activities, but have they become explosive and uncontrollable when interrupted?

ASD and Anxiety Disorders

Prevalence

The estimated prevalence rate of anxiety disorders in U.S. children ages 9–17 is 15–20% (Kessler et al., 2012); estimates are much lower for preschool children, reported to be approximately 1.5% in a recent epidemiological sample from Norway (Wichstrøm et al., 2012). There are several studies evaluating anxiety disorders in ASD. The large NSCH epidemiological study of children with ASD found that 18.8% of preschoolers, 39.4% of school-age children, and 48.9% of adolescents with ASD met criteria for an anxiety disorder (Close et al., 2012)—rates that are all well above the general population risk. A relatively large study (N = 115 children) of consecutive ASD referrals to a developmental disabilities specialty clinic found prevalence rates for 6- to 12-year-olds with ASD of 32% for generalized anxiety disorder and 23% for social phobia (Kaat et al., 2013). Rates of comorbid anxiety disorders in a large sample (*N* = 217) of children with ASD referred to a psychopharmacology clinic were similarly high: specific phobia (37%), separation anxiety disorder (37%), agoraphobia (35%), generalized anxiety disorder (35%), social phobia (28%), and panic disorder (6%; Joshi et al., 2010). Studies have also shown an increased rate of anxiety among first-degree relatives of individuals with ASD (Bolton, Pickles, Murphy, & Rutter, 1998; Hallett, Ronald, et al., 2013).

Diagnostic Criteria and Symptom Expression

The anxiety disorders included in DSM-5 that may co-occur with ASD are generalized anxiety disorder (i.e., persistent and excessive anxiety about a number of issues or activities), panic disorder (i.e., recurrent sudden onset of intense fear), agoraphobia (i.e., fear and avoidance of situations where escape may be difficult), specific phobia (i.e., fear and avoidance of a specified object or situation), social phobia (i.e., fear and avoidance of social or performance situations), and separation anxiety disorder (i.e., anxiety about separation from caregivers).

Anxiety seems to increase with age in ASD (Gadow, DeVincent, Pomeroy, & Azizian, 2005). Symptoms are reported at about the same rate as the general population in preschool-age children with ASD, but appear to increase above population rates in school-age children and adolescents with ASD (Weisbrot, Gadow, DeVincent, & Pomeroy, 2005). Some studies suggest that specific phobias are the most common anxiety disorders in ASD (Joshi et al., 2010; Leyfer et al., 2006). One study found a higher rate of medical, animal, and situational phobias in children with ASD than in children with Down syndrome or typically developing controls (Evans, Canavera, Kleinpeter, Maccubbin, & Taga, 2005). Lainhart (1999) suggested that individuals with ASD may be at greater risk for anxiety disorders because of cognitive impairments—for example, not understanding certain phenomena (e.g., thunderstorms) and therefore experiencing inordinate anxiety about them. Leyfer et al. (2006) have indicated that anxiety varies less over time in children with ASD than in anxious peers without ASD, appearing more trait-like than state-like. In this study, anxiety was more likely to focus on one rather than multiple things (often associated with transitions or environmental changes) and few participants met criteria for generalized anxiety disorder. Irritability is often a component of how anxiety disorders are manifest in children with ASD (Mayes et al., 2011).

In summary, there is ample evidence that anxiety symptoms are elevated in persons with ASD and therefore are important targets of intervention to improve well-being and overall functioning. There are also clear overlaps between core behaviors of ASD and some anxiety disorders, such as social phobia—such overlaps require clinicians to weigh carefully whether additional diagnoses are required.

ASD and Obsessive–Compulsive and Related Disorders

The new DSM-5 category of obsessive–compulsive and related disorders includes a range of conditions such as obsessive-compulsive disorder (OCD; i.e., involuntary thoughts that cause marked anxiety and actions that serve to neutralize the anxiety), body dysmorphic disorder, hoarding disorder, trichotillomania (hair-pulling disorder), and excoriation (skin-picking disorder; American Psychiatric Association, 2013).

Prevalence

No prevalence studies of the co-occurrence of ASD and OCD have been conducted.

Diagnostic Criteria and Symptom Expression

OCD is characterized by the presence of obsessions (persistent thoughts) and or compulsions (repetitive acts that a person feels driven to perform). Key issues remain unresolved regarding the relationship between core ASD symptoms and OCD (Bejerot, 2007). The need for sameness, cognitive inflexibility, sensory-seeking behavior, and repetitive use of objects often seen in ASD can be confused with OCD, although the diagnostic criteria for OCD do not include these symptoms. Differentiating the common ritualistic behaviors seen in ASD from the compulsions of OCD is more difficult. One differentiating feature is the prominent anxiety if a ritual is not completed that is part of OCD—rituals in ASD often appear to bring pleasure, or at least are much less ego dystonic than those in OCD. The repeated touching or tapping of objects, which is sometimes seen in ASD as a sensory-seeking or self-stimulating behavior, could also be viewed as a compulsive behavior. In most cases of ASD, although it can be difficult to assess because of self-report problems, this behavior is not performed to counteract intrusive thoughts or reduce anxiety. Therefore, it should be a rare child who is diagnosed with comorbid ASD and OCD, and this should be done only when obsessions and compulsions that are similar in form to children without ASD are present and cannot be accounted for by the stereotyped and repetitive behavior symptoms of ASD.

ASD and ADHD

Prevalence

The prevalence of ADHD in U.S. children is estimated to be 3–7% (American Psychiatric Association, 2013; Kessler et al., 2012; Merikangas et al., 2010). Dual diagnoses of ADHD and any pervasive developmental disorder were formally excluded by DSM-IV-TR diagnostic rules but widely debated and challenged (Gargaro, Rinehart, Bradshaw, Tonge, & Sheppard, 2011; Goldstein & Schwebach, 2004). DSM-5 concedes that neurodevelopmental disorders frequently co-occur and explicitly allows clinicians to diagnose comorbid ASD and ADHD. The NSCH epidemiological study of children with ASD reported that 21.6% of preschoolers, 44.6% of school-age children, and 52.6% of adolescents with ASD also met criteria for ADHD (Close et al., 2012). In contrast, in a large sample of children and adolescents with ASD from the Simons Simplex Collection (*N* = 1,838), rates were much lower, with a 16% comorbidity rate by parent report (Hanson, Cerban, Slater, Caccamo, Bacic, & Chan, 2013).

Diagnostic Criteria and Symptom Expression

Core features of ADHD include inattention (e.g., failing to pay attention to detail, not listening, difficulty with organization), hyperactivity (e.g., fidgeting, difficulty playing quietly), and impulsivity (e.g., blurting out responses, difficulty waiting a turn), with symptoms present before age 7 (American Psychiatric Association, 2013). Comorbid diagnoses of ASD and ADHD are commonly made in clinical practice—in part because the attention and hyperactivity symptoms can be quite impairing, are not improved by standard treatments for ASD, and do have effective treatments that would not be offered without the comorbid diagnosis. Since the overlap between attentional issues and ASD is covered in detail elsewhere in this book (see Corbett & Iqbal, Chapter 9, this volume), we only briefly discuss a few key issues in the differential diagnosis.

Common features of ADHD in ASD include difficulties in listening to and following instructions, keeping things organized, sitting still, taking turns, talking excessively, and interrupting others. Many of these difficulties can be challenging to differentiate from the core impairments of ASD (Craig et al., 2015; Grzadzinski, Dick, Lord, & Bishop, 2016; Miodovnik, Harstad, Sideridis, & Huntington, 2015)—for example, turn-taking deficits, excessive talking, and interrupting may be secondary to social impairments, while poor organization may be an executive function difficulty. It is critical to examine the pervasiveness of symptoms across settings. It has been suggested that the attention problems that occur in the context of ASD are qualitatively different from those found in ADHD. "Overfocus" of attention and internal distractibility may be more characteristic of ASD, whereas underfocused attention and distractibility by external events and stimuli are the hallmarks of ADHD. It has also been suggested that hyperactivity may be more prominent in children with ASD at younger ages, but that it diminishes with age (as it does in children diagnosed with ADHD alone; Harvey, Lugo-Candelas, & Breaux, 2015), with impulsivity, inattention, and distractibility remaining in adulthood (Tantum, 2003). Others have found that children who met criteria for ASD at one point but lose the diagnosis later in life present very much like children with primary ADHD later in childhood (Blumberg et al., 2016; Fein, Dixon, Paul, & Levin, 2005). Conducting additional tests of attention will provide clarity to differential diagnosis. (Refer to Chapter 9, this volume, for useful assessment measures for ADHD.)

ASD and Tic Disorders

Prevalence

The general population prevalence of Tourette's disorder is reported to be 0.77% and of transient tic disorder to be 3% (Knight et al., 2012). Rates are consistently higher in boys than girls and in children than adults (Knight et al., 2012). Rates of Tourette's disorder appear to be significantly higher in ASD than in the general population, but no epidemiological or community-based studies of children with ASD have yet looked at their co-occurrence using DSM-5 (or DSM-IV) criteria. In a recent large study of clinic-referred children with ASD, 23% met criteria for chronic motor or vocal tic disorder, while 18% met full criteria for Tourette's disorder (Joshi et al., 2010). A study of clinic-referred adults documented that 20% met criteria for chronic tic disorders (Hofvander et al., 2009).

Diagnostic Criteria and Symptom Expression

The childhood onset (mean age 6–7 years) of multiple motor and one or more vocal tics is the hallmark of Tourette's disorder. Tics are sudden, recurrent, stereotyped movements or vocalizations that can be simple (e.g., head or shoulder jerks, eye blinking, throat clearing, sniffing, grunting) or complex (touching, saying words or phrases, echolalia), with a variable course. For full criteria for Tourette's disorder to be met, symptoms must occur often throughout the day for a period of more than 1 year, without a tic-free period of more than 3 consecutive months. Chronic motor or vocal tic disorder is characterized by the presence of either motor or vocal tics, but not both (American Psychiatric Association, 2013).

Common features of ASD-like stereotypies and tic disorders include abnormal motor movements, echolalia, need for sameness, and behavioral rigidity (Baron-Cohen, Mortimore, Moriarty, Izaguirre, & Robertson, 1999). This may make the two conditions appear hard to distinguish, but in fact the similarities are largely superficial. In short, the topography of tics, which are rapid, involuntary, and nonrhythmic, is quite different from the stereotypies of ASD, which tend to be rhythmic (e.g., hand flapping, pacing, rocking), longer in duration, and under some voluntary control. Tics are sudden and rapid, lack a purposeful quality, may interrupt the flow of speech and behavior, and often are preceded by an unpleasant sensation or premonitory urge (Jankovic, 1997; Lainhart, 1999). Whereas complex stereotypies are rhythmical, complex tics are spasmodic. Other features that may assist in differentiating symptoms include (1) ASD motor mannerisms tend to involve the hands, fingers, and whole body, whereas tics typically involve the face, neck, arms, and shoulders; (2) individuals with tics may seem distressed by the behaviors, whereas individuals performing autistic stereotypies are not; and (3) stereotyped movements are less variable over time (not waxing and waning) and less influenced by psychosocial factors (Lainhart, 1999). However, when movements or sounds that are rapid, nonrhythmic or spasmodic, and difficult to control are present in a child with ASD, then the additional diagnosis of a tic disorder is warranted.

Although it has been suggested that children with comorbid Tourette's disorder are higher functioning (Burd, Fisher, Kerbeshian, & Arnold, 1987), Canitano and Vivanti (2007) found a positive relationship between the degree of cognitive impairment and the severity of tics, with higher rates in individuals with moderate to severe intellectual disability.

ASD and Psychosis

Prevalence

The prevalence of schizophrenia spectrum disorders across the lifespan is about 1% (American Psychiatric Association, 2013). Due to the low base rates of both conditions, no epidemiological studies have yet examined rates of schizophrenia spectrum disorders in ASD. Several older studies demonstrated that ASD and psychotic disorders can co-occur, but suggested that the rate is not elevated beyond what would be predicted by the general population prevalence (Lainhart, 1999; Volkmar & Cohen, 1991). More recently, however, there has been renewed interest in the association of the conditions, due to similarities in the risk genes and molecular genetic pathways involved (Guilmatre et al., 2009). A recent study by Joshi et al. (2010) of 217 consecutive referrals to a psychopharmacology clinic found a high (20%) rate of comorbid ASD and psychosis, but caution is required in interpretation, as this sample comprised individuals referred for psychiatric care. Nevertheless, several recent reports have highlighted overlap between the autism and schizophrenia spectra (Hallerback, Lugnegard, & Gillberg, 2012; Rapoport, Chavez, Greenstein, Addington, & Gogtay, 2009). King and Lord (2011) suggest that the relationship between them, previously assumed to be "nonoverlapping and incompatible," may need to be reconsidered through careful prospective follow-up studies.

Diagnostic Criteria and Symptom Expression

Psychotic disorders in DSM-5 include schizophrenia and the schizophrenia spectrum disorders, such as schizoaffective disorder, schizophreniform disorder, delusional disorder, catatonia, brief psychotic disorder, and schizotypal personality disorder. Symptoms and duration vary from condition to condition, but core symptoms include positive symptoms (e.g., delusions, hallucinations, disorganized speech and thought) and negative symptoms (e.g., alogia, flat affect, avolition, asociality; American Psychiatric Association, 2013). Differential diagnosis of the two conditions is often straightforward, relying heavily on the developmental history, age of onset, and specific form of symptoms. Individuals with ASD rarely display positive symptoms of psychosis (Konstantareas & Hewitt, 2001), such as delusions and hallucinations, and when these are present in the context of ASD, it is clear that a comorbid diagnosis of a psychotic disorder is warranted. However, for examiners unfamiliar with ASD, there are superficial similarities between ASD and psychosis that might make comorbidity seem more common than it is (Dossetor, 2007) and lead to misdiagnosis (Van Schalkwyk, Peluso, Qayyum, McPartland, & Volkmar, 2015). The pragmatic language abnormalities in ASD (including poor topic maintenance and reciprocity) may present like thought disorder, the highly focused interests may present like delusions, the unusual sensory interests or sensitivities may appear superficially similar to hallucinations, and the poor social judgment and theory-of-mind skills may present in a manner similar to paranoia. Moreover, lack of motivation and independent initiation of activities can be mistaken for the negative symptoms of schizophrenia (e.g., avolition; Lainhart, 1999).

An additional challenging differential exists between conditions at the boundaries of both the autism spectrum and the schizophrenia spectrum, where there may be true overlap of symptoms. Specifically, the prodrome of schizophrenia may include features that are part of the clinical picture of ASD (Dossetor, 2007; Hallerback et al., 2012). Both groups may present with ritualistic behaviors, unusual verbalizations, affective flattening, and social withdrawal. Consistent with this, studies of children with childhood-onset schizophrenia find a high percentage with a previous diagnosis of ASD (Rapoport et al., 2009; Sporn et al., 2004). At present, it is not clear whether this indicates that ASD can be a risk factor for later development of psychosis, whether the diagnostic criteria are sufficiently broad to encompass heterogeneous clinical presentations that are consistent with both the autism spectrum and the emerging schizophrenia spectrum, or whether shared biologic pathways lead to shared phenotypes. Future research is clearly needed in this emerging and exciting area.

USEFUL INSTRUMENTS FOR ASSESSMENT OF PSYCHIATRIC COMORBIDITIES IN ASD

In this section, we first discuss broad based instruments that measure several different areas of psychopathology, and then present specific tools that may be useful for particular comorbid conditions. In each section, we begin with instruments that have already been used with the ASD population in published studies; we then suggest other measures that may be useful because of certain attributes of each instrument, but have not yet been used in published studies with individuals on the autism spectrum.

General Measures of Psychopathology

The Achenbach System of Empirically Based Assessment (ASEBA) evaluates behavior across the lifespan and includes forms for reporting by the self, parents, and teachers (Achenbach, 2009). It measures symptoms of depression and anxiety, somatic complaints, obsessive–compulsive behaviors, attention problems, social difficulties, aggressive behavior, and atypicalities in thinking. The version for young children ages 1½–5 years also provides diagnostic information specifically related to ASD. Although the developers of the ASEBA did not specifically include children with ASD in their normative sample, its measures have been used in ASD research. Two studies demonstrated that the Child Behavior Checklist (CBCL), the ASEBA's caregiver report form for school-age children, can be used to differentiate ASD from other psychiatric conditions (Duarte, Bordin, de Oliveira, & Bird, 2003; Petersen, Bilenberg, Hoerder, & Gillberg, 2006). Of more relevance to this chapter, the CBCL is also used frequently to study comorbid psychiatric conditions in ASD (e.g., Lohr et al., 2017; Mansour, Dovi, Lane, Loveland, & Pearson, 2017; Stratis & Lecavalier, 2017; Vaillancourt et al., 2017).

The Behavior Assessment System for Children, Third Edition (BASC-3; Reynolds & Kamphaus, 2015) has also been used in children with ASD. Similar to the ASEBA, the BASC-3 evaluates symptoms related to major depressive disorder, generalized anxiety disorder, ADHD, behavior disorders, psychosis, and tic disorders. It also provides clinical information specific to ASD. The BASC-3 can be completed by parents, teachers, or the self. Lindner and Rosén (2006) found that children with ASD had a distinct parent-reported profile on the original BASC—with high scores on the Atypicality and Withdrawn scales, and low scores on Social Skills—when compared with children with other conditions or typical development. Although we have cautioned against high reliance on self-report measures with children with ASD, the BASC-3 self-report form for ages 6–7 (Reynolds & Kamphaus, 2015) may be appropriate to use, as the simple response format (i.e., yes/no answers) is more concrete than the Likert-type scales often used on other self-report forms.

The Aberrant Behavior Checklist—Community (ABC–Community; Aman & Singh, 1994) is a 58-item behavior checklist completed by parents, teachers, or clinicians to evaluate problem behaviors in the past 4 weeks. It was initially designed for use with adults in an institutionalized setting, but was later revised for individuals ages 6 years and older residing in the community. The ABC–Community includes five subscales: Irritability, Socially Withdrawn Behavior and Lethargy, Stereotyped Behavior, Hyperactivity and Noncompliance, and Inappropriate Speech Patterns. The factor structure is similar in ASD samples (Brinkley et al., 2007), and it has been utilized in a number of studies, often as a measure of inclusion or change in clinical trials (Akhondzadeh et al., 2004; King et al., 2001; Linday, Tsiouris, Cohen, Shindledecker, & DeCresce, 2001; Sponheim, Oftedal, & Helverschou, 2002). The Irritability subscale in particular is often used to identify patients with elevated symptoms needing psychopharmacological intervention (Arnold et al., 2000).

The Nisonger Child Behavior Rating Form (NCBRF; Aman, Tasse, Rojahn, & Hammer, 1996) is a parent and teacher rating form that was developed to use with children with developmental disabilities. It evaluates symptoms associated with depression, mania, anxiety, behavioral noncompliance, self-injury, ADHD, and tic disorders. It has 66 items rated on a 4-point scale, grouped into six subscales: Conduct Problems, Insecure/Anxious, Hyperactive, Self-Isolated/Ritualistic, Self-Injury/Stereotypic, and Overly Sensitive (parent version) or Irritable (teacher version). It has been used in a large community sample of children with ASD, with findings of elevated irritability, temper tantrums, and depressive symptoms (Lecavalier, 2006). It has also been used, along with the ABC–Community, to evaluate symptom improvement in a clinical trial of risperidone (Shea et al., 2004).

The Schedule for Affective Disorders and Schizophrenia for School-Age Children—Present and Lifetime Version (KSADS-PL 2013) is considered the gold standard in evaluating psychiatric disorders in childhood and adolescence (Kaufman et al., 1997, 2013). The current edition, adapted for use with DSM-5, consists of a 2- to 3-hour parent and child interview. It initially screens for a number of disorders, including major depression, bipolar disorder, anxiety disorders, ADHD, tic disorders, and psychotic disorders, and now includes a section on assessing core symptoms of ASD. Once screening is completed, the KSADS-PL 2013 follows up on specific issues to clarify clinical diagnoses. The ASD section suggests that greater weight should be given to parent report and clinical observation, due to limitations in insight in individuals with ASD. It also suggests that the examiner take into account whether other psychiatric disorders can better account for symptoms presented.

The Autism Comorbidity Interview—Present and Lifetime Version (ACI-PL; Leyfer et al., 2006) is another measure that can be used to assess the presence of additional psychiatric disorders. Unlike the KSADS-PL 2013, the ACI-PL is conducted via parent interview only. It has been shown to have excellent psychometric properties (Leyfer et al., 2006). It was adapted for use with the ASD population in several ways: There is an emphasis on examining baseline behavior and changes from baseline that might signal the onset of another psychiatric condition, there is explicit acknowledgment of the ways in which symptom manifestation may be different in ASD, and certain symptoms that may require specific cognitive capacities not found in some children with ASD (e.g., guilt) are probed only if a child is capable of demonstrating such symptoms.

Version IV of the Diagnostic Interview Schedule for Children (DISC-IV; Fisher, Lucas, Lucas, Sarsfield, & Shaffer, 2006; Shaffer, Fisher, Lucas, Dulcan, & Schwab-Stone, 2000) evaluates a range of diagnostic conditions in childhood, including mood and anxiety disorders, ADHD, tic disorders, and psychosis by directly interviewing the parent (DISC-IV-P for parents of children ages 6–17) and/or the child (DISC-IV-Y for children ages 9–17). Both traditional paper and computer (C-DISC) administration formats are available. There are few open-ended responses, with most responses limited to "yes," "no," "sometimes," or "somewhat." Muris, Steerneman, Merckelbach, Holdrinet, and Meesters (1998), using an earlier version of the DISC, found high rates of anxiety symptoms in ASD. The DISC has not yet been adapted for DSM-5.

A very useful tool for rapid screening for a variety of forms of psychopathology is the Child and Adolescent Symptom Inventory (CASI), currently in its fifth edition (Gadow & Sprafkin, 2013). It is one of only a few instruments available at the writing of this chapter that has been updated with DSM-5 criteria. Screening cutoffs are provided for all the major DSM-5 conditions that can appear in childhood and adolescence (e.g., ASD, ADHD, oppositional defiant disorder, anxiety and mood disorders, tic disorders, etc.), including all those discussed in this chapter. Separate scoring and norms are provided for school-age children (5–12 years) and adolescents (12–18 years). Several studies of children with ASD have used the CASI to examine psychiatric comorbidities (Bitsika & Sharpley, 2017; Gadow et al., 2005; Hallett, Lecavalier, et al., 2013; Kaat et al., 2013; Lerner, De Los Reyes, Drabick, Gerber, & Gadow, 2017).

Specific Measures of Psychopathology

In addition to the general measures of psychopathology just reviewed, a few instruments focus on specific forms of psychiatric disorders and have been used successfully with individuals on the autism spectrum.

Depression

The Children's Depression Inventory—Second Edition (CDI-2; Kovacs, 2012) taps into five key areas of depression: negative mood, interpretation problems, ineffectiveness, anhedonia, and negative self-esteem. Hedley and Young (2006) used the original CDI to examine depressive symptoms in children with Asperger's disorder. The original version of the CDI was also used to assess mood issues before and after treatment in children ages 8–12 years participating in a social skills group (Solomon, Goodlin-Jones, & Anders, 2004). Although the format of the CDI-2 is self-report, it seems less challenging for children to answer than other self-report instruments, because it provides concrete examples of abstract concepts. It also allows a clinician to read the items (if necessary) to a child while the child follows along.

Obsessive–Compulsive Disorder

The various versions of the Yale–Brown Obsessive Compulsive Scale (Goodman et al., 1989; Scahill et al., 1997)—including a form specifically for children on the autism spectrum, the Children's Yale–Brown Obsessive Compulsive Scale for Pervasive Developmental Disorders (CYBOCS-PDD; McDougle et al., 2005; Scahill et al., 2006)—have been used widely. Children ages 6 and over and their parents are interviewed in a semistructured fashion to evaluate a range of possible OCD phenomena, including symptoms related to contamination, aggression, hoarding/saving, magical thoughts/superstitions, and possible obsessive thoughts (somatic, religious, and other). Symptoms are rated on a scale from "none" to "extremely problematic" in terms of time spent, level of distress, resistance, interference with functioning, and degree of control. The CYBOCS-PDD has an additional five-item severity scale for repetitive and ritualistic behaviors, which helps determine whether symptom clusters are more closely associated with OCD or with ASD. For this reason, it is a promising instrument for making this difficult differential diagnosis.

Attention-Deficit/Hyperactivity Disorder

A number of widely used instruments exist that were designed specifically to assess symptoms of ADHD. Some, such as the Conners' Rating Scales, have been used successfully with children on the autism spectrum (Mansour et al., 2017; Posey et al., 2006). See Chapter 9, this volume, for more information about instruments useful in the assessment of ADHD in ASD.

Tic Disorders

The Yale Global Tic Severity Scale is a semistructured interview that collects information from both parents and children on number, frequency, intensity, complexity, and interference of vocal and motor tics (Leckman et al., 1989). It has been used to evaluate tics in a pediatric ASD sample, with ratings based primarily on parent report and clinical observation, due to limited language and self-reporting skills in the children (Canitano & Vivanti, 2007).

Psychosis

The Brief Psychiatric Rating Scale (BPRS; Ventura, Green, Shaner, & Liberman, 1993), the child version of the BPRS (Lachar et al., 2001), the Scale for the Assessment of Negative Symptoms (SANS; Andreasen, 1984a), and the Positive and Negative Syndrome Scale (PANSS; Kay, Opler, & Fiszbein, 1992) all involve conducting an interview with the patient and the patient's family members/caregivers to evaluate a range of positive and negative symptoms. The SANS, PANSS, and BPRS were used in one clinical trial of children with Asperger's disorder (Rausch et al., 2005) to measure change in negative symptoms (e.g., social withdrawal, affective flattening, and avolition) after treatment with risperidone. The SANS, along with the Scale for the Assessment of Positive Symptoms (SAPS; Andreasen, 1984b) and measures of ASD symptomatology, were helpful in differential diagnosis of psychosis and ASD in another study (Konstantareas & Hewitt, 2001). The Rorschach (Exner, 1986) has been used to examine thought disorder-like symptoms in individuals with ASD (Dykens, Volkmar, & Glick, 1991)—however, it is not recommended for differential diagnosis, given the elevated scores that may be produced by the pragmatic language impairments of ASD. In our opinion, the differential diagnosis of ASD and schizophrenia is best made on the basis of the presence of positive symptoms, since superficial similarities between core symptoms of ASD and negative symptoms of schizophrenia may cause individuals with ASD to score high on measures of negative symptoms.

CONCLUDING REMARKS

Evaluation of comorbidity in ASD challenges the best of clinicians. Functioning is already impaired in individuals with ASD, meaning that a change in behavior may have to be marked to be identifiable (Ozonoff, Goodlin-Jones, & Solomon, 2005). Teasing out core symptoms of ASD from other conditions is a complex matter, for several reasons: the fact that many assessment tools have not been standardized on the population with ASD, the limitations of insight in this population, and the need for reliance on observation and parent/caregiver report. Selection artifacts were likely in many of the studies cited in this chapter, as most used clinically ascertained samples that may well have had higher rates of comorbidity than unselected community-based samples of individuals with ASD. Clinicians must remember that apparent comorbidity may arise from overlapping criteria, artificial subdivision of syndromes, or that one disorder may represent an early manifestation of another disorder (Caron & Rutter, 1991). Care must be taken not to overdiagnose comorbidity. Conversely, it is likely that many instances of true comorbidity are missed, resulting in undertreatment or only partial treatment of the individual's difficulties. Emotional and behavioral problems influence family functioning, impacting levels of parental stress (Herring et al., 2006). With research demonstrating the efficacy of both behavioral and psychopharmacological interventions for psychiatric disorders seen in individuals with ASD (e.g., Fung et al., 2016; Reaven, Blakeley-Smith, Culhane-Shelburne, & Hepburn, 2012; Santomauro, Sheffield, & Sofronoff, 2016), it is critically important to identify and treat additional behavioral or emotional issues. DSM-5 embraces the fact that it is not uncommon for children with ASD to have co-occurring conditions and no longer considers certain diagnoses as exclusion criteria for ASD (e.g., psychosis, ADHD). Measurement remains a central issue, given both the limited normative data and the inadequacies of measurement formats for people on the autism spectrum. Difficulties with insight and self-report are coupled with the inherent difficulty of truly understanding the internal emotional experience of someone else. The development of better methods of assessing comorbid symptoms in an "ASD-friendly" manner is needed. Self-report measures might be administered along with picture cards presenting specific, easy-to-identify emotions (such as the Webber Photo Cards for Emotions; Webber, 2005). Such changes from standardized administration need to be studied, to examine the validity and reliability of the assessment process.

Better understanding of comorbid presentations in ASD may also improve our knowledge of the causes of ASD and etiological heterogeneities (Leyfer et al., 2006). Children who demonstrate multiple disorders may represent subtypes that should be studied separately. Conditions that commonly co-occur may provide clues about shared risk factors or shared underlying neuropathological processes.

It is our hope in writing this chapter that accurate identification of the primary and/or secondary problems that affect the functioning of individuals with ASD will result in improved treatment planning and treatment outcomes. Given the complexities detailed in this chapter, it is clear that additional training and expertise in both traditional mental health conditions and neurodevelopmental disorders are critical in providing the best clinical care possible.

REFERENCES

Abdallah, M. W., Greaves-Lord, K., Grove, J., Nørgaard-Pedersen, B., Hougaard, D. M., & Mortensen, E. L. (2011). Psychiatric comorbidities in autism spectrum disorders: Findings from a Danish Historic Birth Cohort. *European Child and Adolescent Psychiatry, 20*(11–12), 599–601.

Achenbach, T. M.(2009). *The Achenbach System of Empirically Based Assessment (ASEBA)*. Burlington: University of Vermont, Research Center for Children, Youth, and Families.

Akhondzadeh, S., Erfani, S., Mohammadi, M. R., Tehrani-Doost, M., Amini, H., Gudarzi, S. S., et al. (2004). Cyproheptadine in the treatment of autistic disorder: A double-blind placebo-controlled trial. *Journal of Clinical Pharmacy and Therapeutics, 29*(2), 145–150.

Aman, M. G., & Singh, N. N. (1994). *Aberrant Behavior Checklist—Community*. East Aurora, NY: Slosson.

Aman, M. G., Tasse, M. J., Rojahn, J., & Hammer, D. (1996). The Nisonger CBRF: A child behavior rating form for children with developmental disabilities. *Research in Developmental Disabilities, 17*, 41–57.

American Psychiatric Association. (2000). *Diagnostic and statistical manual of mental disorders* (4th ed., text rev.). Washington, DC: Author.

American Psychiatric Association. (2013). *Diagnostic and statistical manual of mental disorders* (5th ed.). Arlington, VA: Author.

Andreasen, N. C. (1984a). *Scale for the Assessment of Negative Symptoms (SANS)*. Iowa City: University of Iowa.

Andreasen, N. C. (1984b). *Scale for the Assessment of Positive Symptoms (SAPS)*. Iowa City: University of Iowa.

Angold, A., Erkanli, A., Costello, E. J., & Rutter, M. (1996). Precision, reliability and accuracy in the dating of symptom onsets in child and adolescent psychopathology. *Journal of Child Psychology and Psychiatry, 37*(6), 657–664.

Arnold, L. E., Aman, M. G., Martin, A., Collier-Crespin, A., Vitiello, B., Tierney, E., et al. (2000). Assessment in multisite randomized clinical trials of patients with autistic disorder: The Autism RUPP Network. *Journal of Autism and Developmental Disorders, 30*, 99–111.

Baron-Cohen, S., Mortimore, C., Moriarty, J., Izaguirre, J., & Robertson, M. (1999). The prevalence of Gilles de la Tourette's syndrome in children and adolescents with autism. *Journal of Child Psychology and Psychiatry, 40*(2), 213–218.

Baron-Cohen, S., O'Riordan, M., Stone, V., Jones, R., & Plaisted, K. (1999). Recognition of faux pas by normally developing children and children with Asperger syndrome or high-functioning autism. *Journal of Autism and Developmental Disorders, 29*(5), 407–418.

Baron-Cohen, S., Tager-Flusberg, H., & Cohen, D. (2000). *Understanding other minds: Perspectives from developmental cognitive neuroscience*. New York: Oxford University Press.

Bejerot, S. (2007). An autistic dimension: A proposed subtype of obsessive–compulsive disorder. *Autism, 11*, 101–110.

Ben Shalom, D., Mostofsky, S. H., Hazlett, R. L., Goldberg, M. C., Landa, R. J., Faran, Y., et al. (2006). Normal physiological emotions but differences in expression of conscious feelings in children with high-functioning autism. *Journal of Autism and Developmental Disorders, 36*(3), 395–400.

Berthoz, S., & Hill, E. L. (2005). The validity of using self-reports to assess emotion regulation abilities in adults with autism spectrum disorder. *European Psychiatry, 20*(3), 291–298.

Bitsika, V., & Sharpley, C. F. (2017). The association between parents' ratings of ASD symptoms and anxiety in a sample of high-functioning boys and adolescents with autism spectrum disorder. *Research in Developmental Disabilities, 63*, 38–45.

Blackshaw, A. J., Kinderman, P., Hare, D. J., & Hatton, C. (2001). Theory of mind, causal attribution and paranoia in Asperger syndrome. *Autism, 5*(2), 147–163.

Blumberg, S. J., Zablotsky, B., Avila, R. M., Colpe, L. J., Pringle, B. A., & Kogan, M. D. (2016). Diagnosis lost: Differences between children who had and who currently have an autism spectrum disorder diagnosis. *Autism, 20*(7), 783–795.

Bolton, P. F., Pickles, A., Murphy, M., & Rutter, M. (1998). Autism, affective and other psychiatric disorders: Patterns of familial aggregation. *Psychological Medicine, 28*(2), 385–395.

Brereton, A. V., Tonge, B. J., & Einfeld, S. L. (2006). Psychopathology in children and adolescents with autism compared to young people with intellectual disability. *Journal of Autism and Developmental Disorders, 36*(7), 863–870.

Brinkley, J., Nations, L., Abramson, R. K., Hall, A., Wright, H. H., Gabriels, R., et al. (2007). Factor analysis of the Aberrant Behavior Checklist in individuals with autism spectrum disorders. *Journal of Autism and Developmental Disorders, 37*(10), 1949–1959.

Burd, L., Fisher, W. W., Kerbeshian, J., & Arnold, M. E. (1987). Is development of Tourette disorder a marker for improvement in patients with autism and other pervasive developmental disorders? *Journal of the American Academy of Child and Adolescent Psychiatry, 26*(2), 162–165.

Canitano, R., & Vivanti, G. (2007). Tics and Tourette syndrome in autism spectrum disorders. *Autism, 11*(1), 19–28.

Caron, C., & Rutter, M. (1991). Comorbidity in child psychopathology: Concepts, issues and research strategies. *Journal of Child Psychology and Psychiatry, 32*(7), 1063–1080.

Close, H. A., Lee, L. C., Kaufmann, C. N., & Zimmerman, A. W. (2012). Co-occurring conditions and change in diagnosis in autism spectrum disorders. *Pediatrics, 129*(2), e305–e316.

Costello, E. J., Foley, D. L., & Angold, A. (2006). 10-year research update review: The epidemiology of child and adolescent psychiatric disorders: II. Developmental epidemiology. *Journal of the American Academy of Child and Adolescent Psychiatry, 45*(1), 8–25.

Craig, F., Lamanna, A. L., Margari, F., Matera, E., Simone, M., & Margari, L. (2015). Overlap between autism spectrum disorders and attention deficit hyperactivity disorder: Searching for distinctive/common clinical features. *Autism Research, 8*(3), 328–337.

Derogatis, L. R. (1983). *Symptom Checklist 90—Revised (SCL-90-R)*. Minneapolis, MN: National Computer Systems.

Dossetor, D. R. (2007). "All that glitters is not gold": Misdiagnosis of psychosis in pervasive developmental disorders—a case series. *Clinical Child Psychology and Psychiatry, 12*, 537–548.

Duarte, C. S., Bordin, I. A., de Oliveira, A., & Bird, H. (2003). The CBCL and the identification of children with autism and related conditions in Brazil: Pilot findings. *Journal of Autism and Developmental Disorders, 33*(6), 703–707.

Dykens, E., Volkmar, F., & Glick, M. (1991). Thought disorder in high-functioning autistic adults. *Journal of Autism and Developmental Disorders, 21*(3), 291–301.

Evans, D. W., Canavera, K., Kleinpeter, F. L., Maccubbin, E., & Taga, K. (2005). The fears, phobias and anxieties of children with autism spectrum disorders and Down syndrome: Comparisons with developmentally and chronologically age matched children. *Child Psychiatry and Human Development, 36*(1), 3–26.

Exner, J. (1986). *The Rorschach: A comprehensive system.* New York: Wiley-Interscience.

Fein, D., Dixon, P., Paul, J., & Levin, H. (2005). Pervasive developmental disorder can evolve into ADHD: Case illustrations. *Journal of Autism and Developmental Disorders, 35*(4), 525–534.

Fisher, P., Lucas, L., Lucas, C., Sarsfield, A., & Shaffer, D. (2006). *DISC Interview manual.* New York: Columbia University, DISC Development Group.

Fung, L. K., Mahajan, R., Nozzolillo, A., Bernal, P., Krasner, A., Jo, B., et al. (2016). Pharmacologic treatment of severe irritability and problem behaviors in autism: A systematic review and meta-analysis. *Pediatrics, 137*(Suppl. 2), S124–S135.

Gadow, K. D., DeVincent, C. J., Pomeroy, J., & Azizian, A. (2005). Comparison of DSM-IV symptoms in elementary school-age children with PDD versus clinic and community samples. *Autism, 9*(4), 392–415.

Gadow, K. D., Guttmann-Steinmetz, S., Rieffe, C., & DeVincent, C. J. (2012). Depression symptoms in boys with autism spectrum disorders and comparison samples. *Journal of Autism and Developmental Disorders, 42,* 1353–1363.

Gadow, K. D., & Sprafkin, J. (2013). *Child and Adolescent Symptom Inventory–5.* Stony Brook, NY: Checkmate Plus.

Gargaro, B. A., Rinehart, N. J., Bradshaw, J. L., Tonge, B. J., & Sheppard, D. M. (2011). Autism and ADHD: How far have we come in the comorbidity debate? *Neuroscience and Biobehavioral Reviews, 35*(5), 1081–1088.

Ghaziuddin, M., Ghaziuddin, N., & Greden, J. (2002). Depression in persons with autism: Implications for research and clinical care. *Journal of Autism and Developmental Disorders, 32*(4), 299–306.

Ghaziuddin, M., & Greden, J. (1998). Depression in children with autism/pervasive developmental disorders: A case-control family history study. *Journal of Autism and Developmental Disorders, 28*(2), 111–115.

Gjevik, E., Eldevik, S., Fjæran-Granum, T., & Sponheim, E. (2011). Kiddie-SADS reveals high rates of DSM–IV disorders in children and adolescents. *Journal of Autism and Developmental Disorders, 41,* 761–769.

Goldstein, S., & Schwebach, A. J. (2004). The comorbidity of pervasive developmental disorder and attention deficit hyperactivity disorder: Results of a retrospective chart review. *Journal of Autism and Developmental Disorders, 34*(3), 329–339.

Goodman, W. K., Price, L. H., Rasmussen, S. A., Mazure, C., Fleischmann, R. L., Hill, C. L., et al. (1989). The Yale–Brown Obsessive Compulsive Scale: I. Development, use, and reliability. *Archives of General Psychiatry, 46*(11), 1006–1011.

Grzadzinski, R., Dick, C., Lord, C., & Bishop, S. (2016). Parent-reported and clinician-observed autism spectrum disorder symptoms in children with attention deficit/hyperactivity disorder: Implications for practice under DSM-5. *Molecular Autism, 7*(1), 7.

Guilmatre, A., Dubourg, C., Mosca, A. L., Legallic, S., Goldenberg, A., Drouin-Garraud, V., et al. (2009). Recurrent rearrangements in synaptic and neurodevelopmental genes and shared biologic pathways in schizophrenia, autism, and mental retardation. *Archives of General Psychiatry, 66*(9), 947–956.

Hallerback, M. U., Lugnegard, T., & Gillberg, C. (2012). Is autism spectrum disorder common in schizophrenia? *Psychiatry Research, 198,* 12–17.

Hallett, V., Lecavalier, L., Sukhodolsky, D. G., Cipriano, N., Aman, M. G., McCracken,

J. T., et al. (2013). Exploring the manifestations of anxiety in children with autism spectrum disorders. *Journal of Autism and Developmental Disorders, 43*(10), 2341–2352.

Hallett, V., Ronald, A., Colvert, E., Ames, C., Woodhouse, E., Lietz, S., et al. (2013). Exploring anxiety symptoms in a large-scale twin study of children with autism spectrum disorders, their co-twins and controls. *Journal of Child Psychology and Psychiatry, 54*(11), 1176–1185.

Hanson, E., Cerban, B. M., Slater, C. M., Caccamo, L. M., Bacic, J., & Chan, E. (2013). Prevalence of attention/deficit hyperactivity disorder among individuals with an autism spectrum disorder. *Journal of Autism and Developmental Disorders, 43(*6), 1459–1464.

Happé, F. (1991). The autobiographical writings of three Asperger syndrome adults: Problems of interpretation and implications for theory. In U. Frith (Ed.), *Autism and Asperger syndrome* (pp. 207–242). New York: Cambridge University Press.

Harvey, E. A., Lugo-Candelas, C. I., & Breaux, R. P. (2015). Longitudinal changes in individual symptoms across the preschool years in children with ADHD. *Journal of Clinical Child and Adolescent Psychology, 44,* 580–594.

Hedley, D., & Young, R. (2006). Social comparison processes and depressive symptoms in children and adolescents with Asperger syndrome. *Autism, 10*(2), 139–153.

Herring, S., Gray, K., Taffe, J., Tonge, B., Sweeney, D., & Einfeld, S. (2006). Behaviour and emotional problems in toddlers with pervasive developmental disorders and developmental delay: Associations with parental mental health and family functioning. *Journal of Intellectual Disability Research, 50*(Pt. 12), 874–882.

Hill, E., Berthoz, S., & Frith, U. (2004). Brief report: Cognitive processing of own emotions in individuals with autistic spectrum disorder and in their relatives. *Journal of Autism and Developmental Disorders, 34*(2), 229–235.

Hofvander, B., Delorme, R., Chaste, P., Nyden, A., Wentz, E., Stahlberg, O., et al. (2009). Psychiatric and psychosocial problems in adults with normal-intelligence autism spectrum disorders. *BMC Psychiatry, 9,* 35–44.

Jankovic, J. (1997). Tourette syndrome: Phenomenology and classification of tics. *Neurologic Clinics, 15*(2), 267–275.

Jolliffe, T., & Baron-Cohen, S. (1999). The Strange Stories Test: A replication with high-functioning adults with autism or Asperger syndrome. *Journal of Autism and Developmental Disorders, 29*(5), 395–406.

Joshi, G., Biederman, J., Petty, C., Goldin, R. L., Furtak, S. L., & Wozniak, J. (2012). Examining the comorbidity of bipolar disorder and autism spectrum disorders: A large controlled analysis of phenotypic and familial correlates in a referred population of youth with bipolar I disorder with and without autism spectrum disorders. *Journal of Clinical Psychiatry, 74*(6), 578–586.

Joshi, G., Petty, C., Wozniak, J., Henin, A., Fried, R., Galdo, M., et al. (2010). The heavy burden of psychiatric comorbidity in youth with autism spectrum disorders: A large comparative study of a psychiatrically referred population. *Journal of Autism and Developmental Disorders, 40*(11), 1361–1370.

Kaat, A. J., Gadow, K. D., & Lecavalier, L. (2013). Psychiatric symptom impairment in children with autism spectrum disorders. *Journal of Abnormal Child Psychology, 41,* 959–969.

Kaufman, J., Birmaher, B., Axelson, D., Percpletchikova, F., Brent, D., & Ryan, N. (2013). *K-SADS-PL 2013.* Unpublished manual, Western Psychiatric Institute and Clinic, Pittsburgh, PA.

Kaufman, J., Birmaher, B., Brent, D., Rao, U., Flynn, C., Moreci, P., et al. (1997). Schedule for Affective Disorders and Schizophrenia for School-Age Children—Present and Lifetime Version (K-SADS-PL): Initial reliability and validity data. *Journal of the American Academy of Child and Adolescent Psychiatry, 36*(7), 980–988.

Kay, S. R., Opler, L. A., & Fiszbein, A. (1992). *Positive and Negative Syndrome Scale (PANSS).* Toronto, ON, Canada: Multi-Health Systems.

Kazdin, A. E. (1993). Replication and extension of behavioral treatment of autistic disorder. *American Journal of Mental Retardation, 97,* 377–378.

Kessler, R. C., Petukhova, M., Sampson, N. A., Zaslavsky, A. M., & Wittchen, H. U. (2012). Twelve-month and lifetime prevalence and lifetime morbid risk of anxiety and mood disorders in the United States. *International Journal of Methods in Psychiatric Research, 21*(3), 169–184.

King, B. H., & Lord, C. (2011). Is schizophrenia on the autism spectrum? *Brain Research, 1380,* 34–41.

King, B. H., Wright, D. M., Handen, B. L., Sikich, L., Zimmerman, A. W., McMahon, W., et al. (2001). Double-blind, placebo-controlled study of amantadine hydrochloride in the treatment of children with autistic disorder. *Journal of the American Academy of Child and Adolescent Psychiatry, 40*(6), 658–665.

Klein, S. B., Chan., R. L., & Loftus, J. (1999). Independence of episodic and semantic self-knowledge: The case from autism. *Social Cognition, 17,* 413–436.

Knight, T., Steeves, T., Day, L., Lowerison, M., Jette, N., & Pringsheim, T. (2012). Prevalence of tic disorders: A systematic review and meta-analysis. *Pediatric Neurology, 47,* 77–90.

Konstantareas, M. M., & Hewitt, T. (2001). Autistic disorder and schizophrenia: Diagnostic overlaps. *Journal of Autism and Developmental Disorders, 31*(1), 19–28.

Kovacs, M. (2012). *Children's Depression Inventory—Second Edition (CDI-2).* North Tonawanda, NY: Multi-Health Systems.

Krueger, R. F., & Markon, K. E. (2006). Reinterpreting comorbidity: A model-based approach to understanding and classifying psychopathology. *Annual Review of Clinical Psychology, 2,* 111–133.

Lachar, D., Randle, S. L., Harper, R. A., Scott-Gurnell, K. C., Lewis, K. R., Santos, C. W., et al. (2001). The Brief Psychiatric Rating Scale for Children (BPRS-C): Validity and reliability of an anchored version. *Journal of the American Academy of Child and Adolescent Psychiatry, 40*(3), 333–340.

Lainhart, J. E. (1999). Psychiatric problems in individuals with autism, their parents and siblings. *International Review of Psychiatry, 11,* 278–298.

Lainhart, J. E., & Folstein, S. E. (1994). Affective disorders in people with autism: A review of published cases. *Journal of Autism and Developmental Disorders, 24,* 587–601.

Lecavalier, L. (2006). Behavioral and emotional problems in young people with pervasive developmental disorders: Relative prevalence, effects of subject characteristics, and empirical classification. *Journal of Autism and Developmental Disorders, 36*(8), 1101–1114.

Leckman, J. F., Riddle, M. A., Hardin, M. T., Ort, S. I., Swartz, K. L., Stevenson, J., et al. (1989). The Yale Global Tic Severity Scale: Initial testing of a clinician-rated scale of tic severity. *Journal of the American Academy of Child and Adolescent Psychiatry, 28*(4), 566–573.

Lerner, M. D., De Los Reyes, A., Drabick, D. A. G., Gerber, A. H., & Gadow, K. D.

(2017). Informant discrepancy defines discrete, clinically useful autism spectrum disorder subgroups. *Journal of Child Psychology and Psychiatry, 58*(7), 829–839.

Leyfer, O. T., Folstein, S. E., Bacalman, S., Davis, N. O., Dinh, E., Morgan, J., et al. (2006). Comorbid psychiatric disorders in children with autism: Interview development and rates of disorders. *Journal of Autism and Developmental Disorders, 36*(7), 849–861.

Linday, L. A., Tsiouris, J. A., Cohen, I. L., Shindledecker, R., & DeCresce, R. (2001). Famotidine treatment of children with autistic spectrum disorders: Pilot research using single subject research design. *Journal of Neural Transmission, 108*(5), 593–611.

Lindner, J. L., & Rosén, L. A. (2006). Decoding of emotion through facial expression, prosody and verbal content in children and adolescents with Asperger's syndrome. *Journal of Autism and Developmental Disorders, 36*(6), 769–777.

Lohr, W. D., Daniels, K., Wiemken, T., Williams, P. G., Kelley, R. R., Kuravackel, G., & Sears, L. (2017). The screen for child anxiety-related emotional disorders is sensitive but not specific in identifying anxiety in children with high-functioning autism spectrum disorder: A pilot comparison to the Achenbach System of Empirically Based Assessment Scales. *Frontiers of Psychiatry, 8,* 138.

Magnuson, K. M., & Constantino, J. N. (2011). Characterization of depression in children with autism spectrum disorders. *Journal of Developmental and Behavioral Pediatrics, 32*(4), 332.

Mansour, R., Dovi, A. T., Lane, D. M., Loveland, K. A., & Pearson, D. A. (2017). ADHD severity as it relates to comorbid psychiatric symptomatology in children with autism spectrum disorders. *Research in Developmental Disabilities, 60,* 52–64.

Matson, J. L., & Cervantes, P. E. (2014). Commonly studied comorbid psychopathologies among persons with autism spectrum disorder. *Research in Developmental Disabilities, 35,* 952–962.

Mayes, S. D., Calhoun, S. L., Murray, M. J., Ahuja, M., & Smith, L. A. (2011). Anxiety, depression, and irritability in children with autism relative to other neuropsychiatric disorders and typical development. *Research in Autism Spectrum Disorders, 5,* 474–485.

Mazefsky, C. A., Kao, J., & Oswald, D. P. (2011). Preliminary evidence suggesting caution in the use of psychiatric self-report measures with adolescents with high-functioning autism spectrum disorders. *Research in Autism Spectrum Disorders, 5,* 164–174.

Mazefsky, C. A., Oswald, D. P., Day, T. N., Each, S. M., Minshew, N. J., & Lainhart, J. E. (2012). ASD, a psychiatric disorder, or both?: Psychiatric diagnoses in adolescents with high-functioning ASD. *Journal of Clinical Child and Adolescent Psychology, 41*(4), 516–523.

McDougle, C. J., Scahill, L., Aman, M. G., McCracken, J. T., Tierney, E., Davies, M., et al. (2005). Risperidone for the core symptom domains of autism: Results from the study by the Autism Network of the Research Units on Pediatric Psychopharmacology. *American Journal of Psychiatry, 162*(6), 1142–1148.

Merikangas, K. R., He, J. P., Brody, D., Fisher, P. W., Bourdon, K., & Koretz, D. S. (2010). Prevalence and treatment of mental disorders among US children in the 2001–2004 NHANES. *Pediatrics, 125*(1), 75–81.

Miodovnik, A., Harstad, E., Sideridis, G., & Huntington, N. (2015). Timing of the diagnosis of attention-deficit/hyperactivity disorder and autism spectrum disorder. *Pediatrics, 136,* e830–e837.

Muris, P., Steerneman, P., Merckelbach, H., Holdrinet, I., & Meesters, C. (1998). Comorbid anxiety symptoms in children with pervasive developmental disorders. *Journal of Anxiety Disorders, 12*(4), 387–393.

Oyane, N. M., & Bjorvatn, B. (2005). Sleep disturbances in adolescents and young adults with autism and Asperger syndrome. *Autism, 9*(1), 83–94.

Ozonoff, S., Garcia, N., Clark, E., & Lainhart, J. E. (2005). MMPI-2 personality profiles of high-functioning adults with autism spectrum disorders. *Assessment, 12*(1), 86–95.

Ozonoff, S., Goodlin-Jones, B. L., & Solomon, M. (2005). Evidence-based assessment of autism spectrum disorders in children and adolescents. *Journal of Clinical Child and Adolescent Psychology, 34*(3), 523–540.

Petersen, D. J., Bilenberg, N., Hoerder, K., & Gillberg, C. (2006). The population prevalence of child psychiatric disorders in Danish 8- to 9-year-old children. *European Child and Adolescent Psychiatry, 15*(2), 71–78.

Piven, J., & Palmer, P. (1999). Psychiatric disorder and the broad autism phenotype: Evidence from a family study of multiple-incidence autism families. *American Journal of Psychiatry, 156*(4), 557–563.

Polimeni, M. A., Richdale, A. L., & Francis, A. J. (2005). A survey of sleep problems in autism, Asperger's disorder and typically developing children. *Journal of Intellectual Disability Research, 49*(Pt. 4), 260–268.

Posey, D. J., Wiegand, R. E., Wilkerson, J., Maynard, M., Stigler, K. A., & McDougle, C. J. (2006). Open-label atomoxetine for attention-deficit/hyperactivity disorder symptoms associated with high-functioning pervasive developmental disorders. *Journal of Child and Adolescent Psychopharmacology, 16*(5), 599–610.

Rapoport, J., Chavez, A., Greenstein, D., Addington, A., & Gogtay, N. (2009). Autism spectrum disorders and childhood-onset schizophrenia: Clinical and biological contributions to a relation revisited. *Journal of the American Academy of Child and Adolescent Psychiatry, 48,* 10–18.

Rausch, J. L., Sirota, E. L., Londino, D. L., Johnson, M. E., Carr, B. M., Bhatia, R., et al. (2005). Open-label risperidone for Asperger's disorder: Negative symptom spectrum response. *Journal of Clinical Psychiatry, 66*(12), 1592–1597.

Reaven, J., Blakely-Smith, A., Culhane-Shelburne, K., & Hepburn, S. (2012). Group cognitive behavior therapy for children with high-functioning autism spectrum disorders and anxiety: A randomized trial. *Journal of Child Psychology and Psychiatry, 53*(4), 410–419.

Regier, D. A., Narrow, W. E., Kuhl, E. A., & Kupfer, D. J. (2009). The conceptual development of DSM-5. *American Journal of Psychiatry, 166,* 645–650.

Reynolds, C. R., & Kamphaus, R. W. (2015). *Behavior Assessment System for Children, Third Edition (BASC-3) manual.* Bloomington, MN: NCS Pearson.

Santomauro, D., Sheffield, J., & Sofronoff, K. (2016). Depression in adolescents with ASD: A pilot RCT of a group intervention. *Journal of Autism and Developmental Disorders, 46*(2), 572–588.

Scahill, L., McDougle, C. J., Williams, S. K., Dimitropoulos, A., Aman, A. G., McCracken, J. T., et al. (2006). The Children's Yale–Brown Obsessive Compulsive Scales modified for pervasive developmental disorders. *Journal of the American Academy of Child and Adolescent Psychiatry, 45*(9), 1114–1123.

Scahill, L., Riddle, M. A., McSwiggin-Hardin, M., Ort, S. I., King, R. A., Goodman, W. K., et al. (1997). Children's Yale–Brown Obsessive Compulsive Scale: Reliability and validity. *Journal of the American Academy of Child and Adolescent Psychiatry, 36*(6), 844–852.

Shaffer, D., Fisher, P., Lucas, C. P., Dulcan, M. K., & Schwab-Stone, M. E. (2000). NIMH Diagnostic Interview Schedule for Children Version IV (NIMH DISC-IV): Description, differences from previous versions, and reliability of some common diagnoses. *Journal of the American Academy of Child and Adolescent Psychiatry, 39*(1), 28–38.

Shea, S., Turgay, A., Carroll, A., Schulz, M., Orlik, H., Smith, I., et al. (2004). Risperidone in the treatment of disruptive behavioral symptoms in children with autistic and other pervasive developmental disorders. *Pediatrics, 114*(5), 634–641.

Sicotte, C., & Stemberger, R. M. (1999). Do children with PDDNOS have a theory of mind? *Journal of Autism and Developmental Disorders, 29*(3), 225–233.

Simonoff, E., Pickles, A., Charman, T., Chandler, S., Loucas, T., & Baird, G. (2008). Psychiatric disorders in children with autism spectrum disorders: Prevalence, comorbidity, and associated factors in a population-derived sample. *Journal of the American Academy of Child and Adolescent Psychiatry, 47,* 921–929.

Solomon, M., Goodlin-Jones, B. L., & Anders, T. F. (2004). A social adjustment enhancement intervention for high functioning autism, Asperger's syndrome, and pervasive developmental disorder NOS. *Journal of Autism and Developmental Disorders, 34*(6), 649–668.

Sovner, R. (1996). Behavioral and affective disturbances in persons with mental retardation: A neuropsychiatric perspective. *Seminars in Clinical Neuropsychiatry, 1*(2), 90–93.

Spicer, D. (1998). Autistic and undiagnosed: A cautionary tale. In E. Schopler, G. B. Mesibov, & L. J. Kunce (Eds.), *Asperger syndrome or high-functioning autism?* (pp. 377–382). New York: Plenum Press.

Sponheim, E., Oftedal, G., & Helverschou, S. B. (2002). Multiple doses of secretin in the treatment of autism: A controlled study. *Acta Paediatrica, 91*(5), 540–545.

Sporn, A. L., Addington, A. M., Gogtay, N., Ordonez, A. E., Gornick, M., Clasen, L., et al. (2004). Pervasive developmental disorder and childhood-onset schizophrenia: Comorbid disorder or a phenotypic variant of a very early onset illness? *Biological Psychiatry, 55*(10), 989–994.

Stahlberg, O., Soderstrom, H., Rastam, M., & Gillberg, C. (2004). Bipolar disorder, schizophrenia, and other psychotic disorders in adults with childhood onset AD/HD and/or autism spectrum disorders. *Journal of Neural Transmission, 111*(7), 891–902.

Stewart, M. E., Barnard, L., Pearson, J., Hasan, R., & O'Brien, G. (2006). Presentation of depression in autism and Asperger syndrome: A review. *Autism, 10*(1), 103–116.

Stratis, E. A., & Lecavalier, L. (2017). Predictors of parent–teacher agreement in youth with autism spectrum disorder and their typically developing siblings. *Journal of Autism and Developmental Disorders, 47*(8), 2575–2585.

Tantum, D. (2003). The challenge of adolescents and adults with Asperger syndrome. *Child and Adolescent Psychiatric Clinics of North America, 12,* 143–163.

Vaillancourt, T., Haltigan, J. D., Smith, I., Zwaigenbaum, L., Szatmari, P., Fombonne, E., et al. (2017). Joint trajectories of internalizing and externalizing problems in preschool children with autism spectrum disorder. *Development and Psychopathology, 29*(1), 203–214.

Van Schalkwyk, G. I., Peluso, F., Qayyum, Z., McPartland, J. C., & Volkmar, F. R. (2015). Varieties of misdiagnosis in ASD: An illustrative case series. *Journal of Autism and Developmental Disorders, 45,* 911–918.

Vannucchi, G., Masi, G., Toni, C., Dell'Osso, L., Erfurth, A., & Perugi, G. (2014). Bipolar disorder in adults with Asperger's syndrome: A systematic review. *Journal of Affective Disorders, 168,* 151–160.

Ventura, M. A., Green, M. F., Shaner, A., & Liberman, R. P. (1993). Training and quality assurance with the Brief Psychiatric Rating Scale: "The drift buster." *International Journal of Methods in Psychiatric Research, 3,* 221–244.

Volkmar, F. R., & Cohen, D. J. (1991). Comorbid association of autism and schizophrenia. *American Journal of Psychiatry, 148*(12), 1705–1707.

Walters, A. S., Barrett, R. P., & Feinstein, C. (1990). Social relatedness and autism: Current research, issues, directions. *Research in Developmental Disabilities, 11*(3), 303–326.

Webber, S. (2005). *Webber Photo Cards: Emotions.* Greenville, SC: Super Duper.

Weisbrot, D. M., Gadow, K. D., DeVincent, C. J., & Pomeroy, J. (2005). The presentation of anxiety in children with pervasive developmental disorders. *Journal of Child and Adolescent Psychopharmacology, 15*(3), 477–496.

Wichstrøm, L., Berg-Nielsen, T. S., Angold, A., LinkEgger, H., Solheim, E., & HamreSveen, T. (2012). Prevalence of psychiatric disorders in preschoolers. *Journal of Child Psychology and Psychiatry, 53*(6), 695–705.

Wiggs, L., & Stores, G. (2004). Sleep patterns and sleep disorders in children with autistic spectrum disorders: Insights using parent report and actigraphy. *Developmental Medicine and Child Neurology, 46*(6), 372–380.

Worley, J. A., & Matson, J. L. (2011). Psychiatric symptoms in children diagnosed with autism spectrum disorder: An examination of gender differences. *Research in Autism Spectrum Disorders, 5,* 1086–1091.

CHAPTER ELEVEN

Assessment of Students with Autism Spectrum Disorder in the Schools

Sandra L. Harris
Carolyn Thorwarth Bruey
Mark Palmieri

The assessment of autism spectrum disorder (ASD) in the schools requires psychologists, behavior analysts, and other service providers to know not only the technical nuances of the specific assessment procedures but to possess a sophisticated understanding of how schools operate as systems, the pressure school administrators and educators find themselves under to offer empirically supported assessment, instructional methods for their students, and to demonstrate accountability of educational outcome based on these interventions. Effective leadership can motivate others in a school to contribute to a positive context for learning (Forman & Selman, 2011). For example, school climate can be established in a way that minimizes "bullying" behavior (Leadbeater, Sukhawathanakul, Smith, & Bowen, 2014).

Schools are complex places in which to operate because of the multiple demands the people working in them face from their many constituents—including students, parents, teachers, taxpayers, school board members, district superintendents, state education officials, and state and national legislators. The child study team that assesses the needs of a student with ASD for special services in the public schools should understand not only the needs of the child with ASD but the educational system and community in which that child is to be served.

The current chapter introduces the reader to some of the issues faced by individuals in schools, by schools as systems, and by schools within their larger social systemic context. We also consider the need for empirically supported assessment and intervention methods to educate students with ASD in schools. The chapter describes the psychological assessment methods currently being employed in a variety of settings that serve learners with ASD in public, university operated, and private settings. We offer an overview of the assessment practices in one such public school model program through the close examination of a single case. We also move beyond traditional psychological diagnostic and assessment methods to include a discussion of the use of functional assessment and analysis procedures within the schools and how these often time-consuming procedures might be made more time efficient and user-friendly when adapted for application in classrooms. A case example based on the findings of Palmieri (2007) illustrates the potential time savings that such an assessment process might provide for many of the problem behaviors arising in the classroom.

THE PUBLIC SCHOOL AS A SYSTEM

As school administrators, classroom teachers, school psychologists, and other professionals who work in schools know well, public schools have their own cultures. In order to be an effective innovator within any school, one must understand how the system of that school operates. A consultant or staff member who fails to join effectively with the teaching staff will find the process of innovation difficult, if not impossible to accomplish. The failure to appreciate the demands of the leadership roles in schools and the political and interpersonal intensity that play out in these settings, such as the pressure on principals and other senior managers, has scuttled more than one effort to introduce new teaching or assessment methods that seem to their innovators a substantial contribution to the welfare of students and which have sound empirical data to back them up. Factors such as "organizational climate" (Glisson & Hemmelgarn, 1998) have a substantial impact on how one goes about introducing change, including new assessment methods, to a school system.

Ringeisen, Henderson, and Hoagwood (2003) discuss the complexities of introducing empirically supported mental health services to children in the public schools. Although their target population, children with mental health challenges, is different from that of children on the autism spectrum, some of the same systemic issues arise in trying to serve both populations. They note that the past 20 years have seen major advances in the empirical knowledge base for identifying and serving children with mental health needs (e.g., Lonigan, Elbert, & Johnson, 1998). A parallel can be seen in the education of children on the autism spectrum, where the past several decades have witnessed major advances in our knowledge of how to assess and support the learning of these youngsters (e.g., National Research Council, 2001). In these cases, researchers have made major advances in both understanding the needs of the population and how to serve it effectively—however, broad-scale implementation of services in the public schools lags behind our empirical knowledge. The gap between empirically based knowledge and broadly disseminated implementation is costly to children, their families, their schools, and the wider community.

The assessment and treatment of children on the autism spectrum, like that of children with mental health needs, has shifted from specialized programs and residential settings to community-based programs, especially the public schools (Ringeisen et al., 2003). In recognition of the growing disconnect between our knowledge of empirically supported treatments for children and the practices often available in community settings, especially the public schools, several federal government reports have offered recommendations for closing this troubling gap between what researchers know and what practitioners do in treating children's mental health needs (e.g., U. S. Public Health Service, 2000) and for evaluating and educating youngsters on the autism spectrum (e.g., National Research Council, 2001).

As Ringeisen et al. (2003) note, these national reports on evidence-based and/or empirically supported practices have paid insufficient attention to the context of the schools and how this environment influences the delivery of services. There has been a lack of sensitivity on the part of researchers to the outcomes that are most salient for schools including, for example, the academic achievements of students or the need for ongoing special education services. If we are to effectively introduce research-based methods for the assessment of children on the autism spectrum, we must be attuned to the needs of the school and ensure that the methods we offer address the needs of educators, and not just those of researchers.

In their reflection on the school as a system, Ringeisen et al. (2003) adopt a three-level model of how schools operate. These key factors are the individual, the organization, and the state and national levels of influence. They give examples of child factors at the individual level, including the child's achievements and peer relationships. Teacher variables such as job-related stress, extent of professional training, and relationships within the school are also individual factors. In addition to the children, their teachers, parents, and others, including administrators and school board members, should be considered at this level as they all may have a role to play in supporting high-quality assessment services.

At the organizational level there are such factors as the size of the school and the number of children on the autism spectrum who require specialized services. Ringeisen et al. (2003) highlight such organizational factors as creating a caring environment with strong cooperation among the students, teachers, and family members, and the availability of technical knowledge, resources, and emotional support for all of the participants. From the state and national levels we find such variables as political issues that may underlie educational funding and standards, and the statewide and national legislation that influences access to services and imposes demands for educational accountability. Ringeisen et al. (2003) also discuss the need for an ongoing feedback loop in which new practices are implemented and the outcomes provide feedback for modifications that may be essential to allowing an innovative model to work in a public school setting. As they note, the sooner practitioners—including teachers, school psychologists, and principals—become part of the conversation about the development of an educational intervention or assessment method, the easier it will be to introduce that model into the schools.

An important aspect of implementing effective educational practices for children with ASD is ensuring the involvement of the school psychologists and teaching staff in the planning. It is these psychologists and educators who know when methods are too complex for them to use without enhanced training in teaching or assessment methods. In the next section in this chapter, we describe one program for involving classroom teachers in doing functional assessments during the school day. The use of these assessment methods is a good example of a situation where a well-trained teaching staff, supervised by a behavior analyst or psychologist, can be crucial to the in-depth assessment of a child's challenging behaviors.

CLASSROOM-BASED FUNCTIONAL ANALYSIS

An excellent example of the need to translate a well-studied and effective assessment tool from a research setting to a typical classroom is found in the challenge of adapting functional analysis methods to the realities of the public schools.

Assessing challenging behavior through data-based collection procedures is a necessary component of applied behavior analysis (ABA; Cooper, Heron, & Heward, 1987; Palmieri, 2012). Functional analysis utilizes defined environmental manipulations to reliably identify maintaining variables of challenging behavior. These procedures then inform treatment planning—facilitating an empirical evaluation of a reliable relationship between the intervention and behavior change. The original research on functional analysis procedures was conducted in highly controlled treatment settings (Carr & Durand, 1985; Cooper & Harding, 1993; Iwata, Dorsey, Slifer, Bauman, & Richman, 1994; Iwata, Pace, Kalsher, Cowdery, & Cataldo, 1990; Powers et al., 2014).

Subsequently, the largest body of research on functional analysis has been done in similarly controlled contexts where stimuli from the participant's natural environment are expected to have minimal influence on assessment conditions. One potential result of this structure is that the functional analysis may suggest a relationship that does not exist in the naturalistic context (Hanley, Iwata, & McCord, 2003). This phenomenon may compromise the social validity of functional analysis findings and thus, undermine the translation of intervention from a specialized setting to the person's daily life.

Over time, research attention has shifted toward evaluating the use of functional analysis in outpatient settings with less precise and sustained control than is the case in many research settings (Cooper & Harding, 1993; Cooper, Wacker, Sasso, Reimers, & Donn, 1990; Harding, Wacker, Cooper, Millard, & Jensen-Kovalan, 1994; Northup et al., 1991; O'Reilly et al., 2009). In this regard, a growing body of research has demonstrated the use of functional analysis procedures in a number of naturalistic treatment settings such as outpatient clinics, schools, and homes (Bloom, Iwata, Fritz, Roscoe, & Carreau, 2011; Lambert, Bloom, & Irvin, 2012; Cooper & Harding, 1993; Cooper et al., 1990; Doggett, Edwards, Moore, Tingstrom, & Wilczynski, 2001; Lohrmann-O'Rourke & Yurman, 2001; Steege, Mace, & Brown-Chidsey, 2007; Umbreit, 1995). This line of research often also includes training procedures that facilitate the use of teachers as therapists in functional analysis conditions. Studies of this nature typically stress the importance of capitalizing on related data collection such as indirect measures and descriptive assessment in order to facilitate an efficient and person-centered approach to the functional analysis.

In a study by Doggett et al. (2001), behavioral consultants assisted general education classroom teachers in conducting an entire functional assessment. The functional analysis component of the assessment was implemented during periods of general classroom instruction. Behavioral consultants trained the teachers and supervised the entire assessment procedure, ensuring that the teachers played a primary role in hypothesis development and data analysis. Similarly, in Umbreit's (1995) research, a teacher was supported in the implementation of a functional analysis that proved successful in identifying a function of the student's challenging classroom behavior. Lohrmann-O'Rourke and Yurman (2001) embedded functional analysis conditions naturalistically into the general classroom routine. Erbas, Tekin-Iftar, and Yucesoy (2006) evaluated a structured protocol for training teachers on functional analysis procedures. This research indicated that teachers could successfully acquire the target skills necessary for developing and implementing functional analyses. The study also found that teacher impressions of the social validity of functional analysis procedures were largely positive following formalized training.

This line of applied research has provided a great deal of support for brief functional analysis as a means of assessing challenging behavior (e.g., Cooper et al., 1992; Derby et al., 1992, 1994). Recent expansions of this research have focused on the development of highly time-efficient models of trial-based functional analysis that can be used in typical educational environments (e.g., Bloom et al., 2011; Lambert et al., 2012). These trial-based models, like those initially outlined by Sigafoos and Saggers (1995), have very brief (often 1- or 2-minute) session durations, with sessions terminating after 1 minute or the first occurrence of the target response. LaRue et al. (2010) completed a comparison of traditional and trial-based models of functional analysis and found correspondence between the models in four out of five cases. The trial-based model, however, was substantially more time efficient. In addition, these brief models, as is emphasized in LaRue et al. (2010), avoid conditions where challenging behaviors are repeatedly reinforced and also require minimal interruption to the student's typical day.

Bloom et al. (2011) implemented a trial-based model consisting of conditions broken into three segments each lasting 2 minutes. The functional analysis was broken down into attention, tangible, demand, and ignore conditions. For each of these segments there was a control condition in the first and third position with a test condition embedded between them. As with other trial-based models, the segment was terminated following the occurrence of problem behavior. In this model, graduate students were the implementers of all conditions and not members of the student's natural teaching community—however, these segments were conducted during ongoing classroom activities. This feature is increasingly becoming a hallmark of brief, naturalistic, models that may be particularly viable within educational settings.

The use of analogue functional analysis procedures is now well understood for its potential beneficial application within applied settings. In particular, these procedures are increasingly sought out by educational teams that are faced with the challenge of developing a function-based behavior support plan for a learner with a complex neurodevelopmental disorder such as ASD. Recent advances in functional analysis methodology have allowed for the introduction of ever more efficient models of analysis, thus further increasing the potential value for its use within natural environments (Bloom et al., 2011; LaRue et al., 2010; Lambert et al., 2012). However, there continue to be significant limitations with successful incorporation of functional analysis methodology within educational settings. Long-standing challenges with educator training are perhaps the most prominent of these limitations. Few procedures have reliably incorporated teachers as therapists when executing the functional analysis (Hanley et al., 2003; Lambert et al., 2012; Palmieri, 2007). This has traditionally then limited the application of functional analyses within schools to highly specialized teams such as university-based research programs or educational consultants.

This line of research has been extended by research teams at the Douglass Developmental Disabilities Center (DDDC). The work of the DDDC has included the study of several models of functional analysis applied within classroom settings (LaRue et al., 2010; Palmieri, 2007). The study by Palmieri (2007) assessed a classroom functional analysis procedure that was based upon the initial conditions described by Iwata et al. (1994). Five students enrolled at the DDDC participated in this study. Analogue functional analyses were run in a private assessment room equipped with a worktable and four chairs. The classroom functional analyses were implemented in each student's natural classroom environment. The order of the two functional analysis procedures was alternated for each participant. This study found that the analogue and classroom-based functional analyses each resulted in identical determination of function. The classroom-based analysis, however, has the benefits of being more time efficient, conducted within the natural educational setting of the student, and executed by those educators who work daily with the learner. A clear asset here is the potential to increase the social validity of the analysis due to its naturalistic application and engagement of the typical community.

In the study by Palmieri (2007), each case incorporated indirect data collection procedures (semistructured interviews, questionnaires), descriptive assessment using antecedent–behavior–consequence (ABC) data collection, preference assessments, analogue functional analysis, and a classroom functional analysis. During the descriptive assessment component data were analyzed for function (attention, escape, tangible, automatic reinforcement) based upon the recorded antecedents and consequences. Immediately preceding each set of functional analysis sessions a multiple stimulus without replacement (MSWO) preference assessment was conducted to identify currently preferred tangible items. The format for the preference assessment followed that outlined by DeLeon and Iwata (1996). The analogue functional analysis was developed based upon the conditions (toy play, alone, social attention, and demand) described by Iwata et al. (1994). Conditions lasted 10 minutes with behavior analysts serving as therapists.

The classroom analysis was conducted with the teacher serving as therapist. The model used 5-minute sessions and implemented the following conditions: toy play (control), social attention, demand, and tangible. Condition parameters were modified from those used in Iwata et al. (1994) for application within the natural classroom environment. Prior to the analysis, the teacher received brief training from a graduate-level behavior analyst. In addition to verbal information, the teacher was given a brief written description of the condition protocols and provided with visual prompts that outlined crucial condition components. All information presented in the classroom functional analysis condition descriptions was specifically reviewed with the teacher, allowing him or her time to ask questions and receive clarifications using case examples. The teachers were equipped with an earpiece that enabled the behavior analyst to communicate from outside the classroom throughout the assessment. Using the earpiece, the teacher was given prompts for establishing the contingencies for each session and for providing reinforcement when necessary. The correspondence among independent raters' evaluations of the functional analysis data indicated that across all cases in this study, 93% yielded full or partial agreement scores between the classroom and analogue functional analyses.

This research methodology has subsequently been replicated and expanded by educational teams in the course of supporting the development of individualized behavior support plans for students enrolled within public schools who are experiencing significant complex and challenging behavior.

Case Example: Matthew

Matthew is a 6-year-old boy diagnosed with ASD. He was diagnosed shortly before his third birthday following parent and pediatrician concerns that he was not reaching his developmental milestones appropriately. Following evaluation he was enrolled in a public school-based preschool program to provide him with educational interventions to address his skill deficits. He participated in this preschool program until transitioning to kindergarten. At this time he was placed within a special education classroom designed to provide intensive interventions using a multidisciplinary and evidence-based approach with all teaching practices aligned with ABA methodologies. This classroom was based within a public school and Matthew's team included special and general educators, his parents, a board certified behavior analyst (BCBA), an inclusion specialist, a speech–language therapist, an occupational therapist, and two paraprofessionals.

Matthew experienced significant social interaction and social communication skill deficits as well as delays with all daily living and learning readiness skills. He was unable to communicate vocally and attempts to establish an alternative functional communication system using either sign or a picture-based exchange were at that time unsuccessful. As a result his most reliable successful method of communication included guiding others to items. Complex challenging behavior significantly limited Matthew's ability to participate safely within the general education community and had fully interrupted his ability to participate in any specialized instruction sessions. As a result he was referred for a functional behavior assessment (FBA) to determine his learning needs with respect to the challenging behavior and develop an intervention to address these needs by teaching him adaptive replacement skills.

At the time of referral his challenging behavior included aggression to self and aggression to others. Aggression to self typically included hitting both his hands to his head while screaming. Aggression to others included biting, scratching (using one hand to clasp and pull on a piece of skin of another), and hitting (using both hands, while positioned as fists, to contact the body of another). These behaviors had been present throughout Matthew's time in preschool—however, upon his transition to kindergarten their intensity increased dramatically. Previous interventions had primarily included general supports such as blocking and redirecting his behavior while attempting to model some form of functional communication. There were no previous functional assessments conducted in order to fully understand Matthew's needs.

The teacher interview revealed that Matthew's aggressions were present throughout his entire school day. His teachers were concerned that the behavior "seemed to come out of nowhere," and his team was unsure how to prevent the behavior at all. There were reports that academic demands seemed to trigger the behaviors—however, they were observed all day long, including periods of low demands. When alone Matthew was reportedly somewhat less likely to engage in the behavior if he also had access to highly preferred materials such as videos or small plastic toys that he enjoyed carrying with him. Further, attempts to redirect him and maintain his safety were failing—that is, the team's attempts to prompt Matthew to engage in safe behavior were typically resulting in longer episodes of challenging behaviors, which were then contributing to the use of crisis intervention procedures.

ABC data were collected on Matthew across a period of 2 weeks during all times and settings of the school day. See Figures 11.1 and 11.2. These data were collected by his inclusion specialist, the BCBA, and the special education teacher. All team members received training from the BCBA on data collection procedures and achieved above 85% reliability with all data collection protocols. The ABC data were not well differentiated in Matthew's case—that is, analysis of the antecedent and consequence events did not suggest prominent or clear triggering events. Rather, multiple types of environmental changes such as demands, attention levels, access to preferred items, and transitions were all associated with the behavior. Further, there were multiple instances where all observers were unable to determine a likely environmental change immediately preceding the behavior. Analysis of the consequence events tended to indicate that his team would prompt a safe response (e.g., hands down) and provide verbal directions. At times team members would also introduce preferred items to him immediately after prompting, "Safe hands."

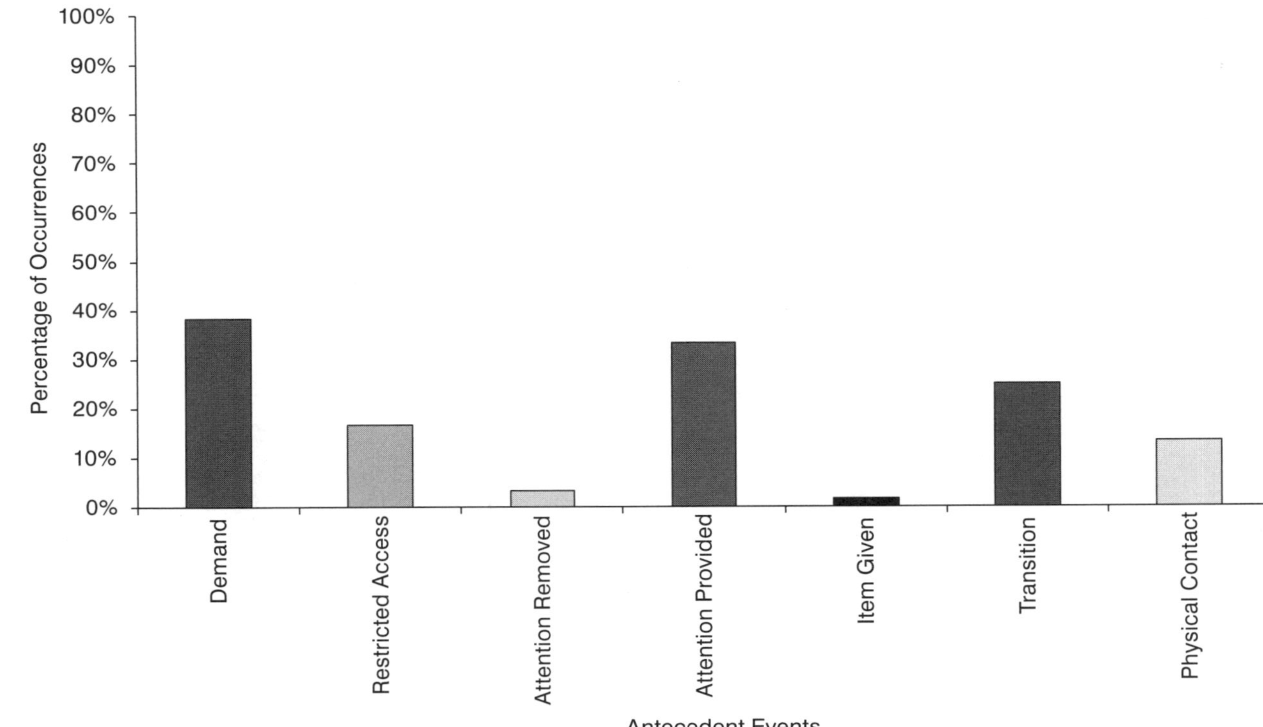

FIGURE 11.1. ABC data collection analysis of antecedents.

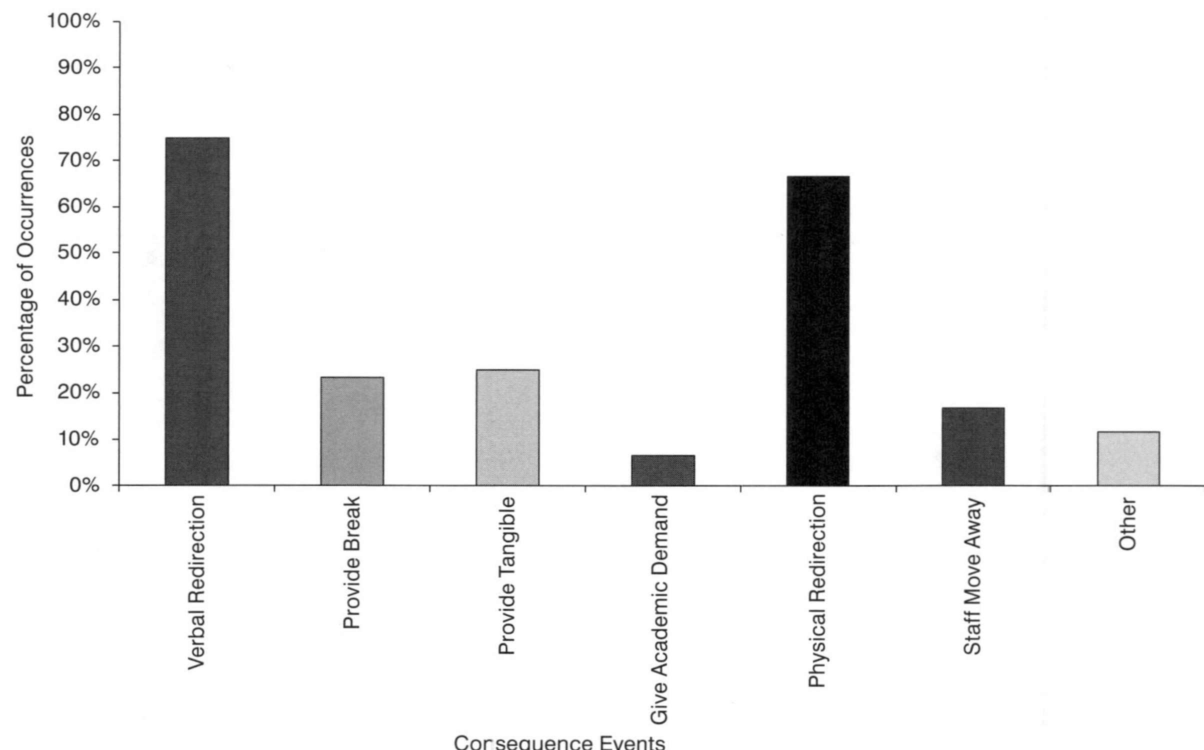

FIGURE 11.2. ABC data collection analysis of consequences.

Given the increasing severity of the aggression and the unclear data achieved through the descriptive assessment, a classroom-based functional analysis was initiated using the same methodology as applied in Palmieri (2007). The analysis was conducted in his special education classroom in the typical areas where Matthew would both work and take breaks during the school day. His special education teacher and paraprofessional team members served as therapists following direct training on implementing the contingencies for each condition. As in Palmieri (2007), MSWO preference assessments were conducted before each classroom-based functional analysis testing session. In Matthew's case, items including Baby Einstein video clips, solid plastic toys that could be held easily in one hand, a trampoline, and a cause-and-effect toy with basic light and sound interactions were consistently identified as highly preferred tangibles. Treatment fidelity checks were executed for 100% of the functional analysis sessions by the BCBA on Matthew's team. His teachers all maintained procedural fidelity above 95% for all components. Interrater reliability data were collected on the topography of each challenging behavior between the BCBA and inclusion specialist and these averaged 91% on head hits, 100% on biting, 92% on scratching, and 96% on hitting.

Matthew's classroom functional analysis consisted of 20 sessions with each of the standard conditions run five times. See Figure 11.3. The sessions required 100 minutes of testing and were spread across four different testing days. During the classroom analysis, the average responses per minute across conditions were toy play (0.00), attention (0.00), demand (0.53), and tangible (0.12). The data strongly indicated that Matthew's aggressions were maintained primarily by negative reinforcement in the form of escape from demands.

The clarity of these data, taken in sharp contrast to the data collected during the descriptive assessment, directly guided the team in intervention planning. Further, the classroom-based functional analysis required far less time to execute than did the ABC data collection. Analysis of the classroom-based functional analysis data allowed the team to see that demands, while often subtle, were layered throughout Matthew's entire day (e.g., any time a teacher approached Matthew) and were triggering his aggressive behavior. The ABC data collection procedures were, in Matthew's case, not sufficiently sensitive to identify this variable due to the inability of the observers to know fully, and from Matthew's perspective, when a demand state had been evoked. Based on the results of the classroom-based functional analysis, Matthew's team was able to develop a behavior support plan that achieved therapeutic gains. This included a sustained reduction in aggression by more than 94% by implementing pairing procedures to reassociate the school environment with positive reinforcement before progressively introducing demands as well as

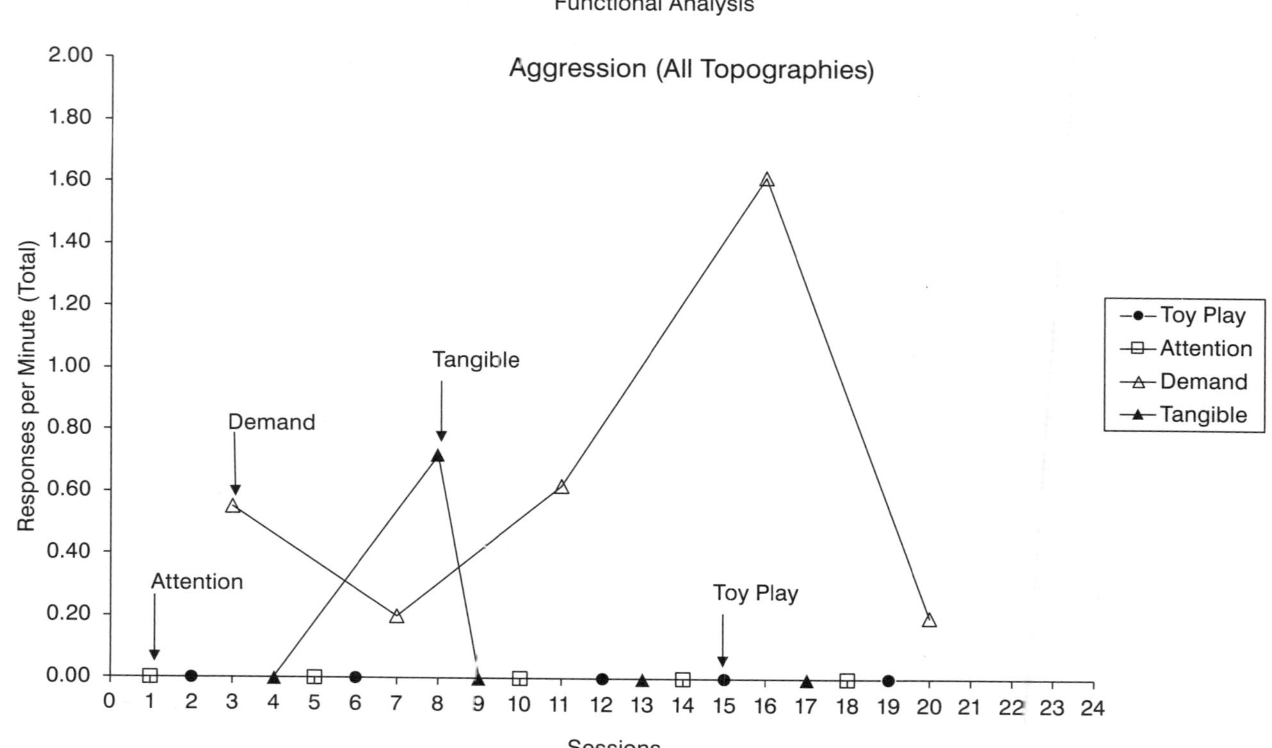

FIGURE 11.3. Functional analysis data on aggression.

intensive functional communication training to teach Matthew to request the termination of demands.

The ability of trained teachers and school-based behavior support staff to serve as therapists during a classroom functional analysis is critical to this procedure's feasibility of incorporation in school settings (Doggett et al., 2001; Lohrmann-O'Rourke & Yurman, 2001; Umbreit, 1995). Team member training in Palmieri's (2007) study and the case illustration above required less than 15 minutes per condition and could be done immediately before the start of the functional analysis sessions. The training components were efficient and provided a general outline and the goals of the functional analysis, and then gave specific instructions for implementing each session. Brief role plays with the teacher and trainer gave a sample of how the conditions would run. The treatment fidelity checks indicated that following training every teacher was able to implement the condition components with appropriate integrity. This training procedure was consistent across staff and applied to teachers and teaching assistants with varying levels of experience. Additionally, the teachers indicated that they felt engaged, highly interested in the process, and very motivated to participate in the development and implementation of the behavior support plans.

Both the interview and descriptive assessment procedures provided meaningful support for conducting comprehensive, individualized, functional analyses. The importance of incorporating descriptive assessment procedures into functional analyses has been stressed repeatedly (Aikman, Garbutt, & Furniss, 2003; Cooper & Harding, 1993; Cooper et al., 1992; Doggett et al., 2001; Powers et al., 2014; Steege et al., 2007; Tiger, Hanley, & Bessette, 2006; Umbreit, 1995). Data from the indirect and descriptive assessments can facilitate the development of clear definitions for the topographies of challenging behavior, identifying likely antecedent and consequence events, relevant individual-specific environmental manipulations, important natural environmental relationships (e.g., divided adult attention with a particular peer), and behavior topographies that tend to covary. However, this does not provide for the level of precise direct analysis that is achieved through functional analyses and can be subject to a variety of confounds inherent to observation-based assessment tools.

School settings are often the first locations where assessments of aberrant behavior are conducted. Brief, naturalistic, and accessible functional analysis procedures may encourage function-driven analyses and treatments to be incorporated more successfully into the client's natural environment. Analyses methods that can be completed in an efficient and socially valid fashion, while maintaining procedural integrity and validity, are the most likely to be adopted into educational settings (Derby et al., 1992; LaRue et al., 2010; Bloom et al., 2011). Brief models that also limit the potential reinforcement of challenging behavior (e.g., LaRue et al., 2010) have a clear benefit of also increasing the likelihood that these procedures will be received as socially valid and viable in the natural environment. Students with complex behavior challenges require access to functional interventions in order to ensure maximum educational benefit and access to the natural learning environment. The use of functional analyses to inform person-centered planning has the potential to markedly expand the impact of high-quality, functional, and evidence-based behavioral interventions within schools.

Case Example: Frankie W.

In addition to adopting empirically supported behavioral assessment methods in the classroom, schools also need to be able to use state-of-the-art tools when conducting traditional psychological assessments. Completing assessments of children who are being considered for classification for special services is an important role for many school psychologists. There are a number of diagnostic tools available for this purpose when one wishes to determine whether a child is on the autism spectrum.

Frankie W. was a 6-year-old boy attending a general education class who was referred by his teacher for a comprehensive assessment. His teacher was concerned because Frankie had been exhibiting unusual and challenging behaviors since entering kindergarten the year before, and these behaviors had increased in frequency and intensity since he started first grade a few months earlier. The school psychologist contacted Mr. and Mrs. W. to request parental permission to conduct the evaluation. Mr. and Mrs. W. were initially hesitant and asked to meet with the school psychologist before giving permission. Recognizing that the parents were likely stressed about the situation, the school psychologist made efforts to set up a meeting for the next day. Such an individualized approach was beneficial in setting the stage for a collaborative relationship between the school and the parents.

During the meeting, the school psychologist and Frankie's teacher started the discussion by noting that Frankie showed clear strengths in various areas. For example, they emphasized that his academic skills were all at grade level and that his fine and gross motor skills were notable. They then outlined their concerns in an objective, supportive manner. They described Frankie's tendency to have prolonged "meltdowns" over apparently minor events (e.g., changes in the class schedule, being asked to participate in show and tell). They stated that Frankie was frequently off task and wanted to discuss *Sponge Bob* episodes at length, becoming upset when the teacher attempted to redirect him back to the task at hand. Due to his tendency to misinterpret others' comments, he often became defensive and argumentative. They were also concerned that Frankie rarely interacted with peers, spending most of recess pacing the outlined boundary of the playground. Although these behaviors were noticed in his half-day kindergarten class, since entering first grade the behaviors had escalated significantly to the point where the school staff believed they were hindering Frankie's learning. As a consequence, they recommended a full assessment in order to obtain a clearer understanding of Frankie's educational and social–emotional needs.

Upon hearing these concerns, Mr. and Mrs. W. acknowledged that Frankie had always been "a bit of a handful" ever since he was a toddler. They described Frankie's meltdowns at home, which were also triggered by seemingly inconsequential events (e.g., if they tried to encourage him to eat a wider variety of foods, or if they rearranged the family room furniture). They reported that he had never appeared interested in peers, but they assumed this was because he was an only child and used to playing alone. They further noted that his interactions with others in the community could be embarrassing in that he would ask socially inappropriate questions such as "Why are you so fat?" He often initiated conversations with strangers, asking them which *Sponge Bob* episode they liked the best before going off on a monologue about his own favorite shows. Mr. and Mrs. W. had attributed many of Frankie's oddities to the fact that he hadn't had much experience interacting with other children or adults since the family home was in a rural area and Frankie had not attended preschool. Given their own concerns as well as those of the school staff, Mr. and Mrs. W. signed the "Permission to Evaluate" form allowing the school to conduct a full assessment. The school team determined that the psychologist, speech–language pathologist, and occupational therapist would all be involved in Frankie's evaluation.

As was typical protocol for their particular school system, the school psychologist took the lead and served as the "hub" for gathering the assessment results and creating the eventual evaluation report. Since Frankie's academic skills all tested at grade level, the school psychologist defined her role as primarily focused on ruling in/out the diagnosis of ASD, as well as to provide information regarding Frankie's behavioral challenges. To this aim, the school psychologist administered two diagnostic tools: the Autism Diagnostic Observation Schedule, Second Edition (ADOS-2; Lord et al., 2012b), with Frankie, and the Autism Diagnostic Interview—Revised (ADI-R; Rutter, Le Couteur, & Lord, 2003) with his parents. In the past, the school psychologist had relied upon checklists such as the Childhood Autism Rating Scale (CARS; Schopler, Reichler, & Renner, 1988)—however, more recent empirical research had shown that administering both the ADOS-2 coupled with the ADI-R was the most valid method for determining whether or not an individual meets criteria for ASD (Garcia-Lavin & Morin, 2012).

The ADOS-2 is a semistructured, standardized assessment of communication, social interaction, play, and imaginative use of materials for individuals who have been referred because of symptomology related to ASD. Standardized, structured activities and materials provide contexts in which social interactions, communication, and other behaviors relevant to ASD are observed. Four different modules are available in the ADOS-2, and the evaluator selects the module that best matches the developmental age and expressive language skills of the child being assessed. Since Frankie was a 6-year-old child with fluent speech, the school psychologist administered Module 3 of the ADOS-2. Results clearly supported the hypothesis that Frankie was on the autism spectrum. His ratings across the Social Affect and Restricted and Repetitive Behavior domains resulted in an ADOS-2 Comparison Score of 7 ("moderate probability of autism spectrum disorder").

The school psychologist then met with Mr. and Mrs. W. in order to score the ADI-R. The ADI-R consists of a wide variety of interview questions targeting both developmental history as well as behaviors specific to ASD. Due to the comprehensive nature of the ADI-R, the structured interview with Frankie's parents required 2 hours of in-depth discussion, including topics such as early development, relationships with peers, speech and language, and the presence of repetitive behaviors or interests. Frankie's scores on the ADI-R across all three domains (Qualitative Abnormalities in Reciprocal Interaction; Qualitative Abnormalities in Communication; and Restricted, Repetitive, and Stereotyped Patterns of Behavior) were just above the designated criteria for ASD. These scores, plus the fact that Frankie's behavioral differences were noted as early as 2 years of age, supported the diagnostic conclusions put forth by the ADOS-2 results.

The school psychologist's next step was to conduct an FBA in order to gain insights as to Frankie's challenging behaviors. Fortunately, she was a BCBA as well as a school psychologist, and was therefore knowledgeable regarding FBAs and data analysis. An unfortunate aspect of the case was that Frankie's current first-grade teacher was a seasoned teacher but she had minimal experience in conducting an FBA in the classroom and was overall less than enthusiastic regarding the time and effort involved. When approached by the school psychologist, the teacher insisted that her chosen profession was "general education, not special education." Although the school psychologist usually relied upon FBA data collected by the teacher, given the teacher's less than receptive stance coupled with the 60 daytime constraints for getting the evaluation completed, the school psychologist determined that she needed to take an individualized and realistic approach. Rather than try to change the teacher's mind, the school psychologist taught one of her school psychology interns how to collect the ABC data and assigned her the task of spending the next 2 weeks in Frankie's classroom. The intern enthusiastically embraced the task and became adept at collecting the data.

Once the FBA data were collected, it became clear that the primary motivation underlying Frankie's challenging behaviors was to avoid or escape nonpreferred tasks. Of special note was the fact that the tasks that were deemed nonpreferred were rarely academic in nature—rather, Frankie was more apt to exhibit challenging behaviors in order to avoid a task that required social and/or communication skills. For example, the frequency of *Sponge Bob* monologues was highest when the teacher asked Frankie to participate in the "morning circle" when students are expected to talk about their own experiences outside the classroom. Similarly, the frequency of pacing during recess was highest immediately after a recess aide had instructed him to play with his classmates. Finally, the FBA revealed that challenging behaviors tended to occur when there was an unexpected change in routine (e.g., a school assembly or other special event)—because the teachers tended to allow Frankie to leave these activities when he became upset, his meltdowns had been inadvertently reinforced.

The school psychologist then gathered the assessment results obtained from the speech–language pathologist as well as the occupational therapist. The speech–language pathologist reported that Frankie showed significant deficits in the social (pragmatic) aspects of communication, while the occupational therapist's assessment reflected no unusual responses to sensory input that significantly impacted his ability to learn. Once the school psychologist combined all of the assessment data into an initial evaluation report, she scheduled a time for the school team to meet with the parents to review the results.

While awaiting the school testing to be completed, Mr. and Mrs. W. had taken Frankie to their local pediatrician to gain his opinion. Although not particularly experienced with children on the autism spectrum, the physician told Mr. and Mrs. W. that Frankie had Asperger's disorder. When Frankie's parents shared the pediatrician's view with the school team, they expressed appreciation for the pediatrician's input. They then took the time to explain to the parents that the American Psychiatric Association's (2013) most recent version of the *Diagnostic and Statistical Manual of Mental Disorders* (DSM-5) no longer included Asperger's disorder as a separate diagnosis—rather, DSM-5 had clustered earlier subcategories into one overall diagnosis of ASD. The school psychologist explained that while professionals were successful in identifying children who were on the autism spectrum, even the most experienced diagnosticians were less effective in teasing out which subcategory of the spectrum was relevant (e.g., especially when differentiating Asperger's disorder, high-functioning autistic disorder, or pervasive developmental disorder not otherwise specified; see Lord et al., 2012a).

In terms of an educational diagnosis, the school psychologist then explained that the federal Individuals with Disabilities Education Improvement Act (IDEIA) denotes a relatively short list of disabilities that must be used in an educational setting, and that Asperger's disorder was never on the IDEIA list. Therefore, prior to DSM-5, even students with a diagnosis of Asperger's disorder were identified with the educational disability of autism within the educational system. The school psychologist then focused the discussion on Frankie's assessment results. She noted that his scores on both the ADOS-2 and ADI-R revealed that an ASD diagnosis was warranted. She acknowledged that given Frankie's intelligence and relatively notable skills, he very well may have been diagnosed with Asperger's disorder if he had been assessed prior to the publication of DSM-5. However, the school psychologist was obligated to use the term "autism spectrum disorder" in order to reflect the current nomenclature.

The speech–language pathologist then reviewed her own assessment results. She noted that although Frankie had a wide vocabulary and could speak in full sentences that were clearly articulated, his test performance revealed significant needs in the area of social communication skills. The speech therapist consequently recommended that Frankie receive 30 minutes of speech therapy per week to address this area. Finally, the occupational therapist discussed her test results and recommended that no occupational therapy was needed at this time.

Once all the data had been reviewed, the team agreed that Frankie was a student with an identified disability of ASD who required specially designed instruction in order to facilitate learning. An individualized education program (IEP) was developed that outlined goals and objectives, as well as evidence-based instructional strategies to support Frankie. The team determined that the goals and objectives could best be implemented within the school's Autistic Support Resource Room, which had a low student:teacher ratio, incorporated evidence-based strategies based on axioms of ABA into their instruction, and had a strong curriculum in the area of social (pragmatic) communication. The school social worker was brought onto the team in order to assist Mr. and Mrs. W. in applying for a community-based behavior support consultant (BSC) to develop behavioral interventions in the home, and this BSC became an active member of the IEP team. The home and school positive behavior support plans were strategically coordinated such that everyone in Frankie's life was supporting him in the exact same way.

On a school system level, the school psychologist and principal recognized the need to address the resistance demonstrated by some of the general education teachers when they were required to work with students on the autism spectrum. Further discussion with these teachers reflected that their resistance was primarily based upon their lack of knowledge rather than any negative feelings toward students on the autism spectrum per se—therefore, the school psychologist and principal developed a full-day staff development program entitled "Autism 101," in which the general education teachers were taught the behavioral characteristics inherent to autism, effective antecedinal strategies, and the steps in conducting an FBA. Once the teachers' skill base increased, they were notably more willing to support students on the autism spectrum.

SUMMARY

In many school settings, there is a troubling disconnect between effective research on demonstrated methods for the assessment and treatment of students on the autism spectrum and actual school-based practice. The responsibility for solving the problem of information transfer resides both with the investigators who develop and attempt to disseminate these innovative tools and the educational personnel whose students could benefit from their application. These are problems best solved by improved two-way communication that begins early in the process of developing the new methods and continues through the successful introduction of the methods in the schools. Accomplishing that goal requires not only good faith effort on the part of the key players including researchers, teachers, school psychologists, and principals but support from school board members, government officials, and others who are in a position to set meaningful and realistic goals for the schools.

REFERENCES

Aikman, G., Garbutt, V., & Furniss, F. (2003). Brief probes: A method for analyzing the function of disruptive behaviour in the natural environment. *Behavioural and Cognitive Psychotherapy, 31,* 215–220.

American Psychiatric Association. (2013). *Diagnostic and statistical manual of mental disorders* (5th ed.). Arlington, VA: Author.

Bloom, S. E., Iwata, B. A., Fritz, J. N., Roscoe, E. M., & Carreau, A. (2011). Classroom application of a trial based functional analysis. *Journal of Applied Behavior Analysis, 44,* 19–31.

Carr, E. G., & Durand, M. V. (1985). Reducing behavior problems through functional communication training. *Journal of Applied Behavior Analysis, 18,* 111–126.

Cooper, J. O., Heron, T. E., & Heward, W. L. (1987). *Applied behavior analysis.* Upper Saddle River, NJ: Prentice Hall.

Cooper, L. J., & Harding, J. (1993). Extending functional analysis procedures to outpatient and classroom settings for children with mild disabilities. In J. Reichle &

D. P. Wacker (Eds.), *Communicative alternatives to challenging behavior: Integrating functional assessment and intervention strategies* (pp. 41–62). Baltimore: Brookes.

Cooper, L. J., Wacker, D. P., Sasso, G., M., Reimers, T. M., & Donn, L. K. (1990). Using parents as therapists to evaluate appropriate behavior of their children: Application to a tertiary diagnostic clinic. *Journal of Applied Behavior Analysis, 23,* 285–296.

Cooper, L. J., Wacker, D. P., Thursby, D., Plagmann, L. A., Harding, J., Millard, T., et al. (1992). Analysis of the effects of task preferences, task demands, and adult attention on child behavior in outpatient and classroom settings. *Journal of Applied Behavior Analysis, 25,* 823–840.

DeLeon, I. G., & Iwata, B. A. (1996). Evaluation of a multiple-stimulus presentation format for assessing reinforcer preferences. *Journal of Applied Behavior Analysis, 29,* 519–533.

Derby, K. M., Wacker, D. P., Peck, S., Sasso, G., DeRaad, A., Berg, W., et al. (1994). Functional analysis of separate topographies of aberrant behavior. *Journal of Applied Behavior Analysis, 27,* 267–278.

Derby, K. M., Wacker, D. P., Sasso, G., Steege, M., Northup, J., Cigrand, K., et al. (1992). Brief functional assessment techniques to evaluate aberrant behavior in an outpatient setting: A summary of 79 cases. *Journal of Applied Behavior Analysis, 25,* 713–721.

Doggett, R. A., Edwards, R. P., Moore, J. W., Tingstrom, D. H., & Wilczynski, S. M. (2001). An approach to functional assessment in general education classroom settings. *School Psychology Review, 30,* 313–328.

Erbas, D., Tekin-Iftar, E., & Yucesoy, S. (2006). Teaching special education teachers how to conduct functional analysis in natural settings. *Education and Training in Developmental Disabilities, 41,* 28–36.

Forman, S. G., & Selman, J. S. (2011). Systems-based service delivery in school psychology. In M. A. Bray & T. J. Kehle (Eds.), *Oxford handbook of school psychology* (pp. 628–646). New York: Oxford University Press.

Garcia-Lavin, B., & Morin, I. (2012). *Agreement among measures of autism spectrum disorders in school-age children.* Fort Lauderdale, FL: Nova Southeastern University. Available from *www.nasponline.org.*

Glisson, C., & Hemmelgarn, A. (1998). The effects of organizational climate and interorganizational coordination on the quality and outcome of children's service systems. *Child Abuse and Neglect, 22,* 401–442.

Hanley, G. P., Iwata, B. A., & McCord, B. E. (2003). Functional analysis of problem behavior: A review. *Journal of Applied Behavior Analysis, 36,* 147–185.

Harding, J., Wacker, D. P., Cooper, L. J., Millard, T., & Jensen-Kovalan, P. (1994). Brief hierarchical assessment of potential treatment components with children in an outpatient clinic. *Journal of Applied Behavior Analysis, 27*(2), 291–300.

Iwata, B. A., Dorsey, M. F., Slifer, K. J., Bauman, K. E., & Richman, G. S. (1994). Toward a functional analysis of self-injury. *Journal of Applied Behavior Analysis, 27,* 197–209. (Original work published 1982)

Iwata, B. A., Pace, G. M., Kalsher, M. J., Cowdery, G. E., & Cataldo, M. F. (1990). Experimental analysis and extinction of self-injurious escape behavior. *Journal of Applied Behavior Analysis, 23,* 11–27.

Lambert, J. M., Bloom, S. E., & Irvin, J. (2012). Trial-based functional analysis and functional communication training in an early childhood setting. *Journal of Applied Behavior Analysis, 45,* 579–584.

LaRue, R. H., Lenard, K., Weiss, M. J., Bamond, M., Palmieri, M., & Kelley, M. E. (2010). Comparison of traditional and trial-based methodologies for conducting functional analyses. *Research in Developmental Disabilities, 31,* 480–487.

Leadbeater, B., Sukhawathanakul, P., Smith, D., & Bowen, F. (2014). Reciprocal associations between interpersonal and values dimensions of school climate and peer victimization in elementary school children. *Journal of Clinical Child and Adolescent Psychology, 43*(3), 1–14.

Lohrmann-O'Rourke, S., & Yurman, B. (2001). Naturalistic assessment of and intervention for mouthing behaviors influenced by establishing operations. *Journal of Positive Behavior Interventions, 3,* 19–27.

Lonigan, C. J., Elbert, J. C., & Johnson, S. B. (1998). Empirically supported psychosocial interventions for children: An overview. *Journal of Clinical Child Psychology, 27,* 138–145.

Lord, C., Petkova, E., Hus, V., Gan, W., Lu, F., Martin, D. M., et al. (2012a). A multisite study of the clinical diagnosis of different autism spectrum disorders. *Archives of General Psychiatry, 69*(3), 306–313.

Lord, C., Rutter, M., DiLavore, P., Risi, S., Gotham, K., & Bishop, S. L. (2012b). *Autism Diagnostic Observation Schedule, Second Edition* (ADOS-2): Manual. Los Angeles: Western Psychological Services.

Mullen, E. M. (1997). *Mullen Scales of Early Learning.* Los Angeles: Western Psychological Services.

National Research Council. (2001). *Educating children with autism.* Washington, DC: National Academy Press.

Northup, J., Wacker, D., Sasso, G., Steege, M., Cigrand, K., Cook, J., et al. (1991). A brief functional analysis of aggressive and alternative behavior in an outpatient clinic setting. *Journal of Applied Behavior Analysis, 24,* 509–522.

O'Reilly, M., Rispoli, M., Davis, T., Machalick, W., Lang, R., Sigafoos, J., et al. (2009). Functional analysis of challenging behavior in children with autism spectrum disorders: A summary of 10 cases. *Research in Autism Spectrum Disorders, 4,* 1–10.

Palmieri, M. J. (2007). *Classroom based functional analysis: A model for assessing challenging behavior within the classroom environment.* Unpublished doctoral dissertation, Rutgers, The State University of New Jersey.

Palmieri, M. J. (2012). Functional analysis. In F. Volkmar, R. Paul, K. Pelphry, & M. D. Powers (Eds.), *The encyclopedia of autism spectrum disorders* (pp. 1370–1371). New York: Springer.

Powers, M. D., Palmieri, M. J., Egan, S. M., Rohrer, J., Nulty, E., & Forte, S. (2014). Behavioral assessment of individuals with autism. In F. Volkmar, S. Rogers, & R. Paul (Eds.), *Handbook of autism and pervasive developmental disorders* (4th ed., pp. 695–736). New York: Wiley.

Ringeisen, H., Henderson, K., & Hoagwood, K. (2003). Context matters: Schools and the "research to practice gap" on children's mental health. *School Psychology Review, 32,* 153–168.

Rutter, M., Le Couteur, A., & Lord, C. (2003). *Autism Diagnostic Interview—Revised (ADI-R) manual.* Los Angeles: Western Psychological Services.

Schopler, E., Reichler, R. J., & Renner, B. R. (1988). *The Childhood Autism Rating Scale.* Los Angeles: Western Psychological Services.

Sigafoos, J., & Saggers, E. (1995). A discrete-trial approach to the functional analysis of aggressive behaviour in two boys with autism. *Australia and New Zealand Journal of Developmental Disabilities, 20*(4), 287–297.

Sparrow, S. S., Balla, D. A., & Cicchetti, D. V. (1984). *Vineland Adaptive Behavior Scales: Interview Edition Survey Form manual.* Circle Pines, MN: American Guidance Service.

Steege, M. W., Mace, F. C., & Brown-Chidsey, R. (2007). Functional evaluation of classroom behavior. In S. Goldstein & R. Brooks (Eds.), *Understanding and managing children's classroom behavior: Creating sustainable, resilient classrooms* (2nd ed., pp. 43–63). New York: Wiley.

Tiger, J. H., Hanley, G. P., & Bessette, K. K. (2006). Incorporating descriptive assessment results into the design of a functional analysis: A case example involving a preschooler's hand mouthing. *Education and Treatment of Children, 29,* 107–124.

Umbreit, J. (1995). Functional assessment and intervention in a regular classroom setting for the disruptive behavior of a student with attention deficit hyperactivity disorder. *Behavioral Disorders, 20,* 267–278.

U.S. Public Health Service. (2000). *Report of the Surgeon General's Conference on Children's Mental Health: A national action agenda.* Washington, DC: U.S. Department of Health and Human Services.

CHAPTER TWELVE

From Assessment to Intervention

Kerry Hogan
Lee M. Marcus

This chapter focuses on how assessment information can be used to help in the individualized programming for students and older persons with autism spectrum disorder (ASD). Historically, formal assessment has been used to generate data about an individual's level of functioning and, at times, to identify a pattern of abilities. There has been less emphasis on the process of translating evaluation data into both general and specific educational suggestions and plans. In this chapter, we address from a conceptual and practical framework what is involved in using assessment information as a starting point for developing meaningful interventions. This framework is grounded in the experience of the Treatment and Education of Autistic and Related Communication Handicapped Children (TEACCH) autism program, one of the first ASD programs to integrate developmental assessment into treatment decision making and planning.

The chapter is organized into the following sections: (1) a brief review of assessment approaches in ASD and how they have been applied to interventions; (2) an overview of the TEACCH approach to assessment; (3) a discussion of using the Psychoeducational Profile (PEP), the primary developmental–behavioral–educational instrument in the TEACCH program, as a vehicle for intervention planning, together with a case example demonstrating the use of the PEP-3; (4) a description and case example of informal assessment, an especially valuable approach in classroom and other nonclinical settings; (5) a brief review of assessment methods and strategies for adolescents and adults, where the emphasis is on functionality of skills in applied settings; and (6) concluding comments.

For the purposes of this chapter, "assessment" is defined as the formal or informal process of gathering data on behavioral and learning/developmental functioning as an aid in developing an initial program and continuing to evaluate its effects over time and settings. This perspective differs from the data-based assessment process. A data-based process focuses on specific goals and objectives, whereas our view of assessment is intended to be broad based and comprehensive. Although data-based monitoring can and should have a role in ASD intervention programs, this chapter addresses the assessment of skills, learning patterns/styles, and ASD-specific behaviors that serve as the basis for individualized programming.

In general, once diagnosis (and, in some cases, prognostic clarification) has been established for a child with ASD, there is a need to understand the child's levels of developmental functioning, including his or her unique pattern of strengths and weaknesses. With a younger child, the assessment profile should be based primarily on guidelines derived from developmental norms, should use developmentally sequenced materials and activities, and should reflect concepts derived from well-established developmental models and themes (such as means–end reasoning, causality, and role-taking perspective). At the adolescent age level and beyond, strictly developmental guidelines may need to be gradually replaced by criterion-based assessment of specific, pragmatic skills. The shift from the more developmentally based approaches to those concerned with assessment of behavior and competence in a functional environment reflects the current efforts of special educators in establishing appropriate secondary-level programs for individuals with severe ASD. Regardless of the fundamental assumptions of the assessment approach, the evaluation and analysis of both abilities and disabilities within and across specific skill areas should be basic objectives.

OVERVIEW OF ASSESSMENT APPROACHES TO INTERVENTION IN ASD

Historically, the link between assessment and intervention in ASD has reflected the philosophical and methodological bases of the treatment model. Not all intervention approaches value assessment—or, at least, not all require a formal or informal assessment process to guide treatment planning. For example, psychodynamic therapies typically operate from a theoretical framework that does not rely on or require an initial systematic assessment leading to a specific treatment plan. Although individualization is possible and adjustments can be made, the intervention is largely based on its conceptual framework. The role and importance of assessment in treatment planning vary: Assessment may be valued as a core, integral, and ongoing part of the intervention process; it may be viewed as a means to jump-start the treatment process, but carried out in either a limited way or not systematically; or it may not be done at all.

In general, tests and other assessment measures that have been standardized on a typical general population have not addressed the unique characteristics of individuals with ASD; nor have they been designed to lead to comprehensive treatment planning. For example, standardized cognitive and achievement tests, although valuable in assessing functioning levels and patterns of strengths and weaknesses, do not lend themselves to being translated into meaningful, individualized intervention goals. These tests were not designed for individuals with ASD, although certain subtest patterns may emerge in those who function in the average range or higher. Such patterns may suggest educational intervention strategies (e.g., for someone with a low verbal score, emphasizing visual methods of instruction), but this test analysis approach is not specific to ASD and is usually secondary to the purpose of the testing.

Researchers have devoted considerable effort to identifying and developing assessment measures that evaluate developmental and behavioral functioning in ASD, especially in the areas of social and communication skills (e.g., Carter, Davis, Klin, & Volkmar, 2005; Tager-Flusberg, Paul, & Lord, 2005; Watson, Lord, Schaffer, & Schopler, 1989). The past few years have seen increasing agreement on and endorsement of many of these measures, based on the factors of validity, reliability, and relevance for the subject population. Some developmental and cognitive tests, such as the Mullen Scales of Early Learning (Mullen, 1995) and the original Differential Ability Scales (Elliott, 1990), have been widely used and are highly regarded in the ASD research field. However, these and other assessment measures used in research are less valuable in generating teaching ideas and strategies, primarily because they were not designed for this purpose and are not specific to ASD. Similarly, widely used and well-standardized diagnostic instruments for ASD, such as the Autism Diagnostic Observation Schedule, Second Edition (Lord et al., 2012), and the Childhood Autism Rating Scale, Second Edition (Schopler & Van Bourgondien, 2010), are used both clinically and in research—they yield valuable information on all aspects of behavioral characteristics seen in ASD across the entire age range. However, they are not intended to serve as a basis for treatment planning, beyond the classification of an individual as having an ASD diagnosis or not.

There are many model ASD intervention programs, which have been reviewed in previous publications (e.g., Dawson & Burner, 2011; Warren et al., 2011; Vismara & Rogers, 2010). All incorporate assessment information to some degree, although with considerable variation in comprehensiveness and in description of how assessment information is organized and translated into treatment goals. All of these, and others not cited, employ explicit data collection methods and have clearly defined philosophies and frameworks, as well as specific approaches. Two groups emerge from among these programs. The first group fully integrates assessment data and considers the assessment process a critical component of intervention planning; the second group appears to be less wedded to assessment as a core component (to judge by published reports), but makes use of these data in treatment planning. Three programs fall into the first group: TEACCH (Boyd et al., 2014; Mesibov & Shea, 2010; Mesibov, Shea, & Schopler, 2005); Social Communication, Emotional Regulation, and Transactional Supports (SCERTS; Prizant, Wetherby, Rubin, Laurent, & Rydell, 2006); and the Developmental, Individual Differences, Relationship-Based Model (DIR; Greenspan & Wieder, 2006). Six programs fall into the second group: the Denver Model/Early Start Denver Model (Rogers & Lewis, 1989; Dawson et al., 2010), the Young Child Project (Lovaas, 1987), the Douglass Developmental Disabilities Center (Harris, Handleman, Arnold, & Gordon, 2001; see Chapter 11, this volume), pivotal response treatment (Cadogan & McCrimmon, 2015; Koegel, Koegel, & McNerney, 2001), Learning Experiences Alternative Program (LEAP; Boyd et al., 2014; Strain & Cordisco, 1994), and the Walden School (McGee, Morrier, Daly, & Jacobs, 2001). As noted earlier, these nine programs are intended to be representative of the range of ASD-specific models cited by the field. They reflect a diversity of frameworks, including developmental, behavioral, eclectic, and social–emotional. The reader is encouraged to review the programs' descriptions in the literature for detailed information about how they incorporate assessment information into treatment and educational planning. The balance of this chapter focuses on the formal and informal assessment methods used in the TEACCH program.

OVERVIEW OF THE TEACCH APPROACH TO ASSESSMENT

Individualized assessment has always been an integral part of the TEACCH program. The rationale for the first version of the PEP included the need for an assessment tool that could reliably measure developmental skills at a time when most professionals believed that children with autism were "untestable," as well as the need to find a systematic method for individualizing educational programs that would meet the needs of children whose learning patterns varied, though they showed the common criteria defining autism (Schopler & Reichler, 1979). The PEP demonstrated that a test that reduced language demands and could be flexibly administered resulted in more accurate developmental information and could help in program planning. By the late 1980s more children were being identified at the preschool age, so the PEP was revised (becoming the PEP-R) to better assess children under age 3. Most recently, the PEP-3 revision (Schopler, Lansing, Reichler, & Marcus, 2005) has brought the test further in line with current concepts of cognitive functioning and psychometric properties (Chen, Chiang, Tseng, Fu, & Hsieh, 2011; De Giacomo et al., 2016; Fulton & D'Entremont, 2013). The strengths of the PEP include its ability to be used with the entire range of preschool- and elementary school-age children with ASD (regardless of the severity of their disorders), its integration of the behavioral and the developmental domains, and its value for educational and home programming. In our work with teachers, we demonstrate how the basic features of the formal PEP assessment instrument can be translated into informal assessment methods in the classroom, and urge them to use these methods to help with day-to-day decision making regarding curriculum and behavior management issues. Specifically, we emphasize the concept of "emerging skills" and the importance of noting each child's interests and learning style, spotting possibly interfering ASD characteristics, and recognizing parents' priorities as they pertain to various curriculum areas.

As a student moves out of childhood and preadolescence and into the teenage years, assessment shifts from the developmental to the functional as the curriculum emphasis changes. The assessment process remains critical, but the focus and location of assessment moves from the classroom to other in-school settings (such as the office or cafeteria) and to actual life space areas in the community (such as work sites). Even for those students who can continue on an academic track, there is a need for functional assessment of communication, social, and work behavior skills. The Adolescent and Adult Psychoeducational Profile (AAPEP; Mesibov, Schopler, Schaffer, & Landrus, 1988) was designed to provide a functional assessment for adolescents and adults with ASD and intellectual disability. It has recently been revised to serve more explicitly as a tool to help with transition planning, becoming the TEACCH Transition Assessment Profile (TTAP; Mesibov, Thomas, Chapman, & Schopler, 2007). An important feature of the AAPEP/TTAP is that it enables a direct and consistent evaluation of a person's skills in a number of functional domains across home, school, and work settings. In addition to the formal assessment instrument that constituted the older AAPEP, the newer TTAP includes an informal measure for older adolescents and adults who are candidates for supported employment services. This instrument, which has been developed and fine-tuned for nearly two decades through our TEACCH Supported Employment program, evaluates the skills and behaviors that are needed in actual work settings (Keel, Mesibov, & Woods, 1997).

The information gathered with these two assessment instruments is used to help with job placement decisions and determining strategies for on-the-job instructional programs. For high-functioning individuals, traditional psychological and achievement tests may also be used to clarify cognitive patterns and strengths and weaknesses. These are supplemented by tasks from neuropsychological tests, as well as by measures of social understanding and expression, theory of mind, and central coherence. Observations and results from all of these measures help pinpoint subtle social and communication problems and specific thinking and learning issues (e.g., literalness, difficulties with perspective taking, and cognitive inflexibility) that may need to be specially addressed in a job setting.

A very important aspect of assessment is gathering and sharing information from and with parents. At the preschool level, the initial assessment process is usually geared to determining a diagnosis and answering questions about its implications (Marcus & Stone, 1993). This time is also used to introduce the parents to our philosophy, approach, and commitment to ongoing support. Because we provide direct follow-up (see below), the initial evaluation serves as a relationship-building experience rather than as the end of an assessment process. Seeking and using parents' observations and opinions are integral to the assessment process, as well as to making such treatment decisions as appropriate school placement, need for medication, and future residential and vocational placements.

THE PEP-3: DESCRIPTION AND CASE EXAMPLE

As noted above, the PEP-3, the most recent revision of the PEP, is a developmental test that helps with diagnosis and individualized programming (De Giacomo et al., 2016; Fulton & D'Entremont, 2013). The test normally can be given in 45–90 minutes and provides multiple opportunities for informal observations of behavior. Covering a developmental age range from about 6 months to 7 years, the PEP-3 includes a direct test and observation scale and a Caregiver Report. The child test scale yields age scores in six developmental areas, three focusing on language skills and the other three focusing on motor skills. Composite scores for these skill areas can be calculated. There are four behavior areas specific to ASD, and the derived standard and percentile scores are based on a sample with ASD. The Caregiver Report allows for an assessment of adaptive skills and specific behaviors. Information from both parts of the instrument can be integrated in formulating a treatment and education plan.

In reviewing the data, the clinician should consider various levels of analysis: examining the child's overall pattern of strengths and weaknesses, analyzing the individual items that were passed or where an "emerging" score was obtained, reviewing the pattern of maladaptive behaviors, and considering the parent's or caregiver's information. Below is a case example based on a PEP-3 assessment.

As part of his 3-year reevaluation, the school psychologist administered the PEP-3 to Sam. Sam was a 5-year-old child with a previous diagnosis of autistic disorder. Previous developmental testing suggested that his level of cognitive development was behind his chronological age by 12–24 months, depending on the area of functioning assessed. According to his performance on the PEP-3, his Communication Skills age equivalent score was at the 40-month level. His Expressive score was higher than his Receptive score; this pattern was related to his strengths in labeling objects and repeating words. His Cognitive Verbal/Preverbal score was at the 48-month level, due to strengths in matching skills and to several emerging skills related to preschool concepts (e.g., identifying numbers, letters, shapes, and colors). Sam's motor skills were more developed than his communication skills. His overall Motor Skills score was 41 months; although this was a lower score than his Communication Skills score, he was at ceiling in Gross Motor Skills. He was at the 45-month level in Fine Motor Skills. Sam was not able to write his name or color in the lines of pictures, but he had emerging skills in copying shapes. He had numerous difficulties with visual–motor imitation tasks because of his limited attention to the examiner.

On the behavioral scales of the PEP-3, Sam's Social Relating Skills were more impaired than those of other children on the autism spectrum. He had a percentile score of 35 in this domain, reflecting his tendency to ignore others, his lack of reciprocity in interactions, and his difficulty in expressing affect appropriate to a situation. By contrast, Sam's Communication Skills (percentile score of 70) were less impaired than those of other children with ASD. Although he demonstrated some unusual uses of language, such as occasional immediate and delayed echolalia, his language development was otherwise delayed but not unusual. Sam's percentile score on the Characteristic Motor Behaviors domain was 75, indicating that he demonstrated fewer unusual motor behaviors than other children with ASD. On the Caregiver Report, Sam's parents noted Personal Self-Care at the 41-month level. His mother reported that she had not previously expected much independence from him in his self-care, and that she would now like to focus on developing these skills at home. His Problem Behaviors outside of school were not severe. In this area, he was at the 80th percentile relative to other children with ASD, and his Adaptive Behavior as measured on the Caregiver Report was also a strength relative to other children with ASD.

Sam's teacher reviewed his PEP-3 developmental performance and noted that he had strengths in visual skills such as matching, communication skills such as labeling, and gross motor skills. To determine appropriate teaching goals, she decided to focus on emerging skills—particularly in Sam's areas of strength—as he was likely to make quicker progress in these areas, which could then be used to develop his areas of weakness. He demonstrated the following emerging abilities: matching letters, counting, naming shapes and colors, and labeling pictures. He had mastered some skills, such as matching objects to picture outlines, and he was interested in books (especially books about vehicles). However, Sam's teacher was concerned about his difficulty in relating to others, especially his lack of attention to other people, as she felt that this difficulty was delaying his development in other areas. For example, she was having a hard time teaching him fine motor movements, such as using scissors, because he did not attend to her demonstrations and resisted physical prompts. She had also discussed Sam's delayed self-care skills with his mother, and had agreed to try to help him develop more independence in daily living activities.

Sam's teacher used all this information to assist her in developing many goals for his individualized education program (IEP). One developmental goal for Sam was to increase his awareness of the math concept of quantity. The teacher planned to use his mastered skill of matching objects to picture outlines to develop his emerging skill of counting. She created several activities to teach him during instructional time, which he could then practice throughout the day. For example, she taught him to attach blocks to cards containing the same number of squares as the numeral written on the card. She also taught him to match pictures of his peers to a number "puzzle" with circles matching the size of the pictures. Once he had mastered these tasks, Sam could practice the block activity during his independent work time and the picture activity during circle time, to help the children count how many students were in class that day.

One of Sam's social goals was to pay more attention to people. Again, the teacher used his mastered skills in matching and his interest in books and vehicles to teach this skill. During her instructional time, she taught Sam several activities. She took pictures of the classroom staff in their cars and the other students in their parents' cars or the buses they rode to school. Using these photographs, she created an adapted book about the people in Sam's school environment and their cars. When looking at the book, Sam had a selection of pictures identical to those in the book, and he matched the pictures to each page in the book so that he had looked at pictures of each person. The teacher also attached pictures of each student to the placemats they used for snacks and to the table at the places where each student usually sat. Sam's job was to pass out placemats, first using the picture cues on the table and then, once he mastered this task, matching each placemat to the person sitting at that place. Sam's teacher also showed this activity to his mother as an example of how she could teach him to be more independent at home.

Sam's teacher thus used the information from the PEP-3 to formulate both social and developmental goals, and to create activities that would allow him to practice these goals throughout his day. Once Sam mastered these goals, she used informal assessment to create new goals. For example, as he mastered the activities created to help him learn the concept of quantity, she began to assess whether he could match blocks to cards with numerals but no outlines. She also assessed whether she could use a number line, so that Sam could match objects to the outlines on the line and then choose the numeral matching that amount. In this way, she combined formal and informal assessment to determine Sam's pattern of learning, strengths, and weaknesses. She also used the concept of emerging abilities to identify areas of readiness, and then based her teaching on all these types of information.

USING INFORMAL ASSESSMENT TO DEVELOP EDUCATIONAL PLANS

The results of standardized intellectual assessments can be used to develop an IEP that is based on an understanding of a student's learning profile. Developmental, vocational, adaptive, and achievement testing are perhaps more directly related to developing intervention goals. But even with the guidance of formal assessment data, teachers are often required to "fill in the gaps" in order to develop effective IEPs. For many reasons, standardized assessments may have limited use for educators. Teachers are often faced with writing goals for students whose records have relatively little assessment information. They may only have access to outdated evaluations. Developmental testing or adaptive assessments contain items that might directly apply to educational goals, but test protocols that indicate performance on specific items are not available to teachers. The general scores in a psychoeducational report provide information about learning profiles that teachers can use to infer goals, but the uneven performance of students with ASD may not be reflected in those goals. All these limitations of formal assessments leave teachers with a need for a method of ongoing assessment to facilitate educational planning throughout the school year. This type of evaluation is called "informal assessment." Informal assessment is based on the student's present performance in the classroom as opposed to his or her performance on a test with standardized administration and scoring.

Informal assessment is a process of presenting novel tasks to a student in order to determine that student's readiness to learn those tasks.

Readiness is determined by observing those areas in which a student demonstrates emerging skills. This type of assessment is intended to be a supplement to, but not a replacement for, formal assessments such as intellectual or achievement testing. In fact, standardized assessment can be a useful starting point for determining the types of skills that might be included in an informal assessment. By identifying a student's current level of performance through informal assessment, a teacher can begin developing specific goals for an IEP.

The advantages of informal assessment in developing an IEP are several. In the TEACCH program, we have observed that activities that have a clear purpose are more readily acquired than tasks where the purpose is not meaningful or is unclear (Mesibov et al., 2005). In informal assessment, a teacher can assess real-life activities or skills presented in a way that is more meaningful to a student than those activities administered in most standardized test instruments. For example, achievement tests may assess reading comprehension by using sentences or paragraphs that have no relation to a student's interests or daily activities. Informal assessment does not have the restrictions of standardized administration, so a teacher can assess comprehension by using materials related to a student's special interest, or sentences with instructions the student would follow in daily life.

Informal assessment also gives the teacher the opportunity to focus on emerging skills where the student is demonstrating readiness to learn. This is one of the most significant advantages of informal assessment over formal educational assessment. Other than the PEP-3 and TTAP, there are no standardized assessment measures that account for emerging abilities. Some measures of adaptive behavior (e.g., the Vineland Adaptive Behavior Scales, Second Edition [Vineland–II]; Sparrow, Cicchetti, & Balla, 2005) provide scores for items that are performed inconsistently. For the most part, though, an examiner is required to identify skills that may be potential learning goals based on items that the student failed during testing, even though the student may not be ready to learn those skills.

Following is a description of how to plan, administer, and interpret informal assessments in order to implement educational goals. The case example that follows this description details the process from start to finish as it might be implemented for a young child with ASD. Figure 12.1 is a graphic representation of this process—beginning with formal assessment; progressing to informal assessment, goal development, and intervention; and then returning to assessment.

Planning an Informal Assessment

For most teachers, determining which activities to assess is the most difficult aspect of an informal assessment. This process can be greatly enhanced

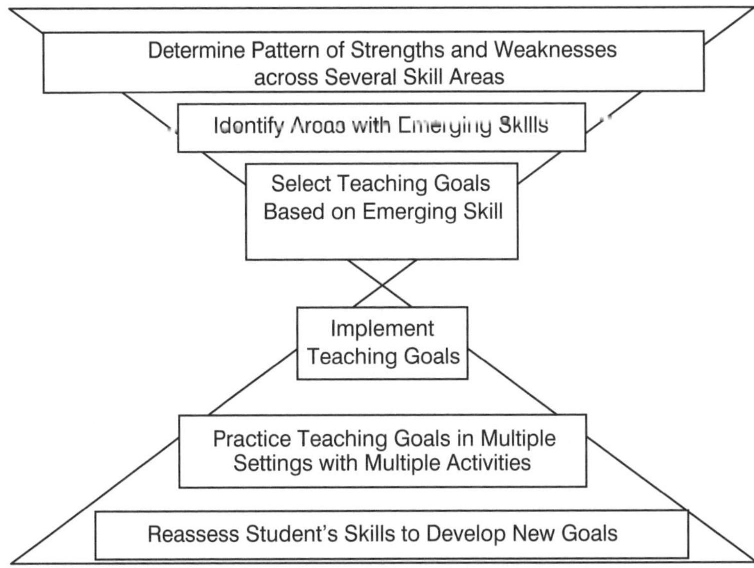

FIGURE 12.1. Process of developing goals from assessment to intervention and back to assessment.

by a good knowledge of typical development, especially for teachers of young children. Understanding developmental norms across a range of skill areas will allow a teacher to determine possible next steps based on developmental test results. Standardized educational and developmental curricula can also provide useful direction to the teacher planning an informal assessment. Norms related to the development of typical students, however, should be used with caution, as the development of students with ASD is likely to be uneven (Joseph, Tager-Flusberg, & Lord, 2002). Teachers should expect that prerequisite skills may not have been mastered even when more advanced skills are present, or that a concept may not have been generalized even if it is demonstrated in one context.

Another source of ideas for informal assessment is task analysis. Teachers of older students especially should have experience with detailed task analysis. During an informal assessment of an adaptive skill, task analysis will assist the teacher in finding those aspects of a task that reflect emerging skills.

Informal assessment should not consist only of tasks that the teacher expects that the student has not learned. Skills that have been acquired in one context should be assessed across a range of contexts. This will assist the teacher in determining whether a skill has generalized to other activities or has been mastered only within the tasks that have been taught.

For example, if a student with ASD has been successfully sorting blocks by color, the teacher may want to assess whether the child can sort other objects by color or match pictures according to color. Until the student has demonstrated competency with that concept in a range of ways, the teacher cannot be confident that the student has mastered that concept. Skills that may have been mastered, therefore, should still be included in an informal assessment.

Skills that the teacher suspects the student would fail are still worth assessing during the informal assessment. This is especially the case if the teacher is aware of particular interests and strengths the student has demonstrated in the past. The uneven skill development of students with ASD results in some students mastering skills even though they appear not to have mastered prerequisite skills. For example, a number of young children with ASD develop some reading skills before they have learned to speak (Craig & Telfer, 2005). A teacher who plans assessments based only on skills expected for a child with a similar developmental level may miss important strengths that were not previously assessed because the child had already met ceiling criteria before reaching that skill in a formal assessment.

Administering the Assessment

Informal assessment can be done at any time. For example, observation of a child's initiations on the playground could be considered an informal assessment of social skills. But informal assessment, despite its name, is not intended to be administered without planning or some structure. It is important for the teacher to be clear about the goals of the assessment and the criteria for passing, emerging, or failing scores. These need not be standardized criteria, but they should be specific enough for the teacher to determine whether skills can be considered as mastered, emerging, or absent.

When the informal assessment is administered, thought should be given to the student's expectations. If the assessment makes use of tabletop activities, then it should be done at a time and place where the student usually works with a teacher, so that it takes place within a familiar work routine. In this way, the student is more likely to be able to give his or her best performance. When the teacher is planning the assessment, a hierarchy of prompts should be considered along with the scoring criteria. For example, a student who is verbal might be presented with the materials and given a brief demonstration. If this prompt is ineffective, then the teacher might give a short verbal instruction. Additional prompts can be used in a systematic fashion. If the teacher is aware of the prompts being used, it will be easier to score the assessment and easier to make decisions about the best teaching techniques.

Monitoring the level of prompting helps the teacher plan a goal, given the student's present performance. The teacher should not, however, confuse exploring prompts with teaching. The assessment is not instructional time, and the teacher should not become sidetracked by teaching. Teaching will not be effective until the emerging skills are identified, and this must be done at the conclusion of the assessment, not during the assessment.

Scoring the Informal Assessment

Identifying "emerging skills," or those skills that a child is most ready to learn, is the goal of informal assessment. If the criterion for each activity is clear, then the student may pass the task, fail it, or complete it partially or with help. If the child can do some part of the task or can complete it with help, this task should be considered an emerging skill. When the teacher is scoring the informal assessment, the primary goal should be to identify emerging abilities.

In addition to identifying emerging abilities, informal assessment is an opportunity for a teacher to observe other aspects of the student's learning style. Because most activities in an informal assessment will be new, the teacher is able to observe the student's problem-solving skills. As in a formal psychoeducational evaluation, all behavior during the assessment is useful information about the student's responses to a variety of materials, his or her patience and persistence with difficult tasks, organizational abilities, and the cues that the student responds to best.

Developing Goals Based on the Informal Assessment

Once the assessment is completed and the teacher has determined which skills reflect emerging abilities, the teacher's task is to design teaching activities that will develop the identified skills. It is important to avoid the trap of designing only one activity to develop each skill. The strengths of students with ASD in the area of memory, and their weaknesses in generalization, often lead to mastery of specific activities through memorization without actually learning the underlying principle.

To develop goals, the teacher should think of times throughout the day when each skill would be used, and then teach activities that correspond to those times of day. Repeated practice in multiple contexts will make the skill more meaningful to a student with ASD and will ensure that when the skill is reassessed, the student will have mastered the concept rather than memorizing a specific task.

Monitoring Goals Based on Informal Assessment

Teachers are required to monitor students' progress on all IEP goals, although planning goals in the manner described above may require types of monitoring that are unfamiliar to some teachers. We suggest that teachers continue to make use of the concepts of "pass," "emerge," and "fail" to assess a student's progress. Some teachers group all of the activities related to a single goal on one data sheet, in order to be able to compare progress on related activities. Most teachers we have worked with prefer to keep activities on data sheets in the order in which they would occur during the day, to promote ease of data collection. With this format, a teacher can record data at the times during the day when memory of a student's performance is freshest. For example, the teacher can keep a record form for each student that has the schedule written in a column on the left, and specific activities related to IEP goals listed to the right of the time of day each one occurs. Following a morning group, a member of the classroom staff can pick up the data sheet for some of the students and circle "pass," "emerge," or "fail" for the skills that were practiced during that time.

After a few days, the teacher may transfer the daily data for each child onto a sheet that groups the activities by goal or curriculum area, to see whether the child is mastering the goal in a variety of areas. Then the teacher is able to observe whether some activities are mastered while others are not. The teacher will also be able to see whether some activities need to be modified because the student's readiness was not what it appeared to be during the original informal assessment. We often find that a teacher needs to restructure activities related to a goal, to help promote more timely progress. Or, if performance is quite different from what the original data suggested, the teacher may need to repeat the assessment.

As the teacher's daily data indicate that a child is consistently passing (or consistently failing) items related to a teaching concept, then the teacher will plan a new informal assessment in order to keep the student's goals in line with his or her progress. Informal assessment, then, is not considered an annual event, but one that will continue throughout the year as the student makes progress. As reflected in Figure 12.1, assessment is always both the beginning and the end of the teaching development process.

Case Example

Susan was a 10-year-old with ASD who completed her mandated reevaluation with the school psychologist. Results indicated that her Wechsler Intelligence Scale for Children—Fourth Edition (WISC-IV; Wechsler, 2003) Full Scale IQ was in the mild range of intellectual disability, with strengths in Perceptual Reasoning. She particularly excelled at WISC-IV Block Design and Matrix Reasoning. On the Woodcock–Johnson III Tests of Achievement (Woodcock, McGrew, & Mather, 2001), she generally performed at the first-grade level, but was at the third-grade level on Math Calculation, Spelling, and Decoding. Her Reading Comprehension, Writing, and Applied Problems were significant weaknesses. The psychologist also completed the Vineland–II with her parents. Susan's Adaptive Behavior Composite was well below her age level, with a standard score of 54. Scores were relatively even across Communication, Daily Living, and Socialization.

Susan's parents were especially interested in seeing that her reading skills advance. Her teacher had observed that, despite her decoding ability, Susan understood words best when they were associated with a practical task or visual image. She decided, therefore, to complete an informal assessment with particular emphasis on Susan's reading comprehension. In the informal assessment, Susan's teacher presented a variety of activities—these included sorting identical words and matching single words to familiar pictures (such as those on her picture schedule or pictures of favorite foods). She also showed Susan sentences and asked her to match the sentences to a picture. To assess her understanding of writing without visual cues, she gave Susan a list of simple written directions, such as "Stand up," to see whether she could follow these directions in a written format. She also gave Susan a list of words and several objects, and asked her to collect all the objects that matched the words on the list. Using simple picture books, Susan's teacher assessed whether she could match pictures to pages of the book containing the same picture, and whether she could match words to pages containing the same word.

During the informal assessment, Susan's teacher observed emerging abilities in the following tasks: matching words to pictures, choosing objects to correspond to a list, matching pictures to sentences, and matching words to pages in a book. Susan's teacher also noticed that she was especially interested in books and pictures about animals. She had observed in the past that Susan enjoyed playing the role of a "helper" at school, and Susan's parents reported that the same was true at home.

Based on this assessment, Susan's teacher planned for her to improve her comprehension skills throughout the day by completing the following activities. During morning group, Susan would match the written names of each student to the picture of each student, to assist in taking attendance. During Susan's work time, her teacher would present file folder activities requiring her to match pictures to words and pictures to short sentences. As Susan mastered these activities, she could practice them during independent work time. Depending on her progress, the teacher could present new folder activities with additional vocabulary and sentence comprehension items during instructional time. Her teacher would make sure that at least a few of the activities involved animals, to maintain Susan's interest in and enjoyment of reading. During her work time with the teacher, Susan would also use adapted books. These books would require her to match words to pictures in the book. The teacher selected several easy books with topics of interest to Susan, in order to expand her repertoire of leisure activities. Once Susan had mastered this skill using these adapted books, her teacher would keep them in the classroom reading center, where Susan could complete them during her free time. All the students in Susan's class took turns completing chores. Susan's teacher had labeled the shelves in the play area, and when it was Susan's turn to clean up, she would practice matching the toys to the written labels. At snack time, Susan would collect supplies to set the table by following brief written directions accompanied by a picture. For example, a direction might be "Put the plates on the table," and there would be a drawing of a person putting plates on the table. Finally, when she was preparing to go home, Susan would pack her school bag, using a written list of single words and checking off each word as she placed that object in her bag.

As indicated by this list of activities, Susan's teacher was following the recommendation of developing a skill by using several activities and having the student practice that skill throughout the day. The specific skills being developed were the comprehension of single written words and short sentences. Rather than learning and practicing this skill in a reading book, Susan would be learning these skills by using her visual strengths. Ideally, Susan's acquisition of these skills would also be promoted by including some of Susan's interests and utilizing her motivation to be helpful to her teacher.

As the teacher taught and then allowed Susan to practice the activities she had created, she noticed that Susan had an exceptional memory and that her performance on some tasks might not reflect her actual comprehension. In particular, she had memorized most of the directions associated with snack time, and she had also memorized where the toys in the play area belong. To accommodate these observations, Susan's teacher changed the position of the toys and their labels once a week, and had Susan begin to practice using written directions for other chores and for a "Simon says" game that the students played during their social group.

As Susan progressed, her teacher noted consistent passing performance on those tasks involving single words and a visual cue. All the words that had been used so far were from the first-grade curriculum. Susan's performance on tasks that included sentences was still inconsistent. So her teacher performed another informal assessment, this time presenting similar tasks with more difficult vocabulary words, longer written checklists, and adapted books that required matching sentences to pictures rather than single words. As the year ended, Susan's teacher noted at the IEP meeting that Susan's reading comprehension had improved, though it was still delayed relative to her decoding skills. Also, because her teacher had selected emerging skills that were within Susan's ability to master without excessive frustration, Susan was more motivated to read and was spending more time in the reading center with her adapted books. She had also begun to explore books that weren't adapted. Susan's parents reported that they had been able to use some of these skills at home. She was now able to follow a written checklist to complete her morning routine independently before school, and to clean up her room. They had also noticed Susan's increased interest in reading, and now saw reading as a potential leisure interest for Susan in the future.

The final step in this process was for Susan's teacher to identify future goals that would build on Susan's newly mastered skills. Susan's teacher planned yet another informal assessment, adding reading activities that were somewhat lengthier and that included number concepts. This allowed her to assess whether Susan was ready to learn adaptive skills such as following a simple recipe.

ASSESSING ADOLESCENTS AND ADULTS

Although the bulk of this chapter examines assessment as it relates to educational goals for younger students with ASD, it is still important to briefly summarize assessment instruments available for those working with older students, and to review their applicability to students with ASD. Not many tests are available for the assessment of adolescents and adults with ASD—those that exist are, however, more closely tied to intervention goals than are many instruments used to test younger children. As students become older, there is more emphasis on adaptive skills within the special education curriculum. Furthermore, the Individuals with Disabilities Education Improvement Act of 2004 (IDEIA) requires that transition plans be developed in adolescence, and this constitutes a legal imperative to assess functional community and vocational skills. Given the functional nature of assessments used with older students, the transition between assessment and intervention is somewhat smoother than it seems with younger students. Although these measures appear to be more practical, they may not always account for the learning styles of individuals with ASD. This shortcoming may lead to educational plans that do not include important goals for students with ASD who are making the transition to adulthood. For example, vocational assessments that focus on basic work skills (e.g., packaging or office work) may neglect work behaviors that limit vocational success in individuals with ASD, such as the ability to cope with transitions or follow verbal instructions.

The instruments most commonly used with adolescents and adults are adaptive interviews, such as the Vineland–II (Sparrow et al., 2005), or adaptive checklists, such as the Adaptive Behavior Assessment System (Harrison & Oakland, 2015). Although these provide general information about adaptive functioning, they do not assess issues specific to adolescent and adult curriculum planning. They also require information from a limited number of sources. Curriculum development for adolescents and adults with ASD requires knowledge about performance across a range of settings—however, limiting information to one or two settings may lead to an incomplete assessment. Checklists that are more specific to the curriculum for adolescents and adults include the Transition Planning Inventory—Updated Version (TPI-UV; Clark & Patton, 2006) and the Becker Work Adjustment Profile—Second Edition (BWAP-2; Becker, 2005). These instruments measure skills related to daily living abilities, community, and vocational functioning. Both instruments also enable information to be obtained from at least two sources. Although interviews and checklists are a useful means of gathering information from multiple sources, their ability to identify emerging skills that are most amenable to instruction is limited. The TPI-UV does contain information for teachers concerning informal assessment. This link between the checklist and specific goals, however, is not a formal component of the assessment.

Some direct assessments also exist, including the Independent Living Scales (ILS; Loeb, 1996) and the Street Survival Skills Questionnaire (SSSQ; Linkenhoker & McCarron, 1993). The ILS contains items that simulate actual living skills, such as managing money, while the SSSQ uses pictures of real-life events to complete the assessment. Both scales assess specific skills that could be easily translated into a transition plan, and the SSSQ has a curriculum guide to facilitate this process. The learning styles of individuals with ASD include poor generalization and difficulties in drawing inferences from abstract stimuli (Mesibov et al., 2005). Assessment instruments containing "real-world" materials are, for individuals with ASD, more likely to provide meaningful information that can be directly transformed into teaching goals.

The only assessment instruments specifically designed for students with ASD who are adolescents or older are the Autism Screening Instrument for Educational Planning—Third Edition (ASIEP-3; Krug, Arick, & Almond, 2008) and the TTAP, described earlier in this chapter (Mesibov et al., 2007). The ASIEP-3 contains items appropriate for adolescents and adults, but was designed for the entire age range from preschool through adult. The ASIEP-3 application to intervention planning for older students is limited by the wide range of skills it is designed to assess. As noted earlier, the TTAP is based on the AAPEP (Mesibov et al., 1998), so it was specifically designed to assess curriculum-related skills for adolescents and adults with ASD. The TTAP has expanded on the AAPEP by adding components that provide for direct assessment in work environments, giving suggestions for developing goals based on test performance, expanding the range of items included in order to facilitate assessment of individuals with a wide range of cognitive abilities, and providing mechanisms for measuring progress as an individual develops his or her skills. The TTAP specifically addresses the characteristics of ASD that can make other assessment instruments less effective when instructors are developing teaching goals for this population. Specifically, it provides for both direct assessment and obtaining interview information from other sources, including caregivers and teachers or work supervisors. Assessing skills across a range of environments and gathering information from other observers will help teachers to determine whether a skill has been acquired and whether it has generalized to a variety of settings. The TTAP also assesses an individual's ability to use a variety of visual supports, such as schedules or visual rules, to determine how the person's visual strengths can be used to improve performance across settings. As with the PEP-3 (Schopler et al., 2005), there are no basal or ceiling rules in administration—this allows for full assessment of the uneven patterns of learning in individuals with ASD. Finally, the TTAP incorporates informal assessment in a variety of school and work environments, to facilitate observation of how different types of job demands interact with the individual's skills and personality. Assessment and instruction in real-world environments will also allow the individual to experience different types of work directly. People with ASD have difficulty making decisions based on abstract or descriptive information; they are better able to make decisions about job preferences when they have experienced different placements firsthand. Making choices based on written or pictured information is less likely to be valid, although this is the typical approach to assessing vocational interests (e.g., the Wide Range Interest and Occupation Test—Second Edition; Glutting & Wilkinson, 2003).

The process of developing curriculum goals based on the TTAP is much like that outlined in Figure 12.1. The pattern of strengths and weaknesses in skill and behavioral development is assessed by direct observation, as well as via caregiver and teacher interviews. From this understanding of the individual's learning profile, and from the identification of emerging skills, specific goals are developed. Those goals are assessed in a variety of environments through the use of informal assessment. Finally, instruction is provided for emerging abilities throughout the areas assessed, and assessment is repeated as skills are mastered. The primary difference when this process is applied to adolescents and adults rather than children is that instruction is more likely to take place in real-life settings than in the classroom. Teaching across several settings is more heavily emphasized, because of the need to prepare adolescents and adults for using their skills in the community.

CONCLUDING COMMENTS

In this chapter, we have described both formal and informal assessment approaches as a basis for planning individualized treatment and education goals and activities for students with ASD. These approaches are largely derived from our experience with the TEACCH model—however, regardless of the model used, psychologists, educators, and other professionals need to view assessment as a continuing process rather than an annual event. Moreover, assessment should be seen as a means of integrating child, home, and school information not just to understand a child's levels of functioning and basic problems but to help determine general and specific needs, and then generate intervention ideas. Being able to communicate with the "end users" (parents, teachers, and other service providers) requires knowledge not only of assessment tools and strategies but also of developmental and educational instruction methods, curricula, and activities. Individuals with ASD and their families, and the professionals who help them, will all be beneficiaries of this effort.

REFERENCES

Becker, R. L. (2005). *Becker Work Adjustment Profile:2*. Columbus, OH: Elbern.

Boyd, B. A., Hume, K., McBee, M. T., Alessandri, M., Gutierrez, A., Johnson, L., et al. (2014). Comparative efficacy of LEAP, TEACCH and non-model-specific special education programs for preschoolers with autism spectrum disorders. *Journal of Autism and Developmental Disorders, 44*(2), 366–380.

Cadogan, S., & McCrimmon, A. W. (2015). Pivotal response treatment for children with autism spectrum disorder: A systematic review of research quality. *Developmental Neurorehabilitation, 18*(2), 137–144.

Carter, A., Davis, N. O., Klin, A., & Volkmar, F. R. (2005). Social development in autism. In F. R. Volkmar, R. Paul, A. Klin, & D. J. Cohen (Eds.), *Handbook of autism and pervasive developmental disorders: Vol. 1* (3rd ed., pp. 312–334). Hoboken, NJ: Wiley.

Chen, K. L., Chiang, F. M., Tseng, M. H., Fu, C. P., & Hsieh, C. L. (2011). Responsiveness of the Psychoeducational Profile—Third Edition for children with autism spectrum disorders. *Journal of Autism and Developmental Disorders, 41*, 1658–1664.

Clark, G. M., & Patton, J. R. (2006). *Transition Planning Inventory—Updated Version: Administration and resource guide*. Austin, TX: PRO-ED.

Craig, H. K., & Telfer, A. S. (2005). Hyperlexia and autism spectrum disorder: A case study of scaffolding language development over time. *Topics in Language Disorders, 25*, 253–269.

Dawson, G., & Burner, K. (2011). Behavioral interventions in children and adolescents with autism spectrum disorder: A review of recent findings. *Current Opinions in Pediatrics, 23*, 616–620.

Dawson, G., Rogers, S., Munson, J., Smith, M., Winter, J., Greenson, J., et al. (2010).

Randomized controlled trial of an intervention for toddlers with autism: The Early Start Denver Model. *Pediatrics, 125,* e17–e23.

De Giacomo, A., Craig, F., Cristella, A., Terenzio, V., Buttiglione, M., & Margari, L. (2016). Can PEP-3 provide a cognitive profile in children with ASD?: A comparison between the developmental ages of PEP-3 and IQ of Leiter–R. *Journal of Applied Research in Intellectual Disabilities, 29*(6), 566–573.

Elliott, C. D. (1990). *Differential Ability Scales.* San Antonio, TX: Psychological Corporation.

Fulton, M. L., & D'Entremont, B. (2013). Utility of the Psychoeducational Profile–3 for assessing cognitive and language skills of children with autism spectrum disorders. *Journal of Autism and Developmental Disorders, 43,* 2460–2471.

Glutting, J. J., & Wilkinson, G. (2003). *Wide Range Interest and Occupation Test—Second Edition.* Austin, TX: PRO-ED.

Greenspan, S. I., & Wieder, S. (2006). *Engaging autism: Helping children relate, communicate and think with the DIR Floortime approach.* Cambridge, MA: Da Capo Press.

Harris, S. L., Handleman, J. S., Arnold, M. S., & Gordon, R. (2001). The Douglass Developmental Disabilities Center. In J. S. Handleman & S. L. Harris (Eds.), *Preschool education programs for children with autism* (2nd ed., pp. 233–260). Austin, TX: PRO-ED.

Harrison, P. L., & Oakland, T. (2015). *Adaptive Behavior Assessment System—Third Edition.* San Antonio, TX: Psychological Corporation.

Individuals with Disabilities Education Improvement Act of 2004, Pub. L. No. 108-446, 118 Stat. 2647 (2004).

Joseph, R. M., Tager-Flusberg, H., & Lord, C. (2002). Cognitive profiles and social–communicative functioning in children with autism spectrum disorder. *Journal of Child Psychology and Psychiatry, 43,* 807–821.

Keel, J. H., Mesibov, G. B., & Woods, A. (1997). TEACCH-supported employment programs. *Journal of Autism and Developmental Disorders, 27,* 3–9.

Koegel, R. L., Koegel, L. K., & McNerney, E. K. (2001). Pivotal areas in intervention for autism. *Journal of Clinical Child Psychology, 30,* 19–32.

Krug, D., Arick, J. R., & Almond, P. (2008). *Autism Screening Instrument for Educational Planning—Third Edition.* Austin, TX: PRO-ED.

Linkenhoker, D., & McCarron, L. (1993). *Street Survival Skills Questionnaire.* San Antonio, TX: Psychological Corporation.

Loeb, P. A. (1996). *Independent Living Scales.* San Antonio, TX: Psychological Corporation.

Lord, C., Rutter, M., DiLavore, P. C., Risi, S., Gotham, K., & Bishop, S. L. (2012). *Autism Diagnostic Observation Schedule, Second Edition (ADOS-2).* Los Angeles: Western Psychological Services.

Lovaas, O. J. (1987). Behavioral treatment and normal educational and intellectual functioning in young autistic children. *Journal of Consulting and Clinical Psychiatry, 55,* 3–9.

Marcus, L. M., & Stone, N. L. (1993). Assessment of the young autistic child. In E. Schopler, M. E. van Bourgondien, & M. Bristol (Eds.), *Preschool issues in autistic and related development of handicaps* (pp. 149–173). New York: Plenum Press.

McGee, G. G., Morrier, M. J., Daly, T., & Jacobs, H. A. (2001). The Walden Early Childhood Programs. In J. S. Handleman & S. L. Harris (Eds.), *Preschool education programs for children with autism* (2nd ed., pp. 157–190). Austin, TX: PRO-ED.

Mesibov, G. B., Schopler, E., Schaffer, B., & Landrus, R. (1988). *Adolescent and Adult Psychoeducational Profile.* Austin, TX: PRO-ED.

Mesibov, G. B., & Shea, V. (2010). The TEACCH program in the era of evidence-based practice. *Journal of Autism and Developmental Disorders, 40,* 570–579.

Mesibov, G. B., Shea, V., & Schopler, E. (2005). *The TEACCH approach to autism spectrum disorders.* New York: Kluwer Academic/Plenum.

Mesibov, G., Thomas, J. B., Chapman, S. M., & Schopler, E. (2007). *TEACCH Transition Assessment Profile—Second Edition.* Austin, TX: PRO-ED.

Mullen, E. M. (1995). *Mullen Scales of Early Learning.* Circle Pines, MN: American Guidance Service.

Prizant, B. M., Wetherby, A. M., Rubin, E., Laurent, A. C., & Rydell, P. J. (2006). *The SCERTS® model: A comprehensive educational approach for children with autism spectrum disorders.* Baltimore: Brookes.

Rogers, S. J., & Lewis, H. (1989). An effective day treatment model for young children with pervasive developmental disorders. *Journal of the American Academy of Child and Adolescent Psychiatry, 28,* 207–214.

Schopler, E., Lansing, M. D., Reichler, R. J., & Marcus, L. M. (2005). *Psychoeducational Profile—Third Edition.* Austin, TX: PRO-ED.

Schopler, E., & Reichler, R. J. (1979). *Individualized assessment and treatment for developmentally disabled children: Vol. 1. Psychoeducational profile.* Baltimore: University Park Press.

Schopler, E., & Van Bourgondien, M. E. (2010). *The Childhood Autism Rating Scale, Second Edition (CARS-2).* Los Angeles: Western Psychological Services.

Sparrow, S. S., Cicchetti, D. V., & Balla, D. A. (2005). *Vineland Adaptive Behavior Scales, Second Edition (Vineland–II).* Circle Pines, MN: American Guidance Service.

Strain, P. S., & Cordisco, L. K. (1994). LEAP Preschool. In S. Harris & J. S. Handleman (Eds.), *Preschool education programs for children with autism* (pp. 225–252). Austin, TX: PRO-ED.

Tager-Flusberg, H., Paul, R., & Lord, C. (2005). Language and communication in autism. In F. R. Volkmar, R. Paul, A. Klin, & D. J. Cohen (Eds.), *Handbook of autism and pervasive developmental disorders* (3rd ed., pp. 335–364). Hoboken, NJ: Wiley.

Vismara, L. A., & Rogers, S. J. (2010). Behavioral treatments in autism spectrum disorder: What do we know? *Annual Review of Clinical Psychology, 6,* 447–468.

Warren, Z., McPheeters, M. L., Sathe, N., Foss-Feig, J. H., Glasser, A., & Veenstra-Vanderweele, J. (2011). A systematic review of early intensive intervention for autism spectrum disorders. *Pediatrics, 127,* e1303–e1311.

Watson, L., Lord, C., Schaffer, B., & Schopler, E. (1989). *Teaching spontaneous communication to autistic and developmentally handicapped children.* Austin, TX: PRO-ED.

Wechsler, D. (2003). *Wechsler Intelligence Scale for Children, Fourth Edition (WISC-IV).* San Antonio, TX: Psychological Corporation.

Woodcock, R. W., McGrew, K. S., & Mather, N. (2001). *Woodcock–Johnson III Tests of Achievement.* Itasca, IL: Riverside.

CHAPTER THIRTEEN

Understanding the Comprehensive Assessment of Autism Spectrum Disorder through Case Studies

Tristyn Teel Wilkerson

The assessment of autism spectrum disorder (ASD) is often challenging even for experienced professionals. Due to the complicated nature of the ASD diagnosis, a comprehensive assessment addressing a wide range of behaviors, development, and emotions must be conducted by an experienced and knowledgeable professional. This is especially true for ASD due to the high rate of comorbidity and related issues (see Chapter 10, this volume). Assessment of ASD may be completed by a number of types of professionals with proper training, including neuropsychologists, psychologists, neurologists, pediatricians, and psychiatrists.

A comprehensive ASD evaluation should include information from a variety of sources. First, it is important to obtain a comprehensive history of the child's development and any relevant symptoms or events that may contribute to diagnostic clarification. Parent interview is essential to understanding at-home and community behavior. Additional historical and observational data may be provided by other adults familiar with the child such as teachers or grandparents through interview or questionnaires. Direct observation of the client is vital to ascertain social functioning and capacity.

Formal standardized evaluation of functioning should be completed in the areas of social functioning, communication ability and behavior, emotional functioning, cognitive and neuropsychological ability, and adaptive behavior and development. By gathering information across a wide variety of relevant areas, a complete diagnostic picture can be obtained. Given that other conditions may be comorbid with ASD, it is important to assess for those conditions using appropriate tools to provide complete diagnostic clarification and relevant recommendations. An extensive body of literature is available to indicate the best instruments to use in the assessment of ASD as reviewed in this volume. Each diagnostician selects those empirically validated instruments that are best suited to his or her practice and diagnostic framework.

At times, referrals to community providers for further assessment and treatment may be indicated. For example, a child with severe motor problems or sensory sensitivity may require assessment by a trained occupational therapist. Speech delays may be assessed by a trained speech and language therapist. A thorough and accurate assessment assists parents, treatment providers, and schools to establish an appropriate course for treatment in an effort to provide the individual with ASD the best possible prognosis given each individual situation. The results of the evaluation should be summarized in a comprehensive written report, including specific and meaningful recommendations for all individuals involved in the child's care and treatment. The evaluation should be concluded with a face-to-face feedback session designed to explain the results, provide recommendations, and answer any questions posed by parents. Additional consultation may be needed with treatment providers and the child's educational team.

The purpose of this chapter is to provide examples of comprehensive assessments to illustrate the decision-making process involved in diagnostic clarification, and to help address common issues that evaluators face. Two cases of clients assessed for possible ASD follow. (All identifying information has been changed to protect confidentiality.)

CASE EXAMPLE 1: RONNIE

Ronnie is a 17-year-old senior in high school. He was referred for evaluation due to social, emotional, and academic concerns. He is currently reportedly failing at school, does not complete assignments, and will not graduate on time. He also struggles socially and lacks motivation and confidence. Ronnie demonstrated a refractory response to trials of psychiatric medications in the past designed to improve attention and focus. Owing to the extent of concerns, a comprehensive evaluation was recommended to better define his current problems and to assist with treatment planning.

This assessment was particularly challenging because Ronnie carried a prior diagnosis of attention-deficit/hyperactivity disorder (ADHD). Parents, teachers, and medical professionals tailored all prior interventions for

Ronnie toward this diagnosis with limited success. The following describes the results of Ronnie's assessment and provides all aspects of a thorough evaluation: background information, adaptive functioning measures, behavioral observations, assessment results and interpretation, diagnostic impressions, and recommendations.

Background Information

Ronnie is the eldest of three siblings. He has a 15-year-old brother who has been diagnosed with depression and ADHD and a 13-year-old sister who struggles with attention problems. His 9-year-old brother also struggles with attention problems and is currently being evaluated for ASD as well.

Ronnie's mother's pregnancy with Ronnie was without complication. After delivery Ronnie experienced cyanosis. It is reported that he aspirated meconium and was placed in the intensive care unit that night for observation and placed on oxygen support. However, no further complications arose. As an infant, Ronnie was described as typical. He was easy to comfort by being held or stroked, enjoyed cuddling, and was regular in terms of sleep and feeding patterns. As a toddler, his activity level was described as normal but he was easily distracted and his persistence and attention were variable depending on the activity.

Ronnie's childhood medical history was overall unremarkable. His parents report significant numbers of stereotyped movements, including twisting his hair and "flipping" his hands. Ronnie currently falls asleep easily and sleeps through the night without disruption. His appetite is reported to have increased in the past 6 months.

Ronnie met all early developmental milestones (walking, speech, etc.) within normal limits. His speech is notable for articulation problems—however, he acquired speech at appropriate times.

Ronnie's mother reported that he struggles to understand directions and situations as well as other adolescents his age. He lacks self-awareness and does not understand social situations and is reported to "lack common sense." Ronnie's mother reported that she was concerned about his ability to succeed in kindergarten because he was a "slow learner"—some early academic skills were noted as delayed (reading, naming coins, etc.). To the best of her knowledge, Ronnie is currently performing at or above grade level in reading, spelling, and math but struggles in academics because he is a "perfectionist" and will not turn in assignments until he is satisfied with them. Ronnie's grades vary anywhere between an A+ and an F, depending on the subject. He does not currently receive special education services but previously received speech therapy services in the school to correct articulation errors and "graduated" from speech therapy in sixth grade. Ronnie's mother reported no behavioral problems in the classroom—however, due to several failing grades, he is required to repeat his 12th-grade year—he is missing math and science credits and has to make them up before he can graduate. Ronnie's mother reported that he "will only do assignments he likes. He has a hard time doing the other ones."

Ronnie seeks friendships with peers but is not often sought out by peers for friendship. He did not have close friends in elementary school. Currently, he has one female friend with whom he attended middle school, but they do not presently attend the same school. He typically spends time only with his siblings. Ronnie's mother reported that he struggles to make friends because he is "too hyper, overdoes everything, scares kids, and doesn't recognize social cues." Ronnie is noted to talk excessively about favorite topics that hold limited interest for others, has difficulty with conversational skills, and does not appear to understand basic social behavior.

At home, Ronnie is described as fidgety. He has difficulty remaining seated, interrupts and intrudes on others, and does not appear to listen to what is being said. At times he has difficulty getting along with his 15-year-old brother—his mother reports that they have a "love/hate relationship." Ronnie's mother stated that Ronnie lacks self-awareness. He has poor self-confidence and self-esteem and, as a result, refuses to express his opinions. His mother reported that he has a current pattern of restricted interests, which includes doll collecting, stating that he is "obsessed" with them. She also reports that most of Ronnie's peers do not share his interest and consider it to be overly feminine, which makes him the target of negative comments and judgments. Discipline used in the home includes discussion of the problem behavior and screen time restriction, which has proven effective in regard to behavioral modification.

Ronnie's main hobbies and interests include doll collecting, video games, texting, and reading books and comic books. His greatest area of accomplishment is playing through an entire soccer season despite difficulty actually playing the sport and poor performance. He dislikes cleaning. When asked what she likes about Ronnie, his mother stated that "he's a very good boy, very compliant, and helps with everything."

Adaptive Functioning Measures

The Conners Comprehensive Behavior Rating Scales (Conners, 2014) was completed by Ronnie's mother and his teacher. For comparative purposes, *T*-scores for the Content and DSM-5 scales appear below (mean = 50, *SD* = 10, high scores indicate problems).

	Parent	Teacher
Content scales		
Emotional Distress	81	43
Upsetting Thoughts	90	48
Worrying	42	—
Social Problems	90	47
Separation Fears	74	47
Social Anxiety	—	42
Defiant/Aggressive Behavior	55	44
Academic Difficulty	57	48
Language	56	51
Math	45	45
Hyperactivity/Impulsivity	90	44
Perfectionistic and Compulsive Behaviors	58	45
Violence Potential	51	44
Physical Symptoms	90	45
DSM-5 scales		
ADHD Inattentive Type	54	42
ADHD Hyperactive–Impulsive Type	50	44
Conduct Disorder	48	44
Oppositional Defiant Disorder	54	42
Major Depressive Episode	90	48
Manic Episode	90	41
Generalized Anxiety Disorder	53	47
Separation Anxiety Disorder	85	47
Obsessive/Compulsive Disorder	90	46
Autism Spectrum Disorder	90	44

Parent report reflects significant concerns in the areas of emotional distress, upsetting thoughts, social problems, separation fears, and physiological symptoms. Teacher report reflects minimal concerns across domains. This is consistent with the parent report that Ronnie is quiet in school and does not attract much negative attention.

Ronnie's parents and teacher were asked to complete the Autism Spectrum Rating Scale (ASRS; Goldstein & Naglieri, 2009). Age-adjusted *T*-scores are as follows (mean = 50, *SD* = 10, high scores indicate problems):

	Parent	Teacher
ASRS scales		
Social Communication	61	65
Unusual Behavior	64	60
Self-Regulation	64	47
DSM-5 scale	66	60
Treatment scales		
Peer Socialization	73	63
Adult Socialization	63	56
Social/Emotional Reciprocity	63	83
Atypical Language	68	59
Stereotypy	68	52
Behavioral Rigidity	49	61
Sensory Sensitivity	71	60
Attention	58	48

Parent report reflects significant symptoms associated with ASD. These include problems with social communication, unusual behaviors, and self-regulation. Ronnie reportedly has problems with peer and adult socialization, social and emotional reciprocity, atypical language, stereotyped behaviors, and sensory sensitivity. Teacher report reflects significant problems with social communication and unusual behaviors, but no difficulties in the area of self-regulation. At school, Ronnie struggles to socialize with peers. He also has problems with social and emotional reciprocity, behavioral rigidity, and sensory sensitivity.

Parent's, teacher's, and Ronnie's responses to the Comprehensive Executive Function Inventory (Naglieri & Goldstein, 2013) placed Ronnie at the following age-adjusted standard scores (mean = 100, *SD* = 15, low scores indicate problems).

	Parent	Teacher	Self-report
Attention	93	115	97
Emotion Regulation	95	112	122
Flexibility	80	119	79
Inhibitory Control	102	119	100
Initiation	99	113	94
Organization	95	111	90
Planning	90	114	94
Self-Monitoring	80	113	76
Working Memory	95	109	96

Ronnie and his mother report behaviors associated with executive functioning in the low-average range overall, with problem areas in flexibility and self-monitoring. Teacher report reflects high-average behaviors associated with executive functioning, with high-average functioning across domains. This is in contrast to both Ronnie's and his mother's reports.

Behavioral Observations

Ronnie, a youth of average size and casual dress, was seen for two assessment sessions in a single day. His behavior in both sessions was similar. Ronnie struggled to maintain appropriate eye contact—he could make eye contact at times but did not sustain it. Receptive and expressive language appeared average. He had some problems with articulation, but it was not difficult to understand him when he spoke. His expression was typically calm and he seemed emotionally stable and was not tearful at any time during the assessment.

Ronnie was alert, attentive, and focused—joint attention and visual and listening response appeared normal. He did not utilize instrumental or informative gestures in order to communicate and the quality of social overture and response was somewhat limited. In the second session, Ronnie was able to speak about some of his specific interests and opened up markedly at that time. However, through the majority of the assessment process, he communicated very minimally.

Ronnie was cooperative and attempted all items set before him. He appeared motivated to do his best, his persistence was normal, and no muscular tension was noted. Ronnie engaged in frequent habitual mannerisms—he often snapped his fingers near his ear repetitively. Activity level was normal and he was occasionally fidgety. He required directions to be repeated on numerous occasions because he was distracted by his need to snap his fingers.

Ronnie appeared moderately confident. He maintained a friendly relationship with this examiner but smiled inconsistently. Overall, his thought processes were logical, focused, and relevant. It was not difficult to establish a working relationship with this pleasant young man.

Assessment Results and Interpretation

Autism

Ronnie participated in the Autism Diagnostic Observation Schedule, Second Edition, Module 4 (Lord & Rutter, 2012). Scores are as follows:

	ADOS score	Autism cutoff	Autism spectrum cutoff
Communication	2	3	2
Social Interaction	6	6	4
Communication + Social Interaction Total	8	10	7
Stereotyped Behaviors and Restricted Interests	3		
ADOS-2 classification: Autism Spectrum			

Ronnie demonstrated numerous behaviors associated with ASD. With regard to language and communication, his affect while speaking tended to be somewhat more flat than is typical for his age. He rarely asked the examiner about her thoughts or feelings. Descriptive conventional, instrumental, informative, emphatic, and emotional gestures were limited in frequency. Ronnie had difficulty with sustained periods of eye contact and was inconsistently able to communicate his own affect. When describing emotions, he tended to be overly formal and practical in the way he expressed himself. He communicated some understanding of emotions and empathy toward others and also demonstrated some insight into typical social situations and relationships. However, he did not appear to understand his role within those relationships. He tended to describe relationships in practical and utilitarian terms rather than in terms of emotions or companionship. The quality of his social overture and response was somewhat limited and the quality of rapport was sometimes comfortable but not sustained. He demonstrated frequent hand and finger mannerisms and repeatedly referenced areas of highly specific topics. His behaviors during this evaluation meet the cutoff for a designation of ASD.

Executive/Neuropsychological Skills

The Cognitive Assessment System, Second Edition (Naglieri, Das, & Goldstein, 2014), was administered as a test of neuropsychological ability. Age-adjusted scaled scores appear below:

	Scaled scores (mean = 10, *SD* = 3)
Planned Codes	9
Planned Connections	9
Planned Number Matching	11
Matrices	13
Verbal–Spatial Relations	12

	Scaled scores (mean = 10, *SD* = 3)
Figure Memory	15
Expressive Attention	10
Number Detection	10
Receptive Attention	10
Word Series	11
Sentence Repetition/Questions	6
Visual Digit Span	9

	IQ (mean = 100, *SD* = 15)	Percentiles (mean = 50)	90% confidence interval
Planning	100	50th	[89, 108]
Simultaneous	120	91st	[125, 113]
Attention	100	50th	[88, 107]
Successive	91	27th	[98, 85]
Executive Functioning without Working Memory	91	27th	[98, 81]
Executive Functioning with Working Memory	100	50th	[107, 93]
Working Memory	94	34th	[101, 88]
Verbal Content	95	37th	[102, 88]
Nonverbal Content	110	74th	[116, 103]
Full Scale	93	32nd	[97, 89]
Visual–Auditory comparison: not significant			

Ronnie's overall neuropsychological functioning is measured within the average range. However, this reflects marked diversity among scores. There is a 29-point difference between highest and lowest composite areas. Ronnie's simultaneous processing is a marked area of strength, which indicates that his problem-solving abilities are intact and indeed superior to the average same-age peer.

Language

The Peabody Picture Vocabulary Test, Fourth Edition (Dunn & Dunn, 2007), was administered as a simple measure of one-word receptive vocabulary. Receptive vocabulary is often considered a good indicator of intellectual potential and growth. Ronnie's performance on this measure yielded a standard score of 107, equivalent to the 68th percentile.

The Expressive Vocabulary Test, Second Edition (Williams, 2007), was administered as a simple synonym measure of expressive language. Ronnie's performance on this measure yielded a standard score of 106, equivalent to the 66th percentile. His receptive and expressive language are measured in the average range.

Verbal Comprehension

Subtests from the Wechsler Adult Intelligence Scale—Fourth Edition (Wechsler, 2008) were administered as a screening of Ronnie's fund of learned verbal knowledge and verbal reasoning. Scaled scores appear below:

	Scaled scores (mean = 10, *SD* = 3)
Similarities	9
Information	11

Ronnie's fund of learned verbal information and verbal reasoning performance is measured in the average range.

Learning and Working Memory

Subtests from the Test of Memory and Learning—Second Edition (Reynolds & Voress, 2007) were administered as an overall screening. Age-adjusted scaled scores are as follows:

	Scaled scores (mean = 10, *SD* = 3)
Verbal subtests	
Memory for Stories	11
Word Selective Reminding	10
Object Recall	11
Paired Recall	11
Nonverbal subtests	
Visual Selective Reminding	13

	Scaled scores (mean = 10, *SD* = 3)	Percentiles
Verbal Memory Index	105	63rd
Learning Index	109	73rd

Ronnie's ability to learn and retain learned information is measured within the average range when compared with same-age peers.

Attention

The Conners Continuous Performance Test II (Conners, 2002) was administered as a computerized measure of Ronnie's ability to sustain attention and inhibit impulsive responding. His performance on this measure yielded a nonclinical profile with a 98.45% confidence interval that Ronnie does not display a clinically significant attention disorder, and he demonstrated good performance (Ronnie's *T*-scores less than 43) across all measured domains.

Motor/Perceptual Functioning

Ronnie appeared right-side dominant and held his pencil in a three-finger pincer grip. Casual observation did not indicate any large motor abnormalities. Fine motor skills for motor speed and coordination, based on the Purdue Pegboard Test (Tiffin, 1948) performance, appeared at the 82nd percentile for the dominant hand, 47th percentile for the nondominant hand, and 56th percentile for both hands.

Ronnie's reproductions of the Rey Complex Figure Test (Osterrieth, 1944) yielded a scaled score of 9, equivalent to the 37th percentile, with immediate recall of the figure yielding a scaled score of 12, equivalent to the 75th percentile.

Academic Functioning

The Woodcock–Johnson IV Tests of Achievement (Schrank, McGrew, & Mather, 2014) were administered as an assessment of academic abilities and fluency.

	Standard scores
Letter/Word Identification	105
Applied Problems	99
Spelling	105
Passage Comprehension	98
Calculation	105
Writing Samples	96
Word Attack	105
Spelling of Sounds	98
Sentence Reading Fluency	101
Math Facts Fluency	109
Sentence Writing Fluency	109
Reading	105
Broad Reading	104
Basic Reading	105
Mathematics	109
Broad Mathematics	100
Math Calculation Skills	109
Written Language	105
Broad Written Language	105
Written Expression	107
Phoneme/Grapheme	100
Academic Skills	105
Academic Fluency	109
Academic Applications	105
Brief Achievement	100
Broad Achievement	101

Ronnie's overall academic performance was measured within the average range when compared with same-age peers. Phoneme/grapheme knowledge, reading, writing, math, academic skills, fluency, and application of academic concepts are all measured within the average range.

Emotional/Personality Skills

Ronnie completed the Reynolds Adolescent Depression Scale (Reynolds, 2002) on which his responses reflected minimal levels of depression.

Ronnie completed the Multidimensional Anxiety Scale for Children, Second Edition (March, 2013). Ronnie's report reflects some elevated anxiety symptoms, particularly in the areas of separation anxiety/phobias and physical symptoms as well as generalized anxiety. He does not report any performance or social anxiety problems.

Ronnie completed the Resiliency Scales for Children and Adolescents (Prince-Embury, 2007). His report reflects reports of low emotional reactivity with average levels of sense of mastery and relatedness to others, such that his report would indicate average resources to deal with stress.

Ronnie also completed the Millon Adolescent Clinical Inventory (Millon, Millon, Davis, & Grossman, 1993). Ronnie's responses on this measure are consistent with youth whose personality profiles are characterized by discomfort with regard to discussing negative or distressing emotions. Adolescents with this personality profile tend to be compliant with social expectation and tend to appear overly cooperative and willingly submit to the expectations and values of authorities. On the surface, these youth tend to express a strong sense of duty to obey those in positions of authority and tend to seek to maintain an image of being mature, responsible, and proper young adults. These youth are not inclined to act out or behave in an impulsive or disruptive manner—they often demonstrate attitudes of personal inadequacy and tend to underplay their strengths and make light of their abilities. Criticism by those in positions of authority or higher social standing can cause considerable distress and humiliation. Youth with this personality profile tend to lack much insight into their own motives, tend to deny negative emotions, and are often disinclined to admit any personal weaknesses. They are often defensive in a guarded way and as a consequence of restraining these feelings, they may complain of stress-related bodily symptoms. These youth also tend to have angry impulses that are rigidly controlled and result in considerable tension—these angry impulses only rarely break through the surface, but when they do, they are notable.

Clinical Interview

Ronnie participated in a brief clinical interview with this examiner. He discussed feelings of anxiety and stated that he worries "for most of the day." His worries extend from fears of the dark, heights, and bugs to performance fears and worries about natural disasters. He also experiences some social anxiety and worries that he will appear stupid or will be unable to stand up for himself if he is bullied. Ronnie stated that he has always perceived himself as somewhat anxious but that worries and fears have increased over the past year—he reported that he constantly feels on edge. He is often so tired by the end of the evening that he falls asleep as soon as his head hits the pillow. "I am always tense and riled up. I get so exhausted feeling that way all day." Ronnie stated that he has difficulty with attention and focus at school and that he finds it difficult to concentrate because he is so worried and nervous and is unable to control these worries. Ronnie denied that this is a significant problem at home, where he feels safe and comfortable.

DSM-5 Diagnostic Overview

- ASD with social communication requiring support, restricted and repetitive behaviors requiring support, without intellectual impairment
- Generalized anxiety disorder

Diagnostic Impressions

Ronnie was referred for evaluation due to problems with academic achievement, rigid and inflexible behavior, anxiety, and social difficulties. His neuropsychological ability is measured within the average range. Ronnie's parent report and self-report indicate significant problems with flexibility and self-monitoring.

Ronnie exhibited many behaviors consistent with ASD—he demonstrates deficits in social reciprocity and communication. Parents reported that he often has difficulty reading the verbal and nonverbal social cues of others. Ronnie reported that he has a single friend and struggles to make friendships at school. During this evaluation he evidenced a lack of gestures for communication and also demonstrated limited empathy and understanding of his own role within relationships. Social overture and response as observed as a part of this evaluation were awkward. At times Ronnie was avoidant—his facial expressions were limited and at times exaggerated. In addition to difficulties with social–emotional reciprocity and communication, Ronnie's parents reported that he has a history of restricted interests and repetitive behavior, which currently includes doll collecting. He demonstrated stereotyped patterns of speech and behavior during this evaluation. Ronnie currently meets DSM-5 criteria for ASD.

Ronnie's parents reported additional mood and anxiety symptoms. His self-report reflects significant generalized, separation, phobic, and physiological aspects of anxiety. He experiences tense muscles and a feeling of being on edge and is easily fatigued as a result of anxiety. His personality profile reflects considerable tension and anxious inhibition of emotional responses. Ronnie's symptoms are described by a DSM-5 diagnosis of generalized anxiety disorder.

Although Ronnie's parents report some history of problems with attention and focus, Ronnie has demonstrated a refractory response to both stimulant and nonstimulant medications in the past. Ronnie reports that he is often preoccupied with worries at school, and misses directions—as a result of poor attention and focus in the classroom, it was important to rule out any clinically significant problems with attention. Ronnie performed well on a test of attention administered as a part of this evaluation. Few problems with executive functioning are reported, as was consistent with Ronnie's strong performance on tasks of planning and attention. At this time, we can rule out a diagnosis of attention deficit. Ronnie's problems with focus are likely due to significant anxiety rather than any attentional deficit.

Recommendations

It is recommended that Ronnie's parents share the results of this evaluation with his primary care provider and his prescribing physician. A trial of medication to reduce anxiety symptoms may be considered. Ronnie's parents may wish to consult with a psychiatrist for medication management, if desired. This examiner is prepared to assist with the collection of behavioral data, as needed, to monitor progress.

Ronnie would benefit from a course of cognitive-behavioral therapy aimed at assisting him in understanding his emotions and developing more appropriate coping strategies when under stress. In addition, therapy should aim to enhance Ronnie's social competence by exploring his thoughts regarding social interaction. His difficulties with attention and poor social motivation may present a barrier to therapy success. His parents may also benefit from therapy designed to teach behavioral strategies in the home. This examiner is prepared to provide referrals as needed.

This evaluation report should be provided to Ronnie's educational team to better understand Ronnie's current functioning. He is currently performing in the average range academically but his grades are below expected and he will not graduate with his class—provision of a guided study period with one-on-one support is recommended. Ronnie may benefit from relaxed deadlines and additional time on tests. He does not turn in assignments that have not been completed and only completes assignments in which he is interested. He reports significant performance anxiety, which should be considered when forming his academic plan. This examiner is prepared to consult with Ronnie's educational team as needed.

Given the extent of Ronnie's difficulties, his parents may wish to consider community- based services, particularly occupational therapy or additional speech therapy. This examiner is prepared to make referrals to community-based providers. Local autism-specific resources will be provided and his parents will be given a list of relevant books that they may find to be a valuable resource.

Should Ronnie choose to pursue post-high school education or training, accommodation will likely need to be made in order for him to experience success. He should be reevaluated prior to enrollment in college to gauge progress, update recommendations, and to consider possible accommodations.

Concluding Discussion

Ronnie's symptom profile is complex. He exhibits problems with social and emotional reciprocity, academic failure, and anxiety. Social learning deficits can often be "explained" away by other diagnoses. It is important that thorough evaluation be completed as anxiety and preoccupations associated with ASD may be responsible for the appearance of inattention rather than any actual attention deficit. It can be very difficult to tease these symptoms apart, as inattention and anxieties are often present in individuals with ASD. In treatment, all symptoms should be addressed. However, for individuals with ASD, the most effective treatments for comorbid diagnoses should be provided by practitioners familiar with ASD.

CASE EXAMPLE 2: AUTUMN

Autumn is a 9-year-old third-grade female. She was referred for evaluation owing to poor academic achievement despite the Americans with Disabilities Act (ADA) 504 plan and accommodations, social problems, learning disabilities, anxiety, and poor attention. Because of the extent of concerns, a comprehensive evaluation was recommended to assist with treatment planning. Autumn was assessed previously when she was 6, and was given a diagnosis of ASD and anxiety. However, her parents sought a second opinion because they felt the diagnosis did not fit their daughter. They originally sought evaluation owing to memory problems and inattention and reported surprise that a diagnosis of ASD was given. Autumn's parents believed that Autumn was generally unresponsive during the first evaluation because she and the psychologist were unable to establish rapport. The following includes the results of Autumn's current evaluation.

Background Information

Autumn is the eldest of three siblings. Autumn's brother (age 5) was diagnosed with ASD and speech delay and her sister (age 3) has a history of separation anxiety. Autumn's mother completed a master's degree and is currently employed at a local women's shelter. She reports a history of post-traumatic stress and depression. Extended family history of ASD is noted. Autumn's father completed a master's degree in engineering. He has a personal history of ADHD and an extended family history of bipolar disorder. Autumn's parents were divorced 2 years ago. Her parents share custody of all three children.

Autumn's mother suffered from preeclampsia during pregnancy. Autumn was born via cesarean section at 37 weeks' gestation and weighed

5 pounds, 6 ounces, at birth. As an infant, Autumn was described as difficult to comfort. She had difficulty sleeping and nursing—she did not sleep unless somebody was sitting up with her until she was approximately 2 years of age. Autumn was described as excessively irritable and restless and also exhibited colic.

As a toddler, Autumn exhibited typical activity level. Transitions were problematic but she dealt well with introduction to new things. Her basic mood was described as engaged and content and her persistence was good.

Autumn's medical history is notable for asthma, diagnosed at age 2. She also has an allergy to peanuts. In addition, she underwent the placement of pressure-equalization tubes in her ear canals at age 2. Currently, Autumn settles down to sleep and sleeps through the night without disruption. Her appetite is described as high—she overeats.

Autumn met most developmental milestones within normal limits with the exception of speech, which developed early. She was noted to talk excessively about favorite topics. She uses words and phrases repetitively, struggles to understand jokes, interprets conversations literally, frequently asks irrelevant questions, and experiences difficulty with conversational skills. Autumn avoids or limits eye contact and exhibits limited facial expression and often misses social cues. She lacks organizational skills and is described as passively inattentive. Autumn's coordination is rated as average to poor—she is average in terms of walking, throwing, catching, shoelace tying, and buttoning, but poor in terms of running, writing, and athletic abilities.

Autumn is reported to have difficulty understanding directions and situations as well as other children her age. She receives "reminders or to have directions explained in many steps." Autumn's mother reported that she was not concerned about her ability to succeed in kindergarten, but in first grade, Autumn started falling behind. She is reportedly performing at grade level in terms of reading and below grade level in terms of spelling and math. She is currently served with an ADA 504 plan and receives small-group instruction in math. In the past, she also had a private tutor for reading.

Autumn's behavior in the classroom is typically good. She is quiet and does not ask for help—it is reported that she is ignored in the classroom. Autumn tends to play with same-age peers. She is reported to enjoy being in charge of younger children and can be bossy. It is reported that she does not often seek out or engage peers, but when she does try she is typically rejected.

At home Autumn is described as very easily frustrated. She does not appear to listen to what is being said and loses items necessary for tasks or activities at home. She often interrupts or intrudes on others. She is described as "very well behaved," and discipline is rarely necessary.

Autumn's main hobbies and interests include the video games Pokémon and Minecraft and reading comics. Her greatest area of achievement is her artistic ability; she is good at painting. She dislikes outdoor activities and group activities. It is reported that Autumn is "sweet and thoughtful. She cares about social justice."

Adaptive Functioning Measures

The Conners Comprehensive Behavior Rating Scales (Conners, 2014) was completed by Autumn's parents and her teacher. For comparative purposes, *T*-scores for the Content and DSM-5 scales appear below (mean = 50, *SD* = 10, high scores indicate problems).

	Father	Mother	Teacher
Content scales			
Emotional Distress	90	90	56
Upsetting Thoughts	46	46	49
Worrying	78	83	–
Social Problems	90	90	82
Separation Fears	50	43	45
Social Anxiety	–	–	65
Defiant/Aggressive Behavior	52	46	52
Academic Difficulties	89	86	68
Language	78	67	63
Math	90	90	80
Hyperactivity/Impulsivity	51	40	48
Perfectionistic and Compulsive Behaviors	49	64	51
Violence Potential	66	51	50
Physical Symptoms	90	90	46
DSM-5 scales			
ADHD Inattentive Type	90	74	78
ADHD Hyperactive–Impulsive Type	51	40	51
Conduct Disorder	49	43	46
Oppositional Defiant Disorder	81	51	67
Major Depressive Episode	63	81	56
Manic Episode	52	52	54
Generalized Anxiety Disorder	85	73	71
Separation Anxiety Disorder	53	42	45
Social Phobia	83	67	68
Obsessive/Compulsive Disorder	45	45	46
Autism Spectrum Disorder	81	87	70

Parent report reflects significant concerns in the areas of emotional distress, worrying, social problems, academic difficulties in both language and math, physical symptoms, and inattention. Teacher report reflects additional concerns in the area of social anxiety. Teacher report also reflects academic difficulties in language and math and inattention in the classroom environment.

Autumn's parents and teacher were asked to complete the ASRS (Goldstein & Naglieri, 2009). Age-adjusted *T*-scores are as follows (mean = 50, *SD* = 10, high scores indicate problems):

	Father	Mother	Teacher
Total scores	62	62	52
ASRS scales			
Social Communication	60	61	51
Unusual Behavior	58	61	49
Self-Regulation	64	50	55
DSM-5 scale	60	62	48
Treatment scales			
Peer Socialization	66	65	45
Adult Socialization	70	62	45
Social/Emotional Reciprocity	58	59	53
Atypical Language	44	54	44
Stereotypy	58	56	51
Behavioral Rigidity	57	53	48
Sensory Sensitivity	56	71	43
Attention	63	62	61

Parent reports reflect some behaviors of concerns associated with ASD. Problems with peer and adult socialization are indicated, as well as attention. However, no social–emotional reciprocity, atypical language, stereotypy, or behavioral rigidity are noted. Teacher report reflects average levels of behaviors associated with ASD.

Parent and teacher responses to the Comprehensive Executive Function Inventory (Naglieri & Goldstein, 2013) placed Autumn at the following age-adjusted standard scores (mean = 100, *SD* = 15, low scores indicate problems):

	Father	Mother	Teacher
Attention	9	95	87
Emotion Regulation	83	91	104
Flexibility	86	98	84
Inhibitory Control	93	109	109
Initiation	74	75	84
Organization	70	75	76
Planning	81	94	94
Self-Monitoring	68	77	75
Working Memory	72	86	86

Parent and teacher reports reflect markedly below-average behaviors associated with executive functioning. This includes difficulties in attention, flexibility, initiation, organization, planning, self-monitoring, and working memory. Initiation of tasks, organization, and self-monitoring appear to be marked areas of weakness.

Home Functioning

Autumn's parents completed the Home Situations Questionnaire (Goldstein, 2016a). Her father indicated that Autumn presents moderate behavioral problems when playing with other children and when visiting the homes of others. Moderate to severe behavioral problems are indicated when Autumn is at school or when asked to do school homework. Her mother indicated mild behavioral problems when Autumn is playing with other children but at no other time.

School Functioning

Autumn's teacher completed the Teacher Observation Checklist (Goldstein, 2016b) indicating that Autumn tends to learn and work very slowly. She usually follows simple instructions but often requires individual help, her approach to problem solving is inexact and careless, and she does not seek extra attention. Autumn demonstrates some enthusiasm for learning—however, she appears to have mild feelings of inadequacy. She adapts easily to new situations, shows some ability to tolerate frustration, and she waits her turn. She demonstrates adequate vocabulary and grammar for her age. Below-average gross- and fine motor coordination is indicated. Autumn is reported to have much difficulty with reversals, directionality, and illegible writing. Achievement is rated as average in terms of reading and very poor in terms of mathematics.

Behavioral Observations

Autumn, a slightly overweight youth of casual dress, was seen for three assessment sessions on three separate days. Behavior in all sessions was similar. Initially, two assessment sessions were scheduled—however, Autumn took a considerable amount of time to complete tasks and, as such, a third assessment session was added. Autumn easily separated from her mother in the waiting room. Her eye contact was good and receptive and expressive articulation, although minimal, was appropriate. She initiated conversation at times and frequently maintained conversation.

Autumn's expression was typically calm. She demonstrated a flat affect. Emotional stability was good and she was not tearful at any time during the assessment.

Autumn was alert and attentive but not always focused. Joint attention, body and object use, and visual and listening response appeared normal. No abnormal sensory behaviors were noted. Autumn demonstrated few instrumental or informative gestures. The quality of her social overture and response, although these were minimal, was appropriate.

Autumn was very cooperative and attempted all items set before her. She appeared motivated to do her best and persistence was normal. No muscular tension or habitual mannerisms were noted.

Autumn was markedly underactive. She moved very slowly and made little spontaneous movement. She was not fidgety—however, she was frequently distracted. She appeared inclined to distrust her abilities. She maintained a positive and friendly relationship with this examiner and smiled appropriately. Overall, her thought processes appeared logical, focused, and relevant. It was not difficult to establish a working relationship with this pleasant young woman. This may be considered a valid estimation of Autumn's overall abilities.

Assessment Results and Interpretation

Autism

The ADOS-2, Module 3 (Lord & Rutter, 2012), was administered as a screening of behaviors associated with autism. Results are as follows:

	ADOS score	Autism cutoff	Autism spectrum cutoff
Social Affect Total	3		
Restrictive and Repetitive Behavior Total	0		
Overall Total	3	9	6
ADOS-2 comparison score	2		
ADOS-2 classification: Nonspectrum			
Level of autism spectrum-related symptoms: minimal to no evidence			

Autumn displayed few behaviors associated with ASD. Previously, Dr. August had given Autumn a diagnosis of autism based on observed behaviors during the ADOS. He noted one specific repetitive behavior: rocking. The most recent version of the ADOS excludes rocking from the classification of repetitive behavior. Dr. August also indicated that Autumn had difficulties in conversation and difficulty with descriptive and communicative gestures. Dr. August indicated that Autumn did not direct facial expressions to communicate and exhibited a very flat affect. However, it is noted that Autumn's mother indicated that she is much more animated in her facial expressions in other settings. Dr. August indicated poor quality of social response, minimal amount of reciprocal social communication, and overall poor quality of rapport. These observations were inconsistent with those made by this examiner during this evaluation.

During the evaluation, Autumn communicated with a flat affect. No immediate echolalia or stereotyped and idiosyncratic use of words or phrases was noted. Autumn frequently offered information about her thoughts, feelings, and experiences. On several occasions, she asked this examiner about my own thoughts, feelings, and experiences. Autumn reported both specific nonroutine and routine events without hesitation. Conversation, although somewhat less in amount than would have been expected given her verbal ability, was appropriate and flowed, building on the examiner's dialogue. It is likely that the frequency of communication was diminished due at least in part to anxiety. Autumn provided leads for this examiner to follow. She demonstrated few descriptive conventional instrumental or informational gestures. However, it should be noted that Autumn demonstrated very little physical activity in general. Her eye contact was appropriate she demonstrated frequent subtle changes in facial expression, and often directed these facial expressions toward this examiner. She exhibited expressions indicative of boredom, irritation, happiness, humor, pleasure, anxiety, and frustration. Linked verbal and nonverbal communication was minimal.

Autumn frequently demonstrated shared enjoyment and interaction. Without prompting, she spontaneously communicated appropriate understanding of various emotions in people and characters and demonstrated appropriate insight into typical social situations and relationships. The quality of her social overture was somewhat minimal but frequently engaged and maintained this examiner's attention. The quality of her social response was also somewhat minimal. Autumn demonstrated appropriate reciprocal social communication, and the quality of rapport was comfortable and sustained. No excessive interest in or references to highly specific topics or repetitive behaviors were noted, nor were any hand-and-finger or other complex mannerisms. Autumn demonstrated no unusual sensory interests. The rocking in her chair that was observed by Dr. August in 2013 was not observed by this examiner. Overall, Autumn's current presentation supports a nonspectrum classification.

Executive/Neuropsychological Skills

The Cognitive Assessment System, Second Edition (Naglieri et al., 2014), was administered as an assessment of neuropsychological ability. Results follow:

	Scaled scores (mean = 10, *SD* = 3)
Planned Codes	6
Planned Connections	5
Planned Number Matching	6
Matrices	13
Verbal–Spatial Relations	9
Figure Memory	11
Expressive Attention	5
Number Detection	9
Receptive Attention	10
Word Series	12
Sentence Repetition/Questions	15
Visual Digit Span	9

	IQ (mean = 100, *SD* = 15)	Percentiles	90% confidence interval
Planning	72	3rd	[81, 68]
Simultaneous	106	66th	[111, 100]
Attention	88	21st	[97, 82]
Successive	112	79th	[118, 104]
Executive Functioning without Working Memory	70	2nd	[83, 66]
Executive Functioning with Working Memory	89	24th	[97, 83]
Working Memory	112	79th	[118, 104]
Verbal Content	109	73rd	[115, 101]
Nonverbal Content	100	50th	[107, 93]
Full Scale	93	32nd	[97, 89]
Visual–auditory comparison: significant for auditory strength			

Autumn's overall neuropsychological ability on the Cognitive Assessment System, Second Edition (Naglieri et al., 2014), is measured in the average range when compared with same-age peers. This includes average simultaneous processing, above-average successive processing, and impaired planning and attention. Children with this pattern of planning and attention weakness struggle to adapt when tasks in school become more complex. They are disorganized learners who have difficulty maintaining attention and focus.

Language

The Peabody Picture Vocabulary Test, Fourth Edition (Dunn & Dunn, 2007), was administered as a simple measure of one-word receptive vocabulary. Autumn's performance on this measure yielded a standard score of 110, equivalent to the 75th percentile. Her receptive vocabulary is measured within the above-average range when compared with same-age peers.

Attention

The Conners Continuous Performance Test II (Conners, 2002) was administered as a computerized measure of Autumn's ability to sustain attention and inhibit impulsive responding. Autumn's performance reflected a 69.35% confidence interval that she is experiencing a clinically significant attention problem. Her performance reflected fast response time (*T*-score 67), numerous commission errors (*T*-score 71), and frequent perseveration (*T*-score 62). She demonstrated poor vigilance over time. Her performance is reflective of inattention, poor vigilance, and impulsive response style.

Motor/Perceptual Functioning

Autumn appeared right-side dominant and held her pencil in a three-finger pincer grip. Casual observation did not indicate any large motor abnormalities. Fine motor skills for motor speed and coordination as measured on the Purdue Pegboard Test (Tiffin, 1948) appeared below the 10th percentile for dominant, nondominant, and both hands. Motor speed and coordination are clearly impaired.

Autumn's reproductions of the figures on the Developmental Test of Visual–Motor Integration (Beery, Buktenica, & Beery, 2010) yielded a standard score of 94, equivalent to the 34th percentile. Autumn's performance on this measure is within the average range when compared with same-age peers.

Academic Functioning

Additional subtests from the Woodcock–Johnson IV Tests of Achievement (Schrank et al., 2014) were administered as an assessment of academic abilities and fluency. Results follow:

	Standard scores
Letter/Word Identification	105
Applied Problems	99
Spelling	82
Passage Comprehension	99
Calculation	85
Writing Samples	99
Word Attack	104
Spelling of Sounds	99
Sentence Reading Fluency	105
Math Facts Fluency	80
Sentence Writing Fluency	100
Reading	101
Broad Reading	101
Basic Reading	105
Mathematics	91
Broad Mathematics	89
Math Calculation Skills	90
Written Language	100
Broad Written Language	99
Written Expression	107
Phoneme/Grapheme	103
Academic Skills	92
Academic Fluency	95
Academic Applications	100
Brief Achievement	99
Broad Achievement	95

Autumn's reading and written language are overall within the average range when compared with same-age peers. Spelling is slightly below average and math is measured in the average to low-average range.

Emotional/Personality Skills

Autumn completed the Reynolds Children's Depression Scale (Reynolds, 1989) on which her responses reflected minimal symptoms of depression.

Autumn completed the Multidimensional Anxiety Scale for Children, Second Edition (March, 2013). *T*-scores appear below (mean = 50, *SD* = 10, high scores indicate problems):

	T-scores
Total Score	48
Anxiety Probability Score	Low
Separation Anxiety/Phobias	41
Generalized Anxiety Disorder Index	49
Social Anxiety Total	50
Humiliation/Rejection	48
Performance Fears	54
Obsessions and Compulsions	49
Physical Symptoms Total	56
Panic	57
Tense/Restless	55
Harm Avoidance	43

Autumn's report on this measure is reflective of low levels of anxiety symptoms. This is markedly different from Autumn's parent report, which reflects elevated levels of anxiety, including problems with worrying, social anxiety, and emotional distress.

Autumn completed the Resiliency Scales for Children and Adolescents (Prince-Embury, 2007). *T*-scores are as follows:

	T-scores (mean = 50, *SD* = 10)
Sense of Mastery	43
Sense of Relatedness to Others	48
Sense of Emotional Reactivity	43
Resource Index	44
Vulnerability Index	49

Autumn's responses on this measure once again reflect minimal concerns.

Clinical Interview

Autumn participated in a brief clinical interview with this examiner. When asked what she would wish for if she could have three wishes, she stated she would wish for (1) a million dollars, (2) a race car for her brother, and (3) a giant stuffed animal for her sister. Autumn spoke about school. She stated that she feels she is good at science and enjoys that subject, but is bad at math—she stated that she finds math frustrating. If allowed to stop going to school, she stated that she would "keep going" because "I like my school."

Autumn discussed emotions. She stated that she enjoys ice-skating and that makes her happy. She is frequently afraid of things, particularly clowns. She stated that she becomes angry when her brother breaks or steals her things. She described the feeling of anger as "feeling like you want to hit something." She stated that it makes her sad when her brother bites her. When queried further about this statement, Autumn stated that this happens when her brother does not like something or when she will not give him her stuffed animal, and so on. She stated that her brother often does things that irritate her. She knows that she is also capable of annoying her brother—this happens particularly when she ignores him.

Autumn reported having a large group of friends—however, she stated that she plays with them primarily at school. She was able to make the distinction between a friend and somebody with whom one just goes to school. She described each of her friends based on a particular characteristic. For example, Ella knows everything about birds, and Margot is "funny."

Autumn also discussed her family. She stated that her mother is "nice and takes care of me." She knows that it makes her mother happy when she listens the first time, and it makes her unhappy when Autumn ignores directives. Autumn spoke about her father and said that he is also nice and "takes care of me too." She indicated that she knows it makes her father happy when she helps her brother and sister, and that it makes him upset when Autumn does "not do what he wants."

DSM-5 Diagnostic Overview

- Unspecified anxiety disorder
- ADHD, predominantly inattentive presentation, moderate
- Significant sensory sensitivity

Diagnostic Impressions

Autumn was referred for evaluation due to social, academic, and emotional concerns at home and in school. Concerns include learning problems, anxiety, inattention, and social problems.

Autumn's neuropsychological profile is characterized by a marked deficit in the areas of planning and attention. Children with this pattern of planning and attention impairment struggle to self-monitor, strategize, understand complex instructions, and complete complex activities. According to parent report, Autumn exhibits behaviors indicative of poor executive functioning skills. Parent and teacher reports place her in the well-below-average to below-average range in the areas of attention, emotion regulation, flexibility, initiation, organization, planning, self-monitoring, and working memory. Autumn does not often think through her decisions, shows poor judgment when making decisions, struggles to regulate her emotional state, does not show initiative in beginning tasks, and is disorganized. She completed an attention measure on which her performance yielded a clinical profile reflecting problems with inattention and impulsivity. Given the presence of inattentive symptoms in the home, poor executive functioning, and performance on measures completed during this evaluation, Autumn qualifies for a DSM-5 diagnosis of ADHD, predominantly inattentive presentation, moderate.

Autumn's neuropsychological profile reflects average ability in the area of successive and simultaneous processing. She demonstrated average overall achievement consistent with her neuropsychological ability. No specific learning disabilities are indicated. Autumn's problems with writing are related to impairments in fine motor speed and coordination.

Of additional concern are Autumn's reported anxiety symptoms. Self-report measures completed by Autumn indicated minimal anxiety—however, during the clinical interview Autumn reported numerous fears. Anxiety was also observed to some extent during this evaluation in terms of performance fears. Parent report indicates elevated levels of emotional distress, worrying, and upsetting thoughts. Autumn's symptoms of mixed anxiety are described by a DSM-5 diagnosis of unspecified anxiety disorder.

Autumn's parents report several behaviors and impairing symptoms that raise concerns of ASD. These include minimal communication of affect, poor interpretation of social cues, literal interpretation of speech, and sensory sensitivity. Autumn was diagnosed with ASD by Dr. August at age 6. However, uncharacteristic of ASD, Autumn is capable of initiating and maintaining conversation. Her overall quality of social overture and response is adequate. She interacted well with this examiner and was able to demonstrate insight into several types of interpersonal relationships and indicated some understanding of her role within those relationships. In addition, Autumn demonstrated an adequate understanding of emotions and communicated that effectively. She also demonstrated empathy and understanding of the emotions of others. Autumn responded appropriately to humor. With regard to communication, she demonstrated adequate nonverbal communication during this assessment and her eye contact was notably good. Autumn's communication of affect through gesture was minimal, but she communicated affect effectively though facial expression despite an overall flat affect.

Although these behaviors and impairing symptoms should be addressed, because Autumn does not exhibit significant problems in the areas of verbal and nonverbal communication, and demonstrates appropriate social and emotional reciprocity, she does not currently meet adequate criteria for a DSM-5 diagnosis of ASD. It is likely that her difficulty in attending to and misinterpretation of social cues is currently a result of inattention and social anxiety rather than a social learning problem.

Recommendations

A copy of this report should be shared with Autumn's pediatrician and other treating medical professionals. Autumn's parents may choose to consider a trial of medication aimed at increasing attention and focus. In addition, her parents may choose to consider a trial of medication to reduce anxiety symptoms. This examiner is prepared to assist with the collection of behavioral data within the home and school settings, as needed, to gauge progress.

A course of individual cognitive-behavioral therapy is recommended for Autumn in order to assist her in addressing unhelpful thoughts that contribute to her anxiety and emotional distress, teach appropriate coping skills, and reduce overall symptoms of anxiety. In addition, therapy may be useful to address problems with social interaction. Autumn may be somewhat resistant to therapy owing to her tendency to minimize emotional concerns. Any therapist working with Autumn must take a significant amount of time to develop trust and rapport before change is likely to occur. This examiner is willing to make referrals as needed.

The results of this evaluation should be shared with Autumn's educational team. She may qualify for services under the Individuals with Disabilities Education Improvement Act of 2004 (IDEIA) classification of Other Health Impairment owing to significant inattention. She is currently within the average range academically, but this is largely owing to significant outside tutoring support. Autumn should be provided with accommodations in the school environment so that her significant attention deficit does not cause her to fall behind. Accommodations that may be considered in the classroom include a quiet space in which to complete work with one-on-one support and frequent assistance, additional time to complete assignments, reduced assignments and/or homework, additional time on tests, provision of a quiet location in which to take tests, and small-group work whenever possible. In addition, Autumn's school team should be aware of her significant anxiety concerns. She is not likely to be disruptive in the classroom and owing, to her significant anxiety, is unlikely to seek support should she require it. Attention should be paid to Autumn's specific needs without the requirement that she seek support independently.

Autumn's parents will be provided with a list of relevant books that they may find to be a valuable resource.

Autumn should be reevaluated in 2 years. At that time, updated evaluation will be useful both to gauge progress and to help her access services and accommodations, as ongoing support is likely to be needed to facilitate Autumn's learning and academic success.

Concluding Discussion

Autumn's case is particularly notable because she had been incorrectly diagnosed with ASD in the past. Given observed behaviors as reported during that evaluation, it is unsurprising that such a conclusion was made. This highlights the immense importance of establishing rapport and a good working relationship during the assessment. Children with attention problems and anxiety may appear to lack appropriate social and emotional reciprocity and understanding—however, once they warm to the examiner, their true abilities can shine. It is important during the assessment process to determine whether the snapshot of behavior that we are able to observe is characteristic of typical functioning or whether it is artificially produced by the assessment process.

CONCLUSION

Both of these case examples presented particular challenges in assessment. As demonstrated above, comprehensive diagnosis required information from a variety of sources. In these cases, information was obtained from parents and educators in addition to self-report from the client. A comprehensive history of the child's development was obtained through parent interview. Direct observation provided additional clinical information. At times, prior assessment provided additional standardized testing data.

Formal evaluation of functioning was completed in regard to social functioning, communication, adaptive behavior and development, emotional functioning, and cognitive and neuropsychological ability. By gathering information across a wide variety of relevant areas, a complete diagnostic picture was obtained. Possible comorbid conditions were included or excluded as appropriate. At the conclusion of each assessment, the examiner met with the family to discuss the results in depth and provided a rationale for recommended treatments. Referrals to community providers for further assessment and treatment were made. Additional academic recommendations were also made to assist the family and school with supporting each child in his or her learning.

Comprehensive ASD assessment is important to provide a tailored treatment path for youth and their families. The first step to intervention is a complete diagnosis. It is not enough to diagnose or rule out ASD. Often, comorbid conditions impact the functioning of the child and need to be addressed as a part of a comprehensive treatment plan. Once an accurate diagnostic picture is obtained, understanding can begin to lead toward treatment, and enhance the likelihood of a positive outcome for our patients and their families.

REFERENCES

Beery K. E., Buktenica, N. A., & Beery N. A. (2010). *The Beery–Buktenica Developmental Test of Visual–Motor Integration: Administration, scoring, and teaching manual* (6th ed.). Minneapolis, MN: Pearson.

Conners, C. K. (2002). *Conners Continuous Performance Test II*. Toronto, ON, Canada: Multi-Health Systems.

Conners, C. K. (2014). *Conners Comprehensive Behavior Rating Scales*. Toronto, ON, Canada: Multi-Health Systems.

Dunn, L. M., & Dunn, D. M. (2007). *Peabody Picture Vocabulary Test, Fourth Edition*. San Antonio, TX: Psychological Corporation.

Goldstein, S. (2016a). *Home Situations Questionnaire*. Salt Lake City, UT: Neurology, Learning and Behavior Center.

Goldstein, S. (2016b). *Teacher Observation Checklist*. Salt Lake City, UT: Neurology, Learning and Behavior Center.

Goldstein, S., & Naglieri, J. (2009). *Autism Spectrum Rating Scale*. Toronto, ON, Canada: Multi-Health Solutions.

Lord, C., & Rutter, M. (2012). *Autism Diagnostic Observation Schedule, Second Edition*. Torrance, CA: Western Psychological Services.

March, J. S. (2013). *Multidimensional Anxiety Scale for Children, Second Edition*. Toronto, ON, Canada: Multi-Health Systems.

Millon, T., Millon, C., Davis, R., & Grossman, S. (1993). *Millon Adolescent Clinical Inventory*. Minneapolis, MN: Pearson.

Naglieri, J., Das, J. P., & Goldstein, S. (2014). *Cognitive Assessment System, Second Edition*. Austin, TX: PRO-ED.

Naglieri, J., & Goldstein, S. (2013). *Comprehensive Executive Function Inventory*. Toronto, ON, Canada: Multi-Health Systems.

Osterrieth, P. A. (1944). *Rey Complex Figure Test*. Lutz, FL: Psychological Assessment Resources.

Prince-Embury, S. (2007). *Resiliency Scales for Children and Adolescents: A profile of personal strength.* San Antonio, TX: Psychological Corporation.

Reynolds, C. R., & Voress, J. K. (2007). *Test of Memory and Learning—Second Edition.* Torrance, CA: Western Psychological Services.

Reynolds, W. (1989). *Reynolds Children's Depression Scale.* Lutz, FL: Psychological Assessment Resources.

Reynolds, W. (2002). *Reynolds Adolescent Depression Scale.* Lutz, FL: Psychological Assessment Resources.

Schrank, F. A., McGrew, K. S., & Mather, N. (2014). *Woodcock–Johnson IV Tests of Achievement.* Itasca, IL: Houghton Mifflin Harcourt.

Tiffin, J. (1948). *Purdue Pegbord Test.* Layfayette, IN: Lafayette Instrument.

Wechsler, D. (2008). *Wechsler Adult Intelligence Scale—Fourth Edition.* San Antonio, TX: Psychological Corporation.

Williams, K. T. (2007). *Expressive Vocabulary Test, Second Edition.* San Antonio, TX: Psychological Corporation.

CHAPTER FOURTEEN

Distinguishing Science and Pseudoscience in the Assessment and Treatment of Autism Spectrum Disorder

Mary E. McDonald
Florence D. DiGennaro Reed

Imagine your child has been diagnosed with an aggressive form of cancer. Your first reaction to this news is, of course, shock and disbelief. Once you move past these initial emotions, you are interested in moving quickly to find a treatment. Where would you look? Most parents would seek answers from doctors and the medical community. While doing your own search for information on treatment you discover two options: (1) a treatment supported by substantial research, the medical community, and physicians treating your child; and (2) an alternative approach with no research support that purports exceptional results in a short period of time, but you must travel to another country and use herbs to treat the cancer.

Now suppose you have a limited amount of time to treat this particularly aggressive cancer. Your child's life is at stake . . . What do you do? The medical community's proposed treatment will be painful and expensive. You also learn it will take time to witness results. The other intervention is much less expensive and simply involves sitting in a room with special herbs boiling near your child. There is no expected pain or hardship with the alternative intervention. Alas, this treatment can be carried out over a 1-week period.

Is it possible to see how a parent might be tempted to choose the alternative treatment rather than the medical community's recommendation?

Fortunately, the treatment for cancer is well researched and many caregivers will seek a science-based medical intervention if presented with this tragic scenario. This is not always the case, surprisingly, even when it comes to cancer. For example, it seems that shark cartilage extract has been proposed as an alternative intervention for the treatment of cancer, which has led to two negative outcomes: a dramatic decrease in the shark population and a diversion of patients from effective treatments (Ostrander, Cheng, Wolf, & Wolfe, 2004). Thankfully, the pursuit of alternative and unsupported treatments for cancer is not the norm, but more often the exception.

How does this type of scenario play out in the autism community in relation to intervention selection for individuals with autism spectrum disorder (ASD)? A number of parallels may be construed here. Parents are also tasked with the difficult decision of choosing an intervention for their children with ASD. They too must face a choice involving a science-based approach or many non-science-based interventions that currently exist. Parents face pressures to act quickly to achieve the most optimal results for their child within a crucial time frame. The decision to adopt a science-based intervention is typically accompanied by years of hard work, a waiting period until desired effects are evident, mounting costs for services, and direct involvement of the parents in treatment. However, alternative interventions are often marketed as miracle cures with immediate effects and less investment financially and personally. Understandably, the latter approach is attractive. Parents may also find it challenging to determine the best course for treatment and adopt a number of strategies to assist with pursuing thc various options. Romanczyk and Gillis (2005) describe seven strategies parents often use to assist them in their decision making:

1. *They know what's best.* Place trust in a service provider and defer to his or her judgment.
2. *Hedge your bets.* Seek several options simultaneously in the hopes a treatment package will be effective.
3. *Fanatical focus.* Pursue a single course with overwhelming intensity and focus.
4. *Hope for the best.* Forgo formal treatment and participate in typical activities that are available.
5. *Cure du jour.* Pursue new treatments as they appear and drop the current program.
6. *A friend told me.* Implement treatment that appeared to work for the child of someone they know or have read about.
7. *Guru selection.* Follow and believe in a single, specific "expert."

The ever increasing incidence of ASD and lack of specific answers regarding causation have given rise to unproven educational interventions and medical treatments. Sadly, parents of newly diagnosed children are often the targets of such interventions, which may boast the promise of a cure or a "quick fix." These interventions may actually cause harm to the child, detract from the use of science-based interventions, and lead parents down a roller coaster ride of hope that is vanquished in the end. The antidote for these unsubstantiated and pseudoscientific interventions is adherence to the scientific method and adoption of scientifically validated assessments and interventions. An understanding of the differences among science, pseudoscience, and antiscience may aid parents in adopting a strategy for assessment and intervention selection that minimizes risks associated with choosing unproven treatments.

DISTINGUISHING SCIENCE, PSEUDOSCIENCE, AND ANTISCIENCE

Three approaches to understanding and explaining phenomena—science, pseudoscience, and antiscience—help provide a framework for categorizing and understanding the myriad options in the assessment and treatment of ASD (Green & Perry, 1999). Moreover, meta-analyses (e.g., Eikeseth, 2009; Eldevik, Hastings, Hughes, Jahr, & Eikeseth, 2010), clinical practice guidelines (e.g., New York State Department of Health Early Intervention Program, 1999), and reviews by independent entities (e.g., National Autism Center, 2009, 2015) have further contributed to our understanding of science-based assessment and treatment by summarizing thorough and critical reviews of published studies that aid in determining which procedures are well established or constitute evidence-based practice (see Chambless & Hollon, 1998).

Science relies on an experimental approach comprising rigorous activities to test hypotheses, rule out alternative explanations for observed findings, and verify effects through replication by independent researchers. Perhaps Michael Shermer captured it best: "Scientific progress is the cumulative growth of a system of knowledge over time, in which useful features are retained and nonuseful features are abandoned, based on the rejection or confirmation of testable knowledge" (2002, p. 31). With respect to autism treatment, scientific research spanning decades has documented improved outcomes resulting from early and intensive behavioral treatment (e.g., Howard, Sparkman, Cohen, Green, & Stanislaw, 2005; Lovaas, 1987; McEachin, Smith, & Lovaas, 1993). As a scientific community, autism researchers developed testable hypotheses about the effects of behavioral treatment, defined relevant variables, and implemented treatments in a carefully planned manner to allow methodologically sound conclusions to be made about the effects of treatment. Additionally, researchers subjected themselves to the peer-review process—wherein experts assessed the scientific rigor of each study before permitting publication—which resulted in dissemination so that others may attempt replication. This gradual accumulation of scientific evidence continuously improves our knowledge about best practices leading to refined treatment procedures and service quality—that is, our understanding about best-practice assessment and treatment changes over time as scientific studies reveal novel findings.

Pseudoscience refers to practices that are mistakenly regarded as being based on the scientific method and purportedly rooted in scientific theory, when in fact they lack supporting evidence (Normand, 2008). Importantly, pseudoscientific practices may not reflect accidental interpretations by laypersons; instead, pseudoscience involves claims described in a way that makes them *appear* to be grounded in science by using jargon or endorsements from individuals who seem to have legitimate credentials (Green & Perry, 1999; Shermer, 2002)—that is, pseudoscience might be best conceptualized as *purposeful misrepresentation* of the state of evidence for a particular practice. Despite lacking scientific support for their effectiveness, numerous treatments are commonly promoted as having empirical evidence whose proponents seek to exploit the vulnerability of hopeful caregivers (Romanczyk, Gillis, White, & DiGennaro, 2008). Through strategic marketing and enticing advertising, ineffective—and sometimes harmful—pseudoscientific treatments may be actively sought by unsuspecting caregivers. For example, dolphin-assisted therapy is a popular, unregulated, and expensive pseudoscientific treatment that involves swimming with dolphins to treat ASD and other disabilities (Romanczyk, Turner, Sevlever, & Gillis, 2015). Although this therapy lacks scientific merit (Marino & Lilienfeld, 2007), proponents argue that touching or swimming with dolphins offers therapeutic benefit and charge hopeful consumers thousands of dollars for a handful of therapy sessions.

Antiscience involves rejection of the scientific method as a mechanism for gaining knowledge for understanding (Green, 1996). In fact, extreme proponents of antiscience fail to recognize the importance or existence of objective facts (Green & Perry, 1999). An example of an antiscientific approach to autism treatment is Miracle Mineral Solution (MMS), which was touted as a cure for ASD and various diseases, such as cancer, Alzheimer's, and human immunodeficiency virus (HIV), by its developer. It was originally developed by former Scientologist Jim Humble, who, according to Gettys (2015), describes himself as a "billion-year-old god from the Andromeda galaxy." MMS has been linked to at least one death and several serious injuries (Russell, 2010). In fact, MMS is not approved to treat any disease as of the date of this writing and has been banned in several countries. Its chemical constituents—sodium chlorite and most any acid—combine to form chlorine dioxide, essentially the same ingredients as bleach (Gettys, 2015). Media reports indicate that parents are told to administer the bleach solution as an enema despite no scientific evidence of its effectiveness and warnings by established and respected entities, such as the Food and Drug Administration (Connett, 2015).

According to Metz, Mulick, and Butler (2005, p. 238), "Fads in the treatment of autism tend to be harmful, fruitlessly expending limited time and monetary resources, falsely raising hopes and expectations, and distracting and detracting from efficacious efforts." They identified the following reasons why parents may gravitate toward such interventions and treatments:

- The nature of ASD is perceived as a severe, lifelong condition, resulting in a poor prognosis.
- Parents, new to the diagnosis, lack knowledge about the disorder, and may be minimally trained in scientific inquiry.
- Parents must deal with conflicting information and competing perspectives from professionals.
- The fads are often presented as quick fixes or cures.
- There is inadequate information about the cause of ASD.
- Medications do not provide a cure; they can only alleviate certain symptoms.

It is true that some interventions may be especially attractive to parents, such as the aforementioned dolphin therapy—who wouldn't want to swim with a dolphin? Interventions may also promise quick results, which can play into the desperation the family is feeling in regard to their child's diagnosis. The interventions may be marketed in a clever or enticing way using the media to promote the results and by sharing convincing testimonials. Moreover, vulnerable parents often believe what other parents tell them about interventions they have used and hope for the same results for their child. Although pseudo- and antiscientific interventions may be attempted by parents of children with ASD at any age, parents of a newly diagnosed child are even more vulnerable to fall prey to alternative interventions that promise cures. Parents frantic to help their children frequently seek guidance on the Internet to find a successful treatment for their child with ASD (McDonald, Pace, Blue, & Schwartz, 2012). Unfortunately, the Internet contains hundreds of examples of pseudoscientific interventions (Romanczyk et al., 2008) that may be challenging to distinguish from science-based interventions.

WARNING SIGNS OF PSEUDOSCIENCE

Awareness of the warning signs of pseudoscience can help professionals be more diligent in selecting interventions and advising parents. The more warning signs a discipline exhibits, the more it begins to resemble pseudoscience rather than science (Herbert, 2000). Lilienfeld, Lynn, and Lohr (2014) and the Association for Science in Autism Treatment (1999) published various warning signs or red flags of which consumers of interventions should be aware. Figure 14.1 summarizes several red flags related to pseudoscience in ASD, which we present in a checklist format for consumer use when confronted with a new or an alternative intervention.

Although we advocate awareness of the possible red flags of pseudoscience, outright dismissiveness of all attempts at new assessments and interventions would undermine progress. All evidence-based practices were considered new procedures early in their development. Nevertheless, a basic tenet of science is that the burden of proof falls squarely on the proponents of an intervention, not the critic (Shermer, 2002). As a consequence, proponents of these techniques are responsible for demonstrating scientifically and convincingly that they work; critics are not responsible for demonstrating the converse (Lilienfeld, Lyn, & Ammirati, 2015).

THE SCIENTIFIC METHOD AND THE EVER-EVOLVING PROCESS

The process by which we acquire knowledge and understand the world is drastically different when it involves the scientific method rather than everyday experiences or commonsense approaches. The *scientific method* is a systematic approach involving several carefully planned activities—observation, prediction, experimentation, explanation, and refining of explanation—in an effort to search for the causes of events (Spata, 2003). This approach requires objectivity and must be based on direct observations with controlled experiments.

An important consideration is that the scientific method is an ever-evolving, self-correcting process. Science allows us to test our assumptions; as knowledge accumulates and we make new discoveries, we can modify our understanding. Science may be prone to mistakes and failed experiments; it is not perfect by any means. Because science is self-correcting, these issues can be addressed in subsequent experiments to inform our understanding.

Science is especially important in the assessment and treatment of ASD. The procedures that constitute "evidence-based" or "science-based" practice evolve as the research advances, which underscores the importance of staying abreast of the scientific literature. Good clinical practice must be informed by carefully designed experiments and the subsequent accumulation of knowledge.

Figure 14.2 depicts the sequence of steps that forms the research process. At the beginning of experimentation, investigators compose a research question informed by casual observations and/or by previous research they

Red flags	Applicable?
High "success" rates are claimed.	
Rapid effects are promised.	
The intervention is said to be effective for many symptoms or disorders.	
The "theory" behind the intervention contradicts objective knowledge (and sometimes common sense).	
An overuse of ad hoc hypotheses designed to immunize claims from falsification.	
The intervention is said to be easy to administer, requiring little training or expertise.	
Other proven treatments are said to be unnecessary, inferior, or harmful.	
Promoters of the intervention are working outside of their area of expertise.	
Promoters benefit financially or otherwise from adoption of the treatment.	
Testimonials, anecdotes, or personal accounts are offered in support of claims about the intervention's effectiveness, but little or no objective evidence is provided.	
Obscurist language is used and prevents consumers from understanding.	
Catchy, emotionally appealing slogans are used in marketing the treatment.	
Belief and faith are said to be necessary for the intervention to "work."	
Skepticism and critical evaluation are said to make the intervention's effects evaporate.	
Promoters resist objective evaluation or scrutiny of the treatment by others.	
Negative findings from scientific studies are ignored or dismissed.	
There is a reversed burden of proof required.	
There is evasion of peer review.	
There is an absence of self-correction.	
Critics and scientific investigators are often met with hostility, and are accused of persecuting the promoters, being "close-minded," or having some ulterior motive for "debunking" the treatment.	

FIGURE 14.1. Red flags checklist for identifying pseudoscience in ASD. Content adapted from Lilienfeld, Lynn, and Lohr (2003) and the Association for Science in Autism Treatment (1999).

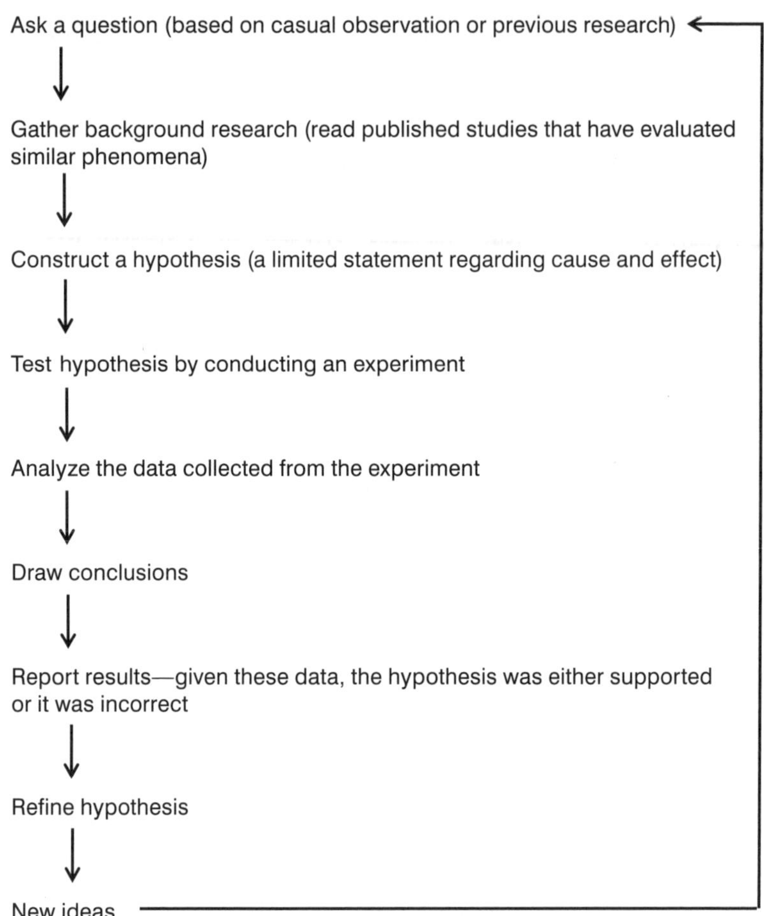

FIGURE 14.2. Steps in the research procss. Adapted from Spata (2003).

or others have conducted. Next, they read published articles that have evaluated phenomena similar to the topic of the present study to help formulate their methodology and study features. After investigators familiarize themselves with the literature, they construct and test a hypothesis—a limited statement of cause and effect—by conducting an experiment. During and after the experiment, the investigators analyze the data collected and draw conclusions about the effects of the independent variable (e.g., intervention) on the dependent variable (e.g., behavior or skills). An important activity in the research process involves disseminating the conclusions by writing scientific papers for scholarly journals and speaking at professional conferences. These activities produce new information and knowledge that allow researchers to refine their hypotheses and understanding, generate new ideas, and pursue future studies so they may add to the literature and subsequently inform practice.

CAUSATION AND PSEUDOSCIENCE IN ASD

Adopting a pseudo- or antiscientific approach can lead caregivers and professionals to draw erroneous conclusions about the causes of ASD or its symptoms. Such incorrect attributions may subsequently result in the pursuit of unsubstantiated and potentially harmful and ineffective assessments and treatments (McDonald et al., 2012). At the very least, these pursuits may delay access to effective intervention. Our history yields numerous examples of these unfortunate and sometimes costly outcomes. For example, the practice of parentectomy, wherein parents are separated from their child with ASD for extended periods of time, developed out of Bruno Bettelheim's unsupported assertion that autism was caused by cold and detached mothers who wished to harm their children (Herbert, Sharp, & Gaudiano, 2002). Imagine the needless suffering parentectomy caused families at that time! Although this inappropriate and antiscientific practice has not been popular for decades, other pseudoscientific treatments abound. Since 2008, the Council on Foreign Relations has documented global outbreaks of measles, mumps, whooping cough, polio, rubella, and other vaccine-preventable diseases (Sifferlin, 2014). The United States has also witnessed an increase in previously eradicated and preventable diseases. What is responsible for these outbreaks? The discredited, but strongly held belief that vaccines cause ASD has incited fear in vulnerable parents who subsequently refuse to vaccinate their children (McDonald et al., 2012). Clearly, the vaccine–autism link is still widely held as Freed, Clark, Butchart, Singer, and Davis (2010) stated that 25% of surveyed parents with a child under the age of 17 believe that vaccines cause ASD in a healthy child. Thousands of families have been impacted—many of whom have been harmed—by the pseudoscientific claim that vaccines cause ASD.

PSEUDOSCIENCE AND ASSESSMENT IN ASD

Less attention has been directed toward pseudoscientific assessment practices, despite their existence. Purposeful misrepresentation of the state of evidence for a particular assessment or inappropriate use of a validated assessment may represent a pseudoscientific approach. Practitioners are generally trained to select interventions based on assessment results, but they may be misguided in their efforts if decisions rely on a flawed or faulty assessment process. Thyer and Pignotti (2010) describe several red flags of pseudoscientific assessment practices, several of which are similar to the warning signs we provided for ASD interventions.

- Inappropriate use of scientific terminology, jargon, or made-up words to describe the assessment.
- A lack of reliability and validity studies on the assessment method.
- Reliance on testimonials and anecdotal evidence to support the assessment's effectiveness and usefulness.
- Claims that the assessment produces remarkable results.
- Use of vivid language in claims of effectiveness (e.g., "unbelievable," "unimaginable").
- Instrument developers that are positioned to make significant amounts of money as a result of selling or otherwise marketing the assessment.
- Practitioners who use the assessment are required to pledge secrecy and refuse to teach others about the assessment.

We urge professionals and parents to exercise caution when considering an assessment practice, particularly when treatment decisions stem from its results.

PSEUDOSCIENCE AND INTERVENTION IN ASD

Researchers have published several comprehensive and high-quality reviews of the scientific literature on autism interventions in the past two decades, many of which are available at low or no cost to consumers (e.g., National Autism Center, 2009, 2015; National Research Council, 2001; New York State Department of Health Early Intervention Program, 1999; Romanczyk et al., 2008; Strock, 2004; U.S. Department of Health and Human Services, 1999). For example, the National Autism Center launched the National Standards Project, which sought to summarize the strength of evidence available for educational and behavioral interventions for individuals with ASD. The reports from 2009 and 2015 also detailed participant ages, diagnoses, and skills/behaviors targeted in the published studies; limitations of the available body of literature; and suggestions for evidence-based practice (National Autism Center, 2009, 2015a, 2015b). Although these varied reviews have provided valuable information to stakeholders, findings also reveal that the number of invalidated interventions far outweighs evidence-based treatment procedures. In 2008, Romanczyk et al. documented that less than 1% of autism interventions could be classified as an evidence-based treatment. Sadly, descriptions of hundreds of pseudo- and antiscientific treatments are still readily marketed on the Internet.

One such pseudoscientific intervention—facilitated communication (FC)—is touted by its proponents as having dramatic benefits without scientific evidence supporting those claims (Tostanoski, Lang, Raulston, Carnett, & Davis, 2014). Individuals who use FC communicate by selecting letters on a keyboard while simultaneously receiving physical, emotional, and other communication supports (Schlosser et al., 2014). However, numerous high-quality studies have experimentally documented that the facilitators providing support actually served as authors of the communications, rather than the users receiving support. Despite the lack of endorsement from national professional organizations (Jacobson, Foxx, & Mulick, 2005) and controlled research refuting proponents' claims and subsequent rejection by the scientific community as early as the 1990s, FC persists and may be increasing in popularity (Lilienfeld, Marshall, Todd, & Shane, 2014). Figure 14.3 displays cumulative records of published research studies on FC since 1999, as well as worldwide Google searches on this topic since 2004. Note that interest in FC has not waned. Its comeback is occurring amid heavy criticism of FC proponents, evidence of harm (e.g., dozens of parents have been falsely accused of sexual abuse by well-meaning, but ill-informed facilitators), and legitimate perceptions that it is a "deceptive and dangerous treatment" (Tostanoski et al., 2014). In fact, concerns are mounting about the recent, but growing interest in the rapid prompting method, which may be conceptualized as an extension of FC (Tostanoski et al., 2014). The primary difference? Rapid prompting entails a facilitator moving a letter board to touch the user's hand, whereas FC involves a facilitator moving the user's hand to touch a letter board.

What are the dangers of FC, rapid prompting, and other pseudoscientific interventions? Individuals who receive ineffective or unsubstantiated treatments are likely to demonstrate little to no progress, which may have a deleterious effect on their learning, adjustment, and quality of life. In fact, the outcomes of FC and rapid prompting have been described as "depriving children with autism of the right to self-expression" (Tostanoski et al., 2014, p. 222), which is countertherapeutic and unethical. Moreover, valuable time is wasted when treatment recipients pursue pseudoscientific treatments in lieu of evidence-based approaches (McDonald et al., 2012). Certainly, some interventions may threaten the user's welfare by increasing the risk of harmful side effects (e.g., toxic effects of MMS, chelation therapies, hyperbaric oxygen therapy) or devastating effects on the individual or family (e.g., FC abuse claims). Additionally, the costs to families and society can reach millions of dollars to cover expenses associated with treatment and litigation. Fortunately, the U.S. Food and Drug Administration has made efforts to address misleading claims of effectiveness by warning

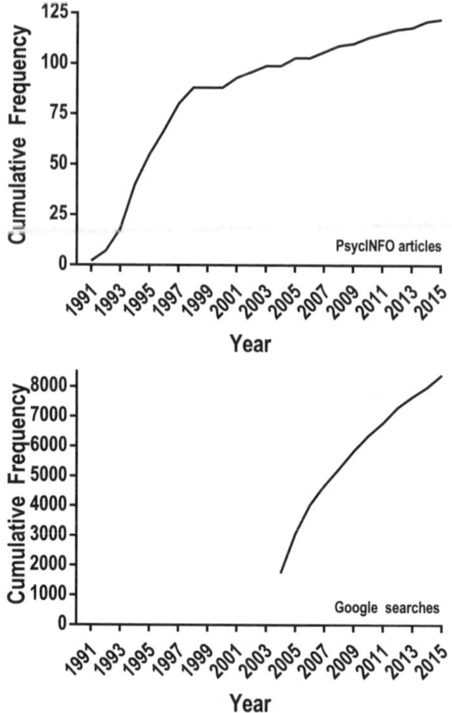

FIGURE 14.3. *Top panel*: A cumulative record of articles published in scholarly journals between 1991 and 2015 using "facilitated communication" and "autism" as keywords. The search was conducted on April 20, 2016, using PsycINFO as the search engine. *Bottom panel*: A cumulative record of worldwide Google searches conducted from 2004 to 2015 for "facilitated communication." The analysis was conducted on April 20, 2016, using Google Trends. *Note*: Google Trends data were not available before 2004, suggesting the findings are an underestimate of total worldwide searches.

companies that they may face legal action if they continue making said claims and by developing outreach materials for families (FDA Consumer Health Information, 2014).

PERSISTENCE OF FADS AND INVALIDATED INTERVENTIONS

Fads and interventions that are not scientifically validated continue to persist even in light of the evidence of science-based interventions. For example, in the area of early intervention where the research has clearly shown that early intensive behavioral intervention is supported for young children with ASD, parents are still choosing complementary or alternative treatments. Research has shown that over 30% of study participants were being treated with such interventions (Green et al., 2006).

Why do interventions persist despite evidence that they are ineffective or even harmful? A number of reasons may explain why such interventions persist. The fact that parents of children with ASD find themselves desperate to find answers and a cure is a strong influence on the persistence of fads and invalidated interventions (Worley, Fodstad, & Neal, 2014). Parents may expose their children to a variety of risks such as not providing inoculations, giving their child transfusions, or exposing their child to chelation. These examples are just three potentially harmful interventions from a long list of interventions currently available. In addition to the potential direct harm, there is also the possibility of indirect harm as a result of the choices made. For example, if parents choose to spend their child's time and their resources on an invalidated intervention, they are often also forgoing a validated intervention (e.g., applied behavior analysis [ABA]). Metz et al. (2005) states that fads in the treatment of ASD tend to be harmful, fruitlessly expending limited time and monetary resources, falsely raising hopes and expectations, and distracting and detracting from efficacious efforts.

The lack of answers regarding the cause of ASD fuels debate about possible causes and interventions (Levy & Hyman, 2003). The fact that we do not know the cause of ASD leaves the possibilities of intervention wide open. When a cause is clearly known, such as with trisomy-21, there is little attention paid to alternative treatments as it would not be expected that they would be effective. However, when the cause in unknown (as it is in ASD), then the families fall prey to the development of a multitude of interventions that are created to fill a perceived need.

The media—including print, films, television, and the Internet—plays a large role in the persistence of invalidated interventions and fads as well. The media is designed to sell; journalists hope to find the next sensational item to attract the attention of the public. In a review of television media portrayal of autism interventions, Schreck and Ramirez (2016) found that mainstream television media stations devoted over 70% of their coverage to non-evidence-based treatments. Often the research lags behind the media's portrayal of an intervention, which can lead to adoption of interventions that lack scientific merit (Smith & Wick, 2008). Although a "healthy skepticism" is warranted when evaluating fantastic claims made to the public about an intervention (Heward, 2009), the promises of a cure can be very tempting and lead parents to select potentially dangerous options. Perhaps Favell (2005, p. 19) captured the phenomenon best:

> Although substantial and well-substantiated progress seen across the decades in dimensions such as the teaching of adaptive skills, treatment of behavior problems, and the overall quality of life of individuals with developmental disabilities, these well-grounded, positive developments have often been eclipsed by the steady appearance of "breakthroughs," "new models," "cures," and "revolutionary strategies" that typically promise results that are more rapid, more beneficial, and easier to achieve than any seen before.

Celebrity endorsement may also play a role in the persistence of invalidated interventions and fads. Humans may be easily influenced by figures considered to be of importance or who hold a prominent place in society. Regardless of their credentials or the lack of science supporting an intervention, a celebrity's endorsement may be appealing to the public and capture their attention just long enough to impact the autism community. One example of this would be Jenny McCarthy's influence on the autism community. McCarthy has a captive audience in parents of children with ASD and has posited that an antivaccine movement is warranted (informed by her perspective that vaccines are responsible for autism, as she believed was the case for her son). To this end, McCarthy has touted a number of biomedical interventions such as a gluten-free diet, vitamins, and detoxification of metals. In regard to her son she stated, "He could not learn while he was frozen in autism" (McCarthy & Carrey, 2008). McCarthy and her story have received a great deal of attention and followers through the years, most often mothers of children with ASD. The dilemma here, of course, is that the biomedical interventions that she promotes are not evidence based and the causal relationship between vaccines and ASD lacks scientific merit. It is easy to see how someone of influence, such as a celebrity, could gain followers even in the absence of any scientific evidence to support the assertions made.

Another possible reason involves the way in which erroneous perceptions of client behavior change can effect the continued use of an invalidated intervention. This perception is typically associated with the clients themselves—however, in the case of autism intervention, this perception could also be observed in the parent of the child receiving the intervention. There are a number of influences that could be attributed to this erroneous perception of intervention effects in ASD. These could include placebo effects, palliative effects, retrospective rewriting of pretreatment functioning, reactivity, or responding to clinician or researcher expectations (Lilienfeld, Ritschel, Lynn, Cautin, & Latzman, 2014).

Finally, the persistence of invalidated interventions may lie with the practitioners, the professionals in our field and related fields. Professionals may offer parents an opportunity to "try" an undocumented approach as an attempt to meet a need in the child. When a credentialed professional utilizes or recommends an intervention it tends to lend credibility to that intervention even though it may not be based in science. Professional organizations may speak out against a popular intervention because it is not evidence based (e.g., ASHA's position paper on FC). Unfortunately, this outcome is rare—typically, professional organizations remain quiet and thereby may also be contributing to the use of treatments based in pseudoscience (Newsom & Hovanitz, 2005).

LEVELS OF EVIDENCE IN AUTISM INTERVENTION

Various levels of evidence exist in regard to interventions used with individuals with ASD. Interventions may show evidence, emerging evidence, no evidence, evidence that shows that the intervention is invalid, or evidence to show that the intervention is harmful. These outcomes may be confusing to a parent of a child with ASD. An intervention with emerging evidence might seem like a viable intervention for a child. Moreover, interventions may appear to have evidence, however, that the research methodology could be flawed or biased. For example, the research may show efficacy of the intervention only when it is combined with other interventions, or several articles might show positive effects of the intervention, but they are all published by the creator of the intervention. So, when it seems that support exists, the evidence must come under scrutiny to determine the efficacy of the research. It is important to evaluate the quality of the research in order to know whether the results are substantiated.

Although it may be clear that the scientific method is an antidote for pseudoscience, the evaluation of the current research base on existing interventions is not always easily accessible to most people. This is especially true in the case of parents of individuals with ASD (Zane, 2005). To this end, a number of professions and organizations have developed research-based resources to assist the public in sifting through the myriad of interventions available and objectively determine their efficacy (National Autism Center, 2009, 2015a, 2015b; Maine Department of Education & Maine Department of Health and Human Services, 2009; Maglione, Gans, Das, Timbie, & Kasari, 2012).

The reviews utilize specific categories of evidence to organize the interventions based on the current research available. For example, the National Autism Center (2015a, 2015b) report described previously adopted the categories of established, emerging, and unestablished. An established intervention was one in which sufficient evidence is available to confidently determine that an intervention produces favorable outcomes for individuals on the autism spectrum—that is, these interventions are established as effective. An emerging intervention was an intervention for which one or more studies suggest that the intervention produces favorable outcomes for individuals with ASD, but additional high-quality studies must consistently show this outcome before we can draw firm conclusions about intervention effectiveness. Finally, the unestablished interventions were interventions for which there is little or no evidence to allow us to draw firm conclusions about intervention effectiveness with individuals with ASD. Additional research may show the intervention to be effective, ineffective, or harmful.

In their research-based reviews of interventions used with individuals with ASD up to age 22, the National Autism Center (2015a, 2015b) categorized 14 treatments as established interventions (e.g., behavioral interventions, modeling), 18 as emerging interventions (e.g., social communication intervention, technology-based intervention), and 13 as unestablished interventions (e.g., developmental, individual-differences, and relationship-based model [DIR/Floortime]; sensory intervention). Unfortunately, their classification system used only three categories of evidence, which limits the ability to see the continuum of levels of evidence. Furthermore, the report categorized some items outside of the expected category. For example, behavioral interventions are listed under established interventions and a number of interventions are included within the behavioral interventions category. However, modeling (established intervention) is listed separately and organized in the behavioral interventions category. This may lead to some possible confusion regarding specific interventions and their respective coding. Despite these concerns, reviews such as the National Autism Center (2015a, 2015b) report can be helpful when looking at the broader picture but must also be critiqued and analyzed accordingly.

One common finding among the systematic reviews that have been conducted is that interventions based on the principles of ABA have a track record of effectiveness when incorporated in well-designed programs for individuals with ASD. A well-designed program requires professionals to implement the framework of evidence-based practice (National Autism Center, 2015a, 2015b). In addition to the previously discussed components, the National Autism Center (2015b) specifically addresses evidence-based practice in schools for students with ASD—it is an educator's guide to assist in providing appropriate interventions to students with ASD. The group also published a manual created specifically as a resource for parents navigating the myriad of autism interventions (National Autism Center, 2011).

Another example of such a review is the state of the evidence report generated by the Maine Administrators of Services for Children with Disabilities (Tweed, Connolly, & Beaulieu, 2009). This comprehensive report was developed to review the research literature on interventions with individuals with ASD and disseminate the information to professionals, policy makers, and families affected by ASD. The report utilized Reichow, Volkmar, and Cicchetti's (2008) validated rubric that focuses on levels of evidence for interventions along five levels. The levels range from proven and effective to demonstrating evidence of harm (see Table 14.1). Although the reviewers appeared to have used a thorough process for reviewing and categorizing the interventions, one must be cautious in accepting the findings at face value. First, the report was published in 2009 and therefore is in need of revision at the time of this writing. To that end, it is possible that some of the emerging interventions may now have enough evidence to be categorized in the established category. Clearly, there continues to be a need for comprehensive and current reviews regarding the state of autism intervention (Wong et al., 2015)

KEY QUESTIONS FOR PARENTS AND PROFESSIONALS TO ASK

It is important for parents and professionals to question interventions and the individuals providing those interventions. But what questions should they ask to divert them from a path of seeking pseudoscientific approaches? To equip parents and professionals with the right questions when faced with a potential new intervention for individuals with ASD, we compiled a list for consumer use (see Table 14.2). Our goal is to provide the consumer with a starting point when attempting to gather information.

RESOURCES FOR PARENTS AND PROFESSIONALS

The Internet is a common place for both parents and professionals to look for information about ASD in our current technological society. Unfortunately, there are no guidelines for finding high-quality websites (Reichow et al., 2012). Reichow and colleagues surveyed participants regarding ASD websites' accuracy of content and whether the content was current. Information was provided blind to the research participants who were also asked to note who they would recommend to use the website. Some of the top websites selected in the research included the Association for Science in Autism Treatment, Wikipedia, Autism Speaks, and the Centers for Disease Control and Prevention. Websites are listed for reference in Table 14.3.

There is also a great deal of information on the Internet about pseudoscience and its impact on decison making. Lilienfeld, Lohr, and Morier (2001) identified a number of websites that could be useful for anyone interested in learning more about pseudoscience. See Table 14.4 for a listing of these websites.

TABLE 14.1. Levels of Evidence by Intervention Category for ASD Treatment

Level 1: Established evidence

The treatment has been proven effective in multiple strong or adequately rated group experimental design studies, single-subject studies, or a combination. Results must be replicated in studies conducted by different research teams.

Category	Interventions
Applied behavior analysis (ABA)	• ABA for challenging behavior • ABA for communication • Early intensive behavioral intervention
Augmentative and alternative communication	Picture Exchange Communication System
Pharmacological approaches	• Halperidol (Haldol) for aggression • Methylphenidate (Ritalin) for hyperactivity • Risperidone (Risperdal) for irritability, social withdrawal, hyperactivity, and stereotypy

Level 2: Promising evidence

The intervention has been shown effective in more than two strong or adequately rated group experimental design studies or at least three single-subject studies. Additional research is needed by separate teams to confirm that the intervention is effective across settings and researchers.

Category	Interventions
ABA	ABA for adaptive living skills
Augmentative and alternative communication	Voice output communication aid (VOCA)
Psychotherapy	Cognitive-behavioral therapy (CBT) for anxiety

Level 3: Preliminary evidence

The intervention has been shown effective in at least one strong or adequately rated group or single-subject design study. More research is needed to confirm results.

Category	Interventions
ABA	• ABA for academics (numeral recognition, reading instruction, grammatical morphemes, spelling) • ABA for vocational skills
Augmentative and alternative communication	Sign language

(continued)

TABLE 14.1. *(continued)*

Developmental, social-pragmatic models	Developmental, social-pragmatic models (eclectic models)
Diet and nutritional approaches	Vitamin C for sensorimotor symptoms (modest effect)
Pharmacological approaches	• Atomoxetine (Strattera) for attention deficit and hyperactivity • Clomipramine (Anafranil) for stereotypy, ritualistic behavior, and social behavior • Clonidine (Catapres) for hyperactivity, irritability, inappropriate speech, stereotypy, and oppositional behavior
Psychotherapy	CBT for anger management
Sensory integration therapy	Touch therapy/massage
Other	Hyperbaric oxygen treatment

Level 4: Studied and no evidence of effect

Numerous (three or more) strong or adequately rated studies have determined that the intervention has no positive effect on the desired outcomes.

Category	Interventions
Pharmacological approaches	Dimethylglycine (DMG) Secretin

Level 5: Insufficient evidence

Conclusions cannot be drawn on the efficacy of the intervention due to a lack of quality research and/or mixed outcomes across several studies.

Category	Interventions
ABA	ABA for academics (cooperative learning groups)
Augmentative and alternative communication	Facilitated communication
Diet and nutritional approaches	• Gluten–casein-free diets • Omega-3 fatty acid supplements • Vitamin B6/magnesium supplements
Developmental, social-pragmatic models	• DIR/Floortime • RDI • SECRETS • Solomon's PLAY model

(continued)

TABLE 14.1. *(continued)*

Pharmacological approaches	• Guanfacine (Tenex) • Intravenous immunoglobin • Melatonin • Naltrexone (Revia) • Selective serotonin reuptake inhibitors: citalopram (Celexa) and fluoxetine (Prozac) • Valproic acid (Depakote) • Intravenous chelation using edetate disodium
Sensory integration therapy	• Auditory integration training • Sensory integration training
Social skills training	• Social skills training • Social stories
Other	TEACCH

Note. Adapted from Tweed, Connolly, and Beaulieu (2009).

TABLE 14.2. Key Questions for Parents and Professionals to Ask

	Parent	Professional
Have I completed the red flags checklist provided in this chapter?	×	×
How does this intervention address assessment results and my child's/the client's needs, desires, and strengths?	×	×
Are there any published research articles in peer-reviewed journals documenting the efficacy or effectiveness of the proposed intervention method? If yes, do they meet the standards of rigor for science?	×	×
Is the proposed intervention solely supported through testimonials and anecdotal reports?	×	×
Does the current setting have the necessary resources to implement the intervention consistent with the procedures documented in the published studies?	×	×
Is there any evidence of harm associated with this intervention? What are the risks? Is there adequate consumer protection?	×	×
What position statements from respected professional organizations support or do not support the intervention?	×	×

(continued)

TABLE 14.2. *(continued)*

	Parent	Professional
Are the intervention procedures consistent with professional guidelines and standards of practice in the interventionist's chosen field (e.g., Behavior Analyst Certification Board, American Psychological Association, National Association of School Psychologists, National Association for the Education of Young Children, Council for Exceptional Children)?	×	×
What are the credentials of the interventionist? What kind of training and supervision would the interventionist need to have before implementing the intervention? Is that particular training and experience documented and substantiated?	×	×
What types of ongoing supervision and professional support is available for the interventionist?	×	×
Does the interventionist pursue continuing education opportunities and, if so, what types?		×
What is the current caseload and commitments of the interventionist? Does he or she have sufficient time and resources to devote to implementing and monitoring the intervention?	×	×
What is the expected outcome? Can the team measure the effects of the intervention and share data regularly to document potential changes, no changes, or worsening outcomes?	×	×
What happens during a typical treatment session?	×	×
How involved are parents and primary caregivers in the day-to-day delivery of my child's intervention?	×	
What activities can I do at home to support the goals of the intervention?	×	
What type of data will the interventionist collect and how often?	×	×
Does every individual with ASD receive the exact same intervention? Will the interventionist modify the intervention and base these decisions on frequent, systematic evaluation of direct observational data?	×	×

Note. These questions were informed by our professional experiences and adaptations from several resources including the Autism Special Interest Group of the Association for Behavior Analysis (2007), the Association for Science in Autism Treatment (n.d.), Autism Spectrum Therapies (n.d.), and Celiberti, Buchanan, Bleecker, Kreiss, and Rosenfeld (2004).

TABLE 14.3. Useful Websites about Autism and Autism Intervention

Website	Description
www.asatonline.org	The website of the Association for Science in Autism Treatment is dedicated to educating the public about the importance of science-based interventions in autism. Reviews of research related to interventions are included on the site.
www.cdc.gov/ncbddd/autism/index.html	This webpage of the Centers for Disease Control and Prevention provides information about screening, diagnosis, treatment, and research.
www.autismspeaks.org	Autism Speaks is an organization that provides information, funding, and resources to the public about ASD and promotes autism awareness.
https://en.wikipedia.org/wiki/Autism	This is an autism-specific Wikipedia page that covers causes, characteristics, and intervention.

Note. Content adapted from Reichow et al. (2012).

TABLE 14.4. Useful Websites for Information about Pseudoscience

Website	Description
www.asatonline.org	The website of the Association for Science in Autism Treatment provides information about the difference between science and pseudoscience and reviews pseudoscience-based interventions as they pertain to the treatment of ASD.
www.skeptic.com	The Skeptics Society webpage includes full-text articles from *The Skeptic.*
www.srmhp.org	The Scientific Review of Mental Health Practice is devoted to distinguishing scientifically supported claims from scientifically unsupported claims in clinical psychology, psychiatry, social work, and allied disciplines.
www.skepticnews.com	The *Skeptic News* webpage provides updates on events and news related to pseudoscience.
www.quackwatch.com	Quackwatch is an international network of people who are concerned about health-related frauds, myths, fads, fallacies, and misconduct.

Note. Content was adapted from Lilienfeld, Lohr, and Morier (2001).

CONCLUSION

The desire for a quick fix or the many interventions that promise cures or rapid results lead parents, professionals, and policy makers toward unproven or ineffective interventions for individuals with ASD. Symptoms of ASD appear early in life and persist throughout the person's lifetime. Although we have seen advances in the treatment of ASD, the cause remains widely unknown and this then leaves autism wide open for the development of a large number of interventions (Worley et al., 2014). The unfortunate truth is that these interventions are most often not subject to scientific inquiry and thereby are often used in the absence of any reported efficacy. Parents and children are potentially subjected to harm and, at the very least, a roller coaster ride of emotions as their hopes are raised and dashed again and again. It is of utmost importance that the public is educated about interventions for individuals with ASD and that interventions based in pseudoscience are not left unchecked and allowed to persist. The antidote to pseudoscience is education, critical thinking, and the use of the scientific method. Consumers must be critical of the "newest fad" touted by celebrities, professionals, or advocates of the intervention (Worley et al., 2014). At this time, it is well documented that treatments based in ABA have the most research support and ideally should receive the most attention and promotion in comparison with the pseudoscientific interventions to which we previously referred. The responsibility of our community lies with the promotion of science-based interventions while educating others to have a critical lens toward unproven interventions.

REFERENCES

Association for Science in Autism Treatment. (1999). Pseudoscientific therapies: Some warning signs. Available from *www.asatonline.org/wp-content/uploads/2014/08/spring99.pdf.*

Autism Special Interest Group of the Association for Behavior Analysis. (2007). Consumer guidelines for identifying, selecting, and evaluating behavior analysts working with individuals with autism spectrum disorders. Available from *www.apbahome.net/downloads/AutGuidelines.pdf.*

Celiberti, D., Buchanan, S., Bleecker, F., Kreiss, D., & Rosenfeld, D. (2004). The road less traveled: Charting a clear course for autism treatment. In *Autism: Basic information* (pp. 17–31). Robbinsville, NJ: Autism New Jersey.

Chambless, D. L., & Hollon, S. D. (1998). Defining empirically supported therapies. *Journal of Consulting and Clinical Psychology, 66,* 17–18.

Connett, D. (2015, November). Autism: Potentially lethal bleach "cure" feared to have spread to Britain. *Independent.* Available from *www.independent.co.uk/life-style/health-and-families/health-news/autism-potentially-lethal-bleach-cure-feared-to-have-spread-to-britain-a6744291.html.*

Eikeseth, S. (2009). Outcome of comprehensive psychoeducational interventions for young children with autism. *Research in Developmental Disabilities, 30,* 158–178.

Eldevik, S., Hastings, R. P., Hughes, J. C., Jahr, E., & Eikeseth, S. (2010). Using participant data to extend the evidence base for intensive behavioral intervention for children with autism. *American Association on Intellectual and Developmental Disabilities, 115*(5), 381–405.

Favell, J. E. (2005). Sifting sound practice from snake oil. In J. W. Jacobson, R. M. Foxx, & J. A. Mulick (Eds.), *Controversial therapies for developmental disabilities: Fad, fashion, and science in professional practice* (pp. 19–30). Mahwah, NJ: Erlbaum.

FDA Consumer Health Information. (2014, April). Beware of false or misleading claims for treating autism. Available from *www.fda.gov/downloads/ForConsumers/ConsumerUpdates/UCM394800.pdf.*

Freed, G. L., Clark, S. J., Butchart, A. T., Singer, D. C., & Davis, M. M. (2010). Parental vaccine safety concerns in 2009. *Pediatrics, 125*(4), 654–659.

Gettys, T. (2015, May). Quack defends bleach enemas to "cure" autism: If it's poison, where is the "sea of dead children"? Available from *www.rawstory.com/2015/05/quack-defends-bleach-enemas-to-cure-autism-if-its-poison-where-is-the-sea-of-dead-children.*

Green, G. (1996). Early behavioral intervention for autism: What does research tell us? In C. Maurice, G. Green, & S. C. Luce (Eds.), *Behavioral intervention for young children with autism: A manual for parents and professionals* (pp. 29–44). Austin, TX: PRO-ED.

Green, G., & Perry, L. (1999). Science, pseudoscience, and anti-science: What's this got to do with my kid? *Science in Autism Treatment.* Available from *www.asatonline.org/pdf/spring99.pdf.*

Green, V. A., Pituch, K. A., Itchon, J., Choi, A., O'Reilly, M., & Sigafoos, J. (2006). Internet survey of treatments used by parents of children with autism. *Research in Developmental Disabilities, 27,* 70–84.

Herbert, J. D. (2000). Defining empirically supported treatments: Pitfalls and possible solutions. *Behaviour Therapist, 23*(6), 113–121.

Herbert, J. D., Sharp, I. R., & Gaudiano, B. A. (2002). Separating fact from fiction in the etiology and treatment of autism: A scientific review of the evidence. Available from *www.srmhp.org/0101/autism.html.*

Heward, W. L. (2009). *Exceptional children: An introduction to special education.* Upper Saddle River, NJ: Pearson.

Howard, J. S., Sparkman, C. R., Cohen, H. G., Green, G., & Stanislaw, H. (2005). A comparison of intensive behavior analytic and eclectic treatments for young children with autism. *Research in Developmental Disabilities, 26*(4), 359–383.

Jacobson, J. W., Foxx, R. M., & Mulick, J. A. (2005). *Controversial therapies for developmental disabilities: Fad, fashion, and science in professional practice.* Mahwah, NJ: Erlbaum.

Levy, S. E., & Hyman, S. L. (2003). Use of complementary and alternative treatments for children with autism spectrum disorders is increasing. *Pediatric Annals, 32,* 685–691.

Lilienfeld, S. O., Lohr, J. M., & Morier, D. (2001). The teaching of courses in the science and pseudoscience of psychology: Useful resources. *Teaching of Psychology, 28*(3), 182–191.

Lilienfeld, S. O., Lynn, S. J., & Ammirati, R. J. (2015). Science versus pseudoscience. In R. L. Cautin & S. O. Lilienfeld (Eds.), *The encyclopedia of clinical psychology* (pp. 1–7). Hoboken, NJ: Wiley.

Lilienfeld, S. O., Lynn, S. J., & Lohr, J. M. (2014). Science and pseudoscience in clinical psychology: Initial thoughts, reflections and considerations. In S. O. Lilienfeld, S. J. Lynn, & J. M. Lohr (Eds.), *Science and pseudoscience in clinical psychology* (pp. 1–38). New York: Guilford Press.

Lilienfeld, S. O., Marshall, J., Todd, J. T., & Shane, H. C. (2014). The persistence of fad interventions in the face of negative scientific evidence: Facilitated communication for autism as a case example. *Evidence-Based Communication Assessment and Intervention, 8*(2), 62–101.

Lilienfeld, S. O., Ritschel, L. A., Lynn, S. J., Cautin, R. L., & Latzman, R. D. (2014). Why ineffective psychotherapies appear to work: A taxonomy of causes of spurious therapeutic effectiveness. *Perspectives on Psychological Science, 9*(4), 355–387.

Lovaas, O. I. (1987). Behavioral treatment and normal educational and intellectual functioning in young autistic children. *Journal of Consulting and Clinical Psychology, 55,* 3–9.

Maglione, M. A., Gans, D., Das, L., Timbie, J., & Kasari, C. (2012). Nonmedical interventions for children with ASD: Recommended guidelines and further research needs. *Pediatrics, 130,* S169–S178.

Marino, L., & Lilienfeld, S. O. (2007). Dolphin-assisted therapy: Flawed data, flawed conclusions. *Anthrozoös, 11*(4), 194–200.

McCarthy, J., & Carrey, J. (2008, April). Jenny McCarthy: My son's recovery from autism. CNN.com. Available from *http://edition.cnn.com/2008/US/04/02/mccarthy.autismtreatment/index.html.*

McDonald, M. E., Pace, D., Blue, E., & Schwartz, D. (2012). Critical issues in causation and treatment of autism: Why fads continue to flourish. *Child and Family Behavior Therapy, 34*(4), 290–304.

McEachin, J., Smith, T., & Lovaas, O. I. (1993). Long-term outcome for children with autism who received early intensive behavioral treatment. *American Journal of Mental Retardation, 97*(4), 359–372.

Metz, B., Mulick, J. A., & Butler, E. M. (2005). Autism: A late 20th century fad magnet. In J. Jacobson, R. Foxx, & J. Mulick (Eds.), *Controversial therapies for developmental disabilities: Fad, fashion, and science in professional practice* (pp. 237–264). Mahwah, NJ: Erlbaum.

National Autism Center. (2009). *National standards report: National standards project. Addressing the need for evidence-based practice guidelines for autism spectrum disorders.* Randolph, MA: Author.

National Autism Center. (2011). *A parent's guide to evidence-based practices and autism: Providing information and resources for families of children with autism spectrum disorders.* Randolph, MA: Author.

National Autism Center. (2015a). *Evidence-based practice and autism in the schools: An educator's guide to providing appropriate interventions to students with autism spectrum disorder* (2nd ed.). Randolph, MA: Author.

National Autism Center. (2015b). *National standards project, phase 2: Findings and conclusions. Addressing the need for evidence-based practice guidelines for autism spectrum disorder.* Randolph, MA: Author.

National Research Council. (2001). *Educating children with autism.* Committee on

Educational Interventions for Children with Autism, Division of Behavioral and Social Sciences and Education. Washington, DC: National Academy Press.

New York State Department of Health Early Intervention Program. (1999). *Clinical practice guideline: Guideline technical report. Autism/pervasive developmental disorder, assessment and intervention for young children (ages 0–3 years), No. 4217.* Albany: New York State Department of Health.

Newsom, C., & Hovanitz, C. A. (2005). The nature and values of empirically validated interventions. In J. W. Jacobson, R. M. Foxx, & J. A. Mulick (Eds.), *Controversial therapies for developmental disabilities: Fad, fashion, and science in professional practice* (pp. 31–44). Mahwah, NJ: Erlbaum.

Normand, M. P. (2008). Science, skepticism, and applied behavior analysis. *Behavior Analysis in Practice, 1,* 42–49.

Ostrander, G. K., Cheng, K. C., Wolf, J. C., & Wolfe, M. J. (2004). Shark cartilage, cancer and the growing threat of pseudoscience. *Journal of Cancer Research, 64,* 8485–8491.

Reichow, B., Halpern, J. L., Steinhoff, T. B., Letsinger, N., Naples, A., & Volkmar, F. R. (2012). Characteristics and quality of autism websites. *Journal of Autism and Developmental Disorders, 42,* 1263–1274.

Reichow, B., Volkmar, F. R., & Cicchetti, D. V. (2008). Development of the evaluative method for evaluating and determining evidence-based practices in autism. *Journal of Autism and Developmental Disorders, 38,* 1311–1319.

Romanczyk, R. G., & Gillis, J. M. (2005). Treatment approaches for autism: Evaluating options and making informed choices. In D. Zager (Ed.), *Autism: Identification, education, and treatment* (3rd ed., pp. 515–536). Hillsdale, NJ: Erlbaum.

Romanczyk, R. G., Gillis, J. M., White, S., & DiGennaro, F. D. (2008). Comprehensive treatment packages for ASD: Effectiveness and cost-benefit. In J. Matson (Ed.), *Autism spectrum disorder: Evidence based assessment and treatment across the lifespan* (pp. 351–381). Burlington, MA: Elsevier Science.

Romanczyk, R. G., Turner, L. B., Sevlever, M., & Gillis, J. M. (2015). The status of treatment for autism spectrum disorders: The weak relationship of science to interventions. In S. O. Lilienfeld, S. J. Lynn, & J. M. Lohr (Eds.), *Science and pseudoscience in contemporary clinical psychology* (pp. 431–465). New York: Guilford Press.

Russell, M. (2010). 'Miracle' elixir linked to death, illness. *The Sydney Morning Herald.* Available from *www.smh.com.au/national/miracle-elixir-linked-to-death-illness-20100821-13a2z.html.*

Schlosser, R. W., Balandin, S., Hemsley, B., Iacono, T., Probst, P., & Vontetzchner, S. (2014). Facilitated communication and authorship: A systematic review. *Augmentative and Alternative Communication, 30*(4), 359–368.

Schreck, K. A., & Ramirez, J. E. (2016). Television's mixed messages: Choose the best and mute the rest. *Behavioral Interventions, 31*(3), 251–264.

Shermer, M. (2002). *Why people believe weird things: Pseudoscience, superstition, and other confusions of our time.* New York: Holt.

Sifferlin, A. (2014). 4 diseases making a comeback thanks to anti-vaxxers. *Time.* Available from *http://time.com/27308/4-diseases-making-a-comeback-thanks-to-anti-vaxxers.*

Smith, T., & Wick, J. (2008). Controversial treatments. In F. R. Volkmar, A. Klin, & K. Chawarska (Eds.), *Autism spectrum disorders in infancy and early childhood* (pp. 243–273). New York: Guilford Press.

Spata, A. V. (2003). *Research methods: Science and diversity.* New York: Wiley.

Strock, M. (2004). Autism spectrum disorders (pervasive developmental disorders) (NIH Publication No. NIH-04-5511). Bethesda, MD: National Institute of Mental Health, National Institutes of Health, U.S. Department of Health and Human Services. Available from *www.nimh.nih.gov/publicat/autism.cfm.*

Thyer, B. A., & Pignotti, M. (2010). Science and pseudoscience in developmental disabilities: Guidelines for social workers. *Journal of Social Work in Disability and Rehabilitation, 9,* 110–129.

Tostanoski, A., Lang, R., Raulston, T., Carnett, A., & Davis, T. (2014). Voices from the past: Comparing the rapid prompting method and facilitated communication. *Developmental Neurorehabilitation, 17*(4), 219–223.

Tweed, L., Connolly, N., & Beaulieu, A. (2009). *Interventions for autism spectrum disorders: State of the evidence.* Augusta: Muskie School of Public Service and the Maine Department of Health and Human Services.

U.S. Department of Health and Human Services. (1999). *Mental health: A report of the Surgeon General.* Rockville, MD: U.S. Department of Health and Human Services, Substance Abuse and Mental Health Services Administration, Center for Mental Health Services, National Institutes of Health, National Institute of Mental Health.

Wong, C., Odom, S. L., Hume, K. A., Cox, A. W., Fettig, A., Kucharczyk, S., et al. (2015). Evidence-based practices for children, youth, and young adults with autism spectrum disorder: A comprehensive review. *Journal of Autism and Developmental Disorders, 45*(7), 1951–1966.

Worley, J. A., Fodstad, J. C., & Neal, D. (2014). Controversial treatments for autism spectrum disorders. In J. Tarbox, D. R. Dixon, P. Sturmey, & J. L. Matson (Eds.), *Handbook of early intervention for autism spectrum disorders* (pp. 487–509). New York: Springer.

Zane, T. (2005). Fads in special education: An overview. In J. Jacobson, R. Foxx, & J. Mulick (Eds.), *Controversial therapies for developmental disabilities: Fad, fashion, and science in professional practice* (pp. 175–192). Mahwah, NJ: Erlbaum.

CHAPTER FIFTEEN

Future Directions in the Assessment and Treatment of Autism Spectrum Disorder

Isaac C. Smith
Cara E. Pugliese
Blythe A. Corbett
Susan W. White

The past two decades have seen tremendous advances in the development and validation of tools to aid accurate diagnosis of autism spectrum disorder (ASD). This has been especially so for young children, such that accurate diagnosis can now be made shortly after the first year of life (Chawarska, Klin, Paul, Macari, & Volkmar, 2009), in the context of fairly robust behavioral profiles being first identifiable at around 12 months (Ozonoff et al., 2010). Identification of ASD so early in life is important given the impact of intensive, early intervention (see Smith & Iadarola, 2015). However, several crucial domains of ASD research remain understudied. The aim of the current chapter is to review components of ASD assessment and treatment, with the most pressing needs for future research in two broad areas: (1) assessment and diagnosis, and (2) treatment development and intervention evaluation. Although identification of all the needs and future directions in these areas are beyond the scope of a single chapter, we focus on assessment and diagnosis needs including differential diagnosis of social communication disorder, sex and gender differences in ASD, and the use of biomarkers to diagnose individuals and predict outcome. Within the treatment domain, research needs include functional assessment of adult outcome, elucidation of mechanisms of change in interventions, and development and usage of sensitive measures of change.

Evidence-based assessment is essential to the practice of solid clinical science (cf. Hunsley & Mash, 2007)—its importance must therefore be emphasized as our field continues to evolve. Without accurate assessment, we can neither understand an individual's presenting problem nor recognize when progress is being made, developmentally or with intervention. In this chapter, we identify gaps in our knowledge of evidence-based assessment, and offer suggestions for future research on assessment, development, and treatment of ASD.

Gaps in our understanding of how to best screen for, and diagnose, comorbid psychiatric conditions among people diagnosed with ASD (see Chapter 10) are critical to address in order to inform intervention science. Likewise, our historically male-centric focus within ASD diagnostics suggests caution be taken in applying diagnostic thresholds to females, especially in light of recent research suggesting possible sex[1] differences in ASD expression (Lai et al., 2011; Van Wijngaarden-Cremers et al., 2014). Although difficulties in saturating samples with girls diagnosed with ASD have thus far precluded a complete understanding of phenotypic differences between males and females, we cannot assume a gender-blind stance with respect to diagnostic thresholds.

A large portion of this chapter addresses considerations related to assessment in the context of intervention. As a field, research on ASD has historically been focused on etiology, identification, and diagnosis. This is important research, and its products have informed clinical practice and policy (e.g., Centers for Disease Control and Prevention [Christensen et al., 2016] early identification). However, as we increasingly appreciate the lifelong and pervasive nature of ASD, the necessity of having tools with which to measure change in core and secondary problems has become clear. This is complicated work, owing in part to the nature of ASD. For instance, in treating the core social deficit, it might not be realistic to use the same criterion for success (e.g., within normal limits on an outcome measure of social function) as we might for a client with some other condition (e.g., attention-deficit/hyperactivity disorder [ADHD]). We also address candidate mechanisms for change, or the core processes that are believed to underlie symptom change during treatment (Lerner, White, & McPartland, 2012). This is timely in light of recent advances in experimental therapeutics (Damiano, Mazefsky, White, & Dichter, 2014) and a heightened emphasis on parsimony in treatment development (e.g., transdiagnostic or unified treatments).

---

[1]While it is important to acknowledge gender nonbinary individuals, the majority of research on differences utilizes parent report of birth-assigned biological sex, and thus the term "sex" will be used rather than "gender" throughout.

ASSESSMENT AND DIAGNOSIS: GAPS AND FUTURE DIRECTIONS

Social (Pragmatic) Communication Disorder

In addition to substantial changes made to the diagnostic classification of the autism spectrum, the advent of the fifth edition of *Diagnostic and Statistical Manual of Mental Disorders* (DSM-5; American Psychiatric Association, 2013) brought with it a new neurodevelopmental disorder: social (pragmatic) communication disorder (SCD). Criteria for a diagnosis of SCD include deficits in the use of communication for social purposes, including social pragmatics, turn taking, and understanding nonliteral language (American Psychiatric Association, 2013). While the diagnostic criteria for SCD and ASD share many common elements, notable in SCD criteria is the absence of restricted and repetitive behaviors. The utility of this new diagnosis must be evaluated within the context of the changes to diagnostic criteria for ASD, which were placed under scrutiny by a number of published studies leading up to and following publication of DSM-5. Some of these studies raised concerns about individuals who might no longer qualify for a diagnosis of ASD under the new criteria. Estimates of the number of individuals no longer qualifying for diagnoses under DSM-5 criteria were as high as 40% (McPartland, Reichow, & Volkmar, 2012). Other studies indicated that the vast majority of individuals would retain diagnoses (Huerta, Bishop, Duncan, Hus, & Lord, 2012). Taken together, the literature on the sensitivity and specificity of the new diagnostic criteria were highly variable (see Kulage, Smaldone, & Cohn, 2014; Smith, Reichow, & Volkmar, 2015, for reviews), though most studies indicated that at least a substantial minority of individuals would fail to qualify for diagnosis under the new criteria. Among those individuals failing to meet the new criteria, the largest subgroup is the pervasive developmental disorder not otherwise specified (PDD-NOS) group, most of whom would not qualify for any diagnosis under DSM-5 (Smith et al., 2015).

These data merit mention here given that some have suggested that SCD will fill the gap left by the former PDD-NOS diagnosis, and will constitute another diagnosis that functionally serves as "not-quite" ASD (Skuse, 2012, p. 345). Researchers expressing concerns regarding those individuals who would lose diagnoses under new DSM-5 criteria have hypothesized that some such individuals may now meet criteria for SCD, though none have attempted to map the symptoms of these individuals onto SCD criteria in order to obtain estimates of rates of SCD.

Differential diagnosis of ASD and SCD will likely prove difficult in clinical practice. In order to diagnose SCD, ASD must be ruled out. Detecting restricted and repetitive behaviors as well as sensory issues and rigidity will therefore be critical in making this diagnostic distinction. The manifestation of restricted and repetitive behaviors has been shown to evolve throughout the developmental trajectory such that they may vary in type and intensity, further complicating differential diagnosis (Seltzer, Shattuck, Abbeduto, & Greenberg, 2004). In contrast to the idea that SCD might become a catchall for those individuals whose restricted and repetitive behavior symptoms are not sufficient for a diagnosis of ASD, some have proposed that the co-occurrence of social communication deficits and restricted and repetitive behaviors as seen in ASD is not universal and that communication deficits may exist on their own (Mandy & Skuse, 2008). This hypothesis predated the DSM-5 work group's proposal of SCD, providing further evidence that SCD is phenotypically distinct from ASD.

Moving forward, it is imperative that diagnostic tools allowing for a reliable diagnosis of SCD be developed and validated. Assessment of social and pragmatic language is much more difficult in practice than assessment of more structured components of language (i.e., vocabulary), given that development and use of social and pragmatic language are dependent on a number of variable factors including social contexts, cultural issues, and consideration of one's audience (Norbury, 2014). Parent- or teacher-report measures have been used widely in assessment of this domain, including the use of the Children's Communication Checklist (CCC) and the Social-Interaction Deviance Composite (SIDC; Norbury, 2014). Quantitative analysis of conversational exchanges has also been pursued as an avenue by which to assess the use of social and pragmatic language. Structured observation may also provide a means by which to evaluate language sufficiently to give a diagnosis of SCD. Assessments in this domain offer the most parallels with current diagnostic measures for ASD, as the Autism Diagnostic Observation Schedule (ADOS; Lord et al., 2000) contains coding items designed to assess reciprocity of conversations, amount and quality of social overtures, and integration of language and nonverbal communication. Further research should be conducted to determine the feasibility of adapting the ADOS or other existing assessments of pragmatic language to assess for SCD diagnoses.

Increasing use of existing reliable and valid assessments of pragmatic language (which may be utilized currently in other disciplines such as speech and language pathology), as well as development of tools aiding in the differential diagnosis of ASD and SCD, should be a priority within the ASD research community moving forward. Few studies characterizing samples of individuals with SCD exist, and no treatment studies have been published to date, despite the diagnosis having been published and put into use over 3 years ago. This lack of new studies may reflect difficulty experienced by researchers in separating ASD from SCD. Furthermore, SCD may also be found to lack the clinical utility to be considered a separate construct from ASD, despite a strong theoretical foundation. Future studies might attempt to determine how, and whether, the use of this new diagnostic category is warranted in the future.

Sex-Differentiated Phenomenology

The consensus that ASD is found four times as often in males as females has been replicated across several studies, and has remained strikingly stable despite evolving diagnostic criteria (Halladay et al., 2015; Werling & Geschwind, 2013; Christensen et al., 2016; Fombonne, 2003, 2005). Males are particularly overrepresented among individuals with ASD and average to above-average cognitive ability, with male to female ratio estimates of 5.7–11:1 (Baird et al., 2006; Fombonne, 2005). Conversely, among individuals with ASD and moderate to severe intellectual disability, the ratio is approximately 2:1 (Fombonne, 1999; Werling & Geschwind, 2013). As a result of the higher prevalence of ASD in males, females with a clinical diagnosis of ASD and average intellectual ability tend to be underrepresented in clinical research (Halladay et al., 2015). Evidence from an epidemiological study indicates that females are diagnosed later than males, and females with average IQ are diagnosed significantly later than both females with below-average IQ and males with average IQ (Shattuck et al., 2009).

There is debate over potential reasons for discrepancy in prevalence of ASD diagnoses, though main hypotheses involve influence of biological factors, ascertainment bias, and common diagnostic criteria and measures used. Some researchers believe that sex differences in genetic, hormonal, and neuroimmune processes lead to phenotypic sex differences (see Lai, Lombardo, Auyeung, Chakrabarti, & Baron-Cohen, 2015; Werling & Geschwind, 2013, for reviews). Other research proposes that an ascertainment bias may lead to an artificially low prevalence in females compared with males based on findings that boys tend to display more externalizing behaviors compared with girls, which might trigger earlier and more frequent diagnostic evaluation (Solomon, Miller, Taylor, Hinshaw, & Carter, 2012; Werling & Geschwind, 2013; Worley & Matson, 2011). Finally, current diagnostic criteria are not sex specific; were developed primarily with males in mind; and may not address differential development of social, communication, and play behaviors that are commonly seen between neurotypical boys and girls (Rivet & Matson, 2011). If this same pattern is replicated in the development of key behaviors in ASD, it may lead to underdiagnosis in females.

Children

Despite the challenges associated with identifying ASD in females, there is ongoing research attempting to identify sex differences in ASD symptoms across a variety of measures, though findings thus far have not been entirely consistent. Many studies have failed to detect sex differences in autism symptomatology among youth with ASD (Carter et al., 2007; Holtmann, Bolte, & Poustka, 2007; Mandic-Maravic et al., 2015; Reinhardt, Wetherby, Schatschneider, & Lord, 2015), though some studies indicate that females demonstrate fewer repetitive behaviors (Hartley & Sikora, 2009; Nicholas et al., 2008) and fewer social communication impairments (Zwaigenbaum et al., 2012) on standardized measures. A recent meta-analysis of 39 studies across 9,005 participants by Register-Brown and colleagues (2016) found sex differences across all age ranges to vary based on the diagnostic instrument used. Males demonstrated more severe communication behaviors on the Autism Diagnostic Interview (ADI; Le Couteur et al., 1989), but not the ADOS or other instruments, and had significantly greater restricted interests and repetitive behaviors on the ADI, ADOS, and other instruments in the 11- to 15-year age range, and in individuals with an IQ greater than 70. Scores on diagnostic questionnaires, such as the Autism Spectrum Rating Scale (ASRS; Goldstein & Naglieri, 2009), also indicate that ASD behaviors are significantly more prevalent among males than females, both for 2- to 5- and 6- to 18-year-old age groups.

In addition to analyzing quantitative sex differences on existing measures, it is also important to assess qualitative differences in ASD behaviors. A retrospective study of youth with ASD with average intelligence diagnosed after the age of 5 found no significant difference between the age of first concern and the age of diagnosis in females compared with males, though parents reported phenotypic differences (Hiller, Young, & Weber, 2016). Females were more likely to engage in complex imitation of others, had a strong desire to be liked by peers, and had a more advanced vocabulary than boys. Boys tended to have more restricted interests and were more isolated or withdrawn in preschool social settings.

Adolescents and Adults

In contrast to the number of studies conducted with children, few have examined sex differences in late adolescence and adulthood. Most studies utilizing older adolescents with ASD and average or above-average cognitive abilities do not report general sex differences. Using widely accepted measures, including a clinician observation measure (ADOS; Lord et al., 2000) and a parent-report interview (ADI/ADI-R; Le Couteur et al., 1989; Lord, Rutter, & Le Couteur, 1994), several studies found no sex differences in ASD behaviors in adolescent samples (Bölte, Duketis, Pouskta, & Holtmann, 2011; Holtmann, Bölte, & Poustka, 2007; Frazier, Georgiades, Bishop, & Hardan, 2014; McLennan, Lord, & Schopler, 1993; Solomon et al., 2012). While differences are not seen for total behaviors, some studies report differences in certain domains. For example, Frazier and colleagues (2014) found higher scores on the ADOS Reciprocal Social,

Communication, and Social Affect domains for the females, but the magnitude of the effect was small. Males, on the other hand, have been found to score higher on the Nonverbal Communication domain on the ADI-R (Park et al., 2012).

To date, only a handful of studies have examined autism behaviors in female adults with average cognitive abilities. Most found no differences in social communication behaviors on the ADI-R (Lai et al., 2011; Wilson et al., 2016), while one found that males had greater childhood restricted interests and repetitive behaviors (Wilson et al., 2016). One study reported no differences in the Social Communication and Restricted and Repetitive Behavior domains on the ADOS (Wilson et al., 2016) with another indicating that females were rated to have fewer autistic behaviors than males on the Social Communication and Restricted and Repetitive Behavior domains. In a recent multisite study of 282 adolescents and adults with ASD without intellectual disability (68 females), Pugliese, Trubanova, et al. (2016) reported that females were rated as less impaired on the following ADOS items: use of immediate echolalia, stereotyped and idiosyncratic words or phrases, offering information, conversation, communication of own affect, and empathy.

In contrast with the above measures, several studies utilizing self-report have demonstrated that females tend to report more ASD behaviors on the Autism Spectrum Quotient and Social Responsiveness Scale (Lai et al., 2015; Lehnhardt et al., 2016) highlighting a potential higher self-awareness of autism traits in females with ASD, which might be explained by differential social expectations for males and females, particularly in regard to the Social Communication domain (Bussey & Bandura, 1999). Alternatively, it could indicate greater real-world impairment in females compared with males. These studies highlight the importance of utilizing self-report measures, in addition to clinician and parent reports, to evaluate sex differences in ASD symptomatology. Due to the differences seen across development, it is necessary to focus the research on the population that has been underrepresented in existing research: adolescent and adult females with no intellectual impairment. Further studies, utilizing larger samples of adolescent and adult females with ASD without intellectual disability, are necessary to fully understand the potential sex differences in ASD diagnosis and behaviors.

Limitations of Current Instruments in Females with ASD

Interpretations of sex differences in ASD are currently limited by diagnostic challenges, etiological considerations, and the methodology that we use to identify and measure ASD behaviors. As a whole, females are underrepresented in research and clinical practice, leading to a biased view of the current ASD literature that is male centric and tends to overlook sex differences. A limitation of our diagnostic classification system is its predominant use of males for behavioral exemplars of ASD. Lai and colleagues (2015) call for clarification on the existence of a "female phenotype" of autism based on anecdotal clinical and autobiographical reports of qualitative differences (such as a greater awareness of the need for social interaction, better imagination), and more "typical" stereotyped interests (such as animals or celebrities) in females compared with males.

Higher demands placed on females to engage in socially appropriate behaviors and known differences in attainment of early sociocommunicative milestones (Rose & Rudolph, 2006) may lead to sex-based differences in the manifestation of ASD and place females at risk for underdiagnosis, particularly among those without co-occurring intellectual disability (ID). An ascertainment bias could be present, whereby females do better than males at "masking" or "camouflaging" their ASD symptoms (Dworzynski, Ronald, Bolton, & Happé, 2012; Gould & Ashton-Smith, 2011) for the short time frame of a diagnostic session. Females with ASD have described this phenomenon:

> One of the biggest things that has been missed . . . has been . . . "the chameleon effect." I was raised, as many women are, to blend in. . . . It's not without a tremendous amount of effort, it was hammered into me as a child, and it's incredibly uncomfortable. (Des Roches Rosa, April 22, 2016)

Compounding this issue, widely used diagnostic and screening tools such as the ADOS, ADI, and the Social Communication Questionnaire (SCQ; Rutter, Bailey, & Lord, 2003) were developed with predominately male normative and clinical samples. They have not been sex normed or evaluated with respect to sex bias and thus may not be adequately capturing the presentation of autism in females. For example, Pugliese, Kenworthy, and colleagues (2015) found that females may need a lower cutoff score than males on the ADOS Module 4. If this finding is replicated in future studies, then clinicians may be missing females with ASD who come into the clinic. Additionally, the ADOS is often used as a threshold for inclusion in research studies. If a lower threshold is indeed needed, then studies may be including more impacted females compared with males, which may skew research results. Finally, it is also possible that subtle differences may emerge on item-level examination of these measurements or that measures are not capturing qualitative sex differences in ASD presentation described anecdotally.

To better understand the unique profile of ASD symptoms in females, it will be necessary to undertake a bottom-up approach through identifying potential diagnostic markers clinicians and researchers may not be currently assessing. This could be achieved through cognitive interviewing of affected females and their families to determine whether our current diagnostic measures are adequately capturing symptom presentation. The use of self-advocates in refining existing measures and creating new measures is critical to accurate diagnosis and subsequent treatment of females with ASD. Based on the extant literature, it is imperative that clinicians not rely solely on standard measures to make a diagnosis in females, but obtain a thorough and nuanced developmental history addressing the development of ASD symptoms across the lifespan, as well as "coping strategies" used by affected individuals.

A further avenue of exploration with regard to sex differences is the incorporation of gender identity into our conceptualization of ASD presentation, which has largely been neglected in the research to date. Gender variance is significantly more common among individuals with ASD relative to the general population (Strang et al., 2014, 2016). These individuals are more likely to identify as transgender, or gender nonbinary, complicating both the process of making psychological diagnoses, as well as the lived experience of being an individual on the autism spectrum. By incorporating this subset of individuals, we can begin to disentangle the contribution of biological and social contributions (e.g., one's sex at birth vs. one's gender identification) to sex differences in ASD presentation.

Biomarkers to Diagnose ASD

Despite considerable advances in the early identification and diagnosis of ASD (Chawarska et al., 2009; Ozonoff et al., 2010), treatment development (e.g., Corbett, Blain, Ioannou, & Balser, 2016; White et al., 2013), and efforts to rigorously measure treatment response (e.g., Lerner et al., 2012; Yoder & Symons, 2010) autism remains a behaviorally based disorder (American Psychiatric Association, 2013; Lord et al., 2012). Currently, there are a plethora of investigations exploring potential biomarkers to aid in diagnosis, treatment, and to serve as targets of engagement. According to the National Institutes of Health Working Group, "a biomarker is objectively measured, and evaluated as an indicator of normal biological processes, pathogenic processes, or pharmacologic responses to a therapeutic intervention" (Biomarker Definitions Working Group, 2001, p. 91). In neurodevelopmental disorders, biomarkers must be reliable across development, must be evident at the individual level, and should be specific to a unit of analysis such as diagnostic status or functional process

(McPartland, 2016). Thus, biomarkers broadly considered may include genes, brain structure and functional activity, metabolites, and discrete behavior. It is clear that the identification and use of biomarkers will play an increasingly pivotal role to include combinations of biomarkers for analyzing the complexity of pharmacologic and behavioral treatment response (Lesko & Atkinson, 2001). To date, studies in ASD have failed to identify consistent biomarkers to aid in the assessment and treatment of this complex, heterogeneous disorder.

Current efforts to assess the physiological and neurological correlates offer the potential to identify biomarkers that might aid in diagnosis and treatment of ASD. Hormones play a vital role in numerous bodily processes, and two key hormones involved in the regulation of social and stress responses—specifically, oxytocin (OT) and cortisol—have been implicated in the neuropathology of autism (e.g., Carter, 2007; Corbett, Mendoza, Abdullah, Wegelin, & Levine, 2006; Corbett, Mendoza, Wegelin, Carmean, & Levine, 2008; Hollander et al., 2003; Insel, O'Brien, & Leckman, 1999). Due to the heightened sensitivity to external and internal stimuli, poor response to novelty, and increased prevalence of anxiety in individuals with ASD, an active and growing area of interest has been the examination of cortisol, a primary stress hormone of the limbic–hypothalamic–pituitary–adrenal (LHPA) axis (Taylor & Corbett, 2014). Current and ongoing research examining the physiological profile of the LHPA axis in children with ASD has revealed a pattern of heightened stress to various benign and novel stimuli (Corbettet al., 2006; Corbett et al., 2008; Richdale & Prior, 1992; Spratt et al., 2012; Tordjman et al., 1997), including natural social conditions (Corbett, Schupp, Simon, Ryan, & Mendoza, 2010; Lopata, Volker, Putnam, Thomeer, & Nida, 2008; Naber et al., 2007). In some studies, elevated cortisol levels in ASD have been associated with self-reported trait anxiety (Bitsika, Sharpley, Sweeney, & McFarlane, 2014; Lopata et al., 2008; Simon & Corbett, 2013). Collectively, research shows that physiological arousal in ASD is on a continuum of responsivity (Taylor & Corbett, 2014) and can affect social interaction patterns (Corbett et al., 2010; Corbett, Schupp, & Lanni, 2012; Schupp, Simon, & Corbett, 2013). In recent years, cortisol measurement has been considered for preventative approaches or interventions, such as depression (Adam, Sutton, Doane, & Mineka, 2008). In regard to ASD treatment, cortisol levels have been associated with changes in clinical features, including social communication (Corbett et al., 2011; Corbett, Swain, Newsom, et al., 2014; Viau et al., 2010) and anxiety (Corbett, Blain, et al., 2016). However, variability of this index suggests that it may assist in identifying subgroups or individual differences (Corbett et al., 2008; Schupp et al., 2013), but may be limited in serving as a consistent biomarker for etiology or as a treatment target.

OT, a hypothalamic peptide, plays a critical role in mediating complex social behavior in nonhuman animals (e.g., Bales & Carter, 2003; Bales, Kim, Lewis-Reese, & Sue Carter, 2004; Carter, 1998; Carter, Grippo, Pournajafi-Nazarloo, Ruscio, & Porges, 2008; Insel et al., 1999; Winslow, Shapiro, Carter, & Insel, 1993; Young, Wang, & Insel, 1998) and humans (Kirsch et al., 2005; Kosfeld, Heinrichs, Zak, Fischbacher, & Fehr, 2005; Teng et al., 2013). Thus, it is not surprising that OT has been associated with the neurobiology of autism (Carter, 2007; Insel, 1997; Insel et al., 1999; Jacob et al., 2007; Miller et al., 2013; Skuse & Gallagher, 2009; Welch & Ruggiero, 2005; Young, Pitkow, & Ferguson, 2002). Individuals with autism reportedly have impaired OT processing, resulting in higher levels of plasma OT-X, a precursor to the normal adult form of OT, and lower levels of OT (Feldman, Golan, Hirschler-Guttenberg, Ostfeld-Etzion, & Zagoory-Sharon, 2014; Green et al., 2001; Modahl et al., 1998; Taurines et al., 2014). Additionally, research has shown genetic associations between the oxytocin receptor gene (*OXTR*) and autism (Ebstein, Knafo, Mankuta, Chew, & Lai, 2012; Egawa et al., 2013; Gregory et al., 2009; Jacob et al., 2007; Lerer et al., 2008; Wermter et al., 2009; Wu et al., 2005; Yrigollen et al., 2008). Emerging findings suggest that OT may be a novel therapeutic target for treating social impairments of autism (Aoki et al., 2015; Bartz & Hollander, 2008; Gordon et al., 2013; Heinrichs & Domes, 2008; Neumann, 2008; Posey, Erickson, & McDougle, 2008) by increasing the salience of social and emotional information (e.g., Anagnostou et al., 2012; Hollander et al., 2007; Aoki et al., 2014; Domes et al., 2010; Marsh, Yu, Pine, & Blair, 2010). Although OT may be a potential pharmaceutical treatment, it may not be a sensitive surrogate biomarker of change for behaviorally based treatment (Corbett et al., 2011), and thus more research is needed.

Advances in neuroimaging have elucidated underlying neuropathological brain processes implicated in ASD, and the hope has been that brain-based data may serve as useful and objective markers (e.g., Dawson et al., 2012). The value of imaging data for neurodevelopmental disorders, such as autism, will ultimately depend on factors such as cost, sensitivity, and the extent to which they are available for wide use (McPartland, 2016). In particular, event-related potential (ERP) methods are objective and permit the measurement of brain activity associated with the processing of relevant information without the requirement of overt behavioral, cognitive, or motivational involvement. ERP studies have the ability to examine individual differences in core features of ASD, such as the extent of processing social versus nonsocial information, and which can be measured across developmental and diagnostic profiles not limited by age or cognitive status (Key & Corbett, 2014). ERPs have been identified as a promising neurophysiological marker for detecting treatment effects (Javitt, Spencer,

Thaker, Winterer, & Hajos, 2008). For example, recent findings from a randomized control trial showed between-treatment group effects on memory for faces, which was measured and corroborated by both neuropsychological and ERP measures (Corbett, Key, et al., 2016). While encouraging, additional research is needed to determine whether ERPs are sensitive or specific enough to serve as reliable indices of disease or treatment status.

The use of respiratory sinus arrhythmia (RSA), an index of the parasympathetic nervous system, has potential as a biomarker of physiological arousal in ASD. While baseline RSA is less stable in very young children (Patriquin, Lorenzi, Scarpa, & Bell, 2014), it stabilizes around age 5 and remains stable throughout childhood and adolescence (El-Sheikh, Arsiwalla, Hinnant, & Erath, 2011). Longitudinal studies show that slight variations in both baseline and RSA reactivity should be accounted for as children still show relatively unstable heart period and vagal tone in response to a task (Bornstein & Suess, 2000). As a marker of diagnostic or functional status, early research supports the use of RSA. For example, RSA has been linked to social–cognitive function in ASD, such that higher baseline RSA has been associated with better social behavior (Patriquin, Scarpa, Friedman, & Porges, 2013). Furthermore, given the close associations between the autonomic nervous system (ANS) and behavior (Benevides & Lane, 2013), assessment of arousal in relation to several ASD behaviors such as anxiety, attention, response inhibition, and social cognition is warranted (Kushki, Brian, Dupuis, & Anagnostou, 2014). Changes in heart rate have been associated with anxiety in ASD (Kushki et al., 2013), and atypical RSA reactivity to social tasks is also observed (Edmiston, Jones, & Corbett, 2016; Kushki et al., 2014). RSA may be useful in directly assessing anxiety in children with ASD, though it may be useful only in a subgroup of those who display significant increases in heart rate following an anxiogenic task (Chiu, Anagnostou, Brian, Chau, & Kushki, 2016). One caveat with RSA could be the significant variability between individuals—thus, change in RSA relative to baseline measurements may be a better marker than individual RSA values (Berntson et al., 1997). The promising, though limited results regarding RSA as a marker of functional status lends support to further research aimed at exploring it as a diagnostic, stratification, or treatment target (McPartland, 2016) biomarker in ASD. Due to the relative ease with which heart rate data can be collected, future research into cardiac ANS regulation and arousal as a marker of ASD should be of great benefit.

Taken together, considerable research is needed in the pursuit to identify physiological and neurological correlates of ASD. The heterogeneity of the disorder, diversity of symptom presentation, and variability in response to treatment admittedly challenges the pursuit to identify objective, consistent, sensitive, and cost-effective markers.

FACTORS AFFECTING DIAGNOSIS, TREATMENT, AND OUTCOME

Functional Assessment of Outcome

Although the previous 20 years have seen substantial advances in sensitive and clinically useful diagnostic tools allowing for earlier and more accurate diagnostic decision making, we lack measures that capture ASD symptoms and their impact multidimensionally (Brugha, Doos, Tempier, Einfeld, & Howlin, 2015). While advances in diagnostic measures allow for improved categorical distinctions of ASD versus non-ASD, parallel advances have not been made to allow for improved assessment of functional outcome. Many measures used in outcome studies that assess for core symptoms of ASD do not capture those outcome variables that might have a more meaningful impact on the lives of individuals with ASD—that is, in determining the long-term outcome or success of an individual with ASD, severity of core symptoms or knowledge of social skills may be less relevant than a more ecologically valid consideration of an individual's functioning. For example, an adult with ASD and high levels of social impairment might have an intense restricted interest, but its nature may be relevant to his or her career field and thus adaptive in terms of financial security and personal fulfillment. Such an individual would appear to have achieved a poor outcome from the perspective of traditional symptom severity measures, but have a relatively higher degree of functional independence and quality of life. Assessment of an individual's achievement in a number of different areas—postsecondary education, employment, adaptive behavior, independent living, engagement in daily activities, peer or romantic relationships, and quality of life—should therefore be used to supplement traditional and well-established outcome measures to provide a complete picture of the functioning of an individual with ASD. Some of these more ecologically valid measures of outcome are briefly explored below.

Educational attainment is a critical factor in that it is related to socioeconomic status and plays a role in eventual positive outcomes and functional independence. However, education remains a primary barrier to competitive employment and functional independence for adults with ASD. Rates of individuals with ASD enrolled in 2-year, 4-year, or trade or vocational secondary education programs are lower than those of typically developing college-age samples and those with specific learning impairments (Shattuck et al., 2012). Emerging adults with ASD, even when cognitively able, do not pursue postsecondary education at rates comparable to peers without ASD, potentially due to interference from deficits in other areas, including time management, executive functioning, and poor adaptive living skills (e.g., White et al., 2016). For those individuals with ASD who do pursue postsecondary education, academic and social difficulties are common, and as a result rates of degree completion have been established to be quite low in comparison to other disabilities and typically developing samples (Taylor, Henninger, & Mailick, 2015). Additionally, the difficulties that these individuals encounter in college settings may persist as they attempt to join the workforce. Individuals with ASD who have degrees are frequently unemployed or underemployed, working in jobs that do not require a college degree (Taylor & Seltzer, 2012).

Compared with individuals with other disabilities, including specific learning impairment, learning disability, or ID, individuals with ASD also demonstrate lower levels of employment (Shattuck et al., 2012). The majority of adults with ASD who are employed work in sheltered settings or community centers where they receive accommodations (Taylor & Seltzer, 2012). Individuals with ASD and without ID were three times more likely to have no daytime activities compared with adults with ASD and ID (Taylor & Seltzer, 2012). In a study of 68 individuals with ASD first evaluated at a mean age of 7 who participated in a follow-up study at a mean age of 29 (Howlin, Goode, Hutton, & Rutter, 2004), less than a third of adults with ASD were competitively employed, and many who were did not earn a living wage. A comparable rate of employment was found in an earlier study conducted in the United States with 103 participants (Ballaban-Gil, Rapin, Tuchman, & Shinnar, 1996). This literature indicates that in addition to low levels of any employment, adults with ASD frequently work in positions that are below their qualifications or which they are ill-suited for, which, along with difficulties in completing a postsecondary degree (e.g., White et al., 2016), may help explain why adults with ASD demonstrate a decreased ability to cultivate a career in their chosen field as well as increased rates of switching between jobs (Baldwin, Costley, & Warren, 2014). Such limitations may contribute to overall poorer functional outcomes.

In addition to taking into account educational attainment and employment outcomes, the Howlin et al. (2004) study described above sought to characterize individuals according to their living situation and social relationships, ultimately creating a composite outcome variable in which each participant was categorized as having achieved a very good, good, fair, poor, or very poor outcome according to their achievement across all domains (Howlin et al., 2004). Such an assessment might be considered a more valid indicator of the success of an individual with ASD than those unidimensional assessments of core symptoms typically used in treatment or outcome studies. Global assessments of functioning determining overall level of interference, such as the Children's Global Assessment Scale, might provide a more complete picture of the extent to which symptoms of ASD are preventing a given individual from achieving functional independence (Shaffer et al., 1983).

Apart from composite measures of outcome that take into consideration education, employment, and peer relationships, an individual's subjective rating of quality of life may provide a valid indicator of outcome. Barneveld, Swaab, Fagel, Van Engeland, and De Sonneville (2014) examined quality of life of adults with ASD compared with age-matched samples with ADHD, disruptive behavior disorders, or affective disorders. Adults with ASD rated their satisfaction with employment, education, and relationships significantly lower than comparison groups. Another study conducted with a smaller sample of males with ASD produced similar results, though in comparison to typically developing individuals as opposed to a group with other disorders (Jennes-Coussens, Magill-Evans, & Koning, 2006). In contrast, a long-term prospective follow-up study of a large sample of adults with ASD demonstrated relatively high ratings of quality of life given low levels of independence (Billstedt, Gillberg, & Gillberg, 2011). While rates of ID were relatively higher among this sample, these results articulate an important point regarding quality of life and outcome more broadly. Quality of life, when conceptualized as a subjective rating of one's satisfaction with his or her circumstances, may not be tied directly to functional outcome. An individual might remain highly dependent on family or institutionalized care, but remain satisfied so long as his or her needs are provided. Such an individual would continue to incur public health costs for continued care that have been determined to be substantial (Barrett et al., 2015; Ganz, 2007). Future attempts to improve outcome should therefore focus on efforts to increase education attainment, competitive employment, meaningful peer relationships, and financial independence. Achievement of these outcomes would likely also facilitate improved quality of life for adults with ASD.

Mechanisms of Change in Intervention

An increasing amount of research has focused on evaluating the efficacy of psychosocial interventions for individuals with ASD. Although publication of these studies has resulted in increased awareness of which interventions offer the most empirical support, the field at large has neglected questions of *how* such interventions achieve their effects. As such, examination of the mechanisms of change in current evidence-based interventions for ASD merits further exploration. Advances in understanding of the mediators of effective treatment would allow for more individualized treatment, whether by targeting the processes that are most likely to result in generalizable change (e.g., improving emotion regulation ability) or identifying likely treatment responders (e.g., those with moderate social motivation) to tailor intervention planning. Lerner et al. (2012) explored a number of potential mechanisms underlying effective treatment, including executive functioning (EF), therapeutic relationship, and social motivation.

The construct of EF—which encompasses a number of cognitive abilities including planning and organization, set shifting, impulse control, response inhibition, and verbal working memory—has been studied extensively as it pertains to treatment of ADHD, a prevalent neurodevelopmental disorder. Indeed, deficits in EF have been hypothesized to be the central feature in ADHD (Barkley, 1997; Willcutt, Doyle, Nigg, Faraone, & Pennington, 2005). The potential role EF plays in treatment for ADHD has been explored, with results suggesting that changes in EF are associated with improvements in ADHD symptoms (Holmes, Gathercole, & Dunning, 2009). Deficits in EF abilities found in individuals with ADHD parallel those found in individuals with ASD (Corbett, Constantine, Hendren, Rocke, & Ozonoff, 2009; Geurts, Verté, Oosterlan, Roeyers, & Sergeant, 2005). EF has been strongly implicated as a core process involved in several areas of deficiency characteristic of ASD, such as adaptive functioning and theory of mind (Pugliese, Anthony, et al., 2015, 2016). Notably, a recently developed intervention targeting EF abilities was demonstrated to improve problem-solving, flexibility, and planning/organizing abilities of a sample of children with ASD significantly more than a comparison group receiving social skills training (Kenworthy et al., 2014). This result provides preliminary evidence that EF may be an effective target for intervention in children with ASD and extend to real-world outcomes such as rule following and transitions in classroom settings.

EF is currently measured in ADHD and ASD literature primarily through the use of behavioral tasks and parent-report measures. Tasks such as the Conners' Continuous Performance Test (CPT-II; Conners, 2000) are frequently used to evaluate response inhibition by requiring individuals to react to some stimuli but not others, and measuring frequency of errors and reaction time. Despite its frequent use in assessing for EF deficits in ADHD, the construct validity of the CPT has been questioned (Edwards et al., 2007; Epstein et al., 2003). Another continuous performance task, the Integrated Visual and Auditory (IVA) CPT, integrates data from multiple sensory modalities and has been shown to detect attention deficits in ASD samples that are comparable to ADHD (Corbett & Constantine, 2006). The Wisconsin Card Sorting Task (WCST) continues to be a widely used assessment for the set-shifting component of EF, and has been used extensively with ASD samples (Westwood, Stahl, Mandy, & Tchanturia, 2016). Response inhibition has also been frequently examined in ASD using color–word interference (i.e., Stroop) tasks, such as the Color–Word Interference Test from the Delis–Kaplan Executive Function System (Adams & Jarrold, 2009; Delis, Kaplan, & Kramer, 2001). Finally, these tests address many of the most salient components of EF, and results from studies using these and other measures suggest that individuals with ASD demonstrate a generalized impairment in EF (Corbett et al., 2009).

In summary, researchers and clinicians have options in selecting valid and reliable behavioral tasks to evaluate EF deficits in individuals with ASD. Despite strong psychometric properties, the majority of available assessment tools for EF are limited in their lack of ecological validity (Kenworthy, Yerys, Anthony, & Wallace, 2008). Computer-based tasks, color–word interference, WCST, trail-making tasks, and other traditional measures of EF consistently demonstrate differences between ASD and typically developing groups, but do not necessarily provide insight into the ways in which these deficits might manifest in an individual's functioning in the real world (Chaytor, Schmitter-Edgecombe, & Burr, 2006). Questionnaire-based assessments of EF, such as the Behavior Rating Inventory of Executive Function (BRIEF; Gioia, Isquith, Guy, & Kenworthy, 2000; Gioia & Isquith, 2004) and its second edition (BRIEF-2; Gioia, Isquith, Guy, & Kenworthy, 2015), were developed in part to address the disconnect between the laboratory- or clinic-based assessment of EF and the ways in which EF is used on a day-to-day basis. Another questionnaire, the Comprehensive Executive Function Inventory (CEFI; Naglieri & Goldstein, 2013) assesses nine subscales of EF, has strong psychometric properties, and has demonstrated significant differences in EF abilities between ASD and non-ASD samples. Newer techniques, including a virtual reality task, have been proposed as tools to assess EF in a more applicable manner than either standard tasks or questionnaires (Renison, Ponsford, Testa, Richardson, & Brownfield, 2012). Other proposed options with greater relevance to daily tasks include classroom observation or a recently developed "Executive Function Challenge Task," a 30-minute, semistructured interview consisting of five activities designed to evaluate a child's flexibility and planning skills within the context of a social interaction (Kenworthy et al., 2014). Future research and clinical work should emphasize the use of EF assessments that are increasingly ecologically valid and therefore more representative of the ways in which EF deficits might manifest in the day-to-day lives of individuals with ASD.

Therapeutic relationship is another potential contributor to treatment effectiveness that has been largely neglected by intervention research in ASD. As such, it is not possible to draw conclusions about the role of the relationship between clinician and client, though studies in related domains of child and adolescent psychopathology may provide some insight. In the broader field of developmental psychopathology intervention research, alliance has been established as an important but historically neglected factor in treatment studies (DiGiuseppe, Linscott, & Jilton, 1996; Green, 2006). Evidence from studies of alliance in cognitive-behavioral therapy (CBT) for child anxiety has suggested that improvement in child–therapist alliance throughout the course of treatment was associated with improved outcomes following treatment completion (Chiu, McLeod, Har, & Wood,

2009). In contrast, other studies have found that neither therapeutic alliance nor treatment adherence predict child outcomes in CBT for anxiety (Liber et al., 2010). While some preliminary work has begun to explore the importance of therapeutic relationship in psychotherapy for ASD (Ramsay et al., 2005), others have suggested that therapeutic relationship should not be emphasized in working with individuals with ASD given characteristic deficits in reciprocal social interaction and communication of emotional content (Anderson & Morris, 2006). Future work in identifying mechanisms of effective treatment in ASD should further examine the potential role of therapeutic relationship.

The social motivation theory of ASD posits that individuals who go on to develop ASD demonstrate diminished motivation to attend to social stimuli early in development, reducing the salience of social stimuli and the extent to which brain networks specialize for processing of social stimuli (Dawson, Webb, & McPartland, 2005). Thus, lack of social motivation may be considered a critically important element of treatment. For example, an individual with low social motivation may also demonstrate low interest and investment in interventions addressing social deficits, ultimately limiting the results of such treatments. Despite its potentially critical role in treatment, we know little about the best ways to assess social motivation. Few studies have addressed the role of social motivation in treatment directly, in part due to want of a reliable and valid means of assessing this construct. From a theoretical perspective, social motivation may moderate treatment effectiveness (e.g., interventions are more effective for individuals who are highly socially motivated), but might also serve as a mediator, in that increasing social motivation is the means by which improvement in core social deficits occurs.

While appreciating the role of social motivation in ASD interventions is a priority, developing a quality measure to assess it constitutes a necessary first step. The Social Responsiveness Scale, Second Edition (SRS-2; Constantino & Gruber, 2012) includes a Social Motivation subscale, but does not comprehensively assess the construct. One ecologically valid approach to examining social motivation from a behavioral perspective is by measuring the extent to which children engage in reciprocal social interaction with peers on a playground (Corbett et al., 2014). Although the cognitive construct of social motivation does not map perfectly onto a behavioral assessment (i.e., a child with ASD may have a cognitive desire to engage and not demonstrate the corresponding behavior), this system constitutes an important attempt to increase ecological validity. The use of implicit association tasks (IATs), long used for assessment of implicit biases in race and gender, may also be useful in identifying the extent to which individuals have implicit negative biases associated with social interaction (Clerkin & Teachman, 2010). Preliminary work has explored the extent to which biomarkers, including salivary cortisol and ERPs, might be used to assess social motivation (Corbett et al., 2014; Key & Corbett, 2014). While these novel means of assessing social motivation—via behavioral observation, assessment of implicit biases, and objective biological measures—are still in the early stages, their use complements existing parent-report measures (e.g., SRS-2) to offer the potential for truly multimodal assessment of the construct. Such comprehensive assessment is rarely utilized in ASD research, and social motivation might therefore offer a model to be replicated in other areas.

Although the development and evaluation of novel and existing interventions to address symptoms of ASD is laudable, the majority of these studies have not attempted to answer the "how" and "for whom" questions that are critical in determining future directions in treatment research. Most ASD intervention research has focused on developing new treatments, replicating existing studies, or adapting existing treatments initially developed for different populations (e.g., upward or downward extensions by age, psychiatric comorbidity). Such pursuits are necessary in order to completely delineate which treatments are most effective and should continue to be studied, elucidating the most effective components of each intervention. Also, the means by which a given intervention is effective will allow for selection of the most effective intervention based on presentation of the individual and development of new treatments that are likely to be productive.

Sensitive Measures of Change in Target Outcomes

In addition to complicating identification of viable biomarkers, the heterogeneity of ASD has proven a challenge to the development of sensitive measures of change with intervention. For instance, a self-report measure of anxiety or depression may be desirable for a verbal and cognitively able child, but impractical for a patient with ID or someone who is minimally verbal. Even with relatively higher-functioning patients, concerns about insight and emotion processing have been levied with the use of self-report measures, a standby in the assessment of internalizing problems in non-ASD populations (e.g., Cook, Brewer, Shah, & Bird, 2013; Mazefsky, Kao, & Oswald, 2011). Similar concerns exist with parent-report measures, which have arguably been most heavily relied upon in the ASD treatment literature. Parents often must make assumptions about the child's motivators (thoughts, feelings) for observable behavior, and it cannot be assumed that such parental interpretation is consistently accurate. For example, heightened repetitive behaviors may be interpreted to reflect anxiety, but the same behavior may also reflect a response to anticipated change that is not anxiety driven or a way to avoid social interaction. Although these concerns apply to diagnosis and case conceptualization, they are critical to address in the context of treatment evaluation—as even our best treatments will not be effective if applied inappropriately or to the wrong target.

Concerns with lack of attention to the measurement of outcomes in the context of intervention are not new to this field (e.g., Matson, 2007). In a recent review, it was found that in 195 prospective clinical trials, no single measure was used in more than 7% of the studies and, on average, intervention studies employed 11 different measures to track treatment response (Bolte & Diehl, 2013). These results underscore lack of consensus regarding outcome evaluation and the need for evidence-based guidelines. The importance of having clinically valid measures of treatment impact must be stressed as the very bedrock of treatment research. We have seen recent advancements in the establishment of such guidelines, including attempts to evaluate the degree to which measurement approach affects observed impact. For example, given the pervasiveness and breadth of social communication impairments, the hallmark of ASD, Yoder, Bottema-Beutel, Woynaroski, Chandrasekhar, and Sandback (2013) suggested that how "proximal" or "distal" the dependent variable is to the intervention target, and the degree to which the outcomes are "bounded" to the intervention parameters, are key variables to consider, in evaluation of outcome variables and measures. The Brief Observation of Social Communication Change (BOSCC; Grzadzinski et al., 2016) is an example of a tool developed as a global assessment of change in the core Social Communication domain—not tied to a particular intervention. The BOSCC originated with the Autism Diagnostic Observation Schedule, Second Edition (ADOS-2; Lord et al., 2012) and is similar in structure; the affected child interacted with an adult using a predefined set of toys, and this interaction is video recorded for later scoring. Consistent with the synthesis of Yoder et al. (2013), a recent study found that while intervention effects were observed with a specific measure of joint attention, such effects were not seen with the more global BOSCC (Nordahl-Hansen, Fletcher-Watson, McConachie, & Kaale, 2016).

Given these concerns, we suggest an increased focus on the development of tools that integrate multiple data sources (e.g., behavioral observation and parent report) to gauge severity of both core and associated symptoms. Although most treatment research has arguably relied on parent-report questionnaires to gauge change (Bolte & Diehl, 2013), one modality that has seen recent advancement is the use of direct observational tools in outcome evaluation (e.g., Handen et al., 2013). Tools such as the Contextual Assessment of Social Skills (CASS; Ratto, Turner-Brown, Rupp, Mesibov, & Penn, 2011), a laboratory-based observational measure of social functioning, are growing in popularity, and emerging research suggests the CASS is sensitive to change and viable to administer in terms of time and cost demands (e.g., White, Scarpa, Conner, Maddox, & Bonete, 2015). Use of observational tools in classroom settings has also been used recently as an ecologically valid means of assessing behavior change as a result of intervention (Kenworthy et al., 2014). In ASD, perhaps more so than any other disorder, the multimodal validation of assessment tools is critical. To expand on the example given above, if a clinician treating anxiety in a youth with ASD incorrectly interprets the observed exacerbation of repetitive behaviors as a manifestation of clinical anxiety, rather than a core ASD symptom (related to attempt to avoid social interaction), one might erroneously infer treatment failure or nonresponse. As such, validation of outcome measures is a necessity for the advancement of treatments in our field. In addition to measure validation, it is critical that clinical scientists understand that how the outcome is measured (e.g., whether tightly bound to the intervention itself, or more general) will impact the strength of any observed treatment effects (e.g., Yoder et al., 2013).

CONCLUSION

The explosion in research surrounding assessment and treatment of ASD in the past few decades has led to a far more comprehensive understanding of the etiology, phenomenology, diagnosis, and treatment of ASD in a variety of settings. Current diagnostic instruments allow for valid and reliable diagnosis before the second year of life. The proliferation of evidence-based treatments for ASD has resulted in many new options for services for families of children with ASD. These improvements in diagnosis and treatment form the foundation for improved long-term outcomes, which unfortunately generally remain poor.

Moving forward, there are several pressing needs for future research in assessment of ASD. The relatively newly defined SCD diagnosis will require clarification, particularly in the ways it can be differentiated from ASD. Examinations of its utility as a construct distinct from ASD, further development of valid and reliable assessment of pragmatic language, and treatment studies directly targeting populations of individuals diagnosed with SCD will be critical in determining whether this new diagnosis remains in subsequent editions of DSM.

Phenomenology of ASD in females represents another substantial gap in the current literature. While substantial numbers of studies have examined differences in core features of ASD, adolescent and adult females with average intellectual ability remain understudied. Within this area, self-report measures should complement parent and clinician ratings of ASD symptoms. In addition, further work is needed to determine the extent to which a female-specific ASD phenotype (i.e., with potentially lower levels of restricted and repetitive behaviors and fewer social communication deficits) might result in underdiagnosis of ASD among females. Differences in the use of diagnostic instruments (e.g., ADOS-2) must be examined to determine whether female-specific norms or reduced cutoffs for females are also warranted. Finally, the use of biomarkers such as cortisol, OT, RSA, and ERP to aid in diagnosis, as well as intervention evaluation, present a promising frontier for future research.

Beyond assessment and diagnosis, the evaluation of new treatments, especially the means by which they effect change, and the real-world impact of ASD throughout the lifespan merit further study. There exists an emerging recognition that unidimensional assessment of core ASD symptoms offers only a limited understanding of what constitutes a successful adult outcome for individuals with ASD. In addition to symptom severity, future research should involve such constructs as adaptive functioning, peer and romantic relationships, educational attainment, employment, and financial independence. Assessment of all these domains might offer a more comprehensive picture of an individual's functioning and the extent to which he or she contributes to society. In terms of treatment evaluation, next steps include continued evaluation of proposed mechanisms of effective interventions. Specifically, EF, social motivation, and therapeutic alliance provide potential avenues for future studies of treatment mediators. Direct assessment of treatment effectiveness must also focus on reducing the number of different measures used to evaluate outcomes across studies as well as ensuring that assessment is multidimensional in nature to provide a comprehensive view of changes resulting from treatment.

An increased emphasis in future research on these as-yet understudied areas could lead to identification of sensitive objective biological measures, an increased understanding of what makes interventions effective, and more ecologically valid means of assessing the ways in which individuals with ASD function throughout adolescence and adulthood. In turn, these advances may increase the frequency with which individuals with ASD achieve optimal long-term outcomes.

REFERENCES

Adam, E. K., Sutton, J. M., Doane, L. D., & Mineka, S. (2008). Incorporating hypothalamic–pituitary–adrenal axis measures into preventive interventions for adolescent depression: Are we there yet? *Developmental Psychopathology, 20*(3), 975–1001.

Adams, N. C., & Jarrold, C. (2009). Inhibition and the validity of the Stroop task for children with autism. *Journal of Autism and Developmental Disorders, 39*(8), 1112–1121.

American Psychiatric Association. (2013). *Diagnostic and statistical manual of mental disorders* (5th ed.). Arlington, VA: Author.

Anagnostou, E., Soorya, L., Chaplin, W., Bartz, J., Halpern, D., Wasserman, S., et al. (2012). Intranasal oxytocin versus placebo in the treatment of adults with autism spectrum disorders: A randomized controlled trial. *Molecular Autism, 3*(1), 16.

Anderson, S., & Morris, J. (2006). Cognitive behaviour therapy for people with Asperger syndrome. *Behavioural and Cognitive Psychotherapy, 34*(3), 293–303.

Aoki, Y., Watanabe, T., Abe, O., Kuwabara, H., Yahata, N., Takano, Y., et al. (2015). Oxytocin's neurochemical effects in the medial prefrontal cortex underlie recovery of task-specific brain activity in autism: A randomized controlled trial. *Molecular Psychiatry, 20*(4), 447–453.

Aoki, Y., Yahata, N., Watanbe, T., Takano, Y., Yuki, K., Kuwabara, H., et al. (2014). Oxytocin improves behavioral and neural deficits in inferring others' social emotions in autism. *Brain, 137,* 3073–3086.

Baird, G., Simonoff, E., Pickles, A., Chandler, S., Loucas, T., Meldrum, D., et al. (2006). Prevalence of disorders of the autism spectrum in a population cohort of children in South Thames: The Special Needs and Autism Project (SNAP). *Lancet, 368*(9531), 210–215.

Baldwin, S., Costley, D., & Warren, A. (2014). Employment activities and experiences of adults with high-functioning autism and Asperger's disorder. *Journal of Autism and Developmental Disorders, 44,* 2440–2449.

Bales, K. L., & Carter, C. S. (2003). Developmental exposure to oxytocin facilitates partner preferences in male prairie voles (*Microtus ochrogaster*). *Behavioral Neuroscience, 117*(4), 854–859. Available from *www.ncbi.nlm.nih.gov/entrez/query.fcgi?cmd=Retrieve&db=PubMed&dopt=Citation&list_uids=12931969.*

Bales, K. L., Kim, A. J., Lewis-Reese, A. D., & Sue Carter, C. (2004). Both oxytocin and vasopressin may influence alloparental behavior in male prairie voles. *Hormones and Behavior, 45*(5), 354–361. Available from *www.ncbi.nlm.nih.gov/entrez/query.fcgi?cmd=Retrieve&db=PubMed&dopt=Citation&list_uids=15109910.*

Ballaban-Gil, K., Rapin, I., Tuchman, R., & Shinnar, S. (1996). Longitudinal examination of the behavioral, language, and social changes in a population of adolescents and young adults with autistic disorder. *Pediatric Neurology, 15*(3), 217–223.

Barkley, R. (1997). Behavioral inhibition, sustained attention, and executive functions: Constructing a unifying theory of ADHD. *Psychological Bulletin, 121*(1), 65–94.

Barneveld, P. S., Swaab, H., Fagel, S., Van Engeland, H., & De Sonneville, L. M. J. (2014). Quality of life: A case-controlled long-term follow-up study, comparing young high-functioning adults with autism spectrum disorders with adults with other psychiatric disorders diagnosed in childhood. *Comprehensive Psychiatry, 55*(2), 302–310.

Barrett, B., Mosweu, I., Jones, C. R., Charman, T., Baird, G., Simonoff, E., et al. (2015). Comparing service use and costs among adolescents with autism spectrum disorders, special needs and typical development. *Autism, 19*(5), 562–569.

Bartz, J. A., & Hollander, E. (2008). Oxytocin and experimental therapeutics in autism spectrum disorders. *Progress in Brain Research, 170,* 451–462. Available from *www.ncbi.nlm.nih.gov/entrez/query.fcgi?cmd=Retrieve&db=PubMed&dopt=Citation&list_uids=18655901.*

Benevides, T. W., & Lane, S. J. (2013). A review of cardiac autonomic measures: Considerations for examination of physiological response in children with autism spectrum disorder. *Journal of Autism and Developmental Disorders, 45*(2), 560–575.

Berntson, G. G., Bigger, J. T., Eckberg, D. L., Grossman, P., Kaufmann, P. G., & Malik, M. (1997). Committee report on heart rate variability: Origins, methods and interpretive caveats. *Psychophysiology, 34,* 623–648.

Billstedt, E., Gillberg, I. C., & Gillberg, C. (2011). Aspects of quality of life in adults diagnosed with autism in childhood: A population-based study. *Autism, 15*(1), 7–20.

Biomarkers Definitions Working Group. (2001). Biomarkers and surrogate endpoints: Preferred definitions and conceptual framework. *Clinical Pharmacology and Therapeutics, 69*(3), 89–95.

Bitsika, V., Sharpley, C. F., Sweeney, J. A., & McFarlane, J. R. (2014). HPA and SAM axis responses as correlates of self- vs parental ratings of anxiety in boys with an autistic disorder. *Physiology and Behavior, 127,* 1–7.

Bolte, E. E., & Diehl, J. J. (2013). Measurement tools and target symptoms/skills used to assess treatment response for individuals with autism spectrum disorder. *Journal of Autism and Developmental Disorders, 43*(11), 2491–2501.

Bölte, S., Duketis, E., Poustka, F., & Holtmann, M. (2011). Sex differences in cognitive domains and their clinical correlates in higher-functioning autism spectrum disorders. *Autism, 15*(4), 497–511.

Bornstein, M. H., & Suess, P. E. (2000). Child and mother cardiac vagal tone: Continuity, stability, and concordance across the first 5 years. *Developmental Psychology, 36*(1), 54–65. Available from *www.ncbi.nlm.nih.gov/pubmed/10645744.*

Brugha, T., Doos, L., Tempier, A., Einfeld, S., & Howlin, P. (2015). Outcome measures in intervention trials for adults with autism spectrum disorders: A systematic review of assessments of core autism features and associated emotional and behavioural problems. *International Journal of Methods in Psychiatric Research, 18*(2), 69–83.

Bussey, K., & Bandura, A. (1999). Social cognitive theory of gender development and differentiation. *Psychological Review, 106*(4), 676–713.

Carter, A. S., Black, D. O., Tewani, S., Connolly, C. E., Kadlec, M. B., & Tager-Flusberg, H. (2007). Sex differences in toddlers with autism spectrum disorders. *Journal of Autism and Developmental Disorders, 37*(1), 86–97.

Carter, C. S. (1998). Neuroendocrine perspectives on social attachment and love. *Psychoneuroendocrinology, 23*(8), 779–818. Available from *www.ncbi.nlm.nih.gov/entrez/query.fcgi?cmd=Retrieve&db=PubMed&dopt=Citation&list_uids=9924738.*

Carter, C. S. (2007). Sex differences in oxytocin and vasopressin: Implications for autism spectrum disorders? *Behavioral Brain Research, 176*(1), 170–186. Available from *www.ncbi.nlm.nih.gov/entrez/query.fcgi?cmd=Retrieve&db=PubMed&dopt=Citation&list_uids=17000015.*

Carter, C. S., Grippo, A. J., Pournajafi-Nazarloo, H., Ruscio, M. G., & Porges, S. W. (2008). Oxytocin, vasopressin and sociality. *Progress in Brain Research, 170,* 331–336.

Chawarska, K., Klin, A., Paul, R., Macari, S., & Volkmar, F. (2009). A prospective study of toddlers with ASD: Short-term diagnostic and cognitive outcomes. *Journal of Child Psychology and Psychiatry and Allied Disciplines, 50*(10), 1235–1245.

Chaytor, N., Schmitter-Edgecombe, M., & Burr, R. (2006). Improving the ecological validity of executive functioning assessment. *Archives of Clinical Neuropsychology, 21*(3), 217–227.

Chiu, A. W., McLeod, B. D., Har, K., & Wood, J. J. (2009). Child–therapist alliance and clinical outcomes in cognitive behavioral therapy for child anxiety disorders. *Journal of Child Psychology and Psychiatry and Allied Disciplines, 50*(6), 751–758.

Chiu, T. A., Anagnostou, E., Brian, J., Chau, T., & Kushki, A. (2016). Specificity of autonomic arousal to anxiety in children with autism spectrum disorder. *Autism Research, 9*(4), 491–501.

Christensen, D. L., Baio, J., Braun, K. V., Bilder, D., Charles, J., Constantion, J. N., et al. (2016). Prevalence and characteristics of autism spectrum disorder among children aged 8 years—Autism and developmental disabilities monitoring network, 11 sites, United States, 2012. *Morbidity and Mortality Weekly Report Surveillance Summaries, 65*(No. SS-3), 1–23.

Clerkin, E. M., & Teachman, B. A. (2010). Training implicit social anxiety associations: An experimental intervention. *Journal of Anxiety Disorders, 24*(3), 300–308.

Conners, C. K. (2000). *Conners' CPT II technical guide and software manual.* North Tonawonda, NY: Multi-Health Systems.

Constantino, J. N., & Gruber, C. P. (2012). *Social Responsiveness Scale, Second Edition.* Los Angeles: Western Psychological Services.

Cook, R., Brewer, R., Shah, P., & Bird, G. (2013). Alexithymia, not autism, predicts poor recognition of emotional facial expressions. *Psychological Science, 24*(5), 723–732.

Corbett, B. A., Blain, S. D., Ioannou, S., & Balser, M. (2016). Changes in anxiety following a randomized control trial of a theatre-based intervention for youth with autism spectrum disorder. *Autism 21*(3), 333–343.

Corbett, B. A., & Constantine, L. J. (2006). Autism and attention deficit hyperactivity disorder: Assessing attention and response control with the Integrated Visual and Auditory Continuous Performance Test. *Child Neuropsychology, 12*(4–5), 335–348.

Corbett, B. A., Constantine, L. J., Hendren, R., Rocke, D., & Ozonoff, S. (2009). Examining executive functioning in children with autism spectrum disorder, attention deficit hyperactivity disorder and typical development. *Psychiatry Research, 166*(2–3), 210–222.

Corbett, B. A., Gunther, J. R., Comins, D., Price, J., Ryan, N., Simon, D., et al. (2011). Brief report: Theatre as therapy for children with autism spectrum disorder. *Journal of Autism and Developmental Disorders, 41*(4), 505–511.

Corbett, B. A., Key, A. P., Qualls, L., Fecteau, S., Newsom, C., Coke, C., et al. (2016). Improvement in social competence using a randomized trial of a theatre intervention for children with autism spectrum disorder. *Journal of Autism and Developmental Disorders, 46*(2), 658–672.

Corbett, B. A., Mendoza, S., Abdullah, M., Wegelin, J. A., & Levine, S. (2006). Cortisol circadian rhythms and response to stress in children with autism. *Psychoneuroendocrinology, 31*(1), 59–68. Available from *www.ncbi.nlm.nih.gov/entrez/query.fcgi?cmd=Retrieve&db=PubMed&dopt=Citation&list_uids=16005570.*

Corbett, B. A., Mendoza, S., Wegelin, J. A., Carmean, V., & Levine, S. (2008). Variable cortisol circadian rhythms in children with autism and anticipatory stress. *Journal of Psychiatry and Neuroscience, 33*(3), 227–234.

Corbett, B. A., Schupp, C. W., & Lanni, K. E. (2012). Comparing biobehavioral profiles across two social stress paradigms in children with and without autism spectrum disorders. *Molecular Autism, 3*(1), 13.

Corbett, B. A., Schupp, C. W., Simon, D., Ryan, N., & Mendoza, S. (2010). Elevated cortisol during play is associated with age and social engagement in children with autism. *Molecular Autism, 1*(1), 13.

Corbett, B. A., Swain, D. M., Coke, C., Simon, D., Newsom, C., Houchins-Juarez, N., et al. (2014). Improvement in social deficits in autism spectrum disorders using a theatre-based, peer-mediated intervention. *Autism Research, 7*(1), 4–16.

Corbett, B. A., Swain, D. M., Newsom, C., Wang, L., Song, Y., & Edgerton, D. (2014). Biobehavioral profiles of arousal and social motivation in autism spectrum disorders. *Journal of Child Psychology and Psychiatry, 55*(8), 924–934.

Damiano, C. R., Mazefsky, C. A., White, S. W., & Dichter, G. S. (2014). Future directions for research in autism spectrum disorders. *Journal of Clinical Child and Adolescent Psychology, 43*(5), 828–843.

Dawson, G., Jones, E. J. H., Merkle, K., Venema, K., Lowy, R., Faja, S., et al. (2012). Early behavioral intervention is associated with normalized brain activity in young children with autism. *Journal of the American Academy of Child and Adolescent Psychiatry, 51*(11), 1150–1159.

Dawson, G., Webb, S. J., & McPartland, J. (2005). Understanding the nature of face processing impairment in autism: Insights from behavioral and electrophysiological studies. *Developmental Neuropsychology, 27*(3), 403–424.

Delis, D. C., Kaplan, E., & Kramer, J. H. (2001). *Delis–Kaplan Executive Function System (D-KEFS).* San Antonio, TX: Psychological Corporation.

Des Roches Rosa, S. (2016). How can we all do better by our autistic girls? Available from *www.thinkingautismguide.com/search?q=how+can+we+do+better+by+our+autistic+girls.*

DiGiuseppe, R., Linscott, J., & Jilton, R. (1996). Developing the therapeutic alliance in child–adolescent psychotherapy. *Applied and Preventive Psychology, 5*(2), 85–100.

Domes, G., Lischke, A., Berger, C., Grossmann, A., Hauenstein, K., Heinrichs, M., et al. (2010). Effects of intranasal oxytocin on emotional face processing in women. *Psychoneuroendocrinology, 35*(1), 83–93.

Dworzynski, K., Ronald, A., Bolton, P., & Happé, F. (2012). How different are girls and boys above and below the diagnostic threshold for autism spectrum disorders? *Journal of the American Academy of Child and Adolescent Psychiatry, 51*(8), 788–797.

Ebstein, R. P., Knafo, A., Mankuta, D., Chew, S. H., & Lai, P. S. (2012). The contributions of oxytocin and vasopressin pathway genes to human behavior. *Hormones and Behavior, 61*(3), 359–379.

Edmiston, E. K., Jones, R. M., & Corbett, B. A. (2016). Physiological response to social evaluative threat in adolescents with autism spectrum disorder. *Journal of Autism and Developmental Disorders, 46*(9), 2992–3005.

Edwards, M. C., Gardner, E. S., Chelonis, J. J., Schulz, E. G., Flake, R. A., & Diaz, P. F. (2007). Estimates of the validity and utility of the Conners' Continuous Performance Test in the assessment of inattentive and/or hyperactive-impulsive behaviors in children. *Journal of Abnormal Child Psychology, 35*(3), 393–404.

Egawa, J., Watanabe, Y., Endo, T., Tamura, R., Masuzawa, N., & Someya, T. (2013). Association between *OXTR* and clinical phenotypes of autism spectrum disorders. *Psychiatry Research, 208,* 99–100.

El-Sheikh, M., Arsiwalla, D. D., Benjamin Hinnant, J. B., & Erath, S. A. (2011). Children's internalizing symptoms: The role of interactions between cortisol and respiratory sinus arrhythmia. *Physiology and Behavior, 103*(2), 225–232.

Epstein, J. N., Erkanli, A., Conners, C. K., Klaric, J., Costello, J. E., & Angold, A. (2003). Relations between Continuous Performance Test performance measures and ADHD behaviors. *Journal of Abnormal Child Psychology, 31*(5), 543–554.

Feldman, R., Golan, O., Hirschler-Guttenberg, Y., Ostfeld-Etzion, S., & Zagoory-Sharon, O. (2014). Parent–child interaction and oxytocin production in pre-schoolers with autism spectrum disorder. *British Journal of Psychiatry, 205*(2), 107–112.

Fombonne, E. (1999). The epidemiology of autism: A review. *Psychological Medicine, 29*, 769–786.

Fombonne, E. (2003). Epidemiological surveys of autism and other pervasive developmental disorders: An update. *Journal of Autism and Developmental Disorders, 33*(4), 365–382.

Fombonne, E. (2005). The changing epidemiology of autism. *Journal of Applied Research in Intellectual Disabilities, 18*(4), 281–294.

Frazier, T. W., Georgiades, S., Bishop, S. L., & Hardan, A. Y. (2014). Behavioral and cognitive characteristics of females and males with autism in the Simons Simplex Collection. *Journal of the American Academy of Child and Adolescent Psychiatry, 53*(3), 329–340.e1–3.

Ganz, M. L. (2007). The lifetime distribution of the incremental societal costs of autism. *Archives of Pediatrics and Adolescent Medicine, 161*(4), 343–349.

Geurts, H. M., Verté, S., Oosterlaan, J., Roeyers, H., & Sergeant, J. A. (2005). ADHD subtypes: Do they differ in their executive functioning profile? *Archives of Clinical Neuropsychology, 20*(4), 457–477.

Gioia, G. A., & Isquith, P. K. (2004). Ecological assessment of executive function in traumatic brain injury. *Developmental Neuropsychology, 25*(1–2), 135–158.

Gioia, G. A., Isquith, P. K., Guy, S. C., & Kenworthy, L. (2000). Behavior Rating Inventory of Executive Function—Self-Report version. *Child Neuropsychology, 6*(3), 235–238.

Gioia, G. A., Isquith, P. K., Guy, S. C., & Kenworthy, L. (2015). *Behavior Rating Inventory of Executive Function, Second Edition*. Lutz, FL: Psychological Assessment Resources.

Goldstein, S., & Naglieri, J. A. (2009). *Autism Spectrum Rating Scale*. Toronto, ON, Canada: Multi-Health Systems.

Gordon, I., Vander Wyk, B. C., Bennett, R. H., Cordeaux, C., Lucas, M. V., Eilbott, J. A., et al. (2013). Oxytocin enhances brain function in children with autism. *Proceedings of the National Academy of Sciences of the USA, 110*(52), 20953–20958.

Gould, J., & Ashton-Smith, J. (2011). Missed diagnosis or misdiagnosis?: Girls and women on the autism spectrum. *Good Autism Practice, 12*(1), 34–41.

Green, J. (2006). Annotation: The therapeutic alliance—a significant but neglected variable in child mental health treatment studies. *Journal of Child Psychology and Psychiatry and Allied Disciplines, 47*(5), 425–435.

Green, L., Fein, D., Modahl, C., Feinstein, C., Waterhouse, L., & Morris, M. (2001). Oxytocin and autistic disorder: Alterations in peptide forms. *Biological Psychiatry, 50*(8), 609–613. Available from *www.ncbi.nlm.nih.gov/entrez/query.fcgi?cmd=Retrieve&db=PubMed&dopt=Citation&list_uids=11690596*.

Gregory, S. G., Connelly, J. J., Towers, A. J., Johnson, J., Biscocho, D., Markunas, C. A., et al. (2009). Genomic and epigenetic evidence for oxytocin receptor deficiency in autism. *BMC Medicine, 7*, 62.

Grzadzinski, R., Carr, T., Colombi, C., McGuire, K., Dufek, S., Pickles, A., et al. (2016). Measuring changes in social communication behaviors: Preliminary development of the Brief Observation of Social Communication Change (BOSCC). *Journal of Autism and Developmental Disorders, 46*(7), 1–16.

Halladay, A. K., Bishop, S., Constantino, J. N., Daniels, A. M., Koenig, K., Palmer, K., et al. (2015). Sex and gender differences in autism spectrum disorder: Summarizing evidence gaps and identifying emerging areas of priority. *Molecular Autism, 6*, 36.

Handen, B. L., Johnson, C. R., Butter, E. M., Lecavalier, L., Scahill, L., Aman, M. G., et al. (2013). Use of a direct observational measure in a trial of risperidone and parent training in children with pervasive developmental disorders. *Journal of Developmental and Physical Disabilities, 25*(3), 355–371.

Hartley, S. L., & Sikora, D. M. (2009). Sex differences in autism spectrum disorder: An examination of developmental functioning, autistic symptoms, and coexisting behavior problems in toddlers. *Journal of Autism and Developmental Disorders, 39*(12), 1715–1722.

Heinrichs, M., & Domes, G. (2008). Neuropeptides and social behaviour: Effects of oxytocin and vasopressin in humans. *Progress in Brain Research, 170*, 337–350. Available from *www.ncbi.nlm.nih.gov/entrez/query.fcgi?cmd=Retrieve&db=PubMed&dopt=Citation&list_uids=18655894*.

Hiller, R. M., Young, R. L., & Weber, N. (2016). Sex differences in pre-diagnosis concerns for children later diagnosed with autism spectrum disorder. *Autism, 20*(1), 75–84.

Hollander, E., Bartz, J., Chaplin, W., Phillips, A., Sumner, J., Soorya, L., et al. (2007). Oxytocin increases retention of social cognition in autism. *Biological Psychiatry, 61*(4), 498–503. Available from *www.ncbi.nlm.nih.gov/entrez/query.fcgi?cmd=Retrieve&db=PubMed&dopt=Citation&list_uids=16904652*.

Hollander, E., Novotny, S., Hanratty, M., Yaffe, R., DeCaria, C. M., Aronowitz, B. R., et al. (2003). Oxytocin infusion reduces repetitive behaviors in adults with autistic and Asperger's disorders. *Neuropsychopharmacology, 28*(1), 193–198. Available from *www.ncbi.nlm.nih.gov/entrez/query.fcgi?cmd=Retrieve&db=PubMed&dopt=Citation&list_uids=12496956*.

Holmes, J., Gathercole, S. E., & Dunning, D. L. (2009). Adaptive training leads to sustained enhancement of poor working memory in children. *Developmental Science, 12*(4), F9–F15.

Holtmann, M., Bölte, S., & Poustka, F. (2007). Autism spectrum disorders: Sex differences in autistic behaviour domains and coexisting psychopathology. *Developmental Medicine and Child Neurology, 49*(5), 361–366.

Howlin, P., Goode, S., Hutton, J., & Rutter, M. (2004). Adult outcome for children with autism. *Journal of Child Psychology and Psychiatry and Allied Disciplines, 45*(2), 212–229.

Huerta, M., Bishop, S. L., Duncan, A., Hus, V., & Lord, C. (2012). Application of DSM-5 criteria for autism spectrum disorder to three samples of children with DSM-IV diagnoses of pervasive developmental disorders. *American Journal of Psychiatry, 169*(10), 1056–1064.

Hunsley, J., & Mash, E. J. (2007). Evidence-based assessment. *Annual Review of Clinical Psychology, 3*(1), 29–51.

Insel, T. R. (1997). A neurobiological basis of social attachment. *American Journal of Psychiatry, 154*(6), 726–735. Available from *www.ncbi.nlm.nih.gov/entrez/query.fcgi?cmd=Retrieve&db=PubMed&dopt=Citation&list_uids=9167498*.

Insel, T. R., O'Brien, D. J., & Leckman, J. F. (1999). Oxytocin, vasopressin, and autism: Is there a connection? *Biological Psychiatry, 45*(2), 145–157. Available from *www.ncbi.nlm.nih.gov/entrez/query.fcgi?cmd=Retrieve&db=PubMed&dopt=Citation&list_uids=9951561*.

Jacob, S., Brune, C. W., Carter, C. S., Leventhal, B. L., Lord, C., & Cook, E. H., Jr. (2007). Association of the oxytocin receptor gene (OXTR) in Caucasian children and adolescents with autism. *Neuroscience Letters, 417*(1), 6–9. Available from *www.ncbi.nlm.nih.gov/entrez/query.fcgi?cmd=Retrieve&db=PubMed&dopt=Citation&list_uids=17383819.*

Javitt, D. C., Spencer, K. M., Thaker, G. K., Winterer, G., & Hajos, M. (2008). Neurophysiological biomarkers for drug development in schizophrenia. *Nature Reviews Drug Discovery, 7*(1), 68–83.

Jennes-Coussens, M., Magill-Evans, J., & Koning, C. (2006). The quality of life of young men with Asperger syndrome: A brief report. *Autism, 10*(4), 403–414.

Kenworthy, L., Anthony, L. G., Naiman, D. Q., Cannon, L., Wills, M. C., Luong-Tran, C., et al. (2014). Randomized controlled effectiveness trial of executive function intervention for children on the autism spectrum. *Journal of Child Psychology and Psychiatry and Allied Disciplines, 55*(4), 374–383.

Kenworthy, L., Yerys, B. E., Anthony, L. G., & Wallace, G. L. (2008). Understanding executive control in autism spectrum disorders in the lab and in the real world, *Neuropsychology Reivew, 18,* 320–338.

Key, A. P., & Corbett, B. A. (2014). ERP responses to face repetition during passive viewing: A nonverbal measure of social motivation in children with autism and typical development. *Developmental Neuropsychology, 39*(6), 474–495.

Kirsch, P., Esslinger, C., Chen, Q., Mier, D., Lis, S., Siddhanti, S., et al. (2005). Oxytocin modulates neural circuitry for social cognition and fear in humans. *Journal of Neuroscience, 25*(49), 11489–11493. Available from *www.ncbi.nlm.nih.gov/entrez/query.fcgi?cmd=Retrieve&db=PubMed&dopt=Citation&list_uids=16339042.*

Kosfeld, M., Heinrichs, M., Zak, P. J., Fischbacher, U., & Fehr, E. (2005). Oxytocin increases trust in humans. *Nature, 435*(7042), 673–676. Available from *www.ncbi.nlm.nih.gov/entrez/query.fcgi?cmd=Retrieve&db=PubMed&dopt=Citation&list_uids=15931222.*

Kulage, K. M., Smaldone, A. M., & Cohn, E. G. (2014). How will DSM-5 affect autism diagnosis?: A systematic literature review and meta-analysis. *Journal of Autism and Developmental Disorders, 44*(8), 1918–1932.

Kushki, A., Brian, J., Dupuis, A., & Anagnostou, E. (2014). Functional autonomic nervous system profile in children with autism spectrum disorder. *Molecular Autism, 5,* 39.

Kushki, A., Drumm, E., Pla Mobarak, M., Tanel, N., Dupuis, A., Chau, T., et al. (2013). Investigating the autonomic nervous system response to anxiety in children with autism spectrum disorders. *PLOS ONE, 8*(4), e59730.

Lai, M.-C., Lombardo, M. V., Auyeung, B., Chakrabarti, B., & Baron-Cohen, S. (2015). Sex/gender differences and autism: Setting the scene for future research. *Journal of the American Academy of Child and Adolescent Psychiatry, 54*(1), 11–24.

Lai, M.-C., Lombardo, M. V., Pasco, G., Ruigrok, A. N. V., Wheelwright, S. J., Sadek, S. A., et al. (2011). A behavioral comparison of male and female adults with high functioning autism spectrum conditions. *PLOS ONE, 6*(6), e20835.

Le Couteur, A., Rutter, M., Lord, C., Rios, P., Robertson, S., Holdgrafer, M., et al. (1989). Autism Diagnostic Interview: A standardized investigator-based instrument. *Journal of Autism and Developmental Disorders, 19*(3), 363–387.

Lehnhardt, F. G., Falter, C. M., Gawronski, A., Pfeiffer, K., Tepest, R., Franklin, J., et al. (2016). Sex-related cognitive profile in autism spectrum disorders diagnosed late in life: Implications for the female autistic phenotype. *Journal of Autism and Developmental Disorders, 46*(1), 139–154.

Lerer, E., Levi, S., Salomon, S., Darvasi, A., Yirmiya, N., & Ebstein, R. P. (2008). Association between the oxytocin receptor (OXTR) gene and autism: Relationship to Vineland Adaptive Behavior Scales and cognition. *Molecular Psychiatry, 13*(10), 980–988.

Lerner, M. D., White, S. W., & McPartland, J. C. (2012). Mechanisms of change in psychosocial interventions for autism spectrum disorders. *Dialogues in Clinical Neuroscience, 14*(3), 307–318. Available from *www.ncbi.nlm.nih.gov/pubmed/23226955.*

Lesko, L. J., & Atkinson, A. J., Jr. (2001). Use of biomarkers and surrogate endpoints in drug development and regulatory decision making: Criteria, validation, strategies. *Annual Review Pharmacology and Toxicology, 41,* 347–366.

Liber, J. M., McLeod, B. D., Van Widenfelt, B. M., Goedhart, A. W., van der Leeden, A. J. M., Utens, E. M. W. J., et al. (2010). Examining the relation between the therapeutic alliance, treatment adherence, and outcome of cognitive behavioral therapy for children with anxiety disorders. *Behavior Therapy, 41*(2), 172–186.

Lopata, C., Volker, M. A., Putnam, S. K., Thomeer, M. L., & Nida, R. E. (2008). Effect of social familiarity on salivary cortisol and self-reports of social anxiety and stress in children with high functioning autism spectrum disorders. *Journal of Autism and Developmental Disorders, 38*(10), 1866–1877.

Lord, C., Risi, S., Lambrecht, L., Cook, E. H., Jr., Leventhal, B. L., DiLavore, P. C., et al. (2000). The Autism Diagnostic Observation Schedule—Generic: A standard measure of social and communication deficits associated with the spectrum of autism. *Journal of Autism and Developmental Disorders, 30*(3), 205–223.

Lord, C., Rutter, M., DiLavore, P. C., Risi, S., Gotham, K., & Bishop, S. L. (2012). *Autism Diagnostic Observation Schedule, Second Edition (ADOS-2).* Torrance, CA: Western Psychological Services.

Lord, C., Rutter, M., & Le Couteur, A. (1994). Autism Diagnostic Interview—Revised: A revised version of a diagnostic interview for caregivers of individuals with possible pervasive developmental disorders. *Journal of Autism and Developmental Disorders, 24,* 659–685.

Mandic-Maravic, V., Pejovic-Milovancevic, M., Mitkovic-Voncina, M., Kostic, M., Aleksic-Hil, O., Radosavljev-Kircanski, J., et al. (2015). Sex differences in autism spectrum disorders: Does sex moderate the pathway from clinical symptoms to adaptive behavior? *Scientific Reports, 5,* 10418.

Mandy, W. P. L., & Skuse, D. H. (2008). Research review: What is the association between the social-communication element of autism and repetitive interests, behaviours and activities? *Journal of Child Psychology and Psychiatry and Allied Disciplines, 49*(8), 795–808.

Marsh, A. A., Yu, H. H., Pine, D. S., & Blair, R. J. (2010). Oxytocin improves specific recognition of positive facial expressions. *Psychopharmacology (Berl), 209*(3), 225–232.

Matson, J. L. (2007). Determining treatment outcome in early intervention programs for autism spectrum disorders: A critical analysis of measurement issues in learning based interventions. *Research in Developmental Disabilities, 28*(2), 207–218.

Mazefsky, C. A., Kao, J., & Oswald, D. P. (2011). Preliminary evidence suggesting caution in the use of psychiatric self-report measures with adolescents with high-functioning autism spectrum disorders. *Research in Autism Spectrum Disorders, 5*(1), 164–174.

McLennan, J. D., Lord, C., & Schopler, E. (1993). Sex differences in higher functioning people with autism. *Journal of Autism and Developmental Disorders, 23*(2), 217–227.

McPartland, J. C. (2016). Considerations in biomarker development for neurodevelopmental disorders. *Current Opinion in Neurology, 29*(2), 118–122.

McPartland, J. C., Reichow, B., & Volkmar, F. R. (2012). Sensitivity and specificity of proposed DSM-5 diagnostic criteria for autism spectrum disorder. *Journal of the American Academy of Child and Adolescent Psychiatry, 51*(4), 368–383.

Miller, M., Bales, K. L., Taylor, S. L., Yoon, J., Hostetler, C. M., Carter, C. S., et al. (2013). Oxytocin and vasopressin in children and adolescents with autism spectrum disorders: Sex differences and associations with symptoms. *Autism Research, 6*(2), 91–102.

Modahl, C., Green, L., Fein, D., Morris, M., Waterhouse, L., Feinstein, C., et al. (1998). Plasma oxytocin levels in autistic children. *Biological Psychiatry, 43*(4), 270–277. Available from *www.ncbi.nlm.nih.gov/entrez/query.fcgi?cmd=Retrieve&db=PubMed&dopt=Citation&list_uids=9513736.*

Naber, F. B., Swinkels, S. H., Buitelaar, J. K., Bakermans-Kranenburg, M. J., van IJzendoorn, M. H., Dietz, C., et al. (2007). Attachment in toddlers with autism and other developmental disorders. *Journal of Autism and Developmental Disorders, 37*(6), 1123–1138.

Naglieri, J. A., & Goldstein, S. (2013). *Comprehensive Executive Functioning Inventory.* Toronto, ON, Canada: Multi-Health Systems.

Neumann, I. D. (2008). Brain oxytocin: A key regulator of emotional and social behaviours in both females and males. *Journal of Neuroendocrinology, 20*(6), 858–865. Available from *www.ncbi.nlm.nih.gov/entrez/query.fcgi?cmd=Retrieve&db=PubMed&dopt=Citation&list_uids=18601710.*

Nicholas, J. S., Charles, J. M., Carpenter, L. A., King, L. B., Jenner, W., & Spratt, E. G. (2008). Prevalence and characteristics of children with autism spectrum disorders. *Annals of Epidemiology, 18*(2), 130–136.

Norbury, C. F. (2014). Practitioner review: Social (pragmatic) communication disorder conceptualization, evidence and clinical implications. *Journal of Child Psychology and Psychiatry and Allied Disciplines, 55*(3), 204–216.

Nordahl-Hansen, A., Fletcher-Watson, S., McConachie, H., & Kaale, A. (2016). Relations between specific and global outcome measures in a social-communication intervention for children with autism spectrum disorder. *Research in Autism Spectrum Disorders, 29–30,* 19–29.

Ozonoff, S., Iosif, A.-M., Baguio, F., Cook, I. C., Hill, M. M., Hutman, T., et al. (2010). A prospective study of the emergence of early behavioral signs of autism. *Journal of the American Academy of Child and Adolescent Psychiatry, 49*(3), 256–266.e1–2.

Park, S., Cho, S.-C., Cho, I. H., Kim, B.-N., Kim, J.-W., Shin, M.-S., et al. (2012). Sex differences in children with autism spectrum disorders compared with their unaffected siblings and typically developing children. *Research in Autism Spectrum Disorders, 6*(2), 861–870.

Patriquin, M. A., Lorenzi, J., Scarpa, A., & Bell, M. A. (2014). Developmental trajectories of respiratory sinus arrhythmia: Associations with social responsiveness. *Developmental Psychobiology, 56*(3), 317–326.

Patriquin, M. A., Scarpa, A., Friedman, B. H., & Porges, S. W. (2013). Respiratory sinus arrhythmia: A marker for positive social functioning and receptive language skills in children with autism spectrum disorders. *Developmental Psychobiology, 55*(2), 101–112.

Posey, D. J., Erickson, C. A., & McDougle, C. J. (2008). Developing drugs for core social and communication impairment in autism. *Child and Adolescent Psychiatry Clinics of North America, 17*(4), 787–801. Available from *www.ncbi.nlm.nih.gov/entrez/query.fcgi?cmd=Retrieve&db=PubMed&dopt=Citation&list_uids=18775370.*

Pugliese, C. E., Anthony, L., Strang, J. F., Dudley, K., Wallace, G. L., & Kenworthy, L. (2015). Increasing adaptive behavior skill deficits from childhood to adolescence in autism spectrum disorder: Role of executive function. *Journal of Autism and Developmental Disorders, 45*(6), 1579–1587.

Pugliese, C. E., Anthony, L. G., Strang, J. F., Dudley, K., Wallace, G. L., Naiman, D. Q., et al. (2016). Longitudinal examination of adaptive behavior in autism spectrum disorders: Influence of executive function. *Journal of Autism and Developmental Disorders, 46*(2), 467–477.

Pugliese, C. E., Kenworthy, L., Bal, V. H., Wallace, G. L., Yerys, B. E., Maddox, B. B., et al. (2015). Replication and comparison of the newly proposed ADOS-2, Module 4 algorithm in ASD without ID: A multi-site study. *Journal of Autism and Developmental Disorders, 45*(12), 3919–3931.

Pugliese, C. E., Trubanova, A., Bascom, J., Kenworthy, L., Wallace, G. L., Yerys, B. E., et al. (2016, May). Gender differences on the newly proposed ADOS-2, module 4 algorithm in ASD without ID: A multi-site study. In A. Ratto (Chair), *What is different about females with autism: Where are we and where do we need to go?* Panel conducted at the International Meeting for Autism Research, Baltimore, MD.

Ramsay, J. R., Brodkin, E. S., Cohen, M. R., Listerud, J., Rostain, A. L., & Ekman, E. (2005). "Better strangers": Using the relationship in psychotherapy for adult patients with Asperger syndrome. *Psychotherapy: Theory, Research, Practice, Training, 42*(4), 483–493.

Ratto, A. B., Turner-Brown, L., Rupp, B. M., Mesibov, G. B., & Penn, D. L. (2011). Development of the Contextual Assessment of Social Skills (CASS): A role play measure of social skill for individuals with high-functioning autism. *Journal of Autism and Developmental Disorders, 41*(9), 1277–1286.

Register-Brown, K., Wallace, G., Ratto, A., Rothwell, C., White, E., Pugliese, C. E., et al. (2016, May). A systematic review and meta-analysis reveals sex differences in RRBIs in school age children with ASD without ID. In A. Ratto (Chair), *What is different about females with autism: Where are we and where do we need to go?* Panel conducted at the International Meeting for Autism Research, Baltimore, MD.

Reinhardt, V. P., Wetherby, A. M., Schatschneider, C., & Lord, C. (2015). Examination of sex differences in a large sample of young children with autism spectrum disorder and typical development. *Journal of Autism and Developmental Disorders, 45*(3), 697–706.

Renison, B., Ponsford, J., Testa, R., Richardson, B., & Brownfield, K. (2012). The ecological and construct validity of a newly developed measure of executive function: The virtual library task. *Journal of the International Neuropsychological Society, 18*(3), 440–450.

Richdale, A. L., & Prior, M. R. (1992). Urinary cortisol circadian rhythm in a group of high-functioning children with autism. *Journal of Autism and Developmental*

Disorders, 22(3), 433–447. Available from *www.ncbi.nlm.nih.gov/entrez/query.fcgi?cmd=Retrieve&db=PubMed&dopt=Citation&list_uids=1400105.*

Rivet, T. T., & Matson, J. L. (2011). Gender differences in core symptomatology in autism spectrum disorders across the lifespan. *Journal of Developmental and Physical Disabilities, 23*(5), 399–420.

Rose, A. J., & Rudolph, K. D. (2006). A review of sex differences in peer relationship processes: Potential trade-offs for the emotional and behavioral development of girls and boys. *Psychological Bulletin, 132*(1), 98–131.

Rutter, M., Bailey, A., & Lord, C. (2003). *The social communication questionnaire: Manual.* Los Angeles: Western Psychological Services.

Schupp, C. W., Simon, D., & Corbett, B. A. (2013). Cortisol responsivity differences in children with autism spectrum disorders during free and cooperative play. *Journal of Autism and Developmental Disorders, 43*(10), 2405–2417.

Seltzer, M. M., Shattuck, P., Abbeduto, L., & Greenberg, S. (2004). Trajectory of development in adolescents and adults with autism. *Mental Retardation and Developmental Disabilities Research Reviews, 10*(4), 234–247.

Shaffer, D., Gould, M. S., Brasic, J., Ambrosini, P., Fisher, P., Bird, H., et al. (1983). A Children's Global Assessment Scale (CGAS). *Archives of General Psychiatry, 40*(11), 1228–1231.

Shattuck, P. T., Durkin, M., Maenner, M., Newschaffer, C., Mandell, D. S., Wiggins, L., et al. (2009). Timing of identification among children with an autism spectrum disorder: Findings from a population-based surveillance study. *Journal of the American Academy of Child and Adolescent Psychiatry, 48*(5), 474–483.

Shattuck, P. T., Narendorf, S. C., Cooper, B., Sterzing, P. R., Wagner, M., & Taylor, J. L. (2012). Postsecondary education and employment among youth with an autism spectrum disorder. *Pediatrics, 129*(6), 1042–1049.

Simon, D. M., & Corbett, B. A. (2013). Examining associations between anxiety and cortisol in high functioning male children with autism. *Journal of Neurodevelopmental Disorders, 5*(1), 32.

Skuse, D. H. (2012). DSM-5's conceptualization of autistic disorders. *Journal of the American Academy of Child and Adolescent Psychiatry, 51*(4), 344–346.

Skuse, D. H., & Gallagher, L. (2009). Dopaminergic–neuropeptide interactions in the social brain. *Trends in Cognitive Science, 13*(1), 27–35.

Smith, I. C., Reichow, B., & Volkmar, F. R. (2015). The effects of DSM-5 criteria on number of individuals diagnosed with autism spectrum disorder: A systematic review. *Journal of Autism and Developmental Disorders, 45*(8), 2541–2552.

Smith, T., & Iadarola, S. (2015). Evidence base update for autism spectrum disorder. *Journal of Clinical Child and Adolescent Psychology, 44*(6), 897–922.

Solomon, M., Miller, M., Taylor, S. L., Hinshaw, S. P., & Carter, C. S. (2012). Autism symptoms and internalizing psychopathology in girls and boys with autism spectrum disorders. *Journal of Autism and Developmental Disorders, 42*(1), 48–59.

Spratt, E. G., Nicholas, J. S., Brady, K. T., Carpenter, L. A., Hatcher, C. R., Meekins, K. A., et al. (2012). Enhanced cortisol response to stress in children in autism. *Journal of Autism and Developmental Disorders, 42*(1), 75–81.

Strang, J. F., Kenworthy, L., Dominska, A., Sokoloff, J., Kenealy, L. E., Berl, M., et al. (2014). Increased gender variance in autism spectrum disorders and attention deficit hyperactivity disorder. *Archives of Sexual Behavior, 43*(8), 1525–1533.

Strang, J. F., Meagher, H., Kenworthy, L., de Vries, A., Menvielle, E., Janssen, A., et al. (2016). Initial clinical guidelines for co-occurring autism spectrum disorder and gender dysphoria in adolescents. *Journal of Clinical Child and Adolescent Psychology, 24,* 1–11.

Taurines, R., Schwenck, C., Lyttwin, B., Schecklmann, M., Jans, T., Reefschlager, L., et al. (2014). Oxytocin plasma concentrations in children and adolescents with autism spectrum disorder: Correlation with autistic symptomatology. *Attention Deficit Hyperactivity Disorder, 6*(3), 231–239.

Taylor, J. L., & Corbett, B. A. (2014). A review of rhythm and responsiveness of cortisol in individuals with autism spectrum disorders. *Psychoneuroendocrinology, 49,* 207–228.

Taylor, J. L., Henninger, N. A., & Mailick, M. R. (2015). Longitudinal patterns of employment and postsecondary education for adults with autism and average-range IQ. *Autism, 19*(7), 785–793.

Taylor, J. L., & Seltzer, M. M. (2012). Employment and post-secondary educational activities for young adults with autism spectrum disorder during the transition to adulthood. *Journal of Autism and Developmental Disorders, 41*(5), 566–574.

Teng, B. L., Nonneman, R. J., Agster, K. L., Nikolova, V. D., Davis, T. T., Riddick, N. V., et al. (2013). Prosocial effects of oxytocin in two mouse models of autism spectrum disorders. *Neuropharmacology, 72,* 187–196.

Tordjman, S., Anderson, G. M., McBride, P. A., Hertzig, M. E., Snow, M. E., Hall, L. M., et al. (1997). Plasma beta-endorphin, adrenocorticotropin hormone, and cortisol in autism. *Journal of Child Psychology and Psychiatry, 38*(6), 705–715. Available from *www.ncbi.nlm.nih.gov/entrez/query.fcgi?cmd=Retrieve&db=PubMed&dopt=Citation&list_uids=9315980.*

Van Wijngaarden-Cremers, P. J. M., Van Eeten, E., Groen, W. B., Van Deurzen, P. A., Oosterling, I. J., & Van Der Gaag, R. J. (2014). Gender and age differences in the core triad of impairments in autism spectrum disorders: A systematic review and meta-analysis. *Journal of Autism and Developmental Disorders, 44*(3), 627–635.

Viau, R., Arsenault-Lapierre, G., Fecteau, S., Champagne, N., Walker, C. D., & Lupien, S. (2010). Effect of service dogs on salivary cortisol secretion in autistic children. *Psychoneuroendocrinology, 35*(8), 1187–1193.

Welch, M. G., & Ruggiero, D. A. (2005). Predicted role of secretin and oxytocin in the treatment of behavioral and developmental disorders: Implications for autism. *International Review of Neurobiology, 71,* 273–315. Available from *www.ncbi.nlm.nih.gov/entrez/query.fcgi?cmd=Retrieve&db=PubMed&dopt=Citation&list_uids=16512355.*

Werling, D. M., & Geschwind, D. H. (2013). Sex differences in autism spectrum disorders. *Current Opinion in Neurology, 26*(2), 146–153.

Wermter, A. K., Kamp-Becker, I., Hesse, P., Schulte-Korne, G., Strauch, K., & Remschmidt, H. (2009). Evidence for the involvement of genetic variation in the oxytocin receptor gene (OXTR) in the etiology of autistic disorders on high-functioning level. *American Journal of Medical Genetics Part B: Neuropsychiatric Genetics, 153B*(2), 629–639.

Westwood, H., Stahl, D., Mandy, W., & Tchanturia, K. (2016). The set-shifting profiles of anorexia nervosa and autism spectrum disorder using the Wisconsin Card Sorting Test: A systematic review and meta-analysis. *Psychological Medicine, 46*(9), 1809–1827.

White, S. W., Elias, R., Salinas, C. E., Capriola, N., Conner, C. M., Asselin, S. B., et al. (2016). Students with autism spectrum disorder in college: Results from a preliminary mixed methods needs analysis. *Research in Developmental Disabilities, 56,* 29–40.

White, S. W., Ollendick, T., Albano, A. M., Oswald, D., Johnson, C., Southam-Gerow, M. A., et al. (2013). Randomized controlled trial: Multimodal Anxiety and Social Skill Intervention for adolescents with autism spectrum disorder. *Journal of Autism and Developmental Disorders, 43*(2), 382–394.

White, S. W., Scarpa, A., Conner, C. M., Maddox, B. B., & Bonete, S. (2015). Evaluating change in social skills in high-functioning adults with autism spectrum disorder using a laboratory-based observational measure. *Focus on Autism and Other Developmental Disabilities, 30*(1), 3–12.

Willcutt, E., Doyle, A., Nigg, J., Faraone, S., & Pennington, B. (2005). Validity of the executive function theory of attention-deficit/hyperactivity disorder: A meta-analytic review. *Biological Psychiatry, 57*(11), 1336–1346.

Wilson, C. E., Murphy, C. M., McAlonan, G., Robertson, D. M., Spain, D., Hayward, H., et al. (2016). Does sex influence the diagnostic evaluation of autism spectrum disorder in adults? *Autism, 20*(7), 808–819.

Winslow, J. T., Shapiro, L., Carter, C. S., & Insel, T. R. (1993). Oxytocin and complex social behavior: Species comparisons. *Psychopharmacological Bulletin, 29*(3), 409–414. Available from *www.ncbi.nlm.nih.gov/entrez/query.fcgi?cmd=Retrieve&db=PubMed&dopt=Citation&list_uids=8121969.*

Worley, J. A., & Matson, J. L. (2011). Psychiatric symptoms in children diagnosed with an autism spectrum disorder: An examination of gender differences. *Research in Autism Spectrum Disorders, 5*(3), 1086–1091.

Wu, S., Jia, M., Ruan, Y., Liu, J., Guo, Y., Shuang, M., et al. (2005). Positive association of the oxytocin receptor gene (OXTR) with autism in the Chinese Han population. *Biological Psychiatry, 58*(1), 74–77. Available from *www.ncbi.nlm.nih.gov/entrez/query.fcgi?cmd=Retrieve&db=PubMed&dopt=Citation&list_uids=15992526.*

Yoder, P. J., Bottema-Beutel, K., Woynaroski, T., Chandrasekhar, R., & Sandback, M. (2013). Social communication intervention effects vary by dependent variable type in preschoolers with autism spectrum disorders. *Evidence Based Communication, Assessment, and Intervention, 6*(4), 150–174.

Yoder, P. J., & Symons, F. J. (2010). *Observational measurement of behavior.* New York: Springer.

Young, L. J., Pitkow, L. J., & Ferguson, J. N. (2002). Neuropeptides and social behavior: Animal models relevant to autism. *Molecular Psychiatry, 7*(Suppl. 2), S38–S39. Available from *www.ncbi.nlm.nih.gov/entrez/query.fcgi?cmd=Retrieve&db=PubMed&dopt=Citation&list_uids=12142945.*

Young, L. J., Wang, Z., & Insel, T. R. (1998). Neuroendocrine bases of monogamy. *Trends in Neuroscience, 21*(2), 71–75. Available from *www.ncbi.nlm.nih.gov/entrez/query.fcgi?cmd=Retrieve&db=PubMed&dopt=Citation&list_uids=9498302.*

Yrigollen, C. M., Han, S. S., Kochetkova, A., Babitz, T., Chang, J. T., Volkmar, F. R., et al. (2008). Genes controlling affiliative behavior as candidate genes for autism. *Biological Psychiatry, 63*(10), 911–916.

Zwaigenbaum, L., Bryson, S., Szatmari, P., Brian, J., Smith, I. M., Roberts, W., et al. (2012). Sex differences in children with autism spectrum disorder identified within a high-risk infant cohort. *Journal of Autism and Developmental Disorders, 2,* 2585–2596.

Index

Note. *f* or *t* following a page number indicates a figure or a table.